Resources for Instructor Success

Instructor's Resource CD

ISBN-10: 0-13-512887-0 / ISBN-13: 978-0-13-512887-9
This CD includes all the textbook resources instructors need to teach
critical care nursing courses:

- **Instructor's Resource Manual**—This manual helps faculty plan and manage the critical care nursing course. Presented in an easy-to-use format, the manual includes
  —Detailed lecture notes organized by learning objectives
  —Suggestions for Classroom Activities
  —Suggestions for Clinical Activities
- **Test Item File** with comprehensive rationales.
- **PowerPoint** presentation integrates lecture slides, images, animations or videos, and other resources.
- **iClicker** questions set in PowerPoint with content provided to make your class more interactive (ask your Prentice Hall representative for more information about hardware to enhance your presentation).
- **Complete Image Gallery** in PowerPoint.
- **TestGen Test Item File** with questions in all NCLEX-RN® format, including questions mapped to the chapter learning outcomes.
- **Link to the Pearson Instructor's Resource Center** for additional resources.

Companion Website www.prenhall.com/perrin

Online Course Management Systems

Pearson Course Cartridges are integrated online resources that bring a variety of resources together in one convenient place for faculty and students using Blackboard and WebCt platforms. Course Cartridges feature everything you need for out-of-class work, conveniently organized to match your syllabus.

- NCLEX-RN® Review questions
- Case studies
- MediaLinks
- MediaLink applications
- Test Item File
- PowerPoint Presentations
- Email
- Discussion board
- Class announcements

For information about adopting one of the online courses to accompany *Understanding the Essentials of Critical Care Nursing*, please contact your Pearson Sales Representative or go to one of the sites below, select "Courses," and then "Nursing."

WebCT: http://cms.prenhall.com/webct/index.html/

BlackBoard: http://cms.prenhall.com/blackboard/index.html/

Brief Contents

Understanding the Essentials of CRITICAL CARE Nursing

Kathleen Ouimet Perrin
PhD, RN, CCRN

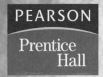

PEARSON

Prentice
Hall

Upper Saddle River, New Jersey 07458

Library of Congress Cataloging-in-Publication Data
Perrin, Kathleen Ouimet.
  Understanding the essentials of critical care nursing / Kathleen Perrin.
    p. cm.
  Includes bibliographical references and index.
  ISBN 978-0-13-172210-1 (alk. paper)
  1. Intensive care nursing. I. Title.
  [DNLM: 1. Critical Care—methods. 2. Critical Illness—nursing.
3. Nursing Care—methods. WY 154 P458u 2009]
  RT120.I5P47 2009
  616.02'8—dc22   2008025189

Notice: Care has been taken to confirm the accuracy of information presented in this book. The authors, editors, and the publisher, however, cannot accept any responsibility for errors or omissions or for consequences from application of the information in this book and make no warranty, express or implied, with respect to its contents.

The authors and publisher have exerted every effort to ensure that drug selections and dosages set forth in this text are in accord with current recommendations and practice at the time of publication. However, in view of ongoing research, changes in government regulations, and the constant flow of information relating to drug therapy and drug reactions, the reader is urged to check the package inserts of all drugs for any change in indications of dosage and for added warnings and precautions. This is particularly important when the recommended agent is a new and/or infrequently employed drug.

Publisher: Julie Levin Alexander
Publisher's Assistant: Regina Bruno
Editor in Chief: Maura Connor
Executive Acquisitions Editor: Pamela Fuller
Editorial Assistant: Jennifer Aranda
Development Editor: Barbara Price
Managing Production Editor: Patrick Walsh
Production Liaison: Cathy O'Connell
Production Editor: Heather Willison, S4Carlisle Publishing Services
Manufacturing Manager: Ilene Sanford
Art Director: Maria Guglielmo
Cover and Interior Designer: Laura Gardner
Director of Marketing: Karen Allman
Senior Marketing Manager: Francisco Del Castillo
Marketing Specialist: Michael Sirinides
Media Project Manager: Stephen Hartner
Director, Image Resource Center: Melinda Patelli
Manager, Rights and Permissions: Zina Arabia
Manager, Visual Research: Beth Brenzel
Manager, Cover Visual Research and Permissions: Karen Sanatar
Image Permission Coordinator: Jan Marc Quisumbing
Composition: S4Carlisle Publishing Services
Printer/Binder: Webcrafters, Inc.
Cover Photo: Steve Allen/Brand X Pictures/Jupiter Inc.
Cover Printer: Phoenix Color

Marked for Online Sales

Pearson Education Ltd., London
Pearson Education Singapore, Pte. Ltd.
Pearson Education Canada, Inc.
Pearson Education—Japan

Pearson Education Australia PTY, Limited
Pearson Education North Asia Ltd., Hong Kong
Pearson Educación de Mexico, S.A. de C.V
Pearson Education Malaysia, Pte. Ltd.
Pearson Education, Upper Saddle River, New Jersey

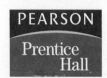

10 9 8 7 6 5 4 3
ISBN: 0-13-172210-7
ISBN-13: 978-0-13-172210-1

About the Author

Kathleen Ouimet Perrin, PhD, RN, CCRN

Kathleen Perrin is a professor of nursing at Saint Anselm College in Manchester, New Hampshire, where she teaches critical care nursing, professional nursing, ethics, and understanding suffering. She received her bachelor's degree from the University of Massachusetts, Amherst; her master's degree from Boston College; and her PhD from Union Institute and University in Cincinnati, Ohio. She has been a practicing critical care nurse for over 30 years and a member of the American Association of Critical Care Nurses (AACN) for nearly as long. Kathleen has served on the board of the Southern New Hampshire AACN and is a past president of the chapter. She is currently president of the Epsilon Tau chapter of Sigma Theta Tau International. She has published and presented in the areas of critical care nursing, nursing ethics, nursing history, suffering experienced by patients as well as health care providers, and conflict among members of the health care team.

Preface

This book is an introduction to critical care. It focuses on elements that are essential for the novice critical care nurse to understand, whether the novice is a student or a new graduate. When I began working as a critical care nurse 30 years ago, I learned about care modalities as I delivered them—but those modalities were in relatively simple, beginning stages. Today, nurses are capable of much more complex care using increasingly complicated care modalities that come with much greater potential for error. Recently, while I was searching for an article about the Pressure-Regulated Volume Control (PRVC) ventilator mode, I found one that began, "Don't even think about reading this until you understand and have worked with the basics of mechanical ventilation." This book provides an understanding of those essential elements of critical care that are the foundation for delivering safe, effective care and the basis for the eventual delivery of sophisticated, expert care.

We are fortunate that nursing practice has changed from my early years, when we learned as we went, experimented with new interventions on our patients, and often relied on intuition to choose those interventions. Our intuition could not be trusted as a basis for practice, and our experiences provided us with too small a sample to draw inferences. Whenever possible, this book relies on evidence-based recommendations for collaborative and nursing practice. It cites individual research studies, but more often cites meta-analyses and evidence-based practice recommendations made by respected professional organizations. When the foundation for practice is based on evidence, it is far more likely to be safe and effective and far less likely to shift as methods of care evolve.

Organization and Key Themes of This Book

The topics for these chapters were chosen after reviewing suggestions for foundational critical care content from a variety of nursing organizations, including the *American Association of Critical Care Nurses* and the *National Council of State Boards of Nursing*. The first chapter addresses what is unique about critical care and critical care nursing, including legal and ethical issues nurses encounter. The second chapter focuses on the needs and concerns that are common to critically ill patients or their families and explores ways nurses might meet those needs. The remaining chapters describe the essentials of providing care to patients with disorders that are commonly seen in critical care settings. There is no attempt to cover all possible content;

rather, the text concentrates on problems that the new critical care nurse is most likely to encounter. Since many patients die in critical care units, or shortly after being transferred out of critical care units, the final chapter discusses care of the dying patient.

A recurrent theme in this book is safe practice. As critical care has become more complex, the potential for error has increased. Chapter 1 includes a discussion of some of the reasons why errors are common in critical care units. Fortunately, there are documented ways in which nurses can prevent or limit health care errors. One of the most effective ways to prevent errors is to improve communication and collaboration among members of the health care team, as described in Chapter 1. In each subsequent chapter, a Safety Initiative feature describes specific recommendations by the *Institute for Health Care Improvement* and other national groups that, when implemented, can limit errors and enhance patient safety.

My father was recently very ill. The skills of his critical care nurses brought him through his illness. They recognized how his needs as a member of the "old, old" population differed from a younger patient, and they adjusted their care accordingly. With the increasing population of people in this age cohort, knowledge of how to care for them must be part of the foundation of critical care practice, so we include information on gerontological patients in each chapter.

In this text, **Nursing Management** is a component of **Collaborative Management**. The content in the Nursing Management sections emphasizes nursing interventions required for safe, effective medical and surgical management of the patient—for example, what are the nursing responsibilities when administering amiodarone, or what nursing assessments are essential after a patient has a cardiac catheterization. In contrast, the **Nursing Care** sections highlight interventions that focus on providing care to a patient and creating a healing environment. Nursing Care sections focus on promoting patient comfort, providing adequate nutrition, and assisting the patient and family to cope with the critical illness or impending death.

Nursing management of critical care patients includes using some of the latest technology developed for the health field. **Building Technology Skills** text sections focus on specific technology that the nurse is most likely to encounter when caring for patients experiencing the conditions discussed in the chapter, and the related skills required to use that technology.

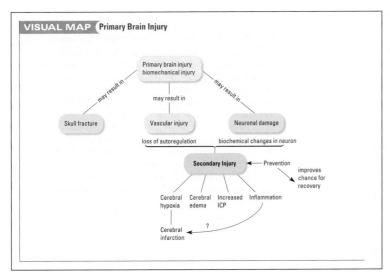

VISUAL MAP | Primary Brain Injury

VISUAL MAPS A critically ill patient is a dynamic system of interrelated factors. In order to help visual learners understand the relationships between and among these factors, each chapter includes visual maps to illustrate the relationships among the disease states, collaborative interventions, and outcomes.

The first map, in the chapter opener, is simple and shows the relationships among major concepts in the disease process or the chapter. Later maps in the chapter are more complex, showing how increasingly detailed information is related. The final map is a summary map, showing how all the pieces are related to patient care.

COMMONLY USED MEDICATIONS

METHYLPREDNISOLONE

Expected Action and Dose: Suppress inflammation and normal immune response. Steroid dosing is generally 30 mg/kg over 15 minutes initially, followed 45 minutes later with 5.4/kg/hr for 23 hours.

Side and Toxic Effects: Depression/euphoria, hypertension, anorexia, peptic ulcer, thromboembolism, decreased wound healing, ecchymoses, and increased likelihood of infection (side effects are more common with high-dose/long-term therapy).

Nursing Responsibilities: The nurse assesses the patient for signs of adrenal insufficiency, monitors intake and output, assesses the patient for changes in level of consciousness and headache, and prevents infection.

COMMONLY USED MEDICATIONS
Medications that are most often prescribed for the conditions addressed in the chapter are highlighted in these boxes. For each medication, information is provided on dosing information, desired effects, nursing responsibilities, and potential side effects.

SAFETY INITIATIVES | Fistula First: National Vascular Access Improvement Initiatives

PURPOSE: To increase the likelihood that every eligible patient will receive the optimal form of vascular access for that patient, usually an AV fistula, and that vascular access complications will be avoided through appropriate access, monitoring, and interventions

RATIONALE: Central venous catheter accesses should be removed as soon as possible. Complications, including infection, catheter failure, thrombosis, inadequate dialysis, and central venous stenosis or occlusion, occur frequently with catheters—and the complication rate rises sharply with duration of use. Studies have also reported that catheter use is associated with an increased risk of mortality.

HIGHLIGHTS OF RECOMMENDATIONS:
Routine CQI review of vascular access
Timely referral to a nephrologist
Early referral to a surgeon for "AVF-only" evaluation and timely placement
Monitoring and maintenance to ensure adequate access functioning
Education for caregivers and patients

Source: Fistula First: National Vascular Access Improvement Initiatives

 Available: http://www.fistulafirst.org/

SAFETY INITIATIVES
Safety is an essential focus in critical care settings. These boxes highlight specific issues related to the content in each chapter. Included are the purpose, the rationale, and highlighted recommendations, with a MediaLink for more information.

GERONTOLOGICAL CONSIDERATIONS Since many of the patients in critical care settings are older adults, this essential information will enhance the effectiveness of critical care nurses.

Gerontological Considerations

AF is the most commonly sustained dysrhythmia in older adults because the incidence of AF increases with age and heart disease. This dysrhythmia results in approximately 24% of strokes in patients aged 80 to 89 years old (Fang, Chen, & Rich, 2007). Stroke prevention is usually accomplished through anticoagulants; however, the elderly are also at increased risk of bleeding from being on anticoagulants because of increased falls, functional impairments, and cognitive dysfunction. Despite their increased risk of bleeding, the benefits of using an anticoagulant generally outweigh the risks in most older adults with AF.

Nursing Diagnoses

PATIENT EXPERIENCING AN INTRACRANIAL DYSFUNCTION

- Decreased intracranial adaptive capacity related to brain injury
- Ineffective tissue perfusion: cerebral related to increased intracranial pressure and decreased cerebral perfusion pressure
- Acute pain related to trauma
- Risk for aspiration related to reduced level of consciousness and depressed cough and gag reflexes
- Risk for injury related to seizure disorder

NURSING DIAGNOSES NANDA Nursing Diagnoses are suggested for the disorders and diseases presented to help the reader categorize the nursing problems that may accompany the medical diagnoses.

CASE STUDY In each chapter, a case study of a real-life patient scenario illustrates the chapter content and provides an example of collaborative and nursing management. Critical thinking questions allow the reader to solve the posed problems. The case studies continue on the Companion Website, offering learners the opportunity to extend the textbook learning and submit responses to their instructors.

CASE STUDY

A 59-year-old male and successful business manager is transported to the hospital after experiencing chest pain at work. Upon arrival to the ED, you notice the patient clutching his chest and moaning. He states that the pain is in the middle of his chest and radiating to his jaw and left arm. You obtain a partial history from the patient.

Subjective data:
- States he has been working overtime for the past week, trying to obtain a multimillion dollar contract for his firm
- States he has been told to lose weight but has not had the time to go on a diet or exercise
- Recently divorced
- He has two children in college and one teenage son
- Is borderline diabetic

Objective data:
- Weight: 250 lb (114 kg)
- Height: 5 feet 11 inches
- Diaphoretic, pale, and short of breath
- BP 170/100
- Pulse 110 bpm and slightly irregular

- Respiratory rate 24
- Temperature 99

Diagnostic studies:
- ECG shows ST elevation in leads V_1–V_4
- Cardiac-specific enzyme troponin I is 12
- Total cholesterol level 275 mg/dL, LDL 120 mg/dL, HDL 35 mg/dL
- Creatinine phosphokinase 300
- Blood glucose 130

1. What are some of the causes of his chest pain?
2. What is the significance of the ECG results?
3. What is the possible pathophysiology of the patient's condition? How is it different from ACS?
4. What factors are contributing to the patient's medical condition?
5. What other lab values would the nurse need to evaluate? Why?
6. What should the immediate management strategies be for this patient? Why?

See answers to Case Studies in the Answer Section at the back of the book.

CRITICAL THINKING QUESTIONS These questions summarize the chapter material, allowing students to test what they have learned.

CRITICAL THINKING QUESTIONS

1. What is an STEMI? How is it differentiated from other causes of ACS?
2. Why is aspirin given to the patient immediately upon arrival to the ED?
3. What is troponin and why is it a useful test in patients with chest pain?
4. What are the electrolyte disturbances the nurse needs to be aware of with the ACS patient? Which is the most important? How is it treated?

5. How is pain managed in the ACS patient?
6. What are the complications of an MI? What are the causes of these complications?
7. What are the advantages of fibrinolytic therapy for the patient?
8. Why would a patient undergo a CABG surgery rather than a PCI?

See answers to Critical Thinking Questions in the Answer Section at the back of the book.

Critical Care Nursing

Critical care nursing is an evolving specialty. *Understanding the Essentials of Critical Care Nursing* is intended to provide novice critical care nurses with a firm foundation so that they are able to understand the complexities of care, and deliver safe, effective care. Eventually, just as understanding basic mechanical ventilation is the basis for understanding the PRVC mode, this foundation in the essentials of critical care nursing should provide the basis for expert practice.

Teaching and Learning Package

To supplement and facilitate active student learning and information provided in the text, a variety of student learning aids and instructor resources are available.

FOR THE STUDENT

Companion Website www.prenhall.com/perrin
This open access online study guide is designed to help students apply the concepts in the book. Each chapter-specific module includes the chapter learning outcomes, the extended case study from the chapter, nursing care plans for priority diagnoses, NCLEX® review questions, MediaLinks to additional resources pertinent to the chapter, MediaLink applications, and interactive exercises.

Online Course Management Systems

Pearson Course Cartridges are integrated online resources that bring a variety of resources together in one convenient place for faculty and students using Blackboard and WebCt platforms. Course Cartridges feature everything you need for out-of-class work, conveniently organized to match your syllabus.

- NCLEX-RN® review questions
- Case studies
- MediaLinks
- MediaLink applications
- Test Item File
- PowerPoint Presentations
- E-mail
- Discussion board
- Class announcements

NCLEX® review questions, MediaLinks to additional resources pertinent to the chapter, MediaLink applications, and interactive exercises.

For information

about adopting one of the online courses to accompany *Understanding the Essentials of Critical Care Nursing,* please contact your Pearson Sales Representative or go to one of the sites below, select "Courses," and then "Nursing."

WEBCT
http://cms.prenhall.com/webct/index.html/

BLACKBOARD
http://cms.prenhall.com/blackboard/index.html/

Acknowledgments

I would like to acknowledge those critical care nurse educators with whom I have worked directly over the past few years and who contributed to this book. June Kasper worked with me to develop the plan for this book. Her insistence on precision and excellence is inspiring. Catherine Fogg serves as a role model of excellence to her students in the clinical and classroom settings every day. Shirley Jackson's wealth of knowledge encompasses the span of critical care; her workdays seem endless and her energy is boundless.

I also appreciate the energy, time, and thought that the authors of all the chapters put into their tasks, giving up weekends and holidays, and persisting despite personal and family difficulties. They brought their expertise in critical care nursing to each of their chapters and their knowledge is one of the foundations of this book.

I could not have completed this task without the assistance and advice of my editors at Pearson/Prentice Hall. From the time Pamela Fuller approached me about the book, she has been incredibly supportive. Barbara Price has been my constant e-mail companion for the past two years, keeping me on track, helping me understand the process of publication, and easing all the chapter authors through the rough spots.

Finally, I need to acknowledge Fred the Cat, who made sure that I was awake and working on the book long before dawn each morning.

Kathleen Ouimet Perrin *Ph. D., RN, CCRN*

Dedication

This book is *dedicated* to my **husband, Robin,** who insisted that I should write this book and provided me with the time and space to do so.

It is also *dedicated* to my **parents, Marie and Charles Ouimet**—especially to my father. His recent illness caused me to experience firsthand how suddenly people can become critically ill, how arduous and long the recovery may be, and how essential critical care nurses are to both patient and family.

Finally, it is *dedicated* to **critical care nurses,** specifically to those nurses who helped my father through his illness and as he began his recovery but also to the countless other nurses who do the same for their patients every day.

Contributors

Text Contributors

LINDA EDELMAN, PhD, BSN
Assistant Professor
University of Utah College of
    Nursing
Salt Lake City, Utah

**CATHERINE FOGG, PhD(C),
    ARNP, BC**
Assistant Professor of Nursing
Saint Anselm College
Manchester, New Hampshire

**SHIRLEY JACKSON, MS, RN,
    CCRN**
Critical Care Clinical Nurse Specialist
Elliot Hospital
Manchester, New Hampshire

JUNE KASPER, MS, RN
Clinical Educator, Endoscopy
Lahey Clinical Medical Center
Burlington, Massachusetts

**MARIANNE L. MATZO, PhD,
    APRN-BC, FAAN**
Professor and Frances E. and A.
    Earl Ziegler Chair in Palliative
    Care Nursing
University of Oklahoma
College of Nursing
Oklahoma City, Oklahoma

**SUSAN MOORE, MSN, PhD,
    MS, BSN**
Assistant Professor
The University of Memphis
Memphis, Tennessee

KATHLEEN SCHULER, MSN, RN
Instructor, ASN Program
Saint Joseph School of Nursing
Nashua, New Hampshire

**SHEILA SULLIVAN, PhD, RN,
    MSN, BSN**
Associate Chief Nurse, Research
Central Arkansas Veterans
    Healthcare System
Little Rock, Arkansas

BETSY SWINNY, MSN, RN
Critical Care Educator
St. Luke's Baptist Hospital
San Antonio, Texas

KELLEY TAYLOR, MSN, RN
Instructor
Saint Anselm College
Manchester, New Hampshire

Supplements Contributors

**ANGELA BALISTRIERIA, RN,
    MSN**
Faculty
Mercy Hospital School of Nursing
Pittsburgh, Pennsylvania

TRACY BLANC, RN BSN
Nursing Instructor
Ivy Tech Community College of
    Indiana
Fort Wayne, Indiana

DONNA BOWLES, RN, MSN, EdD
Associate Professor of Nursing
Indiana University Southeast
Albany, Indiana

**MARYLEE BRESSIE, CCNS,
    CCRN, CEN**
Instructor
Spring Hill College
Mobile, Alabama

**LORI A. BUDD, RN, BS,
    MSN, MBA**
Assistant Professor
John Tyler Community College
Midlothian, Virginia

**MONICA G. CASHIOTTA-MUNN,
    RN, MFT**
Academic and Administrative
    Headquarters Instructor
National University
La Jolla, California

KIM COOPER, RN, MSN
Nursing Department Chair
Ivy Tech Community College
Terre Haute, Indiana

**DIANE DADDARIO, MSN, ACNS-
    BC, RN, BC, CMSRM**
Clinical Instructor, Staff Nurse
Pennsylvania College of Technology
Williamsport, Pennsylvania

**ELIZABETH FRANDER, RN, MSN,
    APRN, FNP-BC**
Associate Professor
Columbus State University
Columbus, Georgia

LINDA FREEMAN, MN, RN
Assistant Professor
John Tyler Community College
Midlothian, Virginia

CARMAN GODFREY, MSN, RN
Instructor, Division of Nursing
Faulkner State College
Bay Minette, Alabama

**THERESE LAHNSTEIN, MSN,
    RN, CCRN**
Associate Professor, Nursing
Columbus State University
Columbus, Georgia

PATTI LALIBERTE, MS, RN
Staff Nurse, Intensive Care Unit
Elliot Hospital
Manchester, New Hampshire

WANDA K. LAWRENCE, PhD,
RNC, MSN
Assistant Professor of Nursing
Winston-Salem State University
Winston-Salem, North Carolina

VIRGINIA LESTER, MSN, RN
(CNS INACTIVE)
Assistant Professor of Nursing
Angelo State University
San Angelo, Texas

SYLVIA LOVE, M.ED, MSN,
ACNP-BC, ANP-BC
Medical Assistant Professor
University of South Alabama
Mobile, Alabama

ANDREA MANN, MSN, RN
Third Level Chair
Frankford Hospital School of
Nursing
Philadelphia, Pennsylvania

KAREN S. MARCH, PhD, RN,
CCRN, ACNS-BC
Associate Professor of Nursing
York College of Pennsylvania
York, Pennsylvania

DAWNA MARTICH, MSN, RN,
Nursing Education Consultant
Pittsburgh, Pennsylvania

ANN MCSWAIN, RN, MSN,
CCNS, CCRN, APRN-BC
Assistant Professor
Lincoln University
Jefferson City, Missouri

NICKOLAUS MIEHL, RN, MSN
Lecturer
Nursing Technology Lab and
Simulation Center Coordinator
Penn State Erie, The Behrend College
Erie, Pennsylvania

DONNA RUSSO, RN, MSN,
CCRN, CNE
Nursing Instructor
Frankford Hospital School of
Nursing
Philadelphia, Pennsylvania

BARBARA KIM STEVENS, MSN,
RN
Assistant Professor
Holzer School of Nursing 113
University of Rio Grande
Rio Grande, Ohio

DOLORES M. ZYGMONT, PhD,
RN
Associate Professor
Interim Director for Graduate
Studies in Nursing
Department of Nursing, College of
Health Professions
Temple University
Philadelphia, Pennsylvania

Reviewers

ANDREA ACKERMAN, PHD, RN, CCRN
Assistant Professor of Nursing
Mount Saint Mary College
Division of Nursing
Newburgh, New York

KATHLEEN ANDREWS, PHD, RN
Chairperson and Associate
 Professor, Department of Nursing
Missouri Western State University
St. Joseph, Missouri

JEANE ASEL, MS/RN, CCRN, APNP-BC
Assistant Clinical Professor
Texas Women's University
Dallas, Texas

DONNA GARBACZ BADER, MA, MSN, BSN, RN, BS, CFS, D-ABMDI
Assistant Professor
School of Nursing & Program
 Coordinator
Bryan LGH College of Health
 Sciences
Lincoln, Nebraska

BRENDA BECKER, BSN, MA, RN
Nursing Faculty
North Hennepin Community
 College
Brooklyn Park, Minnesota

ADRIENNE BERARDUCCI, PHD, ARNP, BC, CCD
Associate Professor
University of South Florida
Tampa, Florida

NANCY BITTNER, PHD, RN, CCRN
Associate Professor, Associate
 Director, School of Nursing
Regis College School of Nursing
 and Health Professions
Weston, Massachusetts

SHIRLEY BRISTOL, JD, RN, MS, CNS
Assistant Professor of Nursing
California State University San
 Bernardino
San Bernardino, California

PAM CHAPMAN, MSN, RN, CCRN
Assistant Professor
La Roche College
Pittsburgh, Pennsylvania

KIM COOPER, RN, MSN
Nursing Department Chair
Ivy Tech Community College
Terre Haute, Indiana

SHERRY COOPER-DYE, RN, MS, APRN, BC
The Ohio State University College
 of Nursing
Columbus, Ohio

KAREN CROUSE, APRN, FNP (BC), CEN
Chair, Department of Nursing
Western CT State University
Danbury, Connecticut

DAVID CURRY, RN-C, PHD, ADULT NP
Associate Professor
SUNY Plattsburgh
Plattsburgh, New York

DIANE DADDARIO, MSN, CNS, RN, BC, CMSRN
Clinical Instructor, Staff Nurse
Pennsylvania College of Technology
Williamsport, Pennsylvania

THERESA DELAHOYDE, MSN, RN
Assistant Professor of Nursing
Bryan LGH College of Health
 Sciences
Lincoln, Nebraska

CAROL DELLARATTA, RN, MS, CCRN
Clinical Assistant Professor
Stony Brook University
Stony Brook, New York

WADDAH DEMEH, RN, PHD(C)
Adjunct Instructor
University of Southern Mississippi
Hattiesburg, Mississippi

DALE DEMILLE, MSN, RN, CCRN, BSN
Adjunct Professor
Quinnipiac University
Hamden, Connecticut

MARY FABICK, MSN, MED, RN, CEN
Associate Professor
Milligan College
Milligan College, Tennessee

CONSTANCE M. FLYNN
Professor of Nursing
Berkshire Community College
Pittsfield, Massachusetts

KATHLEEN L. GILCHRIST, PHD, FNP-C, RN, CCRN, PHN
Professor
California State University Bakersfield
Bakersfield, California

MARGE GINGRICH, RN, MSN
Professor
Harrisburg Area Community College
Harrisburg, Pennsylvania

JONI C. GOLDWASSER, MSN, RN
Assistant Professor
Radford University School of Nursing
Radford, Virginia

CAM HAMILTON, MSN, RN
Instructor
Auburn University Montgomery
Montgomery, Alabama

KARLA HANSON, MS, BSN, RN
South Dakota State University
Brookings, South Dakota

NANCY HAYNES, RN, MN, PhD, CCRN
Assistant Professor
Saint Luke's College
Kansas City, Missouri

LORI HENDRICKX, RN, EdD, CCRN
Associate Professor
South Dakota State University
College of Nursing
Brookings, South Dakota

ROSEANN KAMINSKY, RN, BSEd, BSN, MSN
Associate Professor
Lorain County Community
College
Elyria, Ohio

KATHERINE KELLY, RN, MSN, FNP-C, CEN
Lecturer
Sacramento State University
Sacramento, California

JOAN KING, PhD, RNC, ACNP, ANP
Program Director for the Acute
Care Nurse Practitioner
Program
Vanderbilt University School of
Nursing
Nashville, Tennessee

BONNIE KIRKPATRICK, RN, MS
Auxiliary Clinical Faculty
Ohio State University College of
Nursing
Columbus, Ohio

THERESE M. LAHNSTEIN, RN, MSN, CCRN
Associate Professor, Department of
Nursing
Columbus State University
Columbus, Georgia

PATTI LALIBERTE, MS, RN
Staff Nurse, Intensive Care Unit
Elliot Hospital
Manchester, New Hampshire

ANNE LARSON, RN, BC, PhD
Professor of Nursing
Midland Lutheran College
Fremont, Nebraska

R. SUE LASITER, PhD(C), RN
Assistant Professor
University of Central Missouri
Warrensburg, Missouri

KRISTINE M. L'ECUYER, MSN, RN
Director, Continuing Nursing
Education
Saint Louis University School of
Nursing
St. Louis, Missouri

PAMELA BRINKER LESTER, DNS, ARNP
Adjunct Associate Professor
Florida Atlantic University
Christine E. Lynn College of
Nursing
Boca Raton, Florida

CHRISTINE MARKUT, DNSc, RNC
Associate Professor
Villa Julie College
Stevenson, Maryland

CINDY McCOY, RN, PhD, BC
Associate Professor
School of Nursing
Troy University
Troy, Alabama

ELIZABETH HENDERSON McINTOSH, CRNP, FNP, MSN
Nurse Practitioner, Clinical
Faculty
Auburn University Montgomery
School of Nursing
Montgomery, Alabama

MaryELLEN McMORROW, RN, APN, EdD
Professor
College of Staten Island
Staten Island, New York

ANN MARIE McSWAIN, RN, MSN, CCNS, CCRN, APRN, BC
Assistant Professor
Lincoln University
Jefferson City, Missouri

JANE NORMAN, PhD, RN, CNE
Professor of Nursing/MSN Program
Director
Tennessee State
Nashville, Tennessee

COLLEEN K. NORTON, DNSc, RN, CCRN
Assistant Professor, School of
Nursing and Health
Georgetown University
Washington, D.C.

ELLEN ODELL, DNP, RN
Assistant Professor
University of Arkansas, Fayetteville
Fayetteville, Arkansas

TRACY A. ORTELLI, MS, RN
Adjunct Faculty
Raritan Valley Community College
Somerville, New Jersey

SUDHA C. PATEL, BSN, MN, MA, DNS
Assistant Professor
University of Louisiana
Lafayette, Louisiana

DEBBIE SCHWYTZER, RN, MSN, CEN
Associate Professor of Clinical
Nursing
University of Cincinnati College of
Nursing
Cincinnati, Ohio

GINA M. SEVERINO, RN, MSN, APRN-BC
Assistant Professor of Nursing
Kent State University
Warren, Ohio

SIGRID SEXTON, RN, MSN, CCRN
Associate Professor
Long Beach City College
Long Beach, California

WENDY B. STEWART, BA, RN, BSN, MSN
Professor of Nursing
San Jacinto College-Central
Pasadena, Texas

JEANINE SWAILS, MSN, RN, CNRN
Assistant Professor of Clinical
  Nursing
University of Cincinnati College of
  Nursing
Cincinnati, Ohio

WILLIAM THOMPSON, CRN, MSN
Staff Anesthetist
Society Hill Anesthesia Consultants
Philadelphia, Pennsylvania

SANDRA TURKLESON, MSN, BSN, RN
Assistant Professor
Northern Kentucky University
  School of Nursing and Health
  Professions
Highland Heights, Kentucky

LAURA JEAN WAIGHT, MSN, RN
Instructor of Nursing
West Texas A&M University
Canyon, Texas

DEBRA WALTON, PhD, RN
Associate Professor
Blessing-Rieman College of Nursing
Quincy, Illinois

TAMRA WEIMER, RN, MS, CCRN
Professor School of Nursing
Southwestern Oklahoma State
  University
Weatherford, Oklahoma

JANICE WILCOX, MSN, RN
The Ohio State University College
  of Nursing
Columbus, Ohio

CHRIS WINKELMAN, RN, PhD, CNP, CCRN
Assistant Professor
Frances Payne Bolton School of
  Nursing
Case Western Reserve University
Cleveland, Ohio

CHARLOTTE A. WISNEWSKI, PhD, RN, BC, CDE
Assistant Professor of Nursing
University of Texas Medical Branch,
  School of Nursing
Galveston, Texas

SUSAN L. WOODS, PhD, RN, FAAN, FAHA
Professor and Associate Dean for
  Academic Services
University of Washington
  Seattle, Washington

KAREN ZAPKO, RN, MSN
Assistant Professor
Kent State University
Kent, Ohio

Special Features

Visual Maps

Commonly Used Medications

Nursing Diagnoses

Safety Initiatives

Gerontological Considerations

Contents

What Is Critical Care?

Kathleen Perrin, PhD, RN, CCRN

Learning Outcomes

Upon completion of this chapter, the learner will be able to:

1. Define critical care.

2. State the three levels of care provided in critical care units.

3. Compare and contrast "open" and "closed" critical care units.

4. Explain why critical care units are one of the most common sites for health care errors.

5. Describe the relationship between the patient and the nurse in the AACN's synergy model.

6. Discuss the competencies of critical care nurses as defined by the synergy model.

7. Describe ways to enhance communication and collaboration among members of the health care team.

8. Explain why some health care providers believe that critically ill patients cannot give informed consent.

9. Analyze why moral distress might be a significant concern for critical care nurses.

10. Prioritize measures that a nurse might utilize to prevent compassion fatigue.

Abbreviations

AACN	American Association of Critical-Care Nurses
ANA	American Nurses Association
HRSA	Health Resources and Services Administration
ICU	Intensive Care Unit
IHI	Institute for Healthcare Improvement
IOM	Institute of Medicine
SCCM	Society of Critical Care Medicine

Critical care is the direct delivery of medical care to a critically ill or injured patient. The care is often, but not necessarily, delivered in a specialized unit with advanced technology available. A specially trained team of professionals best meets the complex needs of critically ill patients and their families. When team members use evidence-based practices and collaborate to meet their patients' needs, patient outcomes are significantly better.

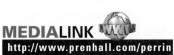

MEDIALINK
http://www.prenhall.com/perrin

See the Companion Website for chapter-specific resources at www.prenhall.com/perrin.

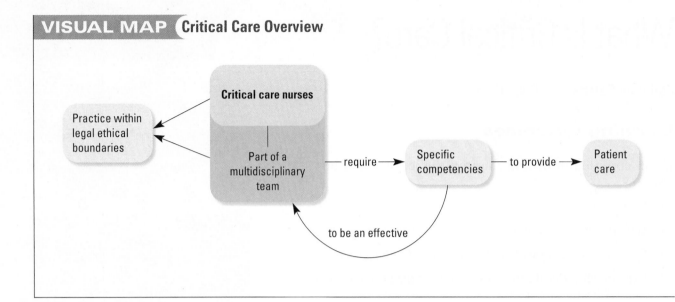

VISUAL MAP Critical Care Overview

Critical Care Defined

Critical care is defined by the Department of Health and Human Services (2001) as the "direct delivery of medical care for a critically ill or injured patient. To be considered critical an illness or injury must acutely impair one or more vital organ systems such that a patient's survival is jeopardized. Critical care is usually but not always given in a critical care area such as a coronary care unit, an intensive care unit, a respiratory care unit, or an emergency care unit."

Trends in Critical Care Units

Although seriously ill patients had historically been grouped together and cared for by a designated nurse, usually near the nurses' station, they were not separated from other patients and placed in critical care units until the early 1950s. At that time the use of mechanical ventilation and cardiopulmonary resuscitation began, and it became more efficient to provide care to gravely ill patients with specially trained nurses in one location in the hospital. By 1958 approximately 25% of community hospitals had an intensive care unit (ICU), and by the late 1960s nearly every hospital in the United States had an ICU.

The number of critical care beds in hospitals has been increasing since 1985, and the number of noncritical care beds has been decreasing. This is partially because critical care has expanded and now includes caring for patients following complicated surgical procedures such as liver transplants. It is also because critical care has become a cost-effective way to treat many patients. The use of noninvasive monitoring and targeted pharmacological therapy has resulted in fewer complications, and, therefore, the cost of caring for some critically ill patients has decreased. This has produced not only cost savings but shortened hospital stays as well, especially for

patients with specific organ system failures such as cardiovascular insufficiency (Society of Critical Care Medicine [SCCM, n.d.]).

According to the SCCM, there are currently more than 5,000 ICUs across the United States. However, there are many differences among the units that are called ICUs. Kirchhoff and Dahl (2006) determined that "unit findings often varied depending on the size of the unit, or size or location of the hospital the unit was in (e.g., urban, suburban, or rural hospitals" (p. 18). In their study, the median number of beds in an ICU was 16 and the average number of admissions was about 2,000 per year. In most critical care units, the length of patient stay was between 2 and 5 days.

Critical care units need to differ because not all hospitals are intended to meet the needs of all types of patients and severity of illness. In 2003, the SCCM endorsed guidelines for critical care services based on three levels of care (Haupt et al., 2003). These guidelines suggested that each hospital provide a level of care appropriate to its mission and the regional needs for critical care services. The recommended levels of care are:

- Level I: comprehensive care for a wide variety of disorders. Sophisticated equipment, specialized nurses, and physicians with specialized preparation are continuously available. Comprehensive support services from pharmacy, nutrition, respiratory, pastoral care, and social work are close at hand. Most of these units are located in teaching hospitals.

- Level II: comprehensive critical care for most disorders but the unit may not be able to care for specific types of patients (e.g., cardiothoracic surgical patients). Transfer arrangements to Level I facilities must be in place for patients with the specific disorders for which the unit does not provide care.

- Level III: initial stabilization of critically ill patients provided but limited ability to provide comprehensive critical care. A limited number of patients who require routine care may remain in the facility but written policies should be in place determining which patients require transfer and where they ought to be transferred.

Critical care units also differ in whether they are "open" or "closed." In an open ICU, nurses, pharmacists, and respiratory therapists are ICU based but the physicians directing patient care may have other obligations. These physicians may or may not choose to consult an intensivist to assist with the management of their ICU patients. In a "**closed ICU**," patient care is provided by a dedicated ICU team that includes a critical care physician. According to Haupt, although patient outcomes appear to be better when patients are cared for in a closed system, the results need to be approached cautiously. The SCCM recommends that "the patient's primary care physician and consultants collaborate in the care of all patients . . . and an intensivist must be given the authority to intervene and direct care for the critically ill patient in urgent and emergent situations" (p. 2682).

Characteristics of the Critical Care Environment

Clearly, the specific nature of the critical care unit and the type of care delivered vary depending on the size and level of the unit. However, over the past 15 years across the level and size of critical care units, there have been more patients receiving care and those patients have been more acutely ill (Kirchoff & Dahl, 2006). It is anticipated that the demand for critical care services will continue to grow over the next 20 years as the baby boom generation ages because Americans over the age of 65 utilize the majority of ICU services.

There are other commonalities among ICUs. The American Hospital Association defines medical and surgical ICUs as "staffed with specially trained nursing personnel and containing monitoring and specialized support equipment for patients who because of shock, trauma, or other life-threatening conditions require intensified, comprehensive observation and care." The qualities of specialized nursing are discussed later in this chapter, but some of the issues associated with specialized equipment and intensified, comprehensive care are discussed next.

Critically ill patients require complex, carefully coordinated care. When a care pattern is complex, failure in one part of the system can unexpectedly affect another. In addition, the care provided to critically ill patients is often coupled, meaning there is little or no buffer between events. Thus, if anything goes wrong, everything can unravel quickly. In addition, when things are tightly coupled even when an error is identified, it can be difficult to prevent the situation from deteriorating, in part because of the complexity and high degree of coupling of care in critical care areas, specifically emergency departments (EDs), ICUs, and operating rooms (ORs), where health care errors most commonly occur.

However, not only do the critically ill patients receive highly complex care, the care they receive is also highly technological. In a foundational study Leape and Brennan (1991) found that 44% of **health care errors** were related to technology, and that all errors were more likely to occur in technologically advanced fields such as vascular, cardiac, and neurosurgery. The Institute of Medicine (Kohn, Corrigan, & Donaldson, 2000) postulates that technology increases errors for several reasons, including:

- Technology changes the tasks people do by shifting the workload and eliminating human decision making.
- Although technology may decrease human workload during nonpeak hours, it often increases it during peak hours or when the system fails or is inadequate (e.g., when medication scanning devices fail without warning and nurses are required to utilize paper systems to dispense medications then must backtrack and redocument when the scanner system is working).
- When the system becomes opaque, users no longer know how to perform a function without it (e.g., when intravenous (IV) pumps are constantly used to calculate doses of continuous medication infusions, nurses can no longer calculate the rate to infuse a drug at a specific dose of mcg/kg/min by hand). Therefore, errors may occur when the system fails.
- When devices are not standardized and demand precision to use (e.g., an ICU uses multiple brands of IV pumps or ventilators), problems can result.

Sandelowski (1997) was concerned about how nurses interact with technology, believing that when nurses focus on interpreting machine-generated texts (like rhythms on an electrocardiogram [ECG] monitor), they may fail to touch patients enough or in the right way. She worried that technology can change the way nurses obtain information from patients and the information they obtain. Thus, the use of technology, although essential to the delivery of critical care, can also predispose to errors in the delivery of care. Each chapter of this text has a selected technology section that explains the technology required to care for a patient.

Safety

The safety of all patients is a concern. However, safety for vulnerable, unstable patients receiving critical care is paramount. Valentin et al. (2006) examined errors that occurred in 205 ICUs worldwide during one 24-hour period.

Only about a quarter of the ICUs reported no errors. The remaining units reported the following types of errors:

- Dislodgment of lines, catheters, and drains
- Medication errors (such as wrong dose, wrong drug, or wrong route)
- Failure of infusion devices
- Failure or dysfunction of a ventilator
- Unplanned extubation while ventilator alarms were turned off

From these data Valentin concluded, "Sentinel events related to medication, indwelling lines, airway, and equipment failure in ICUs occur with considerable frequency. Although patient safety is recognized as a serious issue in many ICUs, there is an urgent need for development and implementation of strategies for prevention and early detection of errors" (p. 1591).

This concern about the frequency of errors and the need to develop preventive strategies is also apparent in a study by Rothschild et al. (2005), who measured the incidence and rates of **adverse events** per 1,000 patient-days in critical care. Twenty percent of the patients they followed experienced at least one adverse event. Of these adverse events, 13% were life threatening or fatal. Most serious medical errors occurred during the ordering or execution of treatments and were skill-based lapses. These lapses could have been prevented with information or technologies that reminded the clinicians of what ought to be done.

Rothschild et al. (2005) concluded that serious errors were common in critical care settings and translated to a rate of 0.8 adverse events and 1.5 serious errors each day for a 10-bed critical care unit. The researchers also noted that these preventable errors were often associated with systemwide problems that caused the errors or near misses by multiple clinicians. They concluded that it is important to find ways to "engineer out" slips and lapses so that treatment is delivered as intended.

Since the release of the Institute of Medicine's (IOM) report, *To Err Is Human* (Kohn et al., 2000), there has been a focus on uncovering systemwide errors and diminishing the potential for errors in hospitals in the United States. To decrease the potential for errors, the report recommends the following:

- Utilizing constraints: An example of a constraint is when the height, weight, and allergies of the patient must be on file to obtain medication for the patient.
- Installing forcing functions or system-level firewalls: An example of a forcing function is that concentrated (undiluted) potassium chloride (KCl) is no longer available on hospital units.
- Avoiding reliance on vigilance: Because humans cannot remain vigilant for a protracted amount of time, checklists, protocols, and rechecking with another professional should be required before major procedures and before potentially dangerous medication administration. Examples are timeouts before surgery or double-checking doses on intensive insulin protocols.
- Simplifying key processes.
- Standardizing key processes.

According to the IOM, safety is more than just the absence of errors; it is an outlook that health care is complex and can be risky. It involves identifying, evaluating, and minimizing hazards in the environment. A safety feature is included in the chapters in this book.

Providers

There are documented ways in which health care providers can enhance safe, effective care and limit risks to critically ill patients. These include developing a multidisciplinary approach to patient care, encouraging a culture of safety, instituting a closed unit, providing adequate staffing, and limiting work hours.

Multidisciplinary Approach to Care

Since the 1986 study by Knaus, Draper, Wagner, and Zimmerman, it has been apparent that when members of various disciplines collaborate in the care of critically ill patients, the patients have better outcomes. Although there is insufficient evidence to recommend a specific model for delivery of critical care, evidence does suggest that care should be delivered by a multidisciplinary team headed by a full-time critical care trained physician and consisting of at least an ICU nurse, a respiratory therapist, and a pharmacist (National Guidelines Clearinghouse, 2003). Outcomes for patients are better when multidisciplinary teams collaborate and work well together. Strategies that encourage teamwork and collaboration among staff members caring for critically ill patients can further improve patient outcomes (Whelan, Burchill, & Tilin, 2003).

Benner (2001) recommends building a moral community and a culture of safety among team members. She defines a culture of safety as the "practice responsibility of all health care team members working together in the moment to provide good health care" (p. 282). In such an environment, practitioners have a responsibility to their patients to make their errors known, have them corrected, and share them with the patient, his family, and other practitioners. This sharing of information benefits the patient but ultimately benefits team members and future patients as well. When providers realize that multiple factors contribute to errors in the complex ICU environment, the focus shifts from one of "shame and blame" for errors to one of practice improvement. With practice improvement as the goal rather than punishment of the health care provider who committed the error, the reporting of errors results in the examination of the factors that contributed to the error and changes in practice patterns.

Henneman (2007) describes a series of errors that occurred one day while she was caring for two critically ill patients. She notes that only one of the errors was a medication dispensing error; it was the only error that was easy to identify and was reported in the traditional pattern. The remainder of the errors resulted from failures of communication or collaboration and breakdowns in the system. These errors were equally harmful to the patient as the medication dispensing error, yet they were not readily identified as errors and were not reported. She believes that she did not report them because "I had become so accustomed to the system failures that I stopped recognizing them as such" (p. 33). If a culture of safety had been established, the breakdowns in communication and collaboration might have been identified as errors and reported. When such system failures are identified, Henneman believes that nurses will no longer have to "work around" them, and patient safety will not continue to be jeopardized.

Instituting a Closed Unit

Although the SCCM was reluctant to state that closed units (units where only intensivists treat patients) improve patient outcomes, the United States government was not. In a report to Congress 2001 on the Critical Care Workforce, the Health Resources and Services Administration (HRSA) suggested that requiring all ICUs to become "closed units" could save the lives of 54,000 of the 360,000 patients who die in critical care units annually. In addition, the report noted economic and quality of life benefits for "closed units."

Ensuring Adequate Staffing

Even the best teamwork and most competent staff will not consistently overcome inadequate staffing. Tarnow-Mordi, Hau, Warden, and Shearer (2000) demonstrated that "patients exposed to high ICU workload were more likely to die than those exposed to lower ICU workload" (p. 188). The three measures of ICU workload most closely tied to mortality in their study were peak occupancy of the ICU, average nursing requirement/occupied bed per shift, and the ratio of occupied to appropriately staffed beds. The American Association of Critical-Care Nurses (AACN) believes that adequate staffing should not be defined as a specific nurse/patient ratio. In its report, *Standards for Establishing and Sustaining Healthy Work Environments: A Journey to Excellence*, the AACN states that the basis for effective staffing is the realization that the needs of critically ill patients fluctuate repeatedly throughout their illness. Instead of mandating a fixed nurse/patient ratio, the

AACN recommends instituting the following measures to ensure adequate staffing:

- The health care organization should have staffing policies that are grounded in ethical principles and support the obligation of nurses to provide quality care.
- Nurses ought to participate in all phases of the staffing process, from education to planning to assigning nurses with the appropriate competencies, to meet the needs of the patients.
- The health care organization should develop a plan to evaluate the effectiveness of staffing decisions and to use the data to develop more effective staffing models.
- The health care organization should provide support and technological services that increase the effectiveness of nursing care delivery and allow nurses to spend their time meeting the needs of the patients and those of the patients' families.

Limiting Hours of Work

The IOM recommended that nurses work no more than 60 hours each week or 12 hours in a 24-hour period (Page, 2004). In 2006, Scott, Rogers, Hwang, and Shang determined that when critical care nurses worked longer than 12 hours, the likelihood of errors and near errors increased and the nurses' vigilance decreased. Unfortunately, in their study of 502 nurses, only one critical care nurse left work on time every day. Most nurses rarely left work on time, even those who were working 12-hour shifts. These extended work hours increased the nurses' potential for errors. In addition, Scott et al. found that two thirds of the nurses struggled to stay awake at least once during the 28-day study period and that 20% fell asleep. Scott et al. summarized their study by affirming the finding of the IOM and saying that to ensure patient safety, extended work shifts should be eliminated.

Defining Critical Care Nursing

According to the AACN, "**critical care nursing** is that specialty that deals specifically with human responses to life threatening problems. A critical care nurse is a licensed professional nurse who is responsible for ensuring that acutely and critically ill patients and their families receive optimal care." The HRSA survey of 2000 found that approximately 25% of nurses employed in hospitals worked more than half their time in a critical care unit (HRSA, 2001). However, critical care nurses work wherever patients with potentially life-threatening problems may be found and that includes EDs, outpatient surgery centers, and even schools.

The AACN believes that critical care nursing should be defined more by the needs of the patients and

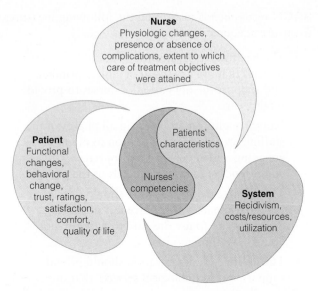

Figure 1-1 Three levels of outcomes delineated by the AACN's Synergy Model for Patient Care: those derived from the patient, those derived from the nurse, and those derived from the health care system.
(Curley, MA. Patient-nurse synergy: optimizing patients' outcomes. *American Journal of Critical Care 1998, 7(1), 64–72.*)

those of their families than by the environment in which care is delivered or the diagnoses of the patients. Therefore, the organization developed the Synergy Model for Patient Care (Figure 1-1). This model is based on the patient's characteristics, the nurses' competencies, and three levels of outcomes derived from the patient, the nurse, and the health care system. An underlying assumption of the synergy model is that optimal patient outcomes occur when the needs of the patient and those of his or her family are aligned with the competencies of the nurse.

Competencies of Critical Care Nurses as Defined by the AACN in the Synergy Model

The synergy model describes each of the competencies of the critical care nurse on a continuum of expertise from 1 to 5, ranging from competent to expert.

Clinical Inquiry

According to the AACN's *Critical Care Nursing Fact Sheet*, the critical care nurse should be engaged in the "ongoing process of questioning and evaluating practice and providing informed practice." One way that critical care nurses might demonstrate this competency would be to provide care based on the best available evidence

rather than on tradition. An expert critical care nurse might be able to evaluate research and develop evidence-based protocols for nursing practice in her agency, whereas a competent nurse might follow evidence-based agency policies and protocols. Critical care nurses (both novice and expert) can develop the mindset that questioning practice is an issue of safety. A safe practitioner is one who wonders, "Why do we do things this way?" or "Why am I being asked to provide this specific type of care to this patient at this moment?"

Clinical Judgment

The AACN fact sheet states that the critical care nurse should engage in "clinical reasoning which includes clinical decision making, critical thinking, and a global grasp of the situation, coupled with nursing skills acquired through a process of integrating formal and experiential knowledge." A competent critical care nurse is able to collect and interpret basic data then follow pathways and algorithms when providing care. She might focus on some specific aspect of care, which a more experienced nurse might recognize as less important. This nurse, when unsure about how to respond, often defers to the expertise of other nurses. An expert nurse is able to use past experience, recognize patterns of patient problems, and "see the big picture." Her previous experience coupled with the ability to see the "big picture" often allows her to anticipate possible untoward events and develop interventions to prevent them.

For example, an ED nurse received a report that a patient with stable vital signs who had had a brick wall fall on his chest would be arriving in the ED in approximately 5 minutes. On arrival the patient was extremely pale with new onset chest pain. The expert ED nurse requested the new graduate get the physician immediately while she prepared for chest tube insertion. By the time the physician arrived the patient was displaying clear signs of a tension pneumothorax. However, the expert nurse had everything prepared for immediate chest tube insertion and decompression and the patient recovered quickly.

Caring

In its fact sheet, the AACN defines caring behaviors as "nursing activities that create a compassionate, supportive, and therapeutic environment for patients and staff, with the aim of promoting comfort and preventing unnecessary suffering." A caring critical care nurse can make an enormous difference in the critical care experience for a frightened patient and family. Whereas a competent nurse might focus on the basic and routine needs of the patient, an expert nurse is able to anticipate patient/family changes and needs, varying her caring approach to meet their needs. For example, a son was frightened and kept leaving the bedside of his dying mother. The expert critical care nurse placed a chair at the mother's bedside and stayed with the son, showing him how to stroke her brow gently and speak to her softly.

Advocacy

The American Nurses Association (ANA) in its *Code of Ethics for Nurses* (2001) states, "The nurse promotes, advocates for, and strives to protect the health, safety, and rights of the patient." In its *Critical Care Nursing Fact Sheet,* the AACN states that "Foremost, the critical care nurse is a patient advocate and defines advocacy as 'respecting and supporting the basic rights and beliefs of the critically ill patient.'" The National Council of State Boards of Nursing lists eight elements for the standard of nurse advocacy for clients. Clearly, nursing professional organizations and the nursing licensure body expect nurses to recognize that their patients may be vulnerable and may require assistance to obtain what they need from the health care system. However, it is sometimes difficult for nurses to advocate for their patients in the current system. Before the nurse can be an effective advocate, she needs to examine some of her own values and beliefs.

A nurse might want to consider the following:

- What types of issues (including end-of-life issues) might arise in the clinical setting for which the patient may need an advocate?

- What is owed to the patient and what are the duties of the nurse in those circumstances?

- If she encountered one of those situations, how would the nurse be able to determine what the patient or family desires or what would be in the patient's best interests?

- Would the nurse be able to differentiate her needs and desires from those of the patient? How certain could she be?

- How would the nurse act for her patient or empower her patient and his family to communicate their needs and desires to the rest of the health care team?

- How would the nurse respond if she thought that the quality of a patient's care was being jeopardized?

- How would the nurse ensure that the discussion was a mutual exploration of concerns and not a confrontation?

According to the AACN, a competent nurse assesses her personal values and patient rights, represents the patient if the patient's needs and desires are consistent with her framework, and acknowledges death as a pos-

sible outcome. However, an expert nurse advocates from the family/patient perspective whether it is similar to or different from her own, empowers the patient and family to speak for or represent themselves, and achieves mutuality in relationships. For example, a patient and his wife wanted to withdraw interventions because the patient was clearly deteriorating and dying. However, their children, who were scattered about the country and had not seen their father during the hospitalization, were unwilling to support the decision. The nurse caring for the patient helped the wife gather the family at the patient's bedside. Then the nurse stayed with the patient and his wife as they explained the patient's condition and their decision to the children.

Systems Thinking

The AACN defines systems thinking as managing the existing environmental and system resources for the benefit of patients and their families. For a vulnerable patient and family, being in an unfamiliar and overwhelming health care system can be intimidating, even frightening. Having a nurse who knows how the system works and explains it to the patient and family, or helps the patient and family obtain what they need, can make the difference between an experience that is overpowering for the family and one that the patient and family believe they can endure. A competent nurse might see himself as a resource for the patient on the specific unit where the patient is receiving care, whereas an expert nurse might know how to negotiate and navigate for the patient throughout the health care system to obtain the necessary or desired care. For example, a patient with ALS requested extubation and discharge home for palliative care. His ICU nurse worked for several days with the hospice and palliative care nurses to prepare his home environment and family for his transition to care at home.

Facilitator of Learning

The AACN states that nurses should be able to facilitate both informal and formal learning for patients, families, and members of the health care team. A competent nurse might follow planned educational programs using standardized materials or see the patient and family as passive recipients of educational materials. An expert nurse would be able to "creatively modify or develop patient/family educational programs and integrate family/patient education throughout the delivery of care." For example, a nurse providing heart failure education realized that many of her patients who could not read would not admit that to her. She discovered that if she showed her patients clearly legible print and asked if the print was okay for them to read, the patients who could not read would readily say that the print was a problem and was too difficult to read. The nurse could then plan appropriate ways to teach her patients.

Response to Diversity

The AACN defines response to diversity as "sensitivity to recognize, appreciate, and incorporate diversity into the provision of care." A competent nurse might recognize the values of the patient but still provide care based on a standardized format. An expert nurse would anticipate the needs of the patient and family based on their cultural, spiritual, or personal values, and would tailor the delivery of care to incorporate these values.

For example, a terrified patient was being rushed to a medical center several hours from his home for an emergent mitral valve replacement. Despite the need for haste, the expert nurse realized the importance of faith to this patient and thus arranged for him to receive the Sacrament of the Sick prior to his transfer.

Collaboration

The AACN defines collaboration as "working with others in a way that promotes each person's contributions toward achieving optimal and realistic patient/family goals." A competent nurse might participate in multidisciplinary meetings and listen to the opinions of various team members. On the other hand, an expert nurse might facilitate the active involvement and contributions of others in meetings and role model leadership and accountability during the meetings. For example, a preceptor encouraged and assisted his orientee to present information on a complex patient with placenta accreda during multidisciplinary rounds and later during nursing grand rounds.

Interdisciplinary Nature of Delivery of Care in Critical Care Environments

For optimum patient outcomes, critical care is delivered by a multidisciplinary team whose members trust each other and communicate and collaborate well.

Communication

In 2005, the AACN declared, "Nurses must be as proficient in communication as they are in clinical skills" (p. 190). Optimal patient care is not possible without skilled communication, and errors are frequent in situations where communication between health care providers and patients and their families is impaired. Rothschild et al. (2005) found that 13.7% of errors in critical care were related to problems communicating clinical information. Meanwhile the Joint Commission on Accreditation of Healthcare Organizations (2006) determined that a breakdown in communication was the leading root factor in sentinel events between 1995

and 2004 and again in 2005. Skilled communication has at least two essential components: the choice and presentation of appropriate content for the message and the way in which the message is conveyed.

Situation Background Assessment Recommendation

The Institute for Healthcare Improvement (IHI) currently advocates a technique borrowed from the military that it believes will improve communication among health care professionals. This technique, called Situation Background Assessment Recommendation (**SBAR**), provides a process for determining what information is appropriate and delivering it in a specific manner. The IHI anticipates that using SBAR will prevent what it describes as "multiple calls to the physician when the record makes clear that the patient is deteriorating but the physician is unaware or does not understand the nurse's statements." On its Web site the IHI provides a document titled "SBAR Report to Physician About a Critical Situation" to guide nurses' communication. The format is:

S: Situation

- I am calling about (patient, name, location).
- The problem I am calling about is (the nurse states specifics).
- I have assessed the patient personally.
- Vital signs are.
- I am concerned about (the nurse states what the specific concern is).

B: Background

- The patient's immediate history is:
- The patient's other physical findings are (e.g., mental status).
- The patient's treatments are (e.g., oxygen therapy):

A: Assessment

- This is what I think the problem is _____.
- Or, I'm not sure what the problem is but the patient is deteriorating.

R: Recommendation

- I suggest (or request) that you (the nurse states the desired course of action).

Two-Challenge Rule

There are times when members of the health care team do not listen and respond to each other even when essential information has been communicated in an appropriate format. Sachs (2005) reported on a 38-year-old woman who experienced a critical illness and fetal demise following numerous errors in communication and planning as well as errors in judgment at Beth Israel Deaconess Medical Center. One of the strategies that the hospital adopted to prevent similar problems in the future was to train everyone to challenge other health care providers, even those senior to them, if they disagreed with the proposed course of action.

The two-challenge rule is a method adapted from the airline industry's crew resource management. When following the two-challenge rule, a nurse who disagrees with another health care provider's proposed intervention would respectfully state his concerns about the intervention twice then would seek a superior as soon as possible and explain his concerns.

Assertive Communication

The essential second element of the two-challenge rule is that the nurse while stating his disagreement should present his concerns respectfully. There is mounting evidence that disrespectful and intimidating communication contributes significantly to health care errors. Connie Barden, past president of the AACN, believes that nurses should speak with a bold voice. According to her, a bold voice is one that does not blame or whine, it does not argue, and it looks past complaints to work with others on solutions (Barden, 2003).

Lindeke and Sieckert (2005) stated that when a nurse needs to make a case for or against a specific action, she should be assertive but not aggressive. To do this the nurse should question the decision calmly and directly rather than hinting. For example, "Dr. Jones, I don't understand why dobutamine is the appropriate medication for Mrs. Green. Would you explain?" The nurse also avoids using disclaimers such as "you might think differently" because that can undermine her position.

Collaboration. According to the National Guidelines Clearinghouse, evidence supports a model of critical care delivery where dedicated intensive care personnel, specifically an intensivist, an ICU nurse, a respiratory care practitioner, and a pharmacist, all work as a team. Since 1986 when Knaus et al. found that outcomes in ICUs were "more related to interaction and coordination of each hospital's intensive care unit staff than to the unit's administrative structure, amount of specialized treatment use, or the hospitals' teaching status," it has been recognized that there is a link between teamwork and patient outcomes in ICUs. Whelan, Burchill, and Tilin concluded that the "evidence is sufficient to warrant the implementation of policies designed to improve the level of communication and collaboration among staff members in intensive care units (2003, p. 527).

Collaboration is a process, not a single event, and it requires that members of the health care team develop a pattern of sharing knowledge and responsibility for pa-

tient care. There are a number of characteristics that influence the degree of collaboration that occurs among members of a health care team. These characteristics are discussed in the sections that follow.

Development of Emotional Maturity. According to Lindeke and Sieckert (2005) emotional maturity is foundational to collaboration because of the positive individual attributes people who are emotionally mature possess. These include being lifelong learners, actively identifying best practices, and keeping their skills current. Emotionally mature people are positive, humble, and willing to take responsibility for their failures and try again. A nurse can begin to develop emotional maturity by mastering her own emotions and recognizing those of others.

Understanding the Perspective of Others. There is evidence that members of the differing health professions have different perspectives on what ought to be communicated as well as what ought to be the goals of patient care. For example, critical care nurses and physicians see the subsets and phases of the illnesses of the same groups of patients differently. The nurse may see only the sickest of a group of patients, whereby only half of the patients survive to hospital discharge. These patients may be severely debilitated at the time of discharge, and the nurse may worry about their ability to survive. The physician or home health nurse, in contrast, may see the same subset of patients on a longer term basis and realize how infrequently they need hospitalization and how well they do afterward. Thus, the physician may realize that the actual outcomes of care are better than the hospital nurse envisions them to be (Shannon, 1997).

When the prognosis is unclear, there is some indication that nurses and physicians use different types of cues to determine what they believe will be the outcome. According to Anspach (1987), physicians are more likely to rely on technological cues, such as lab tests or findings from a physical examination, to determine prognosis, whereas nurses tend to attach more significance to interactive cues, such as when a patient appears depressed, cannot be comforted, or appears to be suffering. Anspach suggests that nurses' reliance on the interactive cues is related to the time they spend caring for and interacting with their patients. There is no current indication that one type of cue is more likely to predict a patient's outcome than the other.

These differences in viewpoints can make collaboration more difficult. However, if health care providers are willing to listen to each other, a holistic view of the patient may be developed. Programs that teach communication and relationship skills have been created to enhance physician-nurse communication in critical care units (Boyle & Kochinda, 2004).

Building the Team

Important to team functioning is the identification of a common goal. In health care that goal is usually patient well-being. Unfortunately, when a patient is critically ill, team members may disagree on what constitutes patient well-being and thus what is in the patient's best interests. Critical care units that have daily multidisciplinary rounds and dialogue about patient prognosis and establishment of patient goals have been demonstrated to have better team functioning and patient outcomes (Narasimhan, Eisen, Mahoney, Acerra, & Rosen, 2006).

Negotiating Respectfully

Nurses encounter a variety of barriers when they attempt to negotiate. The most important one may be that power is often unbalanced in health care negotiations. Lindeke and Sieckert (2005) stated that nurses should therefore contribute to teams from positions of strength by being innovative and by demonstrating integrity in collaboration. In contrast, Gardner (2004) stated that to achieve collaboration there must be some form of power sharing. She identified the informal power bases of information, expertise, and goodwill and recommended that nurses ask for opinions from the quiet, less verbal members of a group as a means of demonstrating goodwill and sharing power.

Managing Conflict Wisely

Encountering conflict can be stressful, but acknowledging it and managing it well is the cornerstone to successful collaboration (Gardner, 2004). Furthermore, when nurses embrace conflict and engage in it assertively yet respectfully, there is an opportunity for growth and innovation in clinical practice. According to Gardner, when encountering conflict the nurse must distinguish between emotional conflict, which arises from relationships, and task conflict, which centers on judgments concerning the best way to achieve an agreed-upon goal. Task conflict, which is easier to manage and is often healthy, can usually be resolved with a discussion of the risks and benefits of each approach. When emotional conflict develops, the nurse manager may need to redirect concerns away from the issue and encourage the disputants to resolve the issue in private.

Ethical and Legal Issues in the Delivery of Critical Care

Nurses who take care of critically ill patients often encounter situations where there is disagreement among the health care team, the patient, and the patient's family about how to proceed. In such circumstances, it is important that the nurse know the legal issues involved as well as how to engage in ethical discourse and decision making.

Ethical Dilemmas

Ethical decision making in critical care takes time, an understanding of the language and concepts of ethics, and an ability to make appropriate distinctions (Perrin & McGhee, 2007). It takes an appreciation of what it is to be human and of the successes and limits of medicine. Further, decision making in nursing ethics takes an ability to communicate with people who are in distress, an awareness of cultural and religious values, and the ability to compromise. Because nurses are intimately involved with patients and families, they may have strong feelings or beliefs about what should be done. Perrin and McGhee believe it is important that nurses learn to translate these feelings and beliefs into ethical discourse so that they can participate in the discussion of what ought to be done for their patients. Nurses are often the people who carry out the interventions, so they ought to believe that acceptable resolutions to the dilemmas have been identified. Nurses should search for morally acceptable alternatives so that they have an alternative to participating in the action if they believe it is not morally justifiable.

Does an Ethical Dilemma Exist?

When a nurse encounters a situation that makes her wonder, "Is this what I ought to be doing to provide care for this patient?" she should explore whether it is an **ethical dilemma**. Ethical dilemmas may exist when there is a conflict between the duties, rights, or values of the people involved in the situation. They may occur when those involved believe that different principles ought to motivate their behavior, or when they believe that considerations of the consequences of their actions should drive their decision making. An ethical dilemma might be defined as a situation that gives rise to conflicting moral claims, resulting in disagreements about choices for action. A cue that a nurse is dealing with an ethical dilemma is the language used to describe the situation. Ethical dilemmas are usually described in terms of right or wrong, duty or obligation, rights or responsibilities, and good or bad. Ethical dilemmas are commonly identified by the question, "What should be done?"

What Information Is Necessary to Make an Informed Decision?

Once it seems apparent that an ethical dilemma exists, the first essential step is the identification of significant information. Without a clear understanding of the particulars of the situation, the nurse will not be able to fully understand the dilemma or choose an action wisely.

It is important that the nurse understand the patient's medical condition. In order to limit potential confusion, it is helpful if the person, family, and all health care providers share an understanding of both the patient's disease state and the goals for his treatment. Disagreement about a patient's prognosis, disease progression, and likely outcome is frequently the reason that health care providers, the patient, and family members are unable to agree on a treatment plan.

Ethical Frameworks That Help Nurses to Understand and Resolve Dilemmas

Utilizing ethical frameworks or perspectives is rather like using a filter. It helps the nurse sort the material and identify what information is important when making her decision. It also assists in identifying appropriate alternatives for action. It is important that the nurse recognize what ethical reasoning system she is using and identify the ethical viewpoints of those involved in the dilemma (Perrin & McGhee, 2007).

Egoist Framework.
One viewpoint that health care providers and families rarely acknowledge they are using is the egoist framework. In an egoist framework, the reasoner (the health care provider or family member) usually chooses the option that is best for the reasoner rather than the patient. For example, a patient with a flail chest might be complaining of pain and asks not to be turned. The nurse might decide that because it was the end of her shift and she was exhausted, the task of turning the patient could wait until the next shift arrived even though she knows that the patient has been lying on his back for several hours.

A nurse might become aware that she was choosing egoist reasoning if she found herself wondering: "What will do me the most good?" or "What action will cause me the least discomfort?"

Consequentialism or Utilitarianism as a Framework.
Another perspective that health care providers might use to make an ethical decision is consequentialism or utilitarianism. Using this framework, a person would ask, "What will bring the greatest good to the greatest number of people?" "What will result in the best consequences to all those directly or indirectly involved?" This system is not concerned with the good of the individual person, but rather what action will benefit the most people. An exhausted nurse caring for a patient with a flail chest injury who uses this ethical reasoning approach would most likely turn the patient. The nurse would decide that if all exhausted nurses did not turn their patients who needed turning, there would not be just one patient with atelectasis or pneumonia but many.

A nurse might recognize that he was using utilitarianism as a framework for ethical reasoning if he found himself wondering: "What would happen to patients if all nurses acted this way?"

Principled Approach.
Many health care providers employ a principled approach when examining ethical dilemmas. This method emphasizes duties and obligations based on rules and principles. The major principles identified in nursing literature include respect for persons with an emphasis on patient autonomy, nonmaleficence often incorporated with beneficence, and justice.

The principled approach, as stressed in respect for persons, stands in opposition to a utilitarian approach because it is concerned with what will benefit each individual person rather than what will bring the greatest good to the most people. This approach emphasizes that people should be treated with empathy and consideration and never approached as a means to an end. Thus, an action is chosen based on a principle or rule rather than on the likely consequences. Unfortunately, there is no agreement on which of the principles should receive priority when two or more are in conflict.

Respect for Persons.
Respect for persons implies that each patient matters. It further implies that each patient should receive full consideration of his concerns and that patients' concerns should be important factors when decisions are made about health care. In fact, if the individual is to be autonomous, he should be the primary decision maker as long as he has the capacity to make the decision. For example, the nurse caring for the patient with the flail chest might have the patient decide when he wanted to be turned but realizes that pain could diminish his capacity to make the decision if he should be turned.

When approaching an ethical dilemma, health care providers guided by the principle of autonomy might ask themselves the following questions:

- Has the patient stated a preference for the management of his care either in the past (advance directive) or currently?

- To whom or how was the preference stated?

- What is the patient's expressed preference?

Beneficence.
Another principle often cited in bioethics is the principle of beneficence, which means attempting to do good for others. Most ethicists believe that it is composed of two parts: beneficence and nonmaleficence. Ethicists argue that nonmaleficence, the principle of avoiding or preventing harm, should take precedence because it is more important to avoid doing harm to patients than it is to attempt to benefit them. If a nurse were utilizing the principle of beneficence to make a decision about turning the patient with the flail chest, she might decide that the patient needs to be turned because leaving him on his back would result in immediate physical harm even though honoring his autonomy and allowing him to make his own decision might incur a moral good.

Questions a nurse utilizing the principles of nonmaleficence or beneficence might ask when making a health care decision include:

- Would the proposed actions result in physical, emotional, or moral harm to the patient?

- What action would result in the least harm to the patient?

- If none of the actions were likely to result in foreseeable harm, what action would offer this patient the most benefit or would be in this patient's best interests?

Justice. Justice may be approached either as one of the cardinal principles of health care ethics or as an ethical theory. Usually the type of justice discussed in health care ethics is distributive justice. Distributive justice deals with the fair distribution of goods and services, which, in this case, are medical and nursing services. This distribution occurs at several levels: the amount of national funds that should be allocated to health care; the allocation of the funds for research, prevention, or illness care within health care; and the allocation of care to individual people.

When considering allocation of care to the individual person, the nurse might ask:

* What is due to this person?
* Is this action fair?
* Does it treat this person like every other and show neither favoritism nor discrimination?

Rights-Based Approaches. In rights-based theories, actions are deemed to be appropriate or not based on selected rights. According to the American Hospital Association, hospitalized patients in the United States have rights to privacy, to confidentiality, and to know their caregiver. Rights may be justified on legal or ethical grounds. Both types of rights can serve as social sanctions and action guides, but only legal rights are enforceable with punishment by the law if they are not followed. A competent person may choose to exercise his rights or forgo them. However, only the holder of the right or his designee can choose to renounce a right. When utilizing a rights-based approach, a nurse might ask the following questions:

* Does the patient have any legal rights in the situation?
* Has the patient chosen to exercise them?
* What is the corresponding duty and whose duty is it?
* Does the patient have any moral rights in the situation?
* What action would best protect the patient's moral and legal rights?

Care-Based Approaches. Benner and Wrubel (1989) have proposed a system of nursing ethics based on care and responsibility. By being "connected" to and by caring about their patients, nurses are able to discern that certain aspects of a situation are relevant. The nurse is able to understand the meaning of the experience to the patient while the patient feels cared for by the nurse and, therefore, develops trust in her. This discernment enables the nurse to identify problems, describe possible solutions, and take action. The process may not be an intellectual activity; rather it may be a rapid, nonreflective understanding of the situation, which Benner calls "embodied intelligence."

A nurse using the caring approach might not need to question how to proceed; rather he might simply know what the patient needs to have done. If, however, a nurse were considering the caring approach, the following questions may arise:

* Have I formed a human connection with this patient?
* Do I know what this experience means to the patient?
* Do I know the person's culture and family and do I appreciate the background meaning?
* Do I know what ought to be done?

All Things Considered, Determining What Ought to Be Done

How should one make a decision and choose a course of action? Most people will state that making any decision should involve clear thinking and consideration of the implications of each of the alternatives. Kuhse (1997) wrote that making an ethical decision is at least "reflective, a social activity, a matter of sound reasoning, impartial, and universal." Moreover, according to Kuhse, making such a decision should not be "a matter of religion, a matter of obedience to authority, what comes naturally, social practice, or just a matter of feelings." When preparing to make a decision, the nurse might ask herself the following questions:

* What ethically justified goals can be identified?
* What are the ethically justified alternatives for action?
* Are there practical constraints to following any of them?
* What arguments can be constructed in favor of these alternatives (this includes considering the probable consequences)?
* How can these arguments be evaluated?
* What ought to be done?
* Is this decision reflective of sound thinking, or is it based on pressures from society, authority, religion, or purely on emotions and feelings?

When the nurse has made a decision she feels prepared to defend, presenting the decision to health care colleagues will allow them to evaluate the decision. This publicity and scrutiny will help to assure all those involved of the soundness of the decision. Besides, most health care decision making is a group process.

Nurses may be represented in the group decision-making process in several ways. First, they may represent their ethical perspective on the situation to a multidisciplinary meeting. For example, many nurses bring complex situations to the ethics committees of the hospitals where they practice. More commonly, nurses serve as the intermediary between patients, families, and health care providers, helping each group to understand the concerns of the others. Nurses often translate the ethical perspectives of their patients for other health care providers and clarify what the providers are saying to patients and families. Less frequently, nurses may act independently on their own moral decisions.

Issues with Both Legal and Ethical Aspects

Critical care nurses regularly encounter a variety of issues that have both ethical and legal implications. Some of the issues are discussed briefly in this chapter and others, such as those concerning end of life, are discussed later in the book. In either case, the content in this book serves merely as an introduction to these complex issues.

Informed Consent

Obtaining **informed consent** has both legal and ethical ramifications. When a patient gives consent, he agrees to the suggested treatment or procedure. Legally, if a nurse treats or touches a patient without consent, it is considered battery, even if the treatment is appropriate and has no negative effects. Consent is usually implied rather than written for "routine" procedures like turning, dressing changes, or most medication administration. It is also implied when a person goes to an ED acutely ill and unresponsive. However, written informed consent should always be obtained before complex procedures such as invasive and surgical procedures, blood administration, and chemotherapy, which might have serious side effects or consequences for the patient.

Informed consent has three components. The decision to permit the treatment or procedure:

- must be made voluntarily
- by a competent adult
- who understands his condition and the possible treatments.

In other words, the patient's decision must be an autonomous choice, not coerced or manipulated by health care providers or family members. In addition, the patient must be capable of rational thought and be able to recognize what the prospective treatment involves.

It is common for health care providers and family members to question the decision-making ability of critically ill patients. Many are intubated and unable to communicate even their most basic needs clearly. Other patients may be experiencing pain or are depressed so that they are not capable of thinking clearly. Such critically ill patients might be determined to lack the capacity to give informed consent. A determination of incapacity does not require a legal proceeding; it is a clinical judgment that can be assessed during conversation with the patient. To determine capacity, the nurse might ask the following questions (Chell, 1998):

- Does the patient understand her medical condition?

- Does the patient understand the options and the consequences of her decision?
- In addition, if the patient is refusing to consent to recommended medical treatment, is her refusal based on rational reasons?

A loss of capacity may be temporary, for example, when a patient has been experiencing pain or is heavily medicated following surgery. During the period of incapacity, a surrogate health care decision maker might be requested to consent to treatment for the patient. Some states allow next of kin to make decisions when a patient is incapacitated. Others require that a decision maker, known as a health care proxy or durable power of attorney for health care purposes, be designated by the patient in an advance directive or appointed by the courts. Often the patient may be critically ill with sepsis and organ failure so the care that the surrogate decision maker is asked to consent to may determine if the patient lives or dies.

If a surrogate decision maker is having difficulty determining what ought to be done, the nurse might explain that there are two common ethically accepted modes for making surrogate decisions. The first is the best interest standard in which the decision maker decides what he believes is in the best interests of the patient. For example, following his wife's stroke a husband might decide that she would consent to administration of rTPA because it would be in her best interests to have minimal neurological impairment. The second method is substituted judgment in which the surrogate decides what he thinks the patient would have decided had she been able to make the decision. For example, a husband might realize that his wife had been in atrial fibrillation and heart failure prior to her stroke and had been saying for months that she could not go on any more. He might decide that she would not have consented to the treatment so he would make that decision for her.

Whether it is the patient who is making the decision for herself or a surrogate who is making the decision for her, it is essential that the decision maker have adequate information about the possible treatment(s) to make a decision. Although the nurse does not usually provide the initial information for the informed consent, it is the nurse who consistently reinforces the teaching and ensures that the decision maker understands:

- The nature and purpose of the proposed treatment or procedure
- The expected outcome and likelihood of success
- The likely risks involved
- The alternatives to treatment
- The risks if no treatment is selected

When the patient is critically ill, the decision maker may be in crisis. So it is imperative that the nurse be willing to explain this information repeatedly and listen to determine that it has been understood. Conflict can develop when health care providers, patients and families, or decision makers do not have a common understanding of the proposed treatment(s) or when they disagree about what the patient would have wanted or what is in the patient's best interests.

End-of-life Issues

There are a number of ethical/legal concerns that surround end-of-life care for the critically ill patient. These include advance directives, limitation of therapy, withdrawal of therapy, euthanasia, and organ donation from deceased donors. They are discussed in detail in Chapter 18. ∞

Issues Related to Organ Transplantation Recipients and Living Donors

As the need for organs for transplant expands, there are concerns about how organs should be allocated and who an appropriate living donor is. These issues are discussed in Chapter 15. ∞

Use of Restraints

In the past it was common practice in the United States to physically restrain confused or frail patients to prevent them from harming themselves. Nurses stated that their primary motive in restraining these patients was beneficence, acting to prevent patients from the harm they might incur if they tried to pull out an endotracheal tube or IV, move around in bed unassisted, or inadvertently disconnect ventilator tubing. However, ethicists have been deeply concerned about the practice. They believe that the principle of nonmaleficence (or not harming a patient) should always take precedence over beneficence (attempting to do good for a patient). As researchers studied restraints, nurses learned that restraining a patient causes physical harm. When people are restrained, they are more likely to become weak, incontinent, constipated, and to develop nosocomial infections. They also recover more s lowly. So there is reason to doubt that the nurses' actions when restraining patients are in fact beneficent. There is also reason to believe that in acting to prevent a potential harm, such as the disconnection of an IV, the nurses may be causing an actual moral harm, such as the deprivation of the patients' autonomy.

However, critically ill patients are not fully aware. According to Bray et al. (2004), there is variability in what patients recall from the experience of being restrained, ranging from patients who remember very little of the experience to patients who describe the event as extremely unpleasant, even frightening. Critically ill patients often perceive the discomfort from an endotracheal tube but lack the capacity to realize its purpose and its necessity. Thus, they are likely to reach up and remove objects that cause them discomfort. How should critical care nurses respond? What is the appropriate balance between keeping a patient safe but possibly leaving them with frightening memories and allowing them freedom of movement? The National Guidelines Clearinghouse lists the following recommendations developed by the American College of Critical Care Medicine Task Force for the use of restraining therapies (2003a):

- Institutions and practitioners should strive to create the least restrictive but safest environment for patients regarding restraint use.
- Restraining therapies should be used only in clinically appropriate situations and not as a routine component of therapy. When restraints are used, the risk of untoward events must outweigh the physical, psychological, and ethical risks of their use.
- Patients must always be evaluated to determine whether treatment of an existing problem would obviate the need for restraint use.
- The choice of restraint should always be the least invasive option capable of optimizing patient safety, comfort, and dignity.
- The rationale for restraint use must be documented in the medical record. Orders for a restraining order should be limited to a 24-hour period. New orders should be written after 24 hours if the restraining orders are to be continued.
- Patients should be monitored for development of complications from restraining therapies every 4 hours, more frequently if they are agitated.
- Patients and their significant others should receive ongoing education as to the need and nature of restraining therapies.

It is nurses who are often left to try to balance their patients' safety needs against their legal and moral rights to be free from physical restraint. This is clearly a difficult balance. Cho, Kim, Kim, and Choi (2006) determined that the main factors in the nurses' decisions to use restraints were the Glasgow Coma Scale score, restless behavior, emotional state, discomfort factors, medical devices, and life-sustaining devices. In their study, 31% of patients were restrained, with more patients being restrained during the night than during the day. Martin and Mathisen (2005) compared the use of restraints in the United States with that in Norway and found dramatic differences. Restraints were used in 40% of patients in the United States, whereas none of the Norwegian patients were restrained. Seven incidents of unplanned removal of an invasive device (either IV or nasogastric tube) occurred, all in restrained patients in the United States.

There were other differences between the care of patients in the two countries. The nurse-patient ratio for the Norwegian sample was 1.05:1, whereas the ratio for the U.S. sample was 0.65:1. In Norway, nursing stations are decentralized and a "norm has prevailed for nurses to remain within a distance that allows for direct visual observation and eye contact with intubated patients, both to avoid isolation and to be alert for behavioral changes" (Martin & Mathisen, 2005, p. 139). However, the Norwegian patients received more sedation and pain medication than the patients in the United States. This may be a concern because patients who are more sedated have been demonstrated to spend more time on a ventilator, in the ICU, and in the hospital.

Cho et al. (2006) concluded that it is important that guidelines on the use of restraints be developed, taught, and followed. Martin and Mathisen (2005) believed, however, that more research is necessary so that nurses can balance sedation, staffing patterns, and physical restraints. Until then nurses need to make the decision to restrain patients carefully, obtain consent if possible, follow available guidelines, and be diligent in their efforts to prevent untoward effects.

Legal Issues

The Nurse Practice Act, which is enacted by the state legislature, defines the practice of nursing in each state and delegates the powers of enforcement for the act to the state Board of Nursing. The Board of Nursing has responsibility for interpreting and implementing the act in each state. Because the act varies from state to state, the critical care nurse needs to be cognizant of the rules and regulations for the practice of nursing of the state in which she is practicing. The easiest way to locate and review the Nurse Practice Act as well as the rules and regulations for any state is to check the Board of Nursing Web site. Most have the information readily available. In order to prevent potential legal problems, it is essential that the nurse know what functions are within the bounds of the practice of professional nursing as defined by the Nurse Practice Act. In addition, the nurse must have the education and experience to competently perform those functions and must perform them in congruence with the policies of the employing institution.

There are two major areas of law: criminal law and civil law. Criminal law involves situations whereby the local, state, or federal government has filed a suit against a nurse. Fortunately these suits are rare for nurses, but they do occur. The most common types of criminal cases are criminal assault and battery, criminal negligence, and murder. The most common types of suits filed against nurses are civil suits involving tort law. Tort law concerns a wrong committed against a person or the person's property. Negligence and assault and battery are examples of torts. When nurses obtain consents from patients or proxies appropriately, before providing care or treatments, they protect themselves against charges of assault and battery.

Negligence

The most common reason for lawsuits against nurses is **negligence**. However, because the nurse is a medical professional, the trend is to call it "malpractice." Critical care nurses are held to the same criteria for negligence or malpractice as any other health care provider. In order to prove negligence all of the following must be demonstrated:

- A duty was owed—A legal duty exists whenever a hospital or health care provider undertakes the care or treatment of a patient.
- The duty was breached—The provider failed to provide care in accordance with the existing, relevant standard of care. The standard of care can be proven by producing an existing standard, an expert testimony, or by obvious error (the thing speaks for itself).
- The breach of the duty was the proximate cause of an injury to the patient.
- Damages—Without harm to the patient (losses that need not be physical or financial but may also be emotional), there is no basis for a claim, regardless of whether or not the medical provider was negligent.

Standards of Care

Nurses are held accountable for practicing in conjunction with the applicable standards of care. This means that critical care nurses should be acquainted with the appropriate standards. There are standards developed by a variety of professional bodies. Perhaps the most appropriate for the critical care nurse are those propagated by the National Council of State Boards of Nursing and the AACN. The standards developed by the AACN are displayed in Table 1–1.

Factors Affecting the Well-being of Critical Care Nurses

Critical care nurses are often placed in situations with higher levels of complexity, uncertainty, and decisional authority than other nurses. Although many critical care nurses derive satisfaction from working in these circumstances, others have the potential of developing moral distress or compassion fatigue. Nurses can utilize specific strategies to enhance their satisfaction with their role.

Moral Distress

In 1984, Jameton described a circumstance that he called "**moral distress**," wherein a nurse would know the right thing to do, yet institutional constraints such as lack of resources or personal authority would prevent her from doing it. Jameton believed that the distress nurses experienced was serious because they were involved in situations that they judged were morally wrong. This state of affairs has not diminished with the passage of years. Recently, Lutzen, Dahlquist, Sriksson, and Norberg (2006) found that nurses facing competing or contradictory moral imperatives felt burdened with a troubled conscience. Elpern and colleagues (2005) studied critical care

TABLE 1–1

Standards of Care for Acute and Critical Care Nursing

Standard of Care I: Assessment
The nurse caring for acute and critically ill patients collects relevant patient health data.

Standard of Care II: Diagnosis
The nurse caring for acute and critically ill patients analyzes the assessment data in determining diagnoses.

Standard of Care III: Outcome Identification
The nurse caring for acute and critically ill patients identifies individualized expected outcomes for the patient.

Standard of Care IV: Planning
The nurse caring for acute and critically ill patients develops a plan of care that prescribes interventions to attain expected outcomes.

Standard of Care V: Implementation
The nurse caring for acute and critically ill patients implements interventions identified in the plan of care.

Standard of Care VI: Evaluation
The nurse caring for acute and critically ill patients evaluates the patients' progress toward attaining expected outcomes.

Standard of Professional Practice I: Quality of Care
The nurse caring for acute and critically ill patients systematically evaluates the quality and effectiveness of nursing practice.

Standard of Professional Practice II: Individual Practice Evaluation
The practice of the nurse caring for acute and critically ill patients reflects knowledge of current professional practice standards, laws, and regulations.

Standard of Professional Practice III: Education
The nurse acquires and maintains current knowledge and competency in the care of acute or critically ill patients.

Standard of Professional Practice IV: Collegiality
The nurse caring for acute and critically ill patients interacts with and contributes to the professional development of peers and other health care providers as colleagues.

Standard of Professional Practice V: Ethics
The nurse's decisions and actions on behalf of acutely and critically ill patients are determined in an ethical manner.

Standard of Professional Practice VI: Collaboration
The nurse caring for acute and critically ill patients collaborates with the team, consisting of patient, family, and health care providers in providing patient care in a healing, humane, and caring environment.

Standard of Professional Practice VII: Research
The nurse caring for acute and critically ill patients uses clinical inquiry in practice.

Standard of Professional Practice VIII: Resource Utilization
The nurse caring for acute and critically ill patients considers factors related to safety, effectiveness, and cost in planning and delivering patient care.

The Standards for Acute and Critical Care Nursing Practice resource is a product and the expanded version is available through the AACN Online Bookstore.

nurses and learned that nurses commonly encounter situations that are associated with high levels of moral distress. In the study, critical care nurses experienced the most distress when providing aggressive care to patients whom the nurses did not believe would benefit from the care. In a study by Gutierrez (2005), 92% of nurses identified overly aggressive treatment as the cause of their distress. Nurses believed that they did not have a voice in the decision making, that they felt powerless, and that they could not find meaning in the patients' or families' suffering.

The AACN believes there is evidence that the moral distress experienced by critical care nurses has a substantial impact on health care. According to their evidence, as many as half of critical care nurses may have left a unit due to moral distress. In addition, nurses who experience moral distress may lose the capacity to care for their patients and experience psychological and physiological problems.

To respond to this concern, the AACN (2004) developed a public policy statement on moral distress, and the Ethics Work Group of the AACN (2006) developed a framework called *Ask-Affirm-Assess-Act: The 4 A's to Rise Above Moral Distress*. The steps of the four A's are discussed in the next sections.

Ask

The nurse asks, "Am I or are members of my team feeling symptoms or showing signs of suffering?" or "Have others noticed these symptoms and behaviors in me?"

Affirm

The nurse recognizes that moral distress is present and makes a commitment to take care of herself, validate her perceptions, and affirm her professional responsibility to act.

Assess

The nurse identifies the sources of her distress by clarifying the circumstances under which the distress occurs. Is it a particular patient care situation? Is it a unit policy or practice? Does it result from lack of collaboration? The nurse next determines the severity of the distress, her readiness to act, and the risks and benefits of any action.

Act

Before acting, the nurse needs to develop an action plan including a self-care plan, a list of sources of support, and possibilities for outside sources of guidance and assistance. Finally, the nurse needs to take actions that will address the specific sources of distress within her work environment using polite but assertive communication. According to the AACN Ethics Work Group the nurse's goal is to preserve her authenticity and integrity.

Gutierrez (2005) also suggested approaches that nurses could utilize on their unit or at the institutional level to respond to moral distress. These include:

- Improving communication between patients, families, and health care providers
- Improving communication between nursing staff and managers
- Providing support to families in their coping
- Developing a forum for ethical discussion
- Promoting moral and ethical dialogue between nursing and medical students
- Facilitating clinical practice guidelines on futility, ethical decision making, and palliative care

Conscientious Refusal

When all else fails, if a nurse believes that he cannot ethically perform an action he is being asked to perform, he may utilize conscientious refusal and ask to be excused from participating in or assisting with the action. In such a situation the supporters of the action can offer a justification for the action and it is legal, but the nurse does not find their reasoning convincing, believes the action is morally wrong, and thinks he would experience moral distress if he participated in it. According to Benjamin and Curtis (1998), a thoughtful nurse would identify his conscientious refusal to participate:

- Based on personal moral standards
- As determined by a prior judgment of rightness or wrongness
- As motivated by personal sanction and not external control

Conscientious refusal is not an option to be chosen without very careful consideration. If the patient and family have developed a relationship with the nurse, they may wish the nurse to remain with them beyond the decision-making phase to see the planned action accomplished and to help them cope with the consequences of their decision.

On the one hand, the nurse must consider the effect that disrupting the nurse-patient relationship will have on the patient and family. On the other hand, the nurse must consider what effect his disapproval of the planned action will have on his ability to deliver quality nursing care to this patient and subsequent similar patients. The nurse must also consider the amount of support he will receive from the administration of the institution. The repercussions for the nurse of employing conscientious refusal may range from nonexistent to dismissal from his nursing position. Institutions vary from being supportive of conscientious refusal and changing their institutional policies to support it, to being legally required by some states to allow nurses to utilize it, to being able to dismiss the nurse who utilizes it.

Compassion Satisfaction/Fatigue

In 1992, Joinson identified the concept of **compassion fatigue** in nurses. In *Compassion Fatigue: An Expert Interview with Charles R. Figley* (Medscape, 2005), Figley further defined the concept and expanded it to others who provide care to suffering individuals. According to Figley, compassion fatigue is a "state of tension and preoccupation with the suffering of those being helped that is traumatizing for the helper." It occurs in care providers who may be so selfless and compassionate that they fail to pay sufficient attention to their own needs. Compassion fatigue differs from burnout in that it may develop suddenly in response to a specific incident of suffering, whereas burnout tends to develop slowly and insidiously in response to various stressors. Compassion fatigue is primarily a response to caring for people who are suffering, whereas burnout is often a response to other stressors such as poor morale in the work environment.

Symptoms

Caregivers who are experiencing compassion fatigue have many symptoms that often parallel the symptoms of the suffering patients with whom they are working. Some of the symptoms of compassion fatigue include:

- Intrusive thoughts or images of patients' situations or traumas
- Difficulty separating work life from personal life
- Lowered tolerance for frustration and/or outbursts of anger or rage
- Dread of working with certain patients
- Depression
- Increase in ineffective and/or self-destructive self-soothing behaviors
- Hypervigilance
- Decreased functioning in nonprofessional situations
- Loss of hope

Nursing professional organizations are realizing how important it is for nurses to care for themselves in order to provide optimal care to their patients. When the ANA Code of Ethics for Nurses was revised in 2001, it added a provision that states, "The nurse owes the same duties to self as to others, including the responsibility to preserve integrity and safety, to maintain competence, and to continue personal and professional growth." There are a variety of self-care practices that critical care nurses should employ primarily for their own health and well-being, but also because they may aid in preventing compassion fatigue.

Standards of Self-Care

The Academy of Traumatology/Green Cross has proposed standards of self-care for caregivers. These standards were described by Figley in an interview with Medscape in 2005. The purpose of the guidelines is twofold: First, to ensure that practitioners do no harm to themselves when helping or treating others and, second, to encourage providers to attend to their own physical, social, emotional, and spiritual needs as a way of ensuring high-quality services to those who look to them for support as a human being (Medscape, 2005).

Included in the proposed guidelines are sections on establishing and maintaining wellness and an inventory of self-care practices. The following are selections from the standard for establishing and maintaining wellness:

- Make a commitment to self-care.
- Develop strategies for letting go of work.
- Develop strategies for acquiring adequate rest and relaxation.
- Plan strategies for practicing effective daily stress reduction.

Next, the proposed standards identify specific ways in which helpers ought to inventory their self-care practices and provide self-care. These are divided into physical, psychological, social/interpersonal, and professional strategies. The standards suggest that caregivers inventory themselves on each of these criteria then develop a prevention plan by selecting one goal from each category and implementing behavior changes.

Caregivers who are experiencing compassion fatigue may have chosen to give up sleep to continue to care for the suffering person or may have engaged in inappropriate self-soothing behaviors such as misuse of alcohol and drugs and either excessive or inadequate intake of nourishment. Assessment and behavior change for physical well-being, therefore, is particularly important.

Strategies for enhancing physical well-being include:

- Monitoring all parts of the body for tension and utilizing appropriate techniques to reduce tension
- Utilizing healthy methods that induce sleep and return to sleep
- Monitoring all food and drink intake with an awareness of their implication for health and functioning

Strategies for enhancing psychological well-being include:

- Sustaining a balance between work and play
- Developing effective relaxation methods
- Maintaining contact with nature or other soothing stimuli
- Developing methods of effective creative self-expression
- Maintaining effective skills for ongoing self-care such as:
  - Assertiveness
  - Stress reduction
  - Interpersonal communication skills
  - Cognitive restructuring
  - Time management

Strategies for enhancing social/interpersonal well-being include:

- Identifying at least five people (a minimum of two at work) who will be highly supportive when called on to deliver help and will respond quickly and effectively
- Knowing when and how to secure help both personally and professionally
- Being involved in addressing and preventing moral harm

Strategies for enhancing professional well-being include:

- Balancing work and home responsibilities: Devoting sufficient time to each without compromising the other
- Establishing boundaries and setting limits concerning:
  - Overworking
  - Therapeutic/professional boundaries
  - Personal boundaries
  - Realism when differentiating between things that one can change and accepting things that one cannot change
- Obtaining support at work from peers, supervisors, and mentors
- Generating work satisfaction by noticing and remembering the joys and achievements of the work

Job Satisfaction

There is evidence that nurses who work with critically ill patients do so because they obtain satisfaction from the type of care they provide. Tummers, van Merode, and Landeweerd (2002) compared the work characteristics and psychological work reactions of nurses employed in critical care with those of nurses employed in nonintensive care nursing. They found that ICU nurses reported

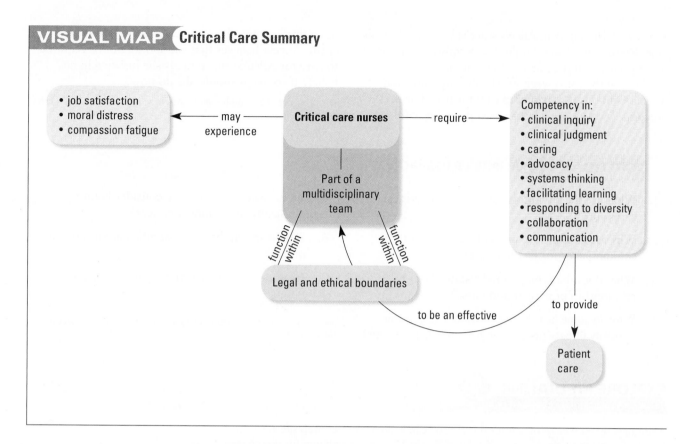

VISUAL MAP Critical Care Summary

- job satisfaction
- moral distress
- compassion fatigue

← may experience ←

Critical care nurses — require →

Competency in:
- clinical inquiry
- clinical judgment
- caring
- advocacy
- systems thinking
- facilitating learning
- responding to diversity
- collaboration
- communication

Part of a multidisciplinary team

function within

Legal and ethical boundaries

to be an effective

to provide

Patient care

---

significantly higher levels of complexity, uncertainty, and decision authority than non-ICU nurses. But although Tummers et al. had anticipated that ICU nurses would experience higher levels of emotional exhaustion in response to these challenges, their study showed that the ICU nurses reported lower levels of exhaustion compared with their non-ICU counterparts. Le Blanc, de Jonge, de Rijk, and Schaufeli (2001) noted that although ICU nurses identified providing nursing and medical care as being very demanding, it also "drove their satisfaction."

CRITICAL CARE SUMMARY

Critical care nurses are an essential part of the team providing care to patients with life-threatening problems. Many critical care nurses experience satisfaction from

In 2007, Ulrich et al. examined how collaboration, communication, leadership, and support for nurses' professional growth related to nurses' satisfaction with their critical care nursing career. They concluded that nurses working in critical care units striving for excellence (as identified by a Beacon Award or Magnet status application or designation) reported healthier work environments and higher job satisfaction. Both healthier work environments for nurses and higher nursing job satisfaction have been associated with better patient outcomes.

the clinical competencies they possess and the care they are able to provide to their patients.

● CASE STUDY

Allen Hale, 27 years old, was admitted to ICU after running a red light in his car and colliding with another car. He is being evaluated for evacuation of a left parietal subdural hematoma. His concomitant injuries include: a flail chest with pulmonary contusions for which he is being ventilated and a fractured femur. His blood alcohol level was 200 mg/dL on admission and there was evidence of marijuana on his toxicology screen. Currently, he is receiving propofol 30 mcg/kg/minute for sedation. He responds to noxious stimuli by withdrawal and his pupils are equal and reactive to light.

The health care team is unable to obtain consent for treatment from him and is unable to reach a next of kin or anyone with health care proxy. How should they proceed?

Two weeks later, Allen is delirious and hallucinating. The physicians have determined that he should have a tracheostomy and a gastrostomy. The social worker has learned that Allen is not from the state, that he does not have a primary care provider, and that he has only one living relative—a sister he has not seen in 5 years. In this state the next of kin may serve as a proxy decision maker. Allen's sister is having a difficult time determining if she should give permission for the surgery. How can the nurse help her to decide?

During the third week of Allen's hospitalization, Angela Gibbons is assigned to care for him. For the previous 2 weeks, Angela has been providing care to the only person in the other car who survived the crash. Angela believes that she should not be required to care for Allen at this time. Is she justified in her belief? If so, what should she do now?

See answers to Case Studies in the Answer Section at the back of the book.

CRITICAL THINKING QUESTIONS

1. What are the advantages of a "closed" critical care unit?

2. Why are critical care units one of the most common sites for health care errors?

3. What does the synergy model state about the relationship of patient and nurse?

4. Why do some health care providers believe that critically ill patients cannot give informed consent?

5. What issues must a nurse consider before physically restraining a patient?

6. Why is moral distress a significant concern for nurses?

7. How can a nurse act to prevent compassion fatigue?

See answers to Critical Thinking Questions in the Answer Section at the back of the book.

EXPLORE MEDIALINK
http://www.prenhall.com/perrin

Additional interactive resources for this chapter can be found on the Web site at http://www.prenhall.com/perrin. Click on "Chapter 1" to select activities for this chapter.

Case Study: Critical Care Nursing

Nursing Care Plan

NCLEX Review Questions

MediaLinks:
- American Association of Critical Care Nurses
- Institute Medicine: To Err Is Human

- Institute for Healthcare Improvement: Critical Care
- Medline Plus: Critical Care
- Medscape: Critical Care
- SBAR technique for communication: a situational briefing model
- Society of Critical Care Medicine

MediaLink Applications

REFERENCES

American Association of Critical-Care Nurses. *The AACN synergy model for patient care.* Retrieved February 13, 2008, from http://web.aacn.org/DesktopModules/Certifications/pages/certifications/general/SynModel.aspx#Basic

American Association of Critical-Care Nurses. (2004). *AACN public policy on moral distress.* Retrieved February 13, 2008, from http://www.aacn.org/aacn/pubpolcy. nsf/Files/MDPS/$file/Moral%20Distress%20_1_7.8.06.pdf

American Association of Critical-Care Nurses. (2005). AACN standards for establishing and sustaining healthy work environments: A journey to excellence. *American Journal of Critical Care, 14*(3), 187–197. Retrieved February 13, 2008, from http://www.aacn.org/aacn/pubpolcy.nsf/Files/HWEStandards/$file/HWEStandards.pdf

American Association of Critical-Care Nurses, Ethics Work Group. (2006). *Ask-affirm-assess-act: The 4A's to rise above moral distress.* Retrieved February 12, 2008, from http://www.aacn.org/AACN/practice.nsf/Files/4as/$file/4A's%20to%20Rise%20Above%20Moral%20Distress.pdf

American Association of Critical-Care Nurses. (n.d.). *Critical care nursing fact sheet.* Retrieved February 12, 2008, from http://www.aacn.org/AACN/practice.nsf/ad0ca3b3bdb4f33288256981006fa692/818297476d23f9628825692900802d92?OpenDocument

American Nurses Association. (2001). *ANA Code of ethics for nurses.* Kansas City, MO: Author.

Anspach, R. R. (1987). Prognostic conflict in life and death decisions. *Journal of Health and Social Behavior, 28,* 215–231.

Barden, C. (2003, May). *Bold voices: Fearless and essential.* Speech delivered at the American Association of Critical-Care Nurses National Teaching Institute and Critical Care Exposition, San Antonio, Texas.

Benjamin, M., & Curtis, J. (1998). *Ethics in nursing* (3rd ed.). New York: Oxford University Press.

Benner, P. (2001). Creating a culture of safety and improvement: A key to reducing medical error. *American Journal of Critical Care, 10*(4), 281–284.

Benner, P., & Wrubel, J. (1989). *The primacy of caring.* Menlo Park, CA: Addison-Wesley.

Boyle, D. K., & Kochinda, C. (2004). Enhancing collaboration communication of nurse and physician leadership in two intensive care units. *Journal of Nursing Administration, 34*(2), 60–70.

Bray, K., Kill, K., Robson, W., Leaver, G., Walker, N., O'Leary, M., et al. (2004). British Association of Critical Care Nurses position statement on the use of restraint in adult critical care units. *Nursing in Critical Care, 9*(5), 199–212.

Chell, B. (1998). Competency: What it is, what it isn't, and why it matters. In J. F.

Monagle & D. C. Thomasima (Eds.), *Health care ethics: Clinical issues for the 21st century* (pp. 116–127). Gaithersburg, MD: Aspen.

Cho, Y., Kim, J., Kim, N., & Choi, H. (2006). Use of physical restraints in intensive care units (ICUs). *American Journal of Critical Care, 15*(3), 341.

Department of Health and Human Services. (2001). *Medicare reimbursement for critical care services.* Retrieved January 4, 2007, from http://www.hhs.gov/oig/oei

Elpern, E. H., Covert, B., & Kleinpell, P. (2005). Moral distress of staff nurses in a medical intensive care unit. *American Journal of Critical Care, 14*(6), 523–530.

Gardner, D. B. (2004). Ten lessons in collaboration. *Online Journal of Issues in Nursing, 10*(1). Retrieved February 13, 2008, from http://www.medscape.com/viewarticle/499266_print

Gutierrez, K. M. (2005). Critical care nurses' perceptions of responses to moral distress. *Dimensions of Critical Care Nursing, 24*(5), 229–241.

Haupt, M. T., Bekes, C. E., Brilli, R. J., Carl, L. C., Gray, A. W., Jastemski, M. S., et al. (2003). Guidelines on critical care service and personnel: Recommendations based on a system of categorization of three levels of care. *Critical Care Medicine, 31*(11), 2677–2683.

Health Resources and Services Administration. (n.d.). *Report to Congress: The critical care workforce: A study of the supply and demand for critical care physicians.* Retrieved February 13, 2008, from http://bhpr.hrsa.gov/healthworkforce/reprots/criticalcare/footnotes.htm

Health Resources and Services Administration (HRSA), Bureau of Health Professions, Division of Nursing. (2001). *The registered nurse population, March 2000: Findings from the national sample survey of registered nurses.* Washington, DC: U.S. Department of Health and Human Services.

Henneman, E. (2007). Unreported errors in the intensive care unit: A case study in the way we work. *Critical Care Nurse, 27*(5), 27–35.

Institute for Health Care Improvement. *SBAR report to physician about a critical situation.* Retrieved June 2007, from http://www.ihi.org/IHI/Topics/PatientSafety/SafetyGeneral/Tools/SBARTechniqueforCommunicationA SituationalBriefingModel.htm

Jameton, A. (1984). *Nursing practice: The ethical issues.* Englewood Cliffs, NJ: Prentice Hall.

Joinson, C. (1992). Coping with compassion fatigue. *Nursing, 22,* 116–120.

Joint Commission on Accreditation of Healthcare Organizations. (2006). *Sentinel event statistics—June 30, 2006.* Retrieved January 4, 2007, from http://www.jointcommision.org/SentinelEvents/Statistics/?HTTP

Kelly, J. (2006). An overview of conflict. *Dimensions of Critical Care Nursing, 25*(1), 22–28.

Kirchhoff, K. T., & Dahl, N. (2006). American Association of Critical Care Nurses' national survey of facilities and units providing critical care. *American Journal of Critical Care, 15*(1), 13–27.

Knaus, W. A., Draper, E. A., Wagner, D. P., & Zimmerman, J. E. (1986). An evaluation of outcome from intensive care in major medical centers. *Annals of Internal Medicine, 104*(3), 410–418.

Kohn, L. T., Corrigan, J. M., & Donaldson, M. S. (Eds.). (2000). *To err is human: Building a safer health system.* Washington, DC: Institute of Medicine: National Academy Press. Retrieved June 4, 2007, from http://www.nap.edu/openbook.php?isbn=0309068371

Kuhse, H. (1997). *Caring: Nurses, women, and ethics.* Oxford: Blackwell.

Leape, L., & Brennan, T. (1991). The nature of adverse events in hospitalized patients. Results of the Harvard Medical Practice Study. *New England Journal of Medicine, 324*(6), 377–384.

Le Blanc, P. M., de Jonge, J., de Rijk, A. E., & Schaufeli, W. B. (2001). Well-being of intensive care nurses (WEBIC): A job analytic approach. *Journal of Advanced Nursing, 36*(3), 460–470.

Lindeke, L. L., & Sieckert, A. M. (2005). Nurse-physician workplace collaboration. *Online Journal of Issues in Nursing, 10*(1). Retrieved February 13, 2008, from http://nursingworld.org/mods/mod775/nrsdrfull.htm

Lutzen, K., Dahlquist, V., Sriksson, S., & Norberg, A. (2006). Developing the concept of moral sensitivity in health care. *Nursing Ethics, 13,* 187–196.

Martin, B., & Mathisen, L. (2005). Use of physical restraints in adult critical care: A bicultural study. *American Journal of Critical Care, 14*(2), 133–142.

Medscape. (2005). *Compassion fatigue: An expert interview with Charles R. Figley.* Retrieved February 13, 2008, from http://www.medscape.com/viewarticle/513615

Narasimhan, M., Eisen, L. A., Mahoney, C. D., Acerra, F. L., & Rosen, M. J. (2006). Improving nurse-physician communication and satisfaction in the intensive care unit with a daily goals worksheet. *American Journal of Critical Care, 15*(2), 217–222.

National Guidelines Clearinghouse. (2003a). *Clinical practice guidelines for the maintenance of patient physical safety in the intensive care unit: Use of restraining therapies.* Retrieved December 14, 2007, from http://www.guideline.gov/summary/summary.aspx?doc_id=4913&nbr=003510&string=restraints

National Guidelines Clearinghouse. (2003b). *Critical care delivery in the intensive care unit: Defining clinical roles and the best practice model.* Retrieved February 13, 2008, from http://guideline.gov/summary/summary.aspx?ss=14&doc_id=5

Page, A. (Ed.). (2004). *Keeping patients safe: Transforming the work environment of nurses.* Washington, DC: The National Academies Press.

Perrin, K., & McGhee, J. (2007). *Ethics and conflict.* Sudbury, MA : Jones and Bartlett.

Rothschild, J. M., Landrigan, C. P., Cronin, J. W., Kaushal, R., Lockley, M., Burdick, et al. (2005). The critical care safety study: The incidence and nature of adverse events and serious medical errors in intensive care. *Critical Care Medicine, 33*(8), 1694–1700.

Sachs, B. P. (2005). A 38-year-old woman with fetal loss and hysterectomy. *Journal of the American Medical Association, 294*(7), 833–840.

Sandelowski, M. (1997). (Ir)reconcilable differences? The debate concerning nursing and technology. *Image: The Journal of Nursing Scholarship, 29*(21), 169–173.

Scott, L. D., Rogers, A. E., Hwang, W., & Shang, Y. (2006). Effects of critical care nurses' work hours on vigilance and patients' safety. *American Journal of Critical Care, 15*(1), 30–45.

Shannon, S. E. (1997). The roots of interdisciplinary conflict around ethical issues. *Critical Care Nursing Clinics of North America, 9,* 13–28.

Society of Critical Care Medicine. (n.d.). History of critical care. Retrieved February 11, 2008, from http://www.sccm.org/AboutSCCM/History_of_Critical_Care/Pages/default.aspx

Tarnow-Mordi, W. O., Hau, C., Warden, A., & Shearer, A. J. (2000). Hospital mortality in relation to staff workload: A 4-year study in an adult intensive care unit. *The Lancet, 356,* 185–189.

Tummers, G. E. R., van Merode, G. G., & Landeweerd, J. A. (2002). The diversity of work: Differences, similarities, and relationships concerning characteristics of the organization, the work and psychological work reactions in intensive care and non-intensive care nursing. *International Journal of Nursing Studies, 39,* 841–855.

Ulrich, B. T., Woods, D., Hart, K. A., Lavandero, R., Leggert, J., & Taylor, D. (2007). Critical care nurses' work environments: Value of excellence in Beacon units and Magnet organizations. *Critical Care Nurse, 27*(3), 68–77.

Valentin, A., Capuzzo, M., Guidet, B., Moreno, R. P., Dolanski, D., Bauer, P., et al. (2006). Patient safety in intensive care: Results from the multinational Sentinel Events Evaluation (SEE) study. *Intensive Care Medicine.* Retrieved January 2, 2007, from http://dx.doi.org/10.1007/s00134-006-0290-7

Whelan, S. A., Burchill, C. N., & Tilin, F. (2003). The link between teamwork and patients' outcomes in intensive care units. *American Journal of Critical Care, 12*(6), 527–534.

chapter 2

Care of the Critically Ill Patient

Kathleen Perrin, PhD, RN, CCRN

Learning Outcomes

Upon completion of this chapter, the learner will be able to:

1. Explain the characteristics of the critically ill patient described in the AACN synergy model.

2. Discuss the concerns expressed by critically ill patients.

3. Describe strategies a nurse might utilize to communicate with a ventilated patient.

4. Explain the use of sedation, pain, and delirium scales with critically ill patients.

5. Evaluate the effectiveness of pharmacological and nonpharmacological management of sedation, pain, and delirium in the critically ill patient.

6. Compare and contrast the use of enteral and parenteral nutrition in the critically ill patient.

7. Discuss ways to identify and meet the needs of families of critically ill patients.

Abbreviations

AACN	American Association of Critical-Care Nurses
BMI	Body Mass Index
CAM-ICU	Confusion Assessment Method of the Intensive Care Unit
CCFAP	Critical Care Family Assistance Program
CCFNI	Critical Care Family Needs Inventory
CPOT	Critical-Care Pain Observation Tool
ICU	Intensive Care Unit
PCA	Patient-Controlled Analgesia
SCCM	Society of Critical Care Medicine
TPN	Total Parenteral Nutrition
VAMASS	Ventilator Adjusted Motor Assessment Scoring Scale

Critically ill patients are at high risk for life-threatening problems, and nurses must often focus on specific life-sustaining treatments. However, critically ill patients have basic needs as well.

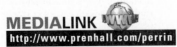

MEDIALINK
http://www.prenhall.com/perrin

See the Companion Website for chapter-specific resources at www.prenhall.com/perrin.

VISUAL MAP Critically Ill Patient Overview

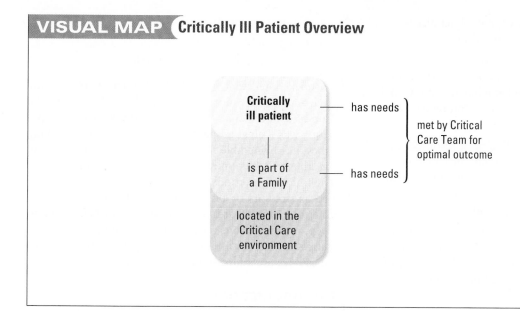

Characteristics of Critically Ill Patients

The American Association of Critical-Care Nurses (AACN) defines **critically ill patients** as "those patients who are at high risk for actual or potential life threatening health problems. The more critically ill the patient is, the more likely he or she is to be highly vulnerable, unstable and complex, thereby requiring intense and vigilant nursing care." As also presented in Chapter 1, ∞ in the synergy model (Figure 2-1), the AACN postulates that when the needs of the patient and family drive the competencies required by the nurse, optimal patient outcomes can be achieved. The AACN continues by identifying and describing eight characteristics of critically ill patients.

The Synergy Model-Patient Characteristics

The characteristics are listed by levels on the health illness continuum from Level 1, which describes a more compromised patient, to Level 5, which indicates a patient who is less compromised. The characteristics are not listed by level on the h-c continuum—rather, each of the synergy model patient characteristics may be scored from 1–5 on the health illness continuum—from Level 1 –

The characteristics are:

- Resiliency: "The ability to bounce back quickly after insult." Patients range along the continuum from being unable to mount a response to having strong reserves.

- Vulnerability: "Susceptibility to actual or potential stressors." Patients range from being fragile to being safe or "out of the woods."

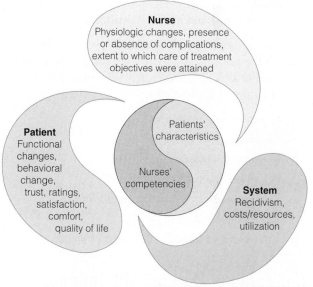

Figure 2-1 Three levels of outcomes delineated by the AACN's Synergy Model for Patient Care: those outcomes derived from the patient are highlighted in this chapter.
(Curley, MA. Patient-nurse synergy: optimizing patients' outcomes. *American Journal of Critical Care 1998, 7(1),* 64–72.)

- Stability: "The ability to maintain a steady state equilibrium." Patients vary from being unresponsive to therapies and at high risk for death to stable and responsive to therapy.

- Complexity: "The intricate entanglement of two or more systems (e.g., body, family)." Patients span the gamut from having atypical presentations of an illness or complex family dynamics to simple clear-cut and typical presentation.

- Predictability: "A characteristic that allows one to predict a certain course of events or course of illness." Patients range from having an unusual or unexpected course of illness to following a critical pathway.

- Resource availability: "Extent of resources the patient, family, and community bring to the situation." Patients may have few of the resources necessary for recovery available to them or may have extensive knowledge and skills.

- Participation in care: "Extent to which patient and/or family engage in care." Patients and families may vary from being unable or unwilling to assist with care to being fully willing and able to participate.

- Participation in decision making: "Extent to which patient and/or family engage in decision making." Patients and families may range from requiring surrogate decision makers to having full capacity and making decisions for themselves.

The synergy model proposes that when these characteristics of the patients are met by the competencies of the nurse (described in Chapter 1), ∞ the patient will have the following outcomes:

- Comfort and healing
- Satisfaction with care
- Absence of complications
- Perceived change in function
- Perceived improvement in quality of life
- Decreased recidivism
- Effective cost resource utilization balance

Concerns of Critically Ill Patients

Critical care nurses have long focused on creating environments conducive to the comfort and healing of their patients. The noise, lights, and alarms in an intensive care unit (ICU) have been assumed to be sources of discomfort to many ICU patients, and nurses have tried to limit these stressors. However, when Cornock (1998) examined what patients in ICUs rated as stressful and compared the findings with what nurses in the same ICUs believed was most stressful for patients, she learned that the environmental factors such as unfamiliar noises and bright lights were not the major sources of stress for patients. Patients described the most stressful items as:

- Being thirsty
- Having tubes in their mouth and nose
- Not being able to communicate

- Being restricted by tubes/lines
- Being unable to sleep
- Not being able to control themselves

Cornock noted that, overall, ICU nurses perceived the environment as more stressful than their patients. Nurses believed that the primary stressor for their patients was being in pain but recognized that having tubes, not being able to control themselves, and not being able to communicate were other areas of concern. The following sections explore some of the issues identified as stressors by both patients and nurses: not being able to communicate, being anxious, not being able to sleep, being delirious (not in control), and being in pain. Nurses' concerns about restraining patients to safeguard tubes/lines are addressed in Chapter 1. ∞

Communication

Critical care nurses and ventilated patients indicate that because communication can be frustrating and difficult, it is one of their major stressors. It does not matter whether the patient is alert or appears to be unresponsive: Studies have documented that ventilated patients need assistance with communication from their health care providers, especially their nurses.

Sedated Patients

Ventilated patients who appear to be sedated and minimally responsive have been shown to recall the communication efforts of their nurses. A common finding among studies of such patients has been the need for effective verbal communication with them by health care providers (Elliot & Wright, 1999). Most studies have demonstrated that ICU nurses spend little time communicating with their sedated patients. Alasad and Ahmad (2005) believed that although nurses know that communication is important, it is easily forgotten in the context of other important patient care needs. Nurses do not ignore patients; rather, they have a tendency to try to anticipate patients' needs and respond to them before they present a problem. Alasad and Ahmad also noted that nurses see communication with ventilated patients as discouraging because it is usually one-way communication. Nonetheless, patients often recall the presence, or absence, of such communication when they awaken.

When nurses communicate with their sedated patients, it is usually for a specific purpose (Elliot & Wright, 1999). Nurses communicate with or around their sedated or unresponsive patients to:

- Provide orientation: Nurses believe that not knowing who is providing care and where the patient is can be stressful to the patient.

- State procedural and task intentions: Studies indicate that nurses communicate more with their sedated patients when the patients are having procedures or tasks done. Patients state that they would prefer to have nurses ask their permission before such tasks and to give them some indication of what they will experience.

- Provide reassurance: Morse (2001) noted that nurses use reassuring words to help a patient hold on and endure a difficult procedure. The nurse might say, "You're doing well—it's almost done" even to a patient who appears unresponsive.

- Apologize and/or recognize discomfort: A nurse might say as he prepares to suction a patient, "I'm sorry, I know this is uncomfortable but I need to clear these secretions now. It is important to help your lungs to heal."

- Obtain a response: Determining if the patient is able to respond to a request is important. However, even when the patient does not respond, it is quite possible he can still hear the request and any other conversation.

- Provide intentional and unintentional distractions: Morse stated that nurses may use intentional distractions as a way of providing some comfort to patients who are undergoing procedures. For example, nurses sometimes sing, hum, or joke with their unresponsive patients while they provide care.

- Provide social information to colleagues: Nurses sometimes have social conversations as they are caring for unresponsive, sedated, or ventilated patients. Patients have identified overhearing such conversations as a source of distress. They have felt removed from the situation and less than human.

As important to patients as the content of communication is the manner in which it is conveyed. Patients identify the need to feel that nurses are "physically present at the bedside" (Patak, Gawlinski, Fung, Doering, & Berg, 2004). Patients see being "physically present" as being kind, patient, and attentive to their needs; offering frequent verbal reassurances; and knowing what information is important and providing it.

Responsive Patients

A majority of responsive, ventilated patients identify communication as highly frustrating (Patak et al., 2004). They frequently modify requests or avoid communication because the activity is so difficult (Magnus & Turkington, 2006). Intubated patients who are severely ill and are probably dying have higher levels of anger and frustration about their inability to communicate than less ill patients (Happ, Tuite, Dobbin, DiVirgilio-Thomas, & Kitutu, J., 2004). Some of the patients' frustrations appear to center around the limited means utilized for them to communicate. Although there are a variety of possible communication adjuncts such as letter boards, speaking valves, and

prosthetic larynxes, they are infrequently used. The most common means of communication used by responsive ventilated patients are head nods in response to yes/no questions, mouthing words, gesturing, and writing. Hand and arm movements are required for both gesturing and writing so the already limited communication from patients is reduced when patients' hands and arms are restrained. Happ et al. recommended limiting the use of such restraints, believing it may be the most effective way to facilitate communication with responsive ventilated patients.

Communication with ventilated patients centers around specific, predictable issues:

- The most common reason for communication between nurses and ventilated patients is the patients' experiences of **pain**.

- Other common reasons for communication are:
  - Identifying patients' emotions
  - Determining patients' symptoms
  - Responding to patients' needs for physical care
  - The physical environment of the ICU
  - The patients' home and family
  - Treatment decision making (Happ et al., 2004)

Patak et al. (2004) recommended five evidence-based interventions to facilitate communication with mechanically ventilated, seriously ill patients. They stated that health care providers should do the following:

- Be educated about the frustration that mechanically ventilated patients experience when they are attempting to communicate their needs and desires.

- When communicating with ventilated patients, they should:
  - Routinely ask patients about their feelings and their state of mind.
  - Ask permission before beginning nursing care and procedures.
  - Evaluate patients' understanding of the information conveyed to them by asking simple yes/no questions.

- Demonstrate attention to the needs of their patients by informing them of their surroundings, plan of care, and when they will return after leaving the bedside.

- Approach each patient with a kind, patient manner; take the time to investigate and understand what the patient is communicating; and respond to the patient's communicated needs.

- Provide writing materials and read the patient's words as they are written, allowing the patient to verify that the reader understands the patient correctly.

Happ, Tate, and Garrett (2006) offered several practical suggestions for communicating with older adults who are intubated. These include the following:

- Provide the patient with his eyeglasses or hearing aids so that it is easier for him to hear or lip read.
- Enunciate slowly and pause while speaking.
- Ask only one question at a time and allow the patient time to respond.
- Establish a series of gestures so that the patient can communicate using them.
- Decide on gestures for yes and no and post them so they are visible to all who wish to communicate with the patient.
- Write out questions with potential answers so the patient can see and hear the question and choices simultaneously then point to his choice.

Comfort

Nurses and families consistently identify pain as one of the major problems for patients in critical care units. Unfortunately, although it is assumed that all patients in critical care will experience some pain or discomfort, pain control is frequently inadequate. Obvious sources of pain are a patient's surgical site or traumatic injury. Many disease processes such as myocardial infarction and subarachnoid hemorrhage are clearly associated with severe pain. However, most critically ill patients also experience discomfort from their monitoring devices and routine nursing care. Immobility may be difficult for patients to endure, especially if they have arthritis. Conversely, turning may be extremely frightening and has been demonstrated to be one of the most painful procedures for critically ill adult patients (Puntillo et al., 2001). Routine procedures such as endotracheal suctioning can be particularly painful. One former patient described her sensations while being suctioned as "a red hot poker being slid down my throat that burned even more as it was withdrawn."

Unresolved pain does not just cause physical and psychic discomfort for the patient. It can impair the patient's recovery from her illness as well. Pain that is not adequately controlled can lead to agitation, interfere with sleep, and contribute to the stress response, causing tachycardia, increased oxygen consumption, immunosuppression, hypercoagulability, and persistent catabolism (London Health Center, n.d.). Unresolved pain can also contribute to pulmonary dysfunction through muscle rigidity and guarding. Thus, it is imperative that critical care nurses assess their patients for pain and manage their pain adequately.

Pain Assessment

Once the critical care nurse recognizes that nearly all her patients will experience some source of discomfort, then one of the nurse's priorities should be to perform a pain assessment on a regular basis. Pain should be assessed and documented at least at the beginning of every shift but usually with each assessment of the patient and each adjustment of pain medication. It has long been established that the most reliable indicator of pain is the patient's self-report of pain. McCaffery's (1968) classic definition of pain is "whatever the person says it is, existing whenever he says it does." Thus, when the patient is able to respond, the nurse should question him concerning his pain. A basic assessment should include at least the intensity and location of pain but, if possible, the nurse should ask the patient to:

- Rate the intensity of the pain on a scale of 0 to 10 with 0 being no pain at all and 10 being the worst pain one can imagine.
- Point to the location of the pain.
- Show where the pain radiates to.
- Describe the characteristics of the pain—Is it burning or aching?
- Indicate if the patient has associated symptoms such as nausea, shortness of breath, or dizziness.
- State what aggravates the pain; for example: Does it hurt more when the patient breathes?
- Consider what alleviates the pain; for example: Does the pain decrease when the head of the bed is elevated?

Because the patient's self-report of pain is the most reliable indicator of the amount and type of pain that a patient is experiencing, the critical care nurse should always attempt to obtain the assessment from the patient. This means always asking the patient even if the nurse thinks the patient may not be able to respond, using simple yes or no questions that only call for a blink of the eye or nod of the head to respond, and allowing adequate time for the patient to respond (Belden, 2006).

Unfortunately, many critically ill patients are unable to communicate their experiences of pain to their nurses. Therefore, critical care nurses must identify other ways to identify pain in these patients. In 1999, McCaffery and Pasero described a hierarchy of pain assessment techniques, including:

- Patient self-report.
- Search for a potential cause of a change in patient behavior.
- Observation of patient behaviors when patient self-report is not possible.
- Surrogate report of a patient's pain or patient's behavior change.
- Attempt of an analgesic trial. If one assumes pain is present, then an analgesic trial may be diagnostic as well as therapeutic (Herr et al., 2006). Attempt of an analgesic trial or use of

bispectral analysis may be the only way of determining the pain needs of a patient who is receiving paralytic agents or is deeply sedated.

With the realization that pain is a persistent problem for critically ill patients and that observation of patient behaviors is a valid approach to pain assessment, there has been a growing emphasis on developing behaviorally based tools for assessment of pain in critically ill patients. Although there are differences among the behaviors that are assessed in the tools, many include:

- Facial expressions: Is the patient showing a relaxed neutral position, or is the patient grimacing?
- Body movements: Is the patient lying completely still, slow and cautious in movement, pulling at tubes, or clenching his fists and rubbing parts of his body?
- Muscle tension: Does the patient resist passive movement?
- Compliance with ventilation: Is the patient ventilating easily or out of synchrony with the ventilator?
- Vocalization: Is the patient speaking normally or crying out with pain?
- Physiologic parameters: What are the patient's vital signs? Is the patient exhibiting diaphoresis or pupil dilation? (Herr et al. [2006] suggested minimizing the emphasis on physiologic parameters, believing they may not be sensitive enough indicators.)

A tool that is currently a source of interest, appears to be valid and reliable, and can be used for both verbal and nonverbal patients is the Critical-Care Pain Observation Tool (CPOT) displayed in Table 2–1 (Gelinas, Fillion, Puntillo, Viens, & Fortier, 2006). Although the choice of a valid, reliable pain assessment tool for a unit is important, it is more important that the critical care nurse develop familiarity with the pain assessment tool utilized on his unit, use it consistently to assess his patients, and medicate his patients for pain in response to their documented pain levels.

Pain Management

Analgesics are the appropriate medication if pain is the cause of a patient's discomfort. Ideally analgesic medications should be administered before pain develops because it is easier to prevent pain than to treat established pain. Thus, the nurse should administer analgesia before a chest tube is removed, for example. However, anticipation of pain is not always possible, so pain medication should be administered as soon as possible after pain begins (Stanik-Hutt, 2003). Stanik-Hutt recommended that whenever possible, the nurse should utilize both opioid and nonopioid medications because

---

TABLE 2–1

Description of the Critical-Care Pain Observation Tool

INDICATOR	DESCRIPTION	SCORE	
Facial expression	No muscular tension observed	Relaxed, neutral	0
	Presence of frowning, brow lowering, orbit tightening, and levator contraction	Tense	1
	All of the above facial movements plus eyelid tightly closed	Grimacing	2
Body movements	Does not move at all (does not necessarily mean absence of pain)	Absence of movements	0
	Slow, cautious movements, touching or rubbing the pain site, seeking attention through movements	Protection	1
	Pulling tube, attempting to sit up, moving limbs/thrashing, not following commands, striking at staff, trying to climb out of bed	Restlessness	2
Muscle tension Evaluation by passive flexion and extension of upper tremities	No resistance to passive movements	Relaxed	0
	Resistance to passive movements	Tense, rigid	1
	Strong resistance to passive movements, inability to complete them	Very tense or rigid	2
Compliance with the ventilator (intubated patients) OR	Alarms not activated, easy ventilation	Tolerating ventilator or movement	0
	Alarms stop spontaneously	Coughing but tolerating	1
	Asynchrony: blocking ventilation, alarms frequently activated	Fighting ventilator	2
Vocalization (extubated patients)	Talking in normal tone or no sound	Talking in normal tone or no sound	0
	Sighing, moaning	Sighing, moaning	1
	Crying out, sobbing	Crying out, sobbing	2
Total, range			0–8

Source: American Association of Critical-Care Nurses (Am J Crit Care www.medscape.com)

COMMONLY USED MEDICATIONS

MORPHINE SULFATE, an Opioid

INTRODUCTION

Morphine has been the gold standard to which all other analgesics are compared and has been the narcotic of choice in critical care. It is potent, has a wide therapeutic range, acts rapidly when given intravenously, and is relatively inexpensive.

Desired Effects: The desired effects, which should become apparent 5 minutes after IV administration and last for 1 1/2 to 2 hours (longer in patients with renal or hepatic impairment), include analgesia, sedation, vasodilation, and relief of air hunger.

Nursing Responsibilities:

- Administration of a bolus dose of morphine for initial pain management. Initial doses are often 2 to 4 mg IV given every 5 minutes until the patient obtains relief. Later, intermittent doses may range from 2.5 to 15 mg every 2 to 4 hours. A dose of 15 mg should be given by IV push over 4 to 5 minutes.

- Initiation of an ongoing morphine infusion if a constant supply of pain medication is needed usually beginning between 1 and 10 mg/hr; however, infusion rates vary greatly depending on the patient's tolerance and level of pain.

- Assessment of the patient's level of discomfort using a valid, reliable pain assessment tool at regular intervals.

- Assessment of the patient's hemodynamic response to the morphine dose.

- Consistent documentation of the patient's symptoms as an indication for additional morphine administration as well as a description of the patient's response to the initial dose and any necessary increases in dose.

- Weaning any ongoing infusion in an appropriate manner such as the following protocol from the London Health Center:
  - If the morphine dose is less than 4 mg/hr, reduce the infusion by 50% and reassess for further weaning in 6 hours.
  - If the morphine dose is greater than 4 mg/hr, reduce the infusion by 25% and reassess in 6 hours.
  - If pain control is inadequate or the patient is agitated, the patient should receive a bolus dose of morphine and the infusion should be returned to the previous rate of infusion.

Side and/or Toxic Effects: Dose reductions are needed in patients with renal failure and in the elderly. Morphine is metabolized by the liver with an active metabolite that produces analgesia and sedation. Because this active morphine metabolite is excreted renally, prolonged analgesia and sedation will occur in patients with renal failure.

   Morphine can produce histamine release, causing vasodilation and hypotension.

COMMONLY USED MEDICATIONS

FENTANYL (SUBLIMAZE), an Opioid

INTRODUCTION

Fentanyl is one hundred times more potent than morphine. It has a faster onset of action than morphine and a shorter duration of action. It is the analgesic of choice in acutely distressed patients and patients with renal dysfunction, morphine allergy, or ongoing hemodynamic instability (National Guidelines Clearinghouse, 2002) because it does not produce histamine release, vasodilation, or hypotension. Fentanyl is metabolized by the liver but none of its metabolites are active analgesics or sedatives. Prolonged drug effect does not occur in renal failure. Fentanyl has a wider margin of safety when compared with older opioids (Taylor, 2005).

Desired Effects: The onset of IV fentanyl is rapid, within 1 to 2 minutes, with a peak in 3 to 5 minutes and a duration of action of 1/2 to 1 hour. The onset of pain relief and sedation should be almost immediate.

Nursing Responsibilities:

- Administration of a bolus dose of fentanyl (IV bolus dose is dependent on the desired effect. For sedation/analgesia in an adult, the dose may range from 0.5 to 1 mcg/kg/dose administered IV over 3 to 5 minutes).

- Starting an intravenous infusion of fentanyl with prn doses for severe breakthrough pain when frequent dosing is required.

- Assessment of the patient's level of discomfort using a valid, reliable pain assessment tool at regular intervals beginning 3 to 5 minutes after the dose.

- Monitoring the patient's respiratory rate and effort as well as his blood pressure throughout therapy.

- Weaning an infusion (if one is needed) in an appropriate manner such as the following protocol from the London Health Center:
  - If the fentanyl dose is less than 50 mcg/hr, reduce infusion by 50% and reassess for further weaning in 6 hours.
  - If the fentanyl dose is more than or equal to 50 mcg/hr, reduce the infusion by 25% and reassess for further weaning in 6 hours.
  - If pain control is inadequate or the patient is agitated, the patient should receive a bolus dose of fentanyl and the infusion should be returned to the previous rate.

Side and/or Toxic Effects: Too rapid administration of fentanyl may result in apnea or respiratory paralysis, muscle rigidity, bradycardia, or hypotension.

   The respiratory depressant effects of fentanyl may outlast its analgesic effects.

they work differently to relieve pain and have complementary effects. Nonsteroidal anti-inflammatory medications and acetaminophen work in the peripheral nervous system to control pain, whereas opioids work in the dorsal horn of the spinal column and in higher levels of the central nervous system. However, for the moderate to severe pain that critically ill patients usually experience, opioids are the drugs of choice and should be used for initial therapy.

General Principles for Administration of Pain or Sedative Medications

- For acute pain, analgesics should be administered intravenously for immediate onset of action.

- "Subsequent doses may be given intravenously or orally on a regular schedule around the clock" (Stanik-Hutt, 2003). The National Guidelines Clearinghouse (2002) states that "scheduled opioid doses or a continuous infusion is preferred over an 'as needed' regimen to ensure consistent analgesia."

- Intravenous infusions of analgesics start to act immediately; however, they will not provide significant analgesia until the infusion reaches "steady state." The time to reach steady state is related to the duration of the effect of the drug, which is measured as a half-life. It generally takes three half-lives to approach steady state and five half-lives to achieve steady state.

- At the initiation of an infusion and when the infusion rate is increased, loading doses must be administered in order to provide immediate analgesia and maintain the desired analgesia until the infusion reaches steady state. Thus, a critically ill patient often will receive an intravenous (IV) bolus of an analgesic followed by an ongoing infusion of the pain medication with intermittent boluses and increases in infusion until the drug attains steady state and the patient experiences pain relief.

- In response to anticipated painful procedures (e.g., turning) the patient might receive an additional bolus. When IV infusion rates are repeatedly increased versus administration of intermittent boluses as a means of responding to acute pain, the risk for excessive analgesia dosing exists (London Health Center, n.d.).

- There are a variety of predictable situations when the doses of pain medications may need to be adjusted.

- Elderly patients and patients with renal insufficiency usually need a decreased dose of medication.

- At the onset of therapy, until comfort is achieved, patients will often require higher doses of pain medication.

- Post-op and post-traumatic injury pain should decrease over time.

According to the London Health Center, there is evidence that daily interruption of continuous infusions of IV analgesics and sedatives results in a reduction in the number of days on a ventilator and the length of stay in ICU. Therefore it recommends that daily weaning of analgesics be automatically attempted when the patient meets the following criteria:

- Pain control is adequate.
- Patient is not receiving neuromuscular blocking agents.

- Patient is hemodynamically stable.
- Patient is stable on the ventilator.

Information concerning the management of pain and promotion of comfort for patients with specific disorders is discussed with each of the disorders. General information about the administration of the most commonly used analgesics follows.

As the patient improves and becomes responsive, he may be switched to patient-controlled analgesia (PCA). Later, using equivalent dosing, the patient may be switched from IV opioids to other medications prior to transfer to another unit or before discharge from the hospital. Details concerning pain management for specific conditions are located in each chapter. Nonpharmaceutical interventions should also be considered as they may reduce or relieve requirements for pain medications. Examples of nonpharmaceutical interventions include back rubs, repositioning, mouth care, music therapy, noise and lighting reduction, family visits, and facilitation of rest and sleep. These should only be utilized as adjunct therapy, however, because of the lack of evidence to support the efficacy of their use for pain management in critically ill patients (Belden, 2006).

Sedation: Guiding Principles

Sedatives are used in the critical care setting to treat **anxiety** and agitation and to provide amnesia. Although the use of sedatives can reduce the stress response and improve the patient's tolerance to interventions, sedatives should be used only after "providing adequate analgesia and treating reversible physiologic causes" (National Guidelines Clearinghouse, 2002). Besides pain, common reversible physiologic causes of anxiety and agitation include:

- Hypoxia
- Hypoglycemia
- Withdrawal
- Sleep deprivation
- Immobility
- Fear

A sedation goal or end point should be established early and redefined regularly for each patient (National Guidelines Clearinghouse, 2002). A goal of care for a sedated patient might be: patient calm, easy to arouse with normal sleep-wake cycles. Some patients—for example, those requiring advanced ventilator therapy—require deeper levels of sedation and their sedation goals would vary accordingly.

COMMONLY USED MEDICATIONS

MIDAZOLAM (VERSED), a Potent Benzodiazepine

INTRODUCTION

Midazolam is indicated for rapid sedation of acutely agitated patients. It has anxiolytic, hypnotic, anticonvulsant, muscle relaxant, and amnestic effects. It has a rapid onset and a short duration of action. This drug is recommended for short-term use because using it longer than 48 to 72 hours can cause accumulation, resulting in unpredictable times to patient awakening and extubation (National Guidelines Clearinghouse, 2002).

Desired Effects: With IV administration, the onset of the drug is within a minute and a half with full anxiolytic and sedative effects being apparent in 3 to 5 minutes.

Nursing Responsibilities:

- For sedation in critically ill patients, a recommended loading dose of 0.01 to 0.05 mg/kg (or 0.5 to 4 mg for an adult) may be given. However, this dose should be reduced by 30% to 50% if the patient is receiving opioid analgesics.

- If possible, a central line should be used for administration; otherwise the IV site should be monitored closely to avoid extravasation.

- Each dose should be administered slowly over 2 to 5 minutes, watching the patient for effects: Mean arterial pressure may be slightly decreased, and heart rate may increase if less than 65 beats per minute (bpm) or decrease if greater than 85 bpm following administration.

- An infusion may be started at 0.02 to 0.1 mg/kg/hr (1 to 7 mg/hr). However, the dose may need to be 30% to 50% less if the patient is receiving an opioid analgesic.

- The dose should be titrated to the patient's level of anxiety/agitation using a sedation assessment scale. The initial infusion rate may be titrated up or down 25% to 50% to attain the patient's goal. The infusion rate may then be decreased by 10% to 25% every few hours to determine the minimum effective infusion rate.

- The use of sedation guidelines or an algorithm is recommended.

- A weaning protocol may be necessary if the patient has been receiving an IV infusion of the drug longer than 72 hours. According to the London Health Center:
  - If the midazolam infusion is less than 4 mg/hr, reduce infusion by 50% and reassess for further weaning in 6 hours.
  - If the midazolam infusion is greater than or equal to 4 mg/hr, reduce infusion by 25% and reassess for further weaning in 6 hours.
  - Discontinue infusion if the rate is less than 1 mg/hr.
  - If the patient's sedation score exceeds the goal or if the patient becomes agitated during sedation weaning, the nurse should administer a midazolam bolus and return to the previous infusion rate.

Side and/or Toxic Effects: Midazolam can cause respiratory depression and hypotension, especially when combined with narcotics.

When used longer than 48 to 72 hours, there may be unpredictable times to patient awakening and prolongation of time to patient extubation.

Withdrawal may develop in patients who receive the drug for a prolonged period and who do not have the dose tapered appropriately.

Numerous side effects are possible, including serious cardiorespiratory events, involuntary movements or hyperactivity, coughing, headache, hiccoughs, nausea, and vomiting.

COMMONLY USED MEDICATIONS

LORAZEPAM (ATIVAN), a Benzodiazepine

INTRODUCTION

Lorazepam has antianxiety, sedative, anticonvulsant effects. It also inhibits the ability to recall events. It has a slower onset but longer duration of action than midazolam. It may be preferred when the duration of sedation is expected to be greater than 48 hours and rapid wakening for neurological assessment is not required. Lorazepam is appropriate for sedation of most patients and may be administered by intermittent or continuous IV dosing (National Guidelines Clearinghouse, 2002). Once steady state is achieved, lorazepam's longer duration of action makes it a more appropriate agent for the maintenance of sedation levels.

Desired Effects: When given by IV bolus, the onset of lorazepam's sedative effects as well as the peak effects should occur in 15 to 30 minutes with a duration of about 8 hours.

Nursing Responsibilities:

- The use of sedation guidelines or an algorithm to initiate and wean doses is recommended.

- Continuous sedation may be achieved by regular bolus doses (e.g., 2 mg IV every 4 hours) or a continuous infusion.

- Lorazepam must be diluted immediately before it is injected with an equal volume of sterile water, dextrose in water, or saline. To ensure that the drug is adequately mixed, the container should be gently inverted repeatedly.

- A 2 mg dose or fraction thereof should be administered slowly over 2 to 5 minutes.

- When given as a continuous infusion, it is usually dissolved in D_5W to avoid crystallization and only enough is prepared for a 12-hour infusion (in plastic) or 24-hour infusion (in glass).

- The dose should be titrated to the patient's level of anxiety/agitation using a sedation assessment scale.

- When administered for longer than 7 days, lorazepam should be weaned according to a protocol to prevent withdrawal. The London Health Center recommends:
  - If the lorazepam dose is less than 2 mg every 4 hours, reduce the dose by 50% and reassess for further weaning in 12 hours.
  - If the lorazepam dose is greater than 2 mg every 4 hours, reduce the dose by 25% and reassess for further weaning in 12 hours.
  - If the sedation scale target is exceeded or if the patient becomes agitated during sedation weaning, the nurse should administer a lorazepam bolus and return to the previous dose.

- A slower weaning protocol recommends that when weaning lorazepam continuous infusion, the infusion rate must be decreased by 10% per day.

- Lorazepam may be discontinued when the intermittent dose is less than 0.5 mg every 4 hours or if the infusion rate is less than 10 mcg/hr.

Side and/or Toxic Effects: According to the London Health Center, use of large parenteral doses (equivalent to 5 to 10 mg/hr) may cause reversible renal tubular necrosis, lactic acidosis, and hyperosmolar states as a result of accumulation of the carrier solvents (polypropylene glycol and polyethylene glycol).

With too rapid IV administration, apnea and cardiac arrest as well as bradycardia and hypotension may occur. The patient may experience dizziness and excessive drowsiness. Both physical and psychological dependence can develop.

Sedation Assessment

Just as it is essential to assess and document pain according to a valid, reliable scale, it is imperative to utilize a comparable scale for assessing agitation and sedation. There are a variety of scales available but there tend to be common factors assessed across sedation scales. According to De Jong et al. (2005) these include:

- Consciousness defined as patient awareness of self and surroundings often assessed by neurological examination. Sedation scales may use the Glasgow Coma Scale or the Reaction Level Scale to evaluate consciousness.

- Agitation defined as patient restlessness characterized by nonpurposeful movement. The most commonly used scales are the Ramsey Sedation Scale and the Riker Sedation/Agitation Scale.

- Anxiety defined as a "subjective feeling of distress and anguish." Critical care nurses have a tendency to focus on the physiologic markers of anxiety (heart rate, blood pressure, and agitation), often failing to ask the patient himself what he was experiencing (Moser et al., 2003). Because anxiety, like pain, is a subjective experience, it is essential to question the patient concerning feelings of anxiety.

- Sleep

- Patient-ventilator synchrony defined as when there is coordination between the respiratory movements of the patient and the ventilator. Although patients are often sedated to ensure patient-ventilator synchrony, there is an association among continuous infusion of sedative, deeper sedation, and a prolonged requirement for ventilator support.

Two examples of sedation assessment scales are included in this chapter. The American Association of Critical-Care Nurses Sedation Assessment Scale is displayed in Table 2–2, and the Ventilator Adjusted Motor Assessment Scoring Scale (VAMASS) is displayed in Table 2–3. Using sedation scales allows objective assessment of patients and hopefully prevents patients from being sedated too deeply or for too long. Excessive sedation of critically ill ventilated patients has been associated with prolonged ventilation and more complications from ventilator therapy.

When caring for a critically ill patient requiring sedation, the critical care nurse should:

- Assess the patient for pain and treat the pain prior to beginning a sedation assessment.

- Assess the patient and administer sedation in response to demonstrated findings on a valid, reliable scale.

- Plan to assess and document the sedation level of each patient at least at the beginning of every shift, every 4 hours unless the patient is sleeping, and whenever there are changes in the patient's level of sedation or agitation.

- Record sedation scale values with any sedative doses.

- Assess for delirium if the patient becomes more confused, disoriented, or agitated with sedation.

- Wean the sedation according to established parameters.

Sedation Administration

The learner should refer to the earlier section, General Principles for Administration of Pain or Sedative Medication, for a brief review of duration, half-life, attaining therapeutic levels of continuous infusions, and intermittent dosing of medications. A specific application of this information for IV sedation is that ultra-short-acting agents such as propofol achieve steady state quickly and require few loading doses, whereas longer acting drugs such as midazolam and lorazepam need more loading doses (London Health Center, n.d.).

Additional general information essential for the critical care nurse to know when providing sedation is that benzodiazepines provide both sedation and amnesia and may provide an analgesic sparing effect. Older patients and those with renal and hepatic failure have slower clearance of benzodiazepines and their metabolites so they will need dosage adjustments. Other patient factors may affect the intensity and duration of these drugs, including previous drug use, alcohol use, age, concurrent pathology, and concurrent drug therapy. Intermittent dosing may be sufficient to achieve sedation goals. However, when consistent levels of sedation are required, infusions may be necessary.

According to the National Guidelines Clearinghouse (2002), the dose of sedatives should be titrated to a defined goal (end point), then systematic tapering of the dose or daily interruption with retitration should be instituted to minimize the effects of prolonged sedation. The London Health Center states similarly that to decrease the potential for excessive sedative administration and prevent prolonged ventilation, daily weaning of sedatives should automatically be attempted when the patient meets the following criteria:

- VAMASS is less than or equal to target VAMASS.

- Sedation is not being used to treat delirium.

- Patient is not receiving neuromuscular blocking agents.

- Patient is hemodynamically stable.

- Patient is stable on the ventilator.

TABLE 2–2

American Association of Critical-Care Nurses Sedation Assessment Scale

DOMAIN OR SUBSCALE	INDICATOR	SCORE BEST 1	2	3	4	WORST 5
Consciousness	Awake and aware of self and environment	Spontaneously opens eyes and initiates interaction with others	Wakens and responds after light verbal or tactile stimuli May return to sleep when stimuli stop	Wakens and responds after strong or noxious verbal or tactile stimuli Returns to sleep when stimuli stop	Displays localization or withdrawal behaviors to noxious stimuli	Displays posturing or no response to strong or noxious stimuli
Agitation	Body movement, patient/staff safety*	Calm body movements and tolerance of treatments and restrictions Movements do not pose a significant risk for safety of patient or staff		Body movements or noncompliance with treatments or restrictions do not pose a significant risk for safety of patient or staff		Body movements or noncompliance with treatments or restrictions poses a significant risk for safety of patient or staff
	Noises of patient	No noises		Frequent moaning or calling out		Shouting, screaming, or other disruptive vocalizations
	Patient's statements†	Very calm				Very restless
Anxiety	Patient's perceived anxiety† (Faces Anxiety Scale‡)	No anxiety				Extreme anxiety
Sleep	Observed sleep	Looks asleep, calm, resting (eyes closed, calm face and body)	Looks asleep, periodically awakens and returns to sleep easily	Awake, naps occasionally for brief periods		Unable to sleep or nap
	Patient's perceived quality of sleep†	I slept well		I slept fair		I slept poorly
Patient-ventilator synchrony	Breathing pattern relative to ventilator cycle	Synchrony of patient and ventilator at all times, patient cooperative and accepting ventilation Coordinated, relaxed chest movement		Occasional resistance to ventilation, or spontaneous breathing is out of synchrony with the ventilator Chest movement occasionally not coordinated with ventilator		Frequent resistance to ventilation, or spontaneous breathing not synchronous with the ventilator Uncoordinated chest and ventilator movements

Source: American Association of Critical-Care Nurses (www.medscape.com)
* This component is assessed in all patients, regardless of the goal of sedation.
† Assumes the patient has the ability to understand directions and communicate his or her perceptions either verbally, in writing, or by pointing to words or pictures. If score is greater than 2 for this subscale, ask the patient if he or she needs something to help him or her relax.
‡ Faces Anxiety Scale reprinted from McKinley et al., with permission of Blackwell Publishing.

TABLE 2-3

Ventilator Adjusted Motor Assessment Scoring Scale (VAMASS)

0	Unresponsive to pain	A	Minimal coughing; few alarms; tolerates movement
1	Opens eyes and/or moves to pain only	B	Coughing, frequent alarms when stimulated; settles with voice or removal of stimulus
2	Opens eyes and/or moves to voice	C	Distressed, frequent coughing or alarms; high RR with normal/ low $PaCO_2$
3	Calm and cooperative	D	Unable to control ventilation; difficulty delivering volumes; prolonged coughing
4	Restless but cooperative; follows commands		
5	Agitated; attempts to get out of bed; may stop behavior when requested but reverts back		
6	Dangerously agitated; pulling at tubes or lines, thrashing about; does not obey commands		

Source: Used by permission: Victoria Hospital Critical Care Trauma Center, London Health Sciences Center London, Ontario

The major reason for this emphasis on daily interruption or automatic weaning is evidence from researchers such as de Wit and Epstein (2003), who stated that patients receiving continuous infusions are more likely to be oversedated.

In contrast to this call for minimal sedation of ventilated patients, Nortvedt, Kvarstein, and Jonland (2005) cautioned that "medical disagreement persists . . . in that the treatment of patients in relation to sedation may be arbitrary and based on personal preferences that lack a sound scientific basis" (p. 533). "We have indications that being awake while undergoing intensive care is not experienced as ordinary wakefulness but as an uneasy feeling of being dizzy and cognitively impaired" (p. 533). There are also some indications that lack of sedation may increase patients' suffering, stress, and hallucinations. Thus, nurses must be aware of ongoing research concerning the effects of sedation. In the meantime, nurses must balance the needs of their critically ill patients for sedation with their needs for adequate ventilation and extubation as soon as possible. In addition, when administering sedation, the nurse must be aware of issues associated with specific sedatives.

Issues related to anxiety and sedation of patients with specific disorders are discussed in the appropriate chapters. General information about the use of specific sedatives in critically ill, ventilated patients follows.

Prevention and Treatment of Delirium

Delirium is very common among critically ill patients, developing in 50% to 80% of severely ill ventilated patients, and 20% to 50% of other ICU patients. Even though delirium is an independent risk factor for morbidity and mortality, only 4% of ICUs had policies requiring regular assessment of all patients for delirium as recently as 2003. This meant that delirium went unrec-ognized in the majority of patients (Truman & Ely, 2003) and probably complicated their recovery. Disorganized thinking, inattention, and a change in level of consciousness characterize delirium.

Predisposing Factors for Delirium

There are three main neurotransmitters involved in the development of delirium: acetylcholine, dopamine, and aminobutyric acid. Dopamine normally excites the brain, whereas the other two counterbalance the dopamine. Delirium probably results from an imbalance among these neurotransmitters in the brain, resulting in unpredictable and inconsistent neurotransmission. Thus, any disease process, medication, or pattern of care that disrupts these neurotransmitters predisposes the patient to delirium. Factors that predispose critically ill patients to delirium include:

- Necessary medical care such as:
  - The use of polypharmacy (patient is receiving three or more drugs)
  - The use of narcotics
  - The use of benzodiazepines (which is particularly important)
- Patient characteristics such as:
  - The presence of infection, especially if the patient develops sepsis
  - Organ dysfunction (especially congestive heart failure) or renal failure with a creatinine greater than 2 mg/dL
  - Electrolyte abnormalities such as hyponatremia
  - Altered vision or hearing
  - Preexisting dementia in the older adult
- Patterns of care provision necessitated by the critical nature of the illness such as:
  - Disruptions in sleep pattern
  - Prolonged immobilization

COMMONLY USED MEDICATIONS

PROPOFOL (DIPRIVAN), a Short-acting General Anesthetic Agent

INTRODUCTION

Propofol has a very short duration of action. It is indicated when sedation is required but rapid awakening to perform neurological assessment or extubation is necessary (National Guidelines Clearinghouse, 2002). It may be utilized for patients with head injuries, although there is conflicting evidence about its ability to reduce intracranial pressure. It has no analgesic properties and appears to provide less amnesia than benzodiazepines.

Desired Effects: The onset of sedation with propofol is 40 seconds with an unknown peak of action and a duration of 3 to 5 minutes.

Nursing Responsibilities:

- A large vein is recommended for the infusion because propofol may result in burning and stinging at the IV site.
- It is administered as a continuous IV infusion due to the short duration of effect.
- The initial infusion dose is often 5 mcg/kg/min. The dose is titrated up slowly (increasing by 5 to 10 mcg/kg/min every 5 minutes) until the sedation goal is reached.
- The patient should be monitored for the development of hypotension, especially during the first 60 minutes.

- The dose should be temporarily reduced (but not stopped) daily to assess neurological and respiratory functioning. Most patients will awaken within 8 minutes.
- An analgesic will be required for pain management because it has no analgesic properties.
- Because propofol is not soluble in water, it is formulated in the same lipid emulsion used for TPN solutions. Therefore:
  - The caloric content of the infusion must be included in the total calories that the patient receives and adjustments should be made to the rate of any feeding to prevent overfeeding.
  - Lipid monitoring is required; triglyceride levels should be monitored after 2 days of propofol infusion.
  - Strict aseptic technique is essential because the lipid solution is an excellent medium for bacterial growth. All bottles must be discarded within 12 hours of being opened. IV tubing must be changed every 12 hours.

Side and/or Toxic Effects: Doses higher than 90 mcg/kg/hr have been associated with a syndrome of lactic acidosis, rhabdomyolysis, and cardiogenic shock. Excessive doses may result in hypotension, which can be managed with fluids, repositioning, or vasopressors. Because the drug contains EDTA, a trace metal chelator, zinc deficiencies may occur in patients who have been receiving the drug for longer than 5 days.

Manifestations of Delirium

Delirium is the sudden onset of disturbances in cognition, attention, and perception that fluctuate over time. Delirium can manifest as hyperactive (agitated), hypoactive (also known as quiet and often not identified at all or misdiagnosed as depression), or mixed. It is likely that the mixed type of delirium is the most prevalent in ICUs (Truman, Gordon, & Ely, 2004).

Delirium Assessment. Every critically ill patient should be screened for delirium at least once each shift. Initially an arousal or sedation/agitation assessment (e.g., VAMASS or Richmond Sedation/Agitation Scale) should be performed. If appropriate, the patient should then be assessed using a delirium assessment scale such as the Confusion Assessment Method of the Intensive Care Unit (CAM-ICU). The CAM-ICU is displayed in Table 2–4, and the instructions for scoring it are available at the ICU delirium Web site. To score positive for delirium on the CAM-ICU, the patient must display:

1) acute changes or a fluctuation in mental status (CAM-ICU Feature 1)
2) accompanied by inattention (Feature 2) and
3) either disorganized thinking (Feature 3) or
4) a level of consciousness other than alert (Feature 4)

Management of Delirium

Treatment of delirium includes the use of medication and environmental and supportive strategies. As soon as delirium is suspected, the patient's medication regimen should be reviewed to determine if it is exacerbating the problem. Treatment with sedatives alone or the combination of sedatives and analgesics can worsen delirium because they do not solve the neurotransmitter imbalance and they can increase agitation. The dosages of any medications thought to be contributing to delirium should be decreased or the drugs should be discontinued.

Guidelines established by the Society of Critical Care Medicine (SCCM) and described by Jacobi et al. (2002) recommend haloperidol (Haldol) for the treatment of delirium, although it has not received FDA approval and it is being used off label when it is administered IV push for delirium. Still the current treatment of delirium is combination therapy using haloperidol and lorazepam. The drugs are usually administered in combination because haloperidol blocks dopamine receptors, whereas lorazepam enhances the action of the inhibitory neurotransmitter GABA. In addition, lorazepam potentiates the tranquilizing effects of haloperidol, so less haloperidol needs to be given to achieve the same effect.

When haloperidol and lorazepam are administered to the delirious patient:

- The haloperidol dose is usually two times the lorazepam dose.
- They are scheduled around the clock.
- The evening dose is larger than the daytime doses to enhance sleep and minimize "sundowning."
- Prn dosing should be available for acute exacerbations.
- The patient needs to be monitored for such adverse effects as QT prolongation and dysrhythmias (torsades de pointes), which can result in sudden death, especially if the drug is administered IV push. Significant extrapyramidal effects may also occur (Truman & Ely, 2003).

TABLE 2-4

CAM-ICU Worksheet

	Positive	Negative
Feature 1: Acute Onset or Fluctuating Course Positive if you answer "yes" to either 1A or 1B.	Positive	Negative
1A: Is the patient different than his/her baseline mental status? Or **1B:** Has the patient had any fluctuation in mental status in the past 24 hours as evidenced by fluctuation on a sedation scale (e.g., RASS), GCS, or previous delirium assessment?	Yes	No
Feature 2: Inattention Positive if either score for 2A or 2B is less than 8. Attempt the ASE letters first. If pt is able to perform this test and the score is clear, record this score and move to Feature 3. If patient is unable to perform this test or the score is unclear, then perform the ASE Pictures. If you perform both tests, use the ASE Pictures' results to score the Feature.	Positive	Negative
2A: ASE Letters: record score (enter NT for not tested) Directions: Say to the patient, *"I am going to read you a series of 10 letters. Whenever you hear the letter A, indicate by squeezing my hand."* Read letters from the following letter list in a normal tone. **S A V E A H A A R T** Scoring: Errors are counted when patients fail to squeeze on the letter "A" and when the patient squeezes on any letter other than "A".	Score (out of 10): _____	
2B: ASE Pictures: record score (enter NT for not tested) Directions are included on the picture packets.	Score (out of 10): _____	
Feature 3: Disorganized Thinking Positive if the combined score is less than 4	Positive	Negative
3A: Yes/No Questions (Use either Set A or Set B, alternate on consecutive days if necessary): Set A Set B 1. Will a stone float on water? 1. Will a leaf float on water? 2. Are there fish in the sea? 2. Are there elephants in the sea? 3. Does one pound weigh more than two pounds? 3. Do two pounds weigh more than one pound? 4. Can you use a hammer to pound a nail? 4. Can you use a hammer to cut wood? Score _____ (Patient earns 1 point for each correct answer out of 4) **3B: Command** Say to patient: "Hold up this many fingers" (Examiner holds two fingers in front of patient) "Now do the same thing with the other hand" (Not repeating the number of fingers). *If patient is unable to move both arms, for the second part of the command ask patient "Add one more finger" Score _____ (Patient earns 1 point if able to successfully complete the entire command)	Combined Score (3A+3B): _____ (out of 5)	
Feature 4: Altered Level of Consciousness Positive if the Actual RASS score is anything other than "0" (zero)	Positive	Negative
Overall CAM-ICU (Features 1 and 2 and either Feature 3 or 4):	Positive	Negative

Source: Copyright © 2002, E. Wesley Ely, MD, MPH and Vanderbilt University, all rights reserved.

Once the patient's confusion has cleared, the doses of haloperidol and lorazepam are usually continued for 3 to 5 days before weaning of the medications is started.

Environmental and supportive strategies may be used as adjunct strategies to prevent and treat delirium. Utilizing some of the nonpharmacological strategies to promote a more restful sleep pattern as described in the next section may help. Limiting unnecessary noise or providing the patient with music to filter out the noise helps some patients. Providing patients with eyeglasses and hearing aids so that they are less likely to misinterpret events in the environment also helps.

The nurse and patient's family will need to reorient the patient to her surroundings frequently. As one patient who was delirious for several days after a motor vehicle crash said, "All the time I was there, I never experienced any pain but the mental anguish I felt was terrible. I wish I could tell my nurses now how they could have helped me. I thought they were part of the Mafia and were trying to do me in at any time. I needed my nurse to say to me every time I woke up, 'You are in _____ Medical Center. You have been in a motor vehicle crash. At the moment, you have a tube in your throat so you can't speak; we have your hands tied to keep you safe so that you do not pull out your tubes. You seem to be seeing and hearing things. These are wild dreams that are caused by the medications we are giving you. Try to remember that you are doing okay and we are trying to help you.'"

Sleep

Sleep disturbances are common in critically ill patients and contribute to delirium and other sources of morbidity. According to Bourne and Mills (2004), there are a multitude of reasons why critically ill patients may have difficulty sleeping, including:

- Environmental factors—An ICU can be a bright, noisy place with alarms sounding and machinery such as ventilators or balloon pumps working appropriately.
- Patient care activities—When a nurse is trying to allow a patient to sleep but needs to monitor vital signs, the tightening of a blood pressure cuff may awaken the patient.
- Discomfort from the acute illness itself such as diaphoresis from a fever may cause sleep disruption.
- Medications—Sedative and analgesic combinations that are commonly used to facilitate mechanical ventilation are among the most sleep disruptive of drugs. Cardiovascular, gastric protective, antiasthma, anti-infective, antidepressant, and anticonvulsant medications have also been reported to cause sleep disorders.
- Withdrawal from prescribed and recreational drugs also may cause sleep disruption.

Sleep disruption is so common in the critically ill that very few mechanically ventilated patients have normal sleep patterns. This is of concern because lack of sleep has been associated with both serious physiologic and psychological effects. The consequences of inadequate sleep include changes in metabolism and immune response and respiratory dysfunction. These may lead to delayed healing and prolong the need for mechanical ventilatory support (Bourne & Mills, 2004). In addition sleep disruption has long been thought to be a factor in the development of ICU psychosis.

Unfortunately, according to Bourne and Mills (2004), the majority of sleep disorders experienced by ICU patients cannot be resolved by the use of medications alone because patients experience disruptions in both the total amount of sleep and the quality of sleep. Critically ill patients suffer particularly from sleep fragmentation and reduced restful sleep. Bourne and Mills believed that there is limited evidence to support the use of drugs to treat sleep disorders in ICU patients and that all the available drugs have potential problems. Therefore, they recommended the following strategies:

- A short course of therapy for any drugs prescribed for acute sleep disturbances
- Appropriate use of sedation, sedation scoring systems, and vigilance for withdrawal syndromes to minimize sleep disturbances

- A combined approach incorporating environmental controls, appropriate treatment of the patient's acute illness, and rational drug use

After noting that it is a nursing challenge to recognize the importance of adequate sleep to critical care patients, Honkus (2003) listed the following methods that can be used to modify the environment and prepare a patient for sleep:

- Assess all intravenous lines for patency and level all transducers, placing the head of the bed in the desired position before the patient is settled for sleep.
- Assess the patient for pain or discomfort and provide medication as needed.
- Provide bedtime comfort: offer a snack if possible, provide a back rub, and arrange pillows and blankets for comfort.
- Decrease noise in the patient's environment as much as possible.
- If it is necessary to disrupt the patient's sleep, try to space procedures so that the patient is able to obtain at least 2 hours of uninterrupted sleep at a time.

Nutrition

Nearly all critically ill patients need a nutritional consult. It may be because they:

- Have had a cardiovascular event and should modify their diet
- Are in renal failure and require adjustment of nutrients in their diet
- Are intubated and require enteral or parenteral nutrition
- Have had surgery and require specialized nutrition for tissue repair
- Have increased caloric and other nutritional needs following trauma or burns

The precise nutritional assessment and requirements for patients with specific disorders are discussed in each of the chapters of this book. A related issue, intensive glucose management for critically ill patients, is discussed in Chapter 13. However, an overview and some general principles concerning nutrition for critically ill adults are discussed in this section.

Although severity of illness is the major factor in determining outcomes of critical illness, the patient's nutritional status and adequacy of nutritional supplementation also contribute to them (Higgins, Daly, Lipson, & Guo, 2006). According to Heyland, Dhaliwal, Drover, Gramlich, and Dodek (2003), the benefits of adequate nutrition in the critically ill patient include:

- Improved wound healing
- Decreased catabolic response to injury

- Improved gastrointestinal function
- Reduction in complications, length of hospital stay, and cost of stay. In addition, it has been postulated that undernourishment of ventilated patients results in diminished ventilatory drive, reduction in the production of surfactant, and difficulty in weaning due to muscle fatigue caused by diaphragmatic and skeletal muscle weakness. This has not been consistently demonstrated in research studies, however (Higgins et al., 2006).

Assessment

The first step in determining a patient's nutritional requirements is doing an assessment. A nutritional assessment includes:

- Obtaining a history
- Reviewing diagnostic studies
- Determining nutritional requirements

The amount of information that the nurse is able to obtain from the history may be limited due to the patient's physical condition. However, it is essential that the nurse learn:

- The patient's current height and weight, and if the patient has recently lost or gained a significant amount of weight
- Information about food allergies, especially allergies to shellfish for patients who may be undergoing studies that require contrast media
- If the patient has been consuming nutritional supplements because some supplements can alter the patient's electrolyte and metabolic balance
- If the patient has had any swallowing difficulties, nausea or vomiting, or constipation or diarrhea
- The amount of alcohol a patient admits to consuming
- Any type of diet the patient may be on, whether medically prescribed or self-determined

The nurse will need to verify the patient's weight and compare it to the patient's previous weights to identify excessive weight gain or loss. It is common for critically ill patients to have weight fluctuations due to fluid imbalances. A change in weight of 2 pounds (or about 1 kg) may represent the loss or retention of approximately a liter of fluid. The patient's weight should also be compared to an ideal body weight, or the patient's body mass index (BMI) should be calculated. (See Table 2–5 for in-

formation about BMI.) Patients who are obese or underweight when admitted to critical care have more complications and longer hospital stays.

A common measure used to identify protein nutritional status in critically ill patients is serum albumin. Critically ill patients often have low serum albumin levels (less than 3.5 g/dL or 35 g/L), most likely reflecting both their nutritional status and the physiologic stress of their illness. Levels of serum prealbumin (normal 20–30 mg/dL) are monitored less frequently but are more immediate indicators of physiologic stress and protein nutritional adequacy (Higgins et al., 2006). Additional studies that are frequently reviewed to determine nutritional adequacy and requirements are serum hemoglobin, magnesium, and phosphorus.

Once the patient's nutritional status has been assessed, the patient's nutritional requirements may be determined.

- A first step is usually to calculate the patient's caloric, protein, and fluid requirements.
- A normal caloric intake is 25 kcal/kg/day for a person who is well nourished, nonstressed, and has a normal albumin level. The nitrogen requirement for the same patient would be 0.8 to 1 g protein/g/day.
- As the stress of the critical illness mounts, the patient will require increasing amounts of calories and may require as much as 1.5 to 2 g/kg/day of protein.
- Fluid intake is closely tied to energy consumption and, normally, a person will require about 1 mL of fluid per calorie. However, fluid requirements are influenced by a wide variety of factors.
- Caloric, protein, and fluid requirements are usually calculated by a nutritionist because both underfeeding and overfeeding patients present problems.

The energy requirements of critically ill, ventilated patients are usually estimated by either a nutritionist or a physician. They may be estimated by using formulas that calculate energy demand based on body size composition, age, and gender, or they may be estimated based on calorimetry. The most commonly used equations to estimate energy requirements for critically ill patients are the Harris-Benedict equations (Table 2–6). Unfortunately, these equations tend to result in unpredictable

TABLE 2–5

Body Mass Index (BMI) Calculation

$$\text{BMI (kg/m}^2) = \frac{\text{Weight (kg)}}{\text{Height (m)}^2}$$

TABLE 2–6

Harris-Benedict Equations for Calculating Basal Energy Expenditure (BEE)

For women, the BEE = 66.5 + (13.75 × kg) + (5.003 × cm) − (6.775 × age)
For men, the BEE = 655.1 + (9.563 × kg) + (1.850 × cm) − (4.676 × age)
The result is multiplied by a stress factor (1.2 to 2.5) for most patients.

errors when used to estimate energy requirements for some patients (Higgins et al., 2006) such as those who are morbidly obese, severely underweight, or have fluid imbalances. Therefore, indirect calorimetry may be utilized instead even though there is not sufficient evidence to recommend it in all circumstances (Heyland et al., 2003).

Indirect calorimetry uses a metabolic chart to measure the heat production, oxygen consumption, and carbon dioxide production of the patient. These values are used to calculate basal energy expenditure in kilocalories. Resting energy requirements are usually calculated so the measurement must occur when the patient has been without food for 2 hours, after the patient has been resting for 30 minutes, and when the patient is in a thermoneutral environment (Higgins et al., 2006). Once a patient's nutritional requirements have been established, a decision can then be made about how to meet them best.

Guidelines for Providing Nutritional Support

Whenever possible, patients should receive oral feedings. However, many critically ill patients are unable to eat and thus require nutritional support. The most recent guidelines suggest that if a critically ill patient is unable to consume adequate nutrition orally within 24 to 48 hours of admission, nutritional support should be started (Heyland et al., 2003). Starting nutritional support early is associated with improved calorie and protein intake, resulting in better nitrogen balance and a trend toward lower mortality. Heyland et al. argued that early nutritional support should be administered enterally if at all possible because it is associated with a much lower risk of infection and better outcomes than parenteral nutrition. They did not recommend using parenteral nutrition in combination with enteral nutrition and stated that when the patient is not tolerating enteral nutrition, there is insufficient evidence to state when parenteral nutrition should be started. They explained that the use of parenteral nutrition is appropriate for patients in whom it would be life sustaining such as patients with short bowel syndrome, perforated gut, or a high-output fistula.

Enteral Nutrition. **Enteral nutrition** is the delivery of nourishment by feeding tube into the gastrointestinal (GI) tract. Initially and for short-term use, enteral feedings may be delivered through a large-bore nasal or oral gastric tube. For long-term use, small-bore feeding tubes or gastrostomies are usually required. Feedings may also be delivered into the small bowel (postpyloric feeding). See Figure 2-2 for information about the various types of feeding tubes and sites.

Enteral feeding is the preferred route for nutritional supplementation because it is associated with significantly lower rates of infection than parenteral nutrition. In part this lower infection rate may occur because enteral feeding prevents translocation of bacteria from the GI tract,

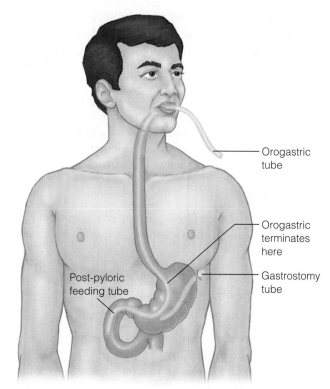

Figure 2-2 Locations of feeding tubes.

which can occur when the GI tract is inactive. Therefore, the recommendation to start feeding early, at 24 to 48 hours after admission, is not only to provide adequate nutrition immediately but also to decrease the likelihood of infection. The most common problems associated with early enteral feeding are:

- High gastric residual volumes
- Bacterial colonization of the stomach
- Increased risk of aspiration pneumonia (Heyland et al., 2003)

Enteral feeding formulas are usually composed of proteins; a source of calories (often lactose free); vitamins; minerals; trace elements; and, possibly, fiber. There are standard formulas and ones that are intended for specific subsets of patients, such as patients with renal failure. The appropriate formula, amount of free water, and any adjuncts for a specific patient are usually determined by the nutritionist in consultation with the physician because patients have differing nutritional needs. For example, the addition of glutamine is recommended for patients with severe burns and trauma. The amount of formula that the patient will require to meet his nutritional requirements is dependent on the chosen product and is calculated by the nutritionist and established as a target dose or goal.

Critical care nurses are responsible for attempting to provide the appropriate amount of nutritional intake while limiting the problems associated with enteral nutrition. Some of the issues associated with enteral feedings and the related nursing interventions are:

- Optimizing delivery of feedings: Most ventilated, enterally fed patients do not receive their energy requirements, primarily because their tube feedings are interrupted frequently (O'Leary-Kelley, Puntillo, Barr, Stotts, & Douglas, 2005). The most common reason for an interruption of a tube feeding is that the patient is about to have a procedure performed, usually either an extubation or an operative one. However, the next most common reason for interruption of tube feedings is the patient developing symptoms of GI intolerance of the feeding tube such as emesis, gastric distention, or high gastric residual.
- Critically ill patients are often started on continuous gastric tube feedings because it is believed continuous feeding may cause less GI intolerance. There are varying philosophies on how best to avoid the development of GI intolerance while ensuring that the patient gets his target dose:
  - To avoid GI distress, some physicians advocate starting at 10 mL/hr and increasing the rate every 6 hours if the tube feeding is tolerated until the patient is at the target dose.
  - In order to attain the target dose more quickly, some physicians advocate starting the feeding at that rate.
  - In the past, to prevent GI distress, nurses checked the patient for gastric residual every 2 to 4 hours and stopped the feeding if the residual was twice the amount of the hourly feeding.
  - According to Heyland et al. (2003) higher residual feeding protocols should be considered as a strategy to optimize patients' nutritional intake.
  - Feeding protocols using higher residual volumes (150 mL to as high as 250 mL) are less likely to result in interruption of gastric feedings. If higher residual protocols are utilized, they are usually accompanied by a motility agent (metoclopramide) and the nurse needs to observe the patient for any indication of GI distress and to stop the feeding for emesis.
  - An alternative to continuous tube feedings are intermittent boluses of tube feeding. According to Heyland et al. (2003), there is insufficient evidence to support the use of one mode of delivery of enteral feeding versus the other. When a bolus dose is delivered, it is usually a larger dose (250–400 mL) and is provided every 4 to 6 hours. Bolus tube feedings have historically been held if the residuals are half of the bolus dose. However, as with continuous

feedings, some advocate administering the bolus as long as the residual is less than the amount described in a protocol (often 150–250 mL) and adding metoclopramide to the regimen if the residuals are high. Patients are more likely to complain of some discomfort such as cramping, bloating, and nausea with bolus doses.

- Prevention of aspiration:
  - Prior to institution of enteral feeding, the nurse must ensure that the nasogastric tube is located in the stomach. Historically this has been accomplished by auscultation for an air bolus over the stomach. However, this method has been demonstrated to be inaccurate. Appropriate methods for identifying placement of the feeding tube in the stomach include:
  - Visualizing the tube in the stomach on an abdominal x-ray
  - Obtaining aspirate from the tube with a pH of less than 5
  - Most authorities now advocate that to prevent aspiration of tube feeding contents and ventilator associated pneumonia, patients receiving gastric feedings be placed in the semirecumbent position (have the head of the bed elevated between 30 and 45 degrees).
- Prevention of bacterial colonization of the stomach:
  - Prepackaged tube feeding products are sterile. Heyland et al. (2003) noted that there was insufficient evidence to recommend the use of closed-system tube feeding systems for enterally fed patients. However, many nursing units are using such closed systems, using sterile water for any additive, and opening the system aseptically. The systems are changed every 24 hours with the expectation that there will be less likelihood of colonization of the stomach.
- Prevention of diarrhea:
  - If the patient is receiving bolus feedings, switching to continuous feedings may decrease the occurrence of diarrhea.
  - If the patient is lactose intolerant, switching to a feeding that does not contain lactose may help.
  - Adequately diluting liquid medications with water may also help.
  - It is unclear whether using *Lactobacillus acidophilus* restores normal flora and decreases the incidence of diarrhea.

Parenteral Nutrition. **Parenteral nutrition** is the infusion of nutrients using a venous catheter located in a large, usually central, vein. According to Simpson and Doig (2005), it is indicated in critically ill patients when nutritional supplementation is needed and enteral feedings cannot be initiated within 24 hours of ICU admission or injury. However, it should be emphasized that enteral nutrition is preferred over parenteral nutrition and that strategies to maximize enteral nutrition should be used before the parenteral route is utilized. Parenteral nutrition solutions usually are formulated by combining dextrose, lipids, protein (in the form of amino acids), electrolytes, water, vitamins, and trace elements. In addition, Heyland et al. (2003) recommended that parenteral nutrition be supplemented with glutamine if at all possible. The specific components of the infusion are prescribed for each patient by his physician and the rate of administration is dependent on the patient's energy requirement. The major risks associated with the administration of parenteral nutrition are:

- Gut mucosal atrophy
- Overfeeding
- Hyperglycemia
- Increased risk of infectious complications
- Increased mortality (Heyland et al., 2003)

Critical care nurses are responsible for maintaining the ongoing infusion while attempting to limit the problems associated with parenteral nutrition. Some of the issues associated with parenteral feedings and the related nursing interventions are:

- Access: Parenteral nutrition is delivered through a catheter with its tip in the superior vena cava or the right atrium.
  - To aid in the prevention of catheter-related sepsis, full barrier precautions should be utilized during insertion of the catheter and the site should be prepped with chlorhexidine.
  - The subclavian vein is the recommended access so a chest x-ray to rule out pneumothorax and to ensure catheter placement is required following catheter insertion and before the IV is utilized.
  - A dedicated line is required for infusion of parenteral nutrition. No other IV infusions or boluses should be administered through the line and no blood should be drawn from it.
  - Policies vary from institution to institution but most require changing the parenteral nutrition solution bag and tubing aseptically every 24 hours.
- Overfeeding: Due to the high concentration of glucose and lipids, overfeeding can occur with parenteral nutrition. Patients who are receiving propofol for sedation should not receive lipids in their parenteral nutrition. Heyland et al. (2003) suggested that all patients could maximize the benefits and minimize the risks of parenteral nutrition by not receiving lipids in the solution.

- Hyperglycemia: Critically ill patients who are receiving parenteral nutrition should be started on intensive glucose management and insulin therapy. This is discussed in detail in Chapter 13. ∞
- Hypoglycemia: A sudden decrease in the rate of infusion of parenteral nutrition can cause the patient's blood sugar to plummet. Therefore, parenteral nutrition is rarely stopped abruptly and it is always infused using an infusion pump.
- Risk of infection:
  - Ensuring that the central line has been inserted utilizing full barrier precautions is the first step in decreasing the risk of infection.
  - Maintaining a dedicated line is the second step. The dressing on the access site should be aseptically applied, securely attached, and changed in accordance with agency policy.
  - Removing lipids from the parenteral nutrition is also helpful in preventing infection because lipids support the growth of many microorganisms.
  - The patient should be monitored for signs of sepsis, including fever, chills, elevated white blood count, and positive blood cultures.
  - If the catheter site is thought to be the source of infection, the catheter is discontinued and the tip is usually sent for culture and sensitivity.

Evaluation of Effectiveness of Nutritional Therapy

The effectiveness of the patient's nutritional therapy can be monitored by:

- Determining the patient's weight daily (expect weight stabilization or ¼ to ½ pound weight gain per day with adequate nutrition)
- Examining the following lab studies:
  - Albumin or prealbumin
  - Hemoglobin and hematocrit
  - Electrolytes, including potassium
  - Magnesium
  - Phosphorus
- Assessing the patient's wounds for granulating tissue

The Needs of the Families of Critically Ill Patients

Molter (1979) did seminal work on the needs of families of patients in critical care, leading to the formation of the Critical Care Family Needs Inventory (CCFNI). Since that time her work has been validated by numerous other researchers. Based on her work, the following have been identified as needs of families of critically ill patients:

- Feel there is hope
- Feel hospital personnel care about the patient

- Have a waiting room near the patient
- Be called at home about changes in the patient's condition
- Know the prognosis
- Have questions answered honestly
- Know specific facts about the patient's prognosis
- Receive information about the patient at least once a day
- Have explanations given in understandable terms
- Be allowed to see the patient frequently

Leske (1991) was one of the researchers who validated Molter's findings, and she grouped the needs of the families into the following five domains:

- Support
- Comfort
- Proximity
- Information
- Assurance

Although these quantitative studies list the needs of the families, it is the qualitative work of other nurse researchers that captures what it is to be a family member of a critically ill patient. Jamerson et al. (1996) described the proximity phase of families' experiences as "hovering." This is a time when family members feel confused and tense as they wait until they can gain access to information about the patient or access to the patient. It has been described by Fulbrook, Allan, Carrol, and Dawson (1999) as maintaining a vigil—a phase during which the family feels a need to watch over the patient because they could not forgive themselves if anything happened while they were away. During this phase, the patient takes precedence and family members want to be with him, to touch him, to talk to him, or even just to sit quietly near him. They want to provide comfort and obtain comfort for the patient.

As the patient's critical illness progresses, the family begins searching actively for information. "Not knowing is the worst part," according to Verhaeghe, Defloor, Van Zuuren, Duijnstee, and Grypndonck (2005), and intensive anxiety can persist until the family believes sufficient information has been obtained. The family may then enter a "tracking phase" in which they observe, analyze, and evaluate the patient's care. It is a phase during which family members want to observe the patient's care and be reassured that he is being cared for appropriately.

How Critical Care Nurses Best Meet the Needs of Patients' Families

Medina (2005) stated, "In the critical care setting, families appear to have a profound beneficial impact on the response of the critically ill patient to the illness" (p. 1005). Families probably confer this beneficial impact by buffering the patient from some of the stress of the environment and illness as well as by serving as a resource for patient care. However, families are not able to perform these important functions if they are under severe stress. Therefore, it is important to the patient, not just the family, that critical care nurses meet the needs of families.

Responses to the Needs of Families of Critically Ill Patients

Health care providers have been attempting to meet the needs of families of critically ill patients since they were identified almost 30 years ago. Some of the families' needs and evidence-based strategies being employed to meet these needs are described next.

Families' Need for Information

Information is the primary need identified by families of critically ill patients (Verhaeghe et al., 2005). The need for information, although important to all families, is even more pronounced for families of patients who are unresponsive. According to Verhaeghe, families want the information to be as accurate and understandable as possible, yet they want it to be provided in such a way that there is room for hope. Most families expect the physician to initiate the explanation with a description of the patient's condition, prognosis, and treatment. They expect the nurse to clarify the information, provide information about the daily care and treatment of the patient, what the role of the family should be, and whether the patient is ready for transfer.

However, families search out information from multiple sources (Nelson, Kinjo, Meier, Ahmad, & Morrison, 2004) so a unified message from all members of the team is important. When choosing a clinician to seek information, families preferred clinicians who spoke to them in understandable terms, were sensitive, honest, and unhurried. They remembered clinicians who talked directly to them and kept their word more than clinicians who had the most information.

Miracle (2006) summarized strategies that might be utilized with families:

- Regular family conferences to discuss patient goals and progress toward the goals can be helpful. If this is not possible, then the family should at least have a daily update from the patient's nurse on the patient's progress.
- Written instructional guides to provide information about the critical care unit, equipment, location of waiting areas, and phone numbers for the unit.
- A way to contact family members and for family members to contact the patient's nurse and primary physician should be established. If the family member has a cell phone this might be utilized; otherwise a pager can be provided.

- If at all possible there should be consistency in the nurse providing care to the patient. Families indicate that it is not only important to receive an update from a nurse but that they prefer to receive it from the same nurse each time.

- Some hospitals provide written and verbal instructions to families to speak with the nurse whenever they have a question they want answered.

Families Need for Proximity

Families consistently state that they would prefer open visiting hours, and patients and families are more satisfied when the unit has flexible rather than limited visiting hours (Sims & Miracle, 2006). Still, only 14% of adult critical care units have open visitation, which allows the family to visit any time they choose. An additional 31% of units are open except during rounds or shift changes (Kirchhoff & Dahl, 2006). It is unclear why restrictions on visiting hours remain because Sims and Miracle stated there is abundant evidence that visitation is not stressful for patients and that it does not impede the delivery of nursing care. In fact, they described the following benefits of open visitation:

- Family members are more satisfied. They can arrange their schedules to their convenience and see the patient whenever they need to. Therefore, families report they are less tired with a flexible visiting policy.

- Communication is facilitated between patient, family, and staff. Families believe they receive more information about the patients' conditions because they see the nurse more frequently and are able to ask questions.

- Open family visitation allows families more opportunity to provide emotional support and reassurance to patients, thus assisting with patients' recoveries.

- There is some evidence that open family visitation may have physiologic benefits for the patient by increasing the amount of patient rest while decreasing the patient's heart rate, blood pressure, and intracranial pressure.

- Flexible visiting hours allow more opportunities for nurse-family interaction and family teaching.

Sims and Miracle (2006) summarized by stating that a liberal visitation policy has been shown to improve patient outcomes. They acknowledged, however, that critical care nurses must remain the gatekeepers for visitors. They recommended a highly individualized visitation policy that is based on the needs of the specific patient at that specific time. It becomes the responsibility of the critical care nurse, not a policy, to determine when a patient is benefiting from a visitor and when the patient would do better without a visitor present.

Some critical care nurses ask family members to leave while a procedure is being performed. However, there is accumulating evidence that it may benefit both the patient and family to have a family member available for the patient during intrusive procedures. The current evidence related to having family members being present during cardiopulmonary resuscitation is discussed in Chapter 18, Care of the Patient at the End of Life. ∞

Families' Needs for Support and Assurance

Henneman and Cardin (2002) explained these needs by saying: families want to believe the patient is being cared for in the 'best way possible' and that everything that ought to be done is being done. When nurses demonstrate competence and caring in their dealings with the patient and family, families are reassured. When a nurse explains what care is being delivered to the patient, focusing on how and why it is expected to help the patient, this offers hope, support, and reassurance to the family.

Families are concerned with the comfort of the patient. They want to be reassured that every effort is being made to keep the patient comfortable. They also have comfort needs of their own. However, most studies indicate that families place their own comfort among the least important of their concerns (Verhaeghe et al., 2005). Issues related to comfort for families are access to telephones and bathrooms, availability of coffee and food while they are waiting, comfortable chairs and sources of distraction in the waiting room, a place to sleep that is in or near the hospital, and information about services available from the hospital.

Continuing Concerns of Families

Unfortunately, despite identifying the needs of families of critically ill patients nearly 30 years ago, critical care personnel have not been able to meet them with uniformity. A variety of gaps in meeting the needs of families still exist. According to Lederer, Goode, and Dowling (2005), the most commonly noted gaps in service include the following:

- There is a discrepancy regarding the amount and adequacy of information shared. Whereas health care providers believe that information is generally available and communication is adequate, family members indicate that communication of patient information is sporadic and inconsistent.

- Family members want more members of the family involved in decisions about patient treatment and care. Health care providers generally prefer fewer family representatives.

- Family members indicate that some support services are not offered or are offered inadequately. Specifically, these include a place for family members to sleep or rest; an opportunity for families of critically ill patients to speak with each other; assistance with travel arrangements; a supply of coffee near the waiting area; and better preparation for home care.

Attempts to Improve Families' Ongoing Concerns

Recognizing that family needs were not being met, the Critical Care Family Assistance Program (CCFAP) was developed. Its goal is to respond to the unmet needs of families of critically ill patients in hospital ICUs through the provision of educational and family support materials (Lederer et al., 2005, p. 69S). CCFAP immediately identified that improvements in communication, environment, and provision of educational and informational materials were required.

Communication. Waiting for news about the patient is time consuming and anxiety provoking for families. Family members wait for long periods of time in a less than pleasant environment just to hear a few words from a doctor or nurse. CCFAP identified several events that consistently caused anxiety and irritation for families: "surgery being cancelled and the family not being informed; an extensive stay in the recovery room after surgery and the family kept unaware of the reason; contradictory information being received from different sources; and the inability to locate or talk to the physician" (Lederer et al., 2005, p. 73S).

Interventions developed by CCFAP units to allay these communication difficulties include:

- Designating specific individuals to be responsible for knowing each family, thus ensuring the family receives necessary information, that questions are answered, and appropriate conferences take place in a timely manner.

- Identifying who is responsible for handling the logistics and scheduling of family or interdisciplinary meetings, especially when several physicians are treating the patient.

- Facilitating weekly group meetings for the families of ICU patients. Some units have meetings that are facilitated by a social worker and a member of the pastoral care team in an attempt to make the ICU environment less frightening. The facilitators offer explanations about equipment, describe medical procedures, identify who the family should.

contact if information is coming too slowly, and provide guidance on ways to be appropriately assertive without being disruptive.

Environmental Changes to Enhance Family Comfort. All of the hospitals involved in CCFAP determined that their waiting areas required improvement (Lederer et al., 2005, p. 73S). They attempted to provide families a more relaxed, less institutional space by expanding the waiting area to make it less cramped, brightening the look of the room, or providing more comfortable furniture. Hospitals also sought to find space for sleeping rooms for families traveling great distances, providing coffee and soft drinks, supplying telephones, and placing televisions or videocassette recorders (VCRs) in the waiting area. Some units also designed and created family consultation rooms for family conferences with physicians and staff.

Education and Information Materials. "The CCFAP model seeks to assist ICUs in the important task of delivering unambiguous, but compassionate, information to families of ICU patients. Families require this information first, to cope with their distress, but primarily to participate in making decisions about family members who cannot speak for themselves about critical care decisions" (Lederer et al., 2005, p. S73). The education provided is of two very different types: general medical information and very specific information about the family member. In addition, many sites supply material to assist family members in becoming familiar with staff so that family members can identify who is caring for the patient, what their responsibilities are, and how to contact the patient's physicians. Also available might be pamphlets with frequently asked questions, information about advance directives, maps and diagrams of the hospital, and simple explanations of the medical and surgical problems most commonly seen in the ICU. This information is also available in an electronic format at an information kiosk. Providing information in a variety of formats allows the family to access it when they are ready and to consult it repeatedly while they are considering their options.

Critical care nurses need to realize that families state they are not receiving adequate, consistent information. This does not mean that health care providers are not providing the information. Rather it means that families may need critical care personnel to repeat information several times and provide it in multiple formats while the family attempts to assimilate it.

CRITICALLY ILL PATIENT SUMMARY

Critically ill patients are physically unstable and require physiologic support. However, the patients have other needs as well, including the needs for comfort, relief of anxiety, and assistance with communication. Families of critically ill patients are often in crisis and have been shown to need as-

surance, information, comfort, support, and proximity to the patient. When nurses' competencies are matched with the patients' needs and the multidisciplinary critical care team functions collaboratively to meet the needs of patients and families, patients' outcomes are enhanced.

(2004). Communication ability, method, and content among nonspeaking nonsurviving patients treated with mechanical ventilation in the intensive care unit. *American Journal of Critical Care, 13*(3), 210–220.

Henneman, E., & Cardin, S. (2002). Family centered critical care: A practical approach to making it happen. *Critical Care Nurse, 22*(6), 12–19.

Herr, K., Coyne, P., Key, T., Manworren, R., McCaffrey, M., Merkel, S., et al. (2006). Pain assessment in the non-verbal patient: Position statement with clinical practice recommendations. *Pain Management Nursing, 7*(2), 44–52.

Heyland, D. K., Dhaliwal, R., Drover, J. W., Gramlich, L., & Dodek, P. (2003). Canadian clinical practice guidelines for nutrition support in mechanically ventilated, critically ill adult patients. *Journal of Parenteral and Enteral Nutrition, 27*(5), 355–373.

Higgins, P., Daly, B. J., Lipson, A. R., & Guo, S. (2006). Assessing nutritional status in chronically critically ill adult patients. *American Journal of Critical Care, 15*(2), 166–176.

Honkus, V. L. (2003). Sleep deprivation in critical care units. *Critical Care Nursing Quarterly, 26*(3), 179–191.

Jacobi, J., Fraser, G., Coursin, D., Riker, R., Fontaine, D., Wittbrodt, E., et al. (2002). Clinical practice guidelines for the sustained use of sedatives and analgesics in the critically ill adult. *Critical Care Medicine, 30*(1), 119–141.

Jamerson, P. A., Scheibmeir, M., Bott, M. J., Crighton, F., Hinton, R. H., & Cobb, A. K. (1996). Experiences in the ICU. The experiences of families with a relative in the intensive care unit. *Heart & Lung, 25*(6), 467–474.

Kirchhoff, K., & Dahl, N. (2006). American Association of Critical Care Nurses' national survey of facilities and units providing critical care. *American Journal of Critical Care, 15*(1), 13–27.

Lederer, M. A., Goode, T., & Dowling, J. (2005). Origins and development: The critical care family assistance program. *Chest, 128*, 65–67.

Leske, J. (1991). Internal psychometric properties of the Critical Care Family Needs Inventory. *Heart & Lung, 20*, 236–242.

London Health Center. (n.d.). *Critical care self directed learning program: Analgesia, sedation, and delirium.* Retrieved February 3, 2008, from http://www.lhscl/critcare/ICU/drugs/drugindex.html

Magnus, V., & Turkington, L. (2006). Communication interaction in ICU—patient and staff experiences and perceptions. *Intensive and Critical Care Nursing, 22*, 167–180.

McCaffery, M. (1968). *Nursing practice patterns related to cognition, bodily pain, and man-environment interactions.* Los Angeles: University of California at Los Angeles Student's Store.

McCaffery, M., & Pasero, C. (1999). Assessment, underlying complexities, misconceptions, and practical tools. In M. McCaffery & C. Pasero (Eds.), *Pain clinical manual* (2nd ed., pp. 35–102). St. Louis, MO: Mosby.

Medina, J. (2005). A natural synergy in creating a patient-focused care environment: The critical care family assistance program and critical care nursing. *Chest, 128*, 99–102.

Miracle, V. (2006). Strategies to meet the needs of families of critically ill patients. *Dimensions of Critical Care Nursing, 25*(3), 121–125.

Molter, N. (1979). Needs of relatives of critically ill patients: A descriptive study. *Heart & Lung, 8*, 332–339.

Morse, J. M. (2001). Toward a praxis of suffering. *Advances in Nursing Science, 24*(1), 47–59.

Moser, D., Chung, M., McKinley, S., Riegel, B., An, K., Cherrington, C., et al. (2003). Critical care nursing practice regarding anxiety assessment and management. *Intensive and Critical Care Nursing, 19*(5), 276–288.

National Guidelines Clearinghouse. (2002). *Clinical practice guidelines for the sustained use of sedatives and analgesics in the critically ill adult.* Retrieved January 6, 2007, from http://www.guidelines.gov/summary/summary/aspx?ss=15&doc_id=171&nbr=2397

Nelson, J. E., Kinjo, K., Meier, D. E., Ahmad, K., & Morrison, R. S. (2004). When critical illness becomes chronic: Informational needs of patients and families. *Journal of Critical Care, 20*, 79–89.

Nortvedt, P., Kvarstein, G., & Jonland, I. (2005). Sedation of patients in intensive care medicine and nursing: Ethical issues. *Nursing Ethics, 12*(5), 522–536.

O'Leary-Kelley, C. M., Puntillo, K., Barr, J., Stotts, N., & Douglas, M. K. (2005). Nutritional adequacy in patients receiving mechanical ventilation who are fed enterally. *American Journal of Critical Care, 14*(3), 222–230.

Patak, L., Gawlinski, A., Fung, N., Doering, L., & Berg, J. (2004). Patients' reports of health care practitioner interventions that are related to communication during mechanical ventilation. *Heart and Lung, 33*(5), 308–318.

Puntillo, K., White, C., Morris, A., Perdue, S., Stanik-Hutt, J., Thompson, C., et al. (2001). Patient perceptions and responses to procedural pain: Results from the Thunder Project II. *American Journal of Critical Care, 10*, 238–251.

Simpson, R., & Doig, G. S. (2005). Parenteral versus enteral nutrition in the critically ill patient: A meta-analysis of trials using the intention to treat principle. *Intensive Care Medicine, 31*(1), 12–23.

Sims, J., & Miracle, V. (2006). A look at critical care visitation: The case for flexible visitation. *Dimensions of Critical Care Nursing, 25*(4), 175–181.

Stanik-Hutt, J. A. (2003). Pain management in the critically ill. *Critical Care Nurse, 23*(2), 99–103.

Taylor, D. R. (2005, December). The pharmacology of fentanyl and its impact on the management of pain. *Medscape Neurology & Neurosurgery, 7*(2). Retrieved February 13, 2008, from http://medscape.com/viewarticle/518441_print

Truman, B., & Ely, E. (2003). Monitoring delirium in critically ill patients: Using the confusion assessment method for the intensive care unit. *Critical Care Nurse, 23*(2), 25–36.

Truman, B., Gordon, S., & Ely, E. (2004). Delirium: A neglected danger in the intensive care unit. *Annals of Long Term Care, 12*(5), 18–22.

Verhaeghe, S., Defloor, T., Van Zuuren, F., Duijnstee, M., & Grypndonck, M. (2005). The needs and experiences of family members of adult patients in an intensive care unit: A review of the literature. *Journal of Advanced Nursing, 14*, 501–509.

Care of the Patient with Respiratory Failure

Sheila Cox Sullivan, PhD, RN, CNE

Learning Outcomes

Upon completion of this chapter, the learner will be able to:

1. Discuss the pathophysiology of ALI/ARDS.

2. Identify the clinical signs and symptoms of ALI/ARDS.

3. Compare and contrast settings for mechanical ventilation, explaining indications or guidelines pertinent to each setting.

4. Analyze a case study using evidence-based guidelines for medical and nursing treatment.

5. Prioritize nursing care for clients with ALI/ARDS.

Abbreviations

ALI	Acute Lung Injury
ARDS	Acute Respiratory Distress Syndrome
ARF	Acute Respiratory Failure
COPD	Chronic Obstructive Pulmonary Disease
CPAP	Continuous Positive Airway Pressure
ERV	Expiratory Reserve Volume
ET	Endotracheal Tube
FiO$_2$	Fraction of Inspired Oxygen
FRC	Functional Residual Capacity
FRV	Functional Residual Volume
HFO	High-Frequency Oscillation
IRV	Inspiratory Reserve Volume
NIV	Noninvasive Mechanical Ventilation
PEEP	Positive End-Expiratory Pressure
PSV	Pressure Support Ventilation
RV	Residual Volume
SIMV	Synchronized Intermittent Mandatory Ventilation
TLC	Total Lung Capacity
VAP	Ventilator-Associated Pneumonia
VC	Vital Capacity
V$_T$	Tidal Volume
VQc	Ventilation Perfusion

Acute Respiratory Failure (ARF) is the failure of the pulmonary system to provide sufficient exchange of oxygen to supply the body's demands (Christie & Goldstein, 2003). ARF is ubiquitous in critical care units, but the most severe respiratory disorder is **acute lung injury (ALI)**, which is considered the pulmonary symptom of multiple organ dysfunction syndrome (MODS). The most severe form of ALI is **acute respiratory distress syndrome (ARDS)**. First identified in 1967 by Ashbaugh, estimates of mortality range as high as 67%, but comorbid factors play a significant role in patient outcomes. The most common treatment for respiratory malfunctions, mechanical ventilation, is the second most commonly implemented intervention in critical care units (Agency for Health Care Policy and Research [AHCPR], 1996).

MEDIALINK
http://www.prenhall.com/perrin

See the Companion Website for chapter-specific resources at www.prenhall.com/perrin.

VISUAL MAP **Acute Lung Injury**

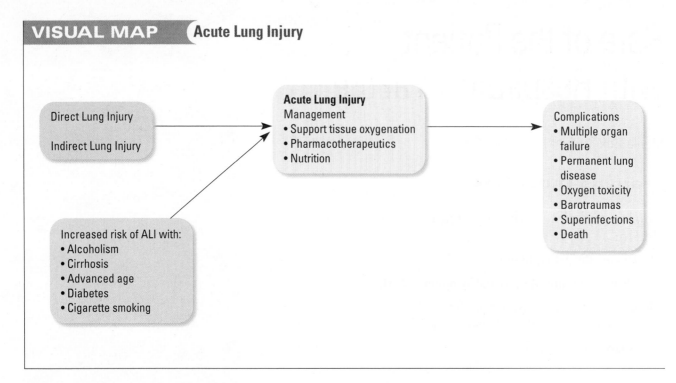

Direct Lung Injury

Indirect Lung Injury

Increased risk of ALI with:
• Alcoholism
• Cirrhosis
• Advanced age
• Diabetes
• Cigarette smoking

Acute Lung Injury
Management
• Support tissue oxygenation
• Pharmacotherapeutics
• Nutrition

Complications
• Multiple organ failure
• Permanent lung disease
• Oxygen toxicity
• Barotraumas
• Superinfections
• Death

Anatomy and Physiology Review

The anatomy of breathing includes the thorax and the airways. Respiratory components contained in the thorax include the rib cage, associated musculature, pleural space, and the lungs (Figure 3-1). The bony rib cage provides protection for the lungs. Although they are roughly the same in size, the right lung has three lobes, whereas the left has only two. The thoracic cavity is lined by the parietal pleura, whereas the lungs are covered by the visceral pleura. These two membranes are separated by a thin layer of pleural fluid, serous in

Figure 3-1 Anterior view of thorax and lungs.

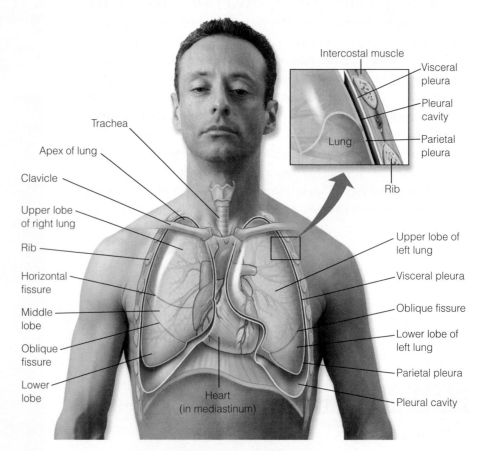

Trachea

Apex of lung

Clavicle

Upper lobe of right lung

Rib

Horizontal fissure

Middle lobe

Oblique fissure

Lower lobe

Intercostal muscle

Visceral pleura

Pleural cavity

Lung

Parietal pleura

Rib

Upper lobe of left lung

Visceral pleura

Oblique fissure

Lower lobe of left lung

Parietal pleura

Pleural cavity

Heart (in mediastinum)

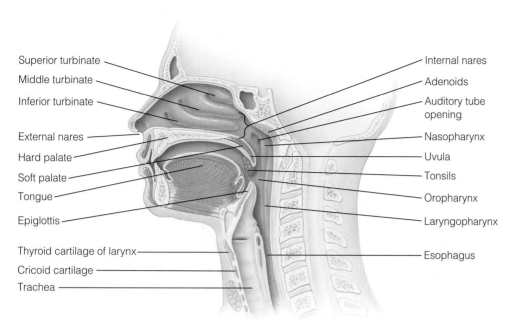

Figure 3-2 Structures of the respiratory system.

Superior turbinate
Middle turbinate
Inferior turbinate

External nares
Hard palate
Soft palate
Tongue
Epiglottis

Thyroid cartilage of larynx
Cricoid cartilage
Trachea

Internal nares
Adenoids
Auditory tube opening
Nasopharynx
Uvula
Tonsils
Oropharynx
Laryngopharynx
Esophagus

nature, which lubricates the pleura, allowing them to slide across one another during the ventilatory cycle. Fluid abnormally collected in this space is termed a pleural effusion. The space between the two lungs is called the mediastinum, and this is where the heart, esophagus, and major vessels are located.

The primary muscle of ventilation is the **diaphragm**, which is the dome-shaped muscle at the base of the lungs. The intercostal muscles pull the ribs up and out, aiding in the increase in thoracic volume. During respiratory distress, use of the intercostal muscles becomes more pronounced, and the sternocleidomastoid and scalenes are recruited to facilitate lung expansion. Normal expiration results from relaxation of the diaphragm and intercostal muscles, but during distress or coughing, the abdominals may assist in forceful exhalation.

Upper airways consist of the naso- and oropharynx and larynx (Figure 3-2). The function of these airways is to warm and cleanse environmental air as it is inhaled, thus protecting the lower airway. The **epiglottis** provides airway protection during ingestion of food and fluids by closing off the tracheal opening during swallowing. The **trachea** is the major tube connecting the upper and lower airways. It is approximately 1 inch in diameter and bifurcates into the mainstem bronchi at the carina, which is located at the fifth thoracic vertebra, or just below the sternal angle.

The lower airway is comprised of the bronchial tree and bronchioles, which branch into ever smaller passages (Figure 3-3). The lower airways are protected by the mucociliary escalator, a complex system of cilia that continuously propel respiratory secretions into the

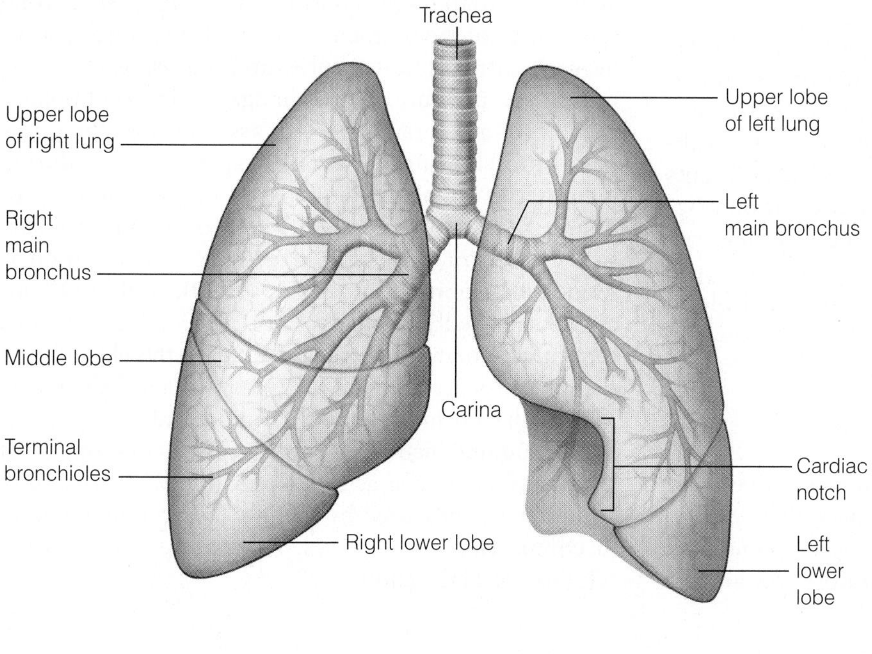

Figure 3-3 Respiratory passages.

Trachea

Upper lobe of right lung
Right main bronchus
Middle lobe
Terminal bronchioles
Right lower lobe

Upper lobe of left lung
Left main bronchus
Carina
Cardiac notch
Left lower lobe

Figure 3-4 Lobule of the lung.

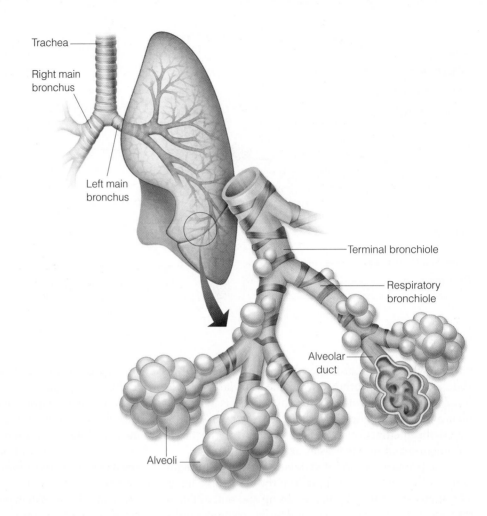

Trachea

Right main bronchus

Left main bronchus

Terminal bronchiole

Respiratory bronchiole

Alveolar duct

Alveoli

upper airways for expulsion. Further protection is provided by the cough reflex, triggered by the presence of foreign substances in the airways. Touching the carina is one method for stimulating this reflex. At the end of the bronchioles are over 300 million **alveoli**. It is within these small balloon-type structures that the exchange of gas between alveoli and capillaries occurs (Figure 3-4).

Bronchial circulation does not participate in gas exchange. The left bronchiole circulation is rooted from the aorta, and right-sided bronchioles are supplied by arteries that originate in the intercostal, subclavian, or internal mammary arteries. Bronchial veins empty into the vena cava. Pulmonary circulation originates from the pulmonary artery, and capillaries arising from these arteries provide the conduits for gas exchange. Venules carry the newly oxygenated blood back to the pulmonary vein for circulation to the rest of the body.

Physiology

It is important for the nurse to discriminate between the two functions of the respiratory system, which are ventilation and respiration. **Ventilation** is the mechanical act of moving air in and out of the respiratory tree and in-

volves primarily the musculoskeletal and nervous systems. **Respiration** involves the transport of oxygen and carbon dioxide between the alveoli and the pulmonary capillaries. Failure in any of these processes results in respiratory failure.

Ventilation

When the diaphragm contracts it flattens, increasing the volume of the thoracic cavity and creating a relative negative intrapulmonary pressure, that is, less than atmospheric pressure. This change in intrapulmonary pressure is potentiated by the assistance of the intercostal muscles during normal respiration, but during distress the use of the intercostals becomes more pronounced, and the scalenes and sternocleidomastoid assist. The effort expended in the act of inspiration is termed the **work of breathing (WOB)**, and WOB increases markedly in clients with chronic lung diseases that affect chest wall structure and/or the elasticity of the lungs. As described in the Gerontological Considerations, the normal changes of aging adversely affect WOB. **Compliance** is a multifaceted component of WOB and is defined as the expansibility of the thorax and lungs as measured by the increase in lung volumes in comparison to increases in intra-alveolar pressure (Guyton & Hall, 2000).

Gerontological Considerations

There are a number of age-related changes in respiratory function. These include:

- Decreased cough and laryngeal reflexes
- Decline in mucociliary escalator function
- Increased VQ mismatches
- Decrease in alveoli
- Increased AP diameter
- Increase in residual volume
- Decrease in respiratory muscle strength

For the healthy older adult, these changes do not appreciably affect normal activities. However, they contribute to a decreased respiratory reserve in the older adult and make it more difficult for the older adult to respond when demand exceeds capacity.

When older adults develop respiratory failure, they often manifest nonspecific symptoms of hypoxemia such as agitation, confusion, disorientation, lethargy, dyspnea, and chest pain.

The chest x-ray of an older adult with ARDs, especially one with preexisting lung disease, may not clear for a period of days to weeks after the ARDs has begun to resolve. Therefore, chest x-rays should not be used to guide therapy.

Historically mortality rates for older adults with ARDs (69% to 80%) were higher than for younger adults. More recently, older adults have not been shown to have significantly higher mortality rates from ARDs unless they have underlying renal, cardiac, and/or neurological disease.

Normal pulmonary volumes and capacities are depicted in Figure 3-5. **Total lung capacity** (TLC) is the maximum volume the lungs can hold. **Tidal volume** (V_T) is the volume of one inhalation/exhalation cycle. **Functional residual capacity** (FRC) is the volume remaining in the lungs after a normal exhalation, whereas inspiratory capacity is the V_T plus the **inspiratory reserve volume** (IRV). IRV is the volume of air one is able to inhale in addition to the V_T. The **residual volume** (RV) is the volume of air that remains in the lungs following forced expiration beyond normal expiration, or the **expiratory reserve volume** (ERV). **Vital capacity** (VC) is the sum of the ERV, V_T, and IRV.

The brainstem controls autonomic respiration, whereas the cerebral cortex controls voluntary ventilatory effort. Central **chemoreceptors** scrutinize the level of the hydrogen ion in the blood, whereas peripheral chemoreceptors monitor oxygen levels as well as carbon dioxide and hydrogen ion levels. The chemoreceptors respond to these changes by stimulating acceleration or slowing of the ventilation rate.

Respiration

Respiration is the process of transporting oxygen (O_2) and carbon dioxide (CO_2) across the alveolar capillary membrane. These gases are transported by the process of diffusion, which causes molecules to move from areas of higher concentration to areas of lower concentration. The elevated concentration of O_2 in the alveoli causes O_2 to diffuse into the capillaries, and the reverse is true for CO_2. This process must occur through the several components of the respiratory membrane (Figure 3-6). Alterations in any of these structures negatively impacts gas exchange.

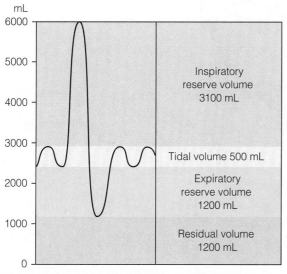
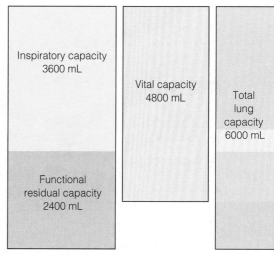

Figure 3-5 Lung volume measurements.

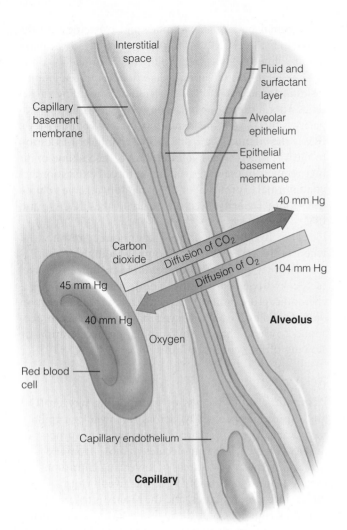

Figure 3-6 Ultrastructure of the respiratory membrane.

Ventilation-Perfusion Relationships

Gas exchange relies on adequate perfusion of the alveoli. Normally, the volume in the conducting airways, such as the trachea and bronchioles, do not participate in gas exchange. This volume is known as anatomical dead space, because these structures are not designed for gas exchange. However, when an alveolus is not perfused, this alveolar cluster is termed an alveolar **dead space unit** because no gas exchange is occurring (Figure 3-7). In dead space units, ventilation exceeds perfusion. Examples include pneumonia or atelectasis. Conversely, when an alveolus is inadequately ventilated in the presence of perfusion, this cluster is referred to as a **shunt unit**. Therefore, in shunt units, perfusion exceeds ventilation, such as with pulmonary embolism or pulmonary infarct. However, when ventilation and perfusion are impaired, the result is a **silent unit**. Silent units occur in severe ARDS or pneumothorax.

Figure 3-7 Ventilation-perfusion relationships. *A,* Normal alveolar-capillary unit with an ideal match of ventilation and blood flow. Maximum gas exchange occurs between the alveolus and blood. *B,* Physiological shunting: A unit with adequate perfusion but inadequate ventilation. *C,* Dead space: A unit with adequate ventilation but inadequate perfusion. In the latter two cases, gas exchange is impaired.

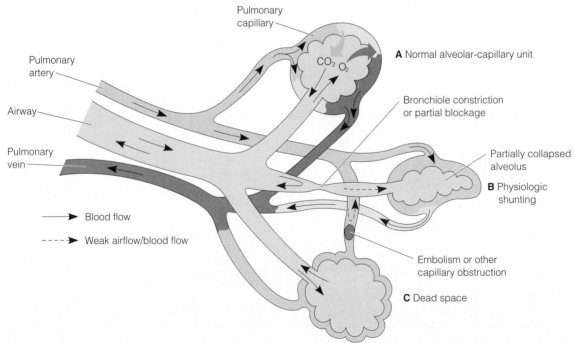

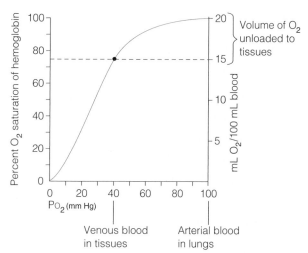

Figure 3-8 Oxygen-hemoglobin dissociation curve. The percent O_2 saturation of hemoglobin and total blood oxygen volume are shown for different oxygen partial pressures (Po_2). Arterial blood in the lungs is almost completely saturated. During one pass through the body, about 25% of hemoglobin-bound oxygen is unloaded to the tissues. Thus, venous blood is still about 75% saturated with oxygen. The steep portion of the curve shows that hemoglobin readily off-loads or on-loads oxygen at Po_2 levels below about 50 mm Hg.

Oxyhemoglobin Dissociation Curve

O_2 is carried in the blood in two ways: about 97% is bound to hemoglobin (Hgb), known as O_2 saturation (SaO_2), and about 3% is dissolved in serum (PaO_2) (Figure 3-8).

The **oxyhemoglobin dissociation curve** depicts the relationship between these two transport methods. A shift in the curve means that the normally predictable affinity of Hgb toward O_2 is altered. This shift means that there is a change in the way O_2 is taken up by the Hgb molecule at the alveolar level as well as a change in the way it is delivered to the tissues. With a shift to the right, there is a decrease in the O_2 saturation for any given PaO_2 (i.e., Hgb has less affinity for O_2). However, this increases O_2 delivery to the tissues (for a brief time) because the hemoglobin Releases the O_2 more Readily.

Factors that shift the curve to the **Right**:

- feveR
- Reduced pH (acidosis)
- hypeRcapnea
- incRease in 2,3 diphosphoglycerate

A shift to the left means there is an increased O_2 saturation for any PaO_2; thus, the delivery of O_2 to the tissues is impaired. In other words, the Hgb hoLds the O_2 to itself.

Factors that shift the curve to the **Left**:

- coLd
- aLkalosis
- Low CO_2
- Low 2,3 diphosphoglycerate

The oxyhemoglobin dissociation curve is clinically important because it helps the clinician understand the client's tissue oxygenation. Further, it reminds the clinician that saturations in excess of 90% do not necessarily guarantee adequate oxygen delivery to the tissues for every patient. It is important to note the steep decrease in PaO_2 once the SaO_2 falls below 90%. These levels of O_2 are unsafe, and the nurse should evaluate the patient closely with the goal of restoring optimal oxygenation as soon as possible. 2,3 Diphosphoglycerate (2,3 DPG) is normally found in red blood cells and increases in response to an acute need for more tissue O_2 (causing the Hgb to release the O_2 more readily). Decreases in 2,3 DPG may be related to septic shock, hypophosphatemia, and blood transfusions from banked blood because some preservatives do not maintain 2, 3 DPG levels (Stacy, 2006a).

Arterial Blood Gases

Arterial blood gases (ABGs) directly measure the pH of the blood, along with the partial pressure of O_2, CO_2, bicarbonate ion, and saturation of Hgb. This information is crucial to adequate treatment of respiratory illness. Interpretation of ABGs is a skill easily mastered with sufficient practice. One should approach ABG with a system for interpretation. One can easily evaluate respiration and acid-base status through this analysis.

Steps for Interpreting Arterial Blood Gases.

Evaluate Oxygenation:

Consider PaO_2 and SaO_2.

Evaluate Acid-Base Status:

Consider pH—Is it alkaline, acidic, or normal?

Consider $PaCO_2$—Is it alkaline, acidic, or normal?

Consider HCO_3—Is it alkaline, acidic, or normal?

Reconsider pH—Has compensation occurred?

EXAMPLE: A client on room air has the following blood gas results:

$$pH = 7.30$$
$$PaCO_2 = 58$$
$$PaO_2 = 95$$
$$HCO_3 = 24$$

In this example, the PaO_2 is greater than 90 and is considered adequate. The pH is less than 7.35 and is thus acidic. The $PaCO_2$ is high, and

Although life saving, endotracheal intubation still presents potential complications, including bronchospasm, laryngeal edema or bleeding from procedural trauma, loss of teeth, and potential infections (pneumonia, sinusitis, or abscess) as well as ulcerations (Stacy, 2006c). In addition, cardiovascular complications can result from prolonged hypoxia during the actual procedure (Charlebois, Earven, Fisher, Lewis, & Merrel, 2005).

Tracheostomy Tubes

Tracheostomy is indicated for long-term mechanical ventilation, and the accepted time frame for performing the procedure is if ventilation time exceeds 2 to 3 weeks (Heffner, 2003). The procedure involves an incision in the neck accessing the trachea and creation of a stoma through which the tracheostomy tube is inserted. The procedure may be done at the bedside or in the operating suite. Advantages of the tracheostomy tube include decreased resistance to airflow and easier secretion clearance, and the patient may resume eating and communication in ways to which they are more accustomed (Heffner, 2003).

The tracheostomy tube is usually constructed of plastic and may have one or two lumens (Figure 3-12). Either type has an inflatable cuff at the distal end of the tube, which is inflated through a pilot balloon. An obturator functions as a stylet to facilitate replacement of the tube should it become dislodged unintentionally. The single lumen provides decreased resistance to airflow, thus allowing the client to breathe with less effort. The double lumen tube consists of an outer cannula that remains in place with a removable inner cannula. This inner cannula is useful in secretion management, as built-up secretions may be removed with the cannula for cleaning or, if disposable, discarded and replaced with a new sterile cannula.

Complications of tracheostomy tubes include infection, bleeding, tube obstruction, and development of fistulas (Stacy, 2006c). Nurses are responsible for providing tracheostomy care according to agency protocol to clean

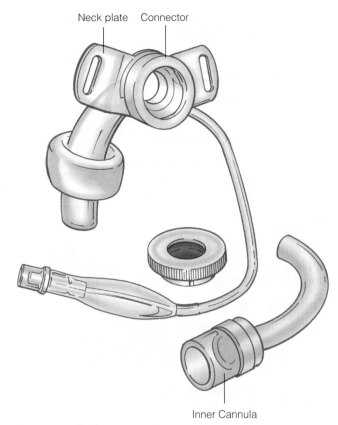

Neck plate   Connector

Inner Cannula

Figure 3-12 Tracheostomy tube.

the stoma and change the dressings or ties as needed. The nurse must remember that the patient will experience a change in body image, and families may struggle to accept this change in the patient's appearance as well. The nurse must assist the family and client to remain positive.

Technological Requirements

Mechanical ventilation is based on four phases of the respiratory cycle: inhalation, switching from inhalation to exhalation, exhalation, and switching from exhalation to inhalation (Table 3–5).

TABLE 3-5

Phases of Mechanical Ventilation

PHASE	VENTILATOR VARIABLE	EXPLANATION
Change from exhalation to inhalation	Trigger	May be flow- or pressure-triggered; inspiratory valve opens and gas begins to flow to patient
Inhalation	Limit/Target	May be related to pressure, flow, or volume; inhalation sustained until target is reached
Change from inhalation to exhalation	Cycle	May be related to pressure, flow, volume, or time; at end of cycle, exhalation valve is opened
Exhalation	Baseline	Exhalation is allowed to a preset level

Source: Adapted from Fenstermacher, D., & Hong, D. (2004). Mechanical ventilation: What have we learned? *Critical Care Nursing Quarterly, 27,* 258–294; Manno, M. S. (2005). Managing mechanical ventilation. *Nursing 2005, 35,* 36–41; and Stacy, K. M. (2006c). Pulmonary therapeutic management. In L. Urden, K. Stacey, & M. Lough (Eds.), *Thelan's critical care nursing.* St. Louis, MO: Mosby.

TABLE 3–6

Settings on Mechanical Ventilators

SETTING	DESCRIPTION	STANDARD RANGE
Oxygen Concentration (FiO_2)	Amount of oxygen in gaseous admixture delivered to client	21% to 100%; desired outcome is SaO_2 over 90%
Tidal Volume (V_T)	Volume of gas delivered in one cycle	10–12 mL/kg If ALI, lung protective levels of 6–8 mL/kg
Rate	Minimal number of breaths per minute	6–20 breaths per minute
Inspiratory: Expiratory Ratio	Ratio of time of inspiration to time of expiration; may be reversed in conditions where lungs are noncompliant	1:2–1:1.5
Flow Rate	Rate at which tidal volume is delivered to client	40–80 liters/minute
Sensitivity	The negative inspiratory pressure or flow a patient must generate in order to trigger the ventilator to deliver a breath	Pressure: 0.5–1.5 cm H_2O below baseline Flow: 1–3 liters/minute below baseline
High Pressure Limit	Ventilator will not exceed this pressure in delivering volume; pop-off mechanism prevents excessive pressure	10–20 cm H_2O above peak inspiratory pressure
Pressure Support	Positive pressure used to decrease client's work of breathing	5–10 cm H_2O
Positive End-Expiratory Pressure (PEEP)	Positive pressure left in lungs at end of expiration; prevents atelectasis and may enhance oxygenation at higher levels	3–5 cm H_2O

Source: Adapted from Fenstermacher, D., & Hong, D. (2004). Mechanical ventilation: What have we learned? *Critical Care Nursing Quarterly, 27,* 258–294; Manno, M. S. (2005). Managing mechanical ventilation. *Nursing 2005, 35,* 36–41; and Stacy, K. M. (2006c). Pulmonary therapeutic management. In L. Urden, K. Stacey, & M. Lough (Eds.), *Thelan's critical care nursing.* St. Louis, MO: Mosby.

Ventilators have a variety of settings with which the nurse must be familiar in order to provide safe, effective care. Table 3–6 summarizes these settings. The first is the fraction of inspired oxygen, or FiO_2. This represents the percentage of O_2 in the mix of air delivered to clients. The FiO_2 of room air is 21% or 0.21. Although commonly expressed as a percentage, FiO_2 is also expressed as a decimal. In room air, nitrogen makes up 78% of air, and numerous other gases comprise the remaining 1%. The nurse should remember that O_2 is a drug and should be titrated by physician order or according to standing orders.

The next setting is the tidal volume, or V_T, which is the volume of gas delivered in one ventilatory cycle. V_T is normally 7 mL/kg of body weight or around 500 mL. In mechanical ventilation, the volume is increased to 8 to 10 mL/kg in order to provide moderate distention without causing trauma. In ALI, volumes are decreased to protect the lungs, to 6 to 8 mL/kg. The rate is the number of breaths the ventilator provides in 1 minute. The mode heavily affects this setting and is discussed momentarily. The client's CO_2 levels also factor into determining the best rate; if elevated, the rate may be elevated to allow the client to "blow off" excess.

The inspiratory:expiratory ratio compares the time spent in inspiration to that in expiration. Normally, a person spends twice as much time in exhalation as in inspiration, so the ratio would be 1:2. In ALI, where the

lungs are "stiff" or noncompliant, the I:E ratio may be reversed in order to allow a slower delivery of the V_T. This more gradual introduction permits the lungs to adjust to the distention while decreasing the risk of barotrauma. Called inverse ratio ventilation, this setting is very uncomfortable for the client, and nurses should ensure the clients are adequately sedated.

The flow rate of the ventilator determines the speed at which the V_T is delivered. Normal rates are 40 to 80 LPM, generally estimating the peak flow at four times the minute volume. Minute volume is determined by totaling the V_{Ts} over 1 minute and is indicative of readiness to wean. When patients are experiencing ventilator dyssynchrony, adjusting the peak flow may increase comfort and improve ventilator tolerance.

Sensitivity determines how much negative pressure the client must generate before the ventilator will deliver a breath. This setting prevents the ventilator from hyperventilating a patient taking very shallow breaths and also helps synchronize the client's intrinsic respiratory rate with mechanical support. This synchrony increases the patient's tolerance of the ventilator.

The high-pressure limit sets a cap on the amount of pressure that can be delivered to the lungs in a breath. If this set amount of pressure is increased, whether by secretions, coughing, or lung compliance, a pop-off valve allows the excess pressure to escape to the atmosphere. This safety setting is very important for protecting the client's lungs from barotrauma. High-pressure alarms should signal the nurse to check the patient to determine if suctioning is needed, whether the patient is biting the tube or has rolled onto it, and to determine if a client is experiencing bronchospasm or mucous plug.

PEEP is just what it sounds like: positive pressure left in the lungs at the end of expiration. This setting usually ranges from 3 to 5 cmH$_2$O, and the pressure helps keep the alveoli open, preventing atelectasis. Higher levels of PEEP, up to 20 cmH$_2$O, can be used to aid in gas exchange. This higher pressure distends the alveolus, providing a greater surface area for gas exchange. Nurses must monitor client blood pressure during increases in PEEP as the increased intrathoracic pressure may cause compression of the vena cava. This compression may decrease right ventricular preload, thus decreasing blood pressure.

Whereas PEEP is at the end of expiration, pressure support occurs at the beginning. To understand PEEP, one might envision blowing up a party balloon and remember how hard it is to do so before the pressure inside the balloon exceeds atmospheric pressure. But once enough air is pushed into the balloon and atmospheric pressure is overcome, the balloon becomes much easier to inflate. The lungs are very similar in that the majority of the work of breathing coincides with moving the ribs and overcoming atmospheric resistance to chest expansion. By providing positive pressure at the beginning of inspiration, the work of breathing decreases, allowing the client to expand the chest more fully while expending less energy. Pressure support is commonly prescribed during the weaning process.

Ventilator Modes

When positive-pressure mechanical ventilation began, microprocessors were not available, and the machines were much bulkier and harder to manipulate. At this time, clients placed on mechanical ventilators were given a set number of breaths at a set volume, no more and no less. It was hoped they would tolerate these settings! Clearly, this was less than optimal patient care, and the controlled mode is extremely rare in critical care at this time.

However, as technology improved, other modes of ventilation (Table 3–7) such as assist control were developed. In this mode, the client regains some control of the rate of breathing. While still receiving a set V_T, the client is able to take additional breaths over the set rate as desired. However, with each breath, the ventilator will deliver the set V_T. One downside of this seemed to be that once it was time to wean a patient, the respiratory muscles had weakened from disuse, prolonging ventilation days.

Therefore, synchronized intermittent mandatory ventilation (SIMV) became available. In this mode, the client again sets the rate independently; however, when breathing in excess of the set rate, the client will only receive the V_T she can pull using her own strength. Now the client is controlling rate as well as volume, but the ventilator serves as a "backup." The client is not allowed

---

TABLE 3–7

Modes of Mechanical Ventilation

MODE	DESCRIPTION	TARGET POPULATION	NURSING IMPLICATIONS
Control Ventilation	Delivers gas at predetermined rate and volume independent of patient effort; rarely used	Apneic patients; neurotrauma patients with no respiratory drive	Patients may be sedated or have induced paralysis
Assist-Control Ventilation (AC)	Delivers gas at a predetermined volume or pressure in response to patient effort; if patient fails to breathe at predetermined time, ventilator will deliver a breath	Patients able to breathe spontaneously with weak respiratory muscles	Patient is able to hyperventilate if volume controlled or may become hypercapneic if pressure controlled
Synchronized Intermittent Mandatory Ventilation (SIMV)	Delivers a preset tidal volume or pressure and rate while allowing spontaneous breaths between; synchronizes with patient effort	Patients who cannot sustain spontaneous ventilation for extended periods	Useful as a weaning mode; increases work of breathing
Continuous Positive Airway Pressure	Applies positive pressure during spontaneous breaths	Effective as a weaning trial or training mode	Patient must be monitored for respiratory distress
Independent Lung Ventilation	Each lung ventilated independently	Patients with unilateral lung disease or fistulas	Requires double-lumen endotracheal tube or two tubes, two ventilators, and sedation
High-Frequency Ventilation	Small volumes of gas delivered at a rapid rate	Useful in patients whose hemodynamic status cannot tolerate conventional ventilation	Requires sedation and/or pharmacological paralysis

Source: Adapted from Manno, M. S. (2005). Managing mechanical ventilation. *Nursing 2005, 35,* 36–41; and Stacy, K. M. (2006c). Pulmonary therapeutic management. In L. Urden, K. Stacey, & M. Lough (Eds.), *Thelan's critical care nursing.* St. Louis, MO: Mosby.

to breathe at less than the set rate, ensuring an adequate minute volume. This feature explains the "intermittent" in the name of the mode. The mode is called synchronized because if the client chooses to initiate a breath when it is almost time for a set volume breath, the ventilator will synchronize with the patient's respiratory effort. This prevents the machine from trying to deliver a breath at the same time a client is trying to exhale.

Continuous positive airway pressure is used as an adjunct to weaning. In this mode, positive pressure is continually applied to the airway. This mode increased functional residual capacity by opening up alveoli. In this mode, the client controls both rate and volume; in other words, the client is essentially breathing on her own. So the modes progress from total control to gradually returning the ability to manage respiratory effort to the client as she is able.

The physician prescribes ventilator settings, but in some facilities, respiratory therapists adjust settings following a physician-approved protocol. Regardless, the health care professional making setting changes should clearly document the alteration in a single, easily accessible location to enhance communication between nurses, respiratory therapists, and physicians.

Weaning Patients from Mechanical Ventilation.
Weaning is the process of determining the patient's readiness to resume spontaneous breathing and concluding mechanical support. The weaning process accounts for up to 40% of the time spent on the ventilator (Manno, 2005). Weaning should not be attempted until the reason for the initiation of ventilation is properly addressed; however, prolonged ventilation is also detrimental to patients (Byrd, Eggleston, Takubo, & Roy, 2006; Tobin, 2001). Numerous indicators are suggested for determining a patient's readiness to wean, including vital capacity, negative inspiratory pressure, hemodynamic status, and the ratio of spontaneous respiratory rate to tidal volume (Manno, 2005). It should be noted that studies indicate that weaning protocols managed by multidisciplinary teams may decrease time on the ventilator (Byrd et al., 2006; Springhouse, 2007).

Physicians currently use four methods to wean patients from mechanical ventilation (Manno, 2005; Tobin, 2001). The first is a spontaneous breathing trial using a T-tube or T-piece. Corrugated tubing is connected to the endotracheal tube perpendicularly (hence, the T), and the patient breathes without any mechanical assistance for increasing time periods. One advantage is the patient is not extubated, and failure to tolerate the procedure does not result in emergent reintubation. This method is favored in patients with weakened respiratory muscles (Manno, 2005).

The second method is using the SIMV mode on the ventilator. This mode allows the client to become increasingly independent as the basal rate decreases. This method is preferred for patients with cardiovascular disease because they adapt to decreases in intrathoracic pressure, and thus increased venous return, more slowly (Manno, 2005). Again, the endotracheal tube remains in place until the patient has demonstrated tolerance of the weaning.

The third method is using continuous positive airway pressure (CPAP) via the ventilator. The patient remains intubated and retains control of the volume and rate of his respirations. The fourth method, pressure support ventilation (PSV), is commonly used in conjunction with CPAP and SIMV (Manno, 2005). The purpose of these methods is to withdraw support gradually, allowing the patient to adapt until minimal assistance is being given, indicating that the patient can breathe unaided. Unfortunately, that optimal level remains undefined empirically (Tobin, 2001).

Complications of Mechanical Ventilation

Mechanical ventilation can cause several complications. The most significant is **ventilator-associated pneumonia (VAP)**, defined as a new lung infection developing within 48 hours of intubation. The mortality rate of VAP ranges from 33% to 50%, and up to 25% of ventilated patients experience VAP (Byrd et al., 2006). Nursing plays an important role in the prevention of VAP; the reader is referred to the discussion of VAP in Chapter 17. ∞ However, nurses may employ specific interventions to assist in prevention of VAP as noted in Table 3–8.

Direct lung injury can result from excessive pressure (barotrauma) or excessive volume (volutrauma). The damage caused to the alveoli by these excesses can result in air leakage into the surrounding structures and may cause subcutaneous emphysema up to pneumothorax or pneumopericardium, both of which are potentially lethal (Chatila & Criner, 2002; Manno, 2005). Measures to prevent these injuries include monitoring V_T and PEEP and being prepared to assist with emergent interventions.

TABLE 3-8

Strategies to Prevent VAP

The key components of the IHI ventilator bundle are:
- Elevation of the head of the bed
- Daily "sedation vacations" and assessment of readiness to extubate
- Peptic ulcer disease prophylaxis
- Deep venous thrombosis prophylaxis

Additional interventions recommended to prevent VAP include:
- Washing hands before and after contact with each patient
- Use of a continuous-suctioning endotracheal tube
- Change of the ventilator circuit no more often than every 48 hours or no longer routinely changing the patient's ventilator circuit
- Preventing oral-tracheal contamination

Another complication of mechanical ventilation is cardiovascular compromise. The presence of positive pressure in the thorax, particularly in the presence of higher levels of PEEP, may decrease venous return, thus decreasing cardiac output. The nurse must monitor cardiac output as well as be vigilant for signs of hepatic or renal dysfunction secondary to decreased blood flow (Manno, 2005). The GI system may also suffer from the positive pressure spilling into the stomach, causing distention and emesis (Manno, 2005), and the stress of ventilation may increase the incidence of ulcer disease (Byrd et al., 2006). Further, side effects of sedation and consequences of immobility facilitate the development of constipation and decreased bowel motility (Chatila & Criner, 2002).

Another common complication is lack of synchrony between the client and the ventilator. This lack of coordination between the perceived need and the function of the ventilator may be caused by anxiety or altered mental status. Working with the respiratory therapist, the nurse may be able to adjust the ventilator settings and alleviate problems such as excessive V_T or insufficient expiratory time. If nonpharmacological emotional support still does not help, the physician may need to order mild sedation to facilitate tolerance of the ventilator (Manno, 2005).

Nursing Care

Caring for the mechanically ventilated client requires the nurse to be vigilant and aware of potential complications. Nurses must also carry out independent nursing interventions designed to minimize time on the ventilator as well as preventing complications. The mechanically ventilated patient requires an interdisciplinary team to maximize outcomes, and the nurse must have full participation on the team. The nurse should ensure that a manual resuscitation bag and alternate O_2 supply is available at the bedside at all times. The bedside stock should contain an adequate supply of suction and oral care supplies.

Routine nursing assessments should include the level of the tube at the patient's lip line, oxygen saturation levels, level of consciousness (or sedation), breath sounds, tolerance of the ventilator, and vital signs. When suctioning or moving the client, the nurse must monitor O_2 saturations and modify activities to ensure adequate oxygenation at all times. The nurse should analyze ABGs (if ordered) and evaluate the adequacy of gas exchange in order to ensure the patient is receiving optimal ventilation and oxygenation. The nurse should verify that the prescribed settings are being delivered via the ventilator, that tubing is free of kinks, and work with respiratory therapists to maintain appropriate temperature of the delivered gas. The nurse should ensure that the ventilator is connected to an emergency electrical outlet, so that if the power fails, the ventilator will receive power from an alternate power source. The Centers for Disease Control and Prevention (CDC) now recommends that ventilator circuits only be changed if they are visibly soiled or malfunctioning, so the nurse should notify the therapist if such concerns arise (Manno, 2005). Sputum should be monitored for color, consistency, odor, and amount, and documentation must reflect these characteristics. The nurse should monitor the mouth or nose for signs of ulceration from tube pressure. Where possible, nurses should also evaluate the daily chest x-ray for tube position and the appearance of potential complications. Common nursing diagnoses are listed in the Nursing Diagnoses feature.

Airway Maintenance

Intubated patients cannot close the glottis, creating an inability to cough effectively (Newmarch, 2006). To facilitate airway patency, the nurse must suction the patient's endotracheal tube to clear secretions as needed. Indications that the patient needs suctioning include adventitious breath sounds, increases in airway pressures, decreased O_2 saturations (Newmarch, 2006), visualization of secretions in the tube, and coughing or gagging. Complications of suctioning include hypoxemia, dysrhythmias, and hemodynamic instability (Demir & Dramali, 2005). Closed suction catheters have not been shown to have an effect on decreasing VAP (Dodek et al., 2004; Zeitoun, de Barros, & Diccini, 2003); however, closed suction catheters are more effective in preventing hypoxia and maintaining PEEP levels (Newmarch, 2006). Using 100% O_2 to preoxygenate the patient before suctioning is a commonly accepted practice; however, in closed suction, no significant changes in SaO_2 and PaO_2 were detected if preoxygenation did not occur (Demir & Dramali, 2005). Instilling normal saline to break up viscous secretions is another debated strategy. The VAP bundle suggests avoiding this practice, and studies have shown that normal saline instillation can prolong the recovery of decreased PaO_2 and SaO_2 values (Akgul & Akyolcu, 2002). Frequency of suctioning should not be on a "routine" basis, but rather driven by patient needs in order to prevent mucosal damage (Blackwood, 1999).

Use of Restraints

Many facilities use protocols to provide care for mechanically ventilated patients, and these protocols frequently include the use of restraints to prevent accidental extubation. Nurses believe they face a choice of "protecting the airway" or restraining a patient when evidence suggests that the opposite is true. The reader is referred to the discussion of physical restraints in Chapter 2. ∞

Communication

One of the most frustrating aspects of caring for a mechanically ventilated patient is the inability to ascertain what the patient is trying to say. Lip reading can be challenging for the most experienced nurse, and the presence of an oral endotracheal tube renders lip reading even more difficult. Patients experience discomfort and frustration when they cannot communicate their needs to staff (Bergbom-Engberg & Haljamae, 1989). Establishing a means of communication is essential to providing good nursing care. A common strategy is blinking eyes (one blink for yes, two for no) or hand squeezes. Once a strategy has been established, it should be communicated among all caregivers to eliminate confusion for the patient. Picture and letter boards can be helpful in decreasing frustration and conserving patient energy. For those patients who are able, providing a pen and clipboard with paper expedites communication. Nurses must always strive to maintain a trusting relationship with the patient, and communication of procedures or interventions before they occur can facilitate this trust (Newmarch, 2006).

Patient and Family Education

Patients and families need to understand why mechanical ventilation is necessary as well as the potential risks of consenting to or refusing the therapy. Explaining why suctioning causes the patient to gag may not make it less uncomfortable, but understanding that it is "normal" may decrease the anxiety. Establishing an emergency stop signal may also be valuable in helping the patient feel some sense of control. Explaining the alarm systems for the ventilator, ECG monitoring, and infusion pumps may decrease anxiety related to the noise for patients and families. Families need to understand that intubated patients are able to hear and why they cannot speak. Many families are afraid to talk to patients, and encouraging them to touch and speak to the patients is very important. If the patient is going home with a tracheostomy, nurses can begin to teach family members tracheostomy care while in the critical care area. Visitation regulations may need to be adapted to allow the family access to the patient and promote psychological health of both the patient and family.

Nutrition

The role of adequate nutrition in critical care cannot be understated. Adequate nutrition facilitates weaning by supporting the hybercarbic and hypoxic ventilatory responses (Newmarch, 2006), and unfed muscles will not work as effectively to help the patient wean. Nurses must again play a role on the multidisciplinary team, and a nutritional consult is an important start to ensuring that the patient receives adequate nutritional support.

The gastrointestinal (GI) tract, if functioning, is the preferred route for providing nutrition to the mechanically ventilated client. The presence of the feeding preserves mucosal integrity, improves intestinal blood flow, and limits complications of sepsis (Raper & Maynard, 1992). Patients can be fed through an NG tube, but the risk of aspiration is increased in gastric feedings. The preferred method is use of a small-bore transpyloric tube that empties into the duodenum. Some facilities limit the role of inserting these tubes to the physician as tracheal intubation or esophageal puncture can result. Radiographic confirmation of the tube's presence in the duodenum should be required before feedings are begun. Nurses can use these tubes to administer medications and must be very aware of what medications can be safely crushed. Nurses should consult with physicians or pharmacists to supply liquid forms of medication when available. Pill form medications must be thoroughly crushed and the tube well flushed after administration.

Numerous nutritional supplements are on the market designed to address compromised organ systems. Protein supplements are also available to meet additional protein

---

SAFETY INITIATIVES   **Prevent Ventilator-Associated Pneumonia**

PURPOSE: To reduce the incidence of postoperative and ventilator-associated pneumonia in hospitalized patients

RATIONALE: "Applying IHIs ventilator bundle in the care of ventilated patients can markedly reduce the incidence of VAP. We have observed an average 45% reduction in the incidence of VAP in a recent ICU collaborative improvement project at IHI. Moreover, there is a trend toward greater success among teams that comply more fully with the terms of the bundle. That is, teams that unfailingly accomplish *every bundle element on every patient every time* have gone months without a single case of pneumonia associated with the ventilator. In the 100,000 Lives Campaign, over 30 hospitals reported more than one year of data with no VAP in their measured population." (IHI Web site)

HIGHLIGHTS OF RECOMMENDATIONS:
The ventilator bundle has four key components:

1. Elevation of the head of the bed to between 30 and 45 degrees
2. Daily "sedative interruption" and daily assessment of readiness to extubate
3. Peptic ulcer disease (PUD) prophylaxis
4. Deep venous thrombosis (DVT) prophylaxis (unless contraindicated)

Source: Institute for Healthcare Improvement
Available: http://www.ihi.org/IHI/Programs/Campaign/VAP.htm

requirements for healing. Feedings may be administered as bolus feedings or continuously. The nurse must monitor the patient's tolerance of the feedings by monitoring for diarrhea, gastric residual as appropriate, and hyperosmolar dehydration. The head of the bed should be elevated to at least 30 degrees during feedings and discontinued during turning or suctioning. If enteral feedings cannot be tolerated, parenteral feedings must be considered.

Acute Lung Injury and Acute Respiratory Distress Syndrome

Acute lung injury (ALI) is defined as a systemic event connected to multiple organ dysfunction syndrome and the syndrome's effect on the pulmonary system (Khadaroo & Marshall, 2002). The American–European Consensus Committee on ARDS established the following criteria to define ALI: The dysfunction must be acute in onset, the client must have bilateral infiltrates on chest radiography, have a ratio of PaO_2 to FiO_2 ″ 300 mm Hg, and PAOP ″ 18 mm Hg. The most deadly form of ALI is acute respiratory distress syndrome (ARDS), delineated by a PaO_2 to FiO_2 ratio of ″ 200 mm Hg (Neff, 2003). Schuster (1995) argues that rather than depending on the PaO_2 to FiO_2 ratio, researchers must use definitions that depend on the diffuse alveolar damage and alterations in gas exchange that are the hallmarks of the syndrome. These diseases have similar pathologic progression and treatment. Incidence of ALI in the United States is higher than in other developed countries and ranges between 17 and 64 per 100,000 person-years, and mortality varies between 34% and 58% (MacCallum & Evans, 2005).

ALI antecedents may be classified as either direct or indirect (Table 3–9). A direct injury represents a

direct assault on pulmonary tissue, whereas an indirect injury results from biochemical mediators resulting from injuries not directly related to the pulmonary system. Sepsis is the most common cause of ARDS, with ARDS developing in 43% of septic patients, and multiple emergency transfusions correlated with development of ARDS in 40% of clients (Hudson, Milberg, Anardi, & Maunder, 1995). ARDS follows aspiration pneumonitis in one third of cases. Other comorbid conditions associated with increased risk of ARDS include alcoholism, cirrhosis, advanced age, diabetes, and cigarette smoking.

Pathophysiology

The initiating sequence of ALI/ARDS is commonly the systemic inflammatory response syndrome or sepsis, and many of the initiating mechanisms of ALI can be traced in that sequence. The progression of events specific to ALI is frequently divided into three stages: exudative, proliferative, and fibrotic. During these stages, a complex series of extreme immune and inflammatory responses damages the alveolar capillary membrane (ACM). This injury results in a cascade of cellular mediators and an amassing of neutrophils, macrophages, and platelets in the damaged ACM. Humoral mediators follow the cellular mediators, resulting in further damage to the ACM. (How this process results in damage to the endothelial and alveolar membranes is further described in Chapter 17 ∞ and displayed in Figure 17-1.)

Disruption of ACM permeability is at the crux of ALI pathophysiology (Figure 3-13). During the first phase, known as the exudative phase, the capillary membrane begins to leak, and protein-rich fluid fills the alveoli, profoundly disrupting gas exchange (Kane & Galanes, 2004). The movement of fluid across the alveolar capillary membrane multiplies 10-fold during the acute phase, which lasts approximately 4 days, and fluid movement remains accelerated for the next 7 days (Kaplan, Calandrino, & Schuster, 1991). This fluid appears on radiography as bilateral infiltrates, but because ALI does not affect left ventricular function directly, pulmonary occlusive pressures stay below 18 mm Hg. As capillary permeability continues to worsen, neutrophils begin to attach to the damaged membrane and may cross into the alveoli, further impairing gas exchange. A key to this stage is the formation of hyaline membranes in the alveoli and conduction airways.

The proliferative phase begins 7 to 10 days after onset and is characterized by the production of type II pneumocytes, macrophage-mediated destruction of hyaline membranes, and resolution of neutrophilic-mediated inflammation (Moss & Ingram, 2001). Type II alveolar cells sustain damage, limiting the production of **surfactant**, resulting in further loss of alveolar function.

TABLE 3–9

Antecedents of ALI

Direct injury:
- Chest trauma
- Pneumonia
- Aspiration of pneumonitis
- Pulmonary contusion
- Near drowning
- Inhalation injury
- Pulmonary embolus
- Radiation
- Eclampsia of pregnancy

Indirect injury:
- Sepsis
- Burns
- Severe trauma with multiple blood transfusions
- Drug overdose
- Cardiopulmonary bypass
- Acute pancreatitis
- Intracranial hypertension
- Drug overdose

Acute respiratory distress syndrome (ARDS) is a severe form of acute respiratory failure that occurs in response to pulmonary or systemic insults. ARDS is characterized by noncardiogenic pulmonary edema caused by inflammatory damage to alveolar and capillary walls. Many disorders may precipitate ARDS, although sepsis is the most common.

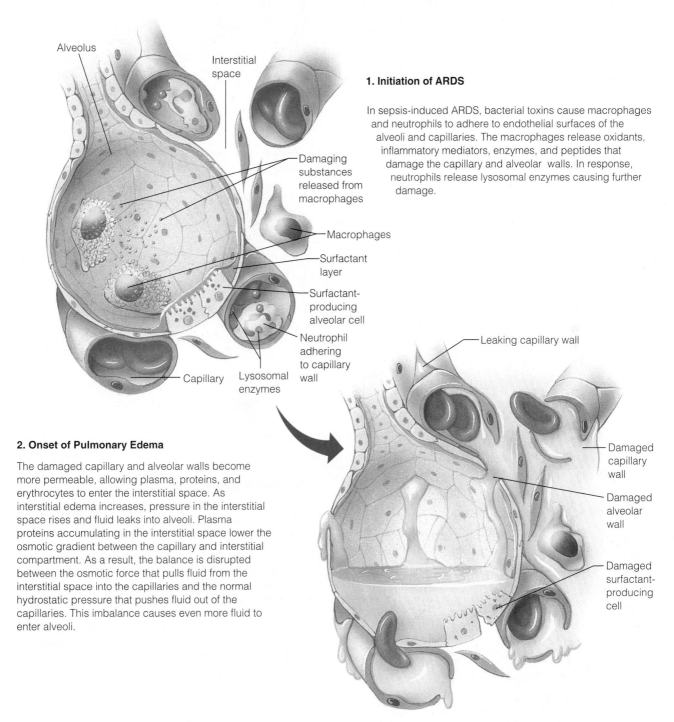

1. Initiation of ARDS

In sepsis-induced ARDS, bacterial toxins cause macrophages and neutrophils to adhere to endothelial surfaces of the alveoli and capillaries. The macrophages release oxidants, inflammatory mediators, enzymes, and peptides that damage the capillary and alveolar walls. In response, neutrophils release lysosomal enzymes causing further damage.

2. Onset of Pulmonary Edema

The damaged capillary and alveolar walls become more permeable, allowing plasma, proteins, and erythrocytes to enter the interstitial space. As interstitial edema increases, pressure in the interstitial space rises and fluid leaks into alveoli. Plasma proteins accumulating in the interstitial space lower the osmotic gradient between the capillary and interstitial compartment. As a result, the balance is disrupted between the osmotic force that pulls fluid from the interstitial space into the capillaries and the normal hydrostatic pressure that pushes fluid out of the capillaries. This imbalance causes even more fluid to enter alveoli.

Figure 3-13 Acute respiratory distress syndrome.

(continued)

4. End-Stage ARDS

Fibrin and cell debris from necrotic cells combine to form hyaline membranes, which line the interior of the alveoli and further reduce alveolar compliance and gas exchange. Because CO_2 cannot diffuse across hyaline membranes, $PaCO_2$ levels now begin to rise while PaO_2 levels continue to fall. Rising $PaCO_2$ levels can lead to respiratory acidosis. Without respiratory support, respiratory failure will develop. Even with aggressive treatment, almost 50% of clients with ARDS die.

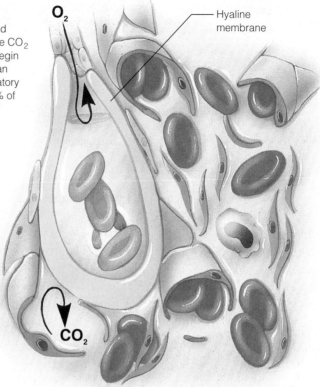

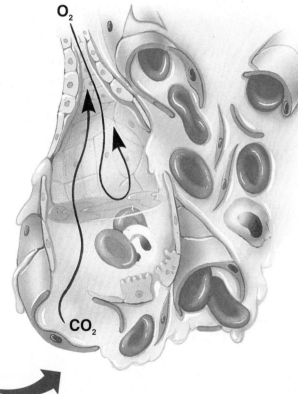

Figure 3-13 (*continued*).

3. Alveolar Collapse

Protein-rich fluid accumulates in the alveoli, inactivating surfactant and damaging type II alveolar cells that produce surfactant. (Surfactant is important in maintaining alveolar compliance—the ability of tissue to stretch or distend.) As active surfactant is lost, the alveoli stiffen and collapse, leading to atelectasis, which increases breathing effort.

Decreased alveolar compliance, atelectasis, and fluid-filled alveoli interfere with gas exchange across the alveolar-capillary membrane. Blood oxygen (PaO_2) levels fall. Because carbon dioxide diffuses more readily than oxygen, however, blood carbon dioxide ($PaCO_2$) levels also fall initially as tachypnea causes more CO_2 to be expired.

TABLE 3-10

Stages of ALI, Associated Pathophysiology, and Assessment Findings

PHASE	PATHOPHYSIOLOGY	ASSESSMENT FINDINGS
Exudative Phase	Capillary membranes leak Protein-rich fluid fills alveoli Gas exchange is disrupted Type I alveolar cells are destroyed Hyaline membranes are formed	Chest x-ray may be normal or show dependent infiltrates Tachypnea and dyspnea Use of accessory muscles but lung sounds may be clear PAWP may be less than 18 mm Hg Change in level of consciousness
Proliferative Phase	Type II alveolar cells are damaged Surfactant production declines Peak inspiratory pressure increases Compliance declines Decreased FRC Further loss of alveolar function Ventilation/perfusion mismatch	Chest x-ray shows diffuse bilateral infiltrates and elevated diaphragm Refractory hypoxemia with hypercarbia despite hyperventilation Dramatically increased WOB Crackles on auscultation PA and PAWP pressures increase RA pressure increases Right-sided heart failure develops Agitation
Fibrotic Phase	Development of fibrotic tissue in the ACM resulting in alveolar disfigurement Decreased lung compliance Worsening pulmonary hypertension Increased dead space ventilation	Leukocytosis and fever Worsening infiltrates on chest x-ray Worsening hypoxemia and hypercarbia Decreased tissue perfusion Increasing heart rate with decreasing blood pressure Lactic acidosis End-organ dysfunction

This decrease in available alveolar surface area results in a ventilation perfusion (VQ) mismatch and hypoxemia. Clients struggle for air due to an increase in the work of breathing, which results from decreases in FRC and lung compliance. Hypoxemia becomes increasingly severe as the increased work of breathing contributes to alveolar hypoventilation. The client also develops pulmonary hypertension due to the structural damage suffered by the alveoli. The resultant increase in right ventricular afterload contributes to right-sided failure. This phase of ARDS may last as long as 1 month.

The final phase is called the fibrotic phase because the altered healing process results in development of fibrotic tissue in the alveolar capillary membrane. The resulting alveolar disfigurement contributes to decreased lung compliance and worsening pulmonary hypertension (Fein & Clallang-Colucci, 2000). Clinical manifestations of this phase include leukocytosis, continuing infiltrates, and fever (Matthay et al., 2003). Not all patients follow this final course, and comorbid factors are a major predictor of outcome (Rocco et al., 2001). The phases of ARDS are correlated with the physical symptoms in Table 3–10.

Client History and Assessment

Due to the severity of the client's illness, the collection of history depends on review of extant records and accounts of significant others. However, an accurate history is crucial in the identification and removal of potential causative factors. Further, the time committed to fully understanding the client may provide quality time with significant others, establishing a basis for a therapeutic relationship during a time of crisis (Van Soeren, 2005).

Initial clinical assessment may reveal a client with tachypnea, tachycardia, and increases in heart rate and respiration that seem incongruent with the remainder of the exam. Such findings should trigger the nurse to perform a detailed assessment for ARDS and notify the physician in order to begin treatment promptly. Additional early symptoms of ARDS include:

- Dyspnea and tachypnea
- Rapid, shallow respiratory pattern
- Use of accessory muscles
- Mottling or cyanosis of skin
- Abnormal breath sounds
- Dry cough
- Change in level of consciousness
- Confusion
- Restlessness
- Retrosternal discomfort
- Tachycardia
- Fever

Diagnostic confirmation will require ABGs and chest radiography but may include a computerized tomography (CT) exam. ABG results confirm hypoxemia and respiratory alkalosis in early phases and may be indicative of the evolution of the disease process (Kane & Galanes, 2004; Laffey et al., 2004). The hypoxemia of ARDs is commonly referred to as **refractory hypoxemia** because the PaO_2 does not respond to increases in FiO_2, responds poorly to standard intervention, and is often disproportionate to radiographic changes (Kane & Galanes, 2004).

Early radiographic results may be normal or reveal some dependent infiltrates, but serial analysis reveals increasingly diffuse bilateral infiltrates. Continuing radiographic exams throughout the course of illness can reveal and document the severity of fibrosis the client suffers (Kane & Galanes, 2004). Inclusion of CT examinations in diagnostic testing for ARDS has been met with increasing favor. In addition to allowing earlier diagnosis, the scans provide the health care team with more detailed information regarding illness severity and response to treatment. Studies have demonstrated distinctions between clients with ARDS resulting from direct versus indirect injury, with indirect injury clients demonstrating more diffuse pulmonary edema (Goodman et al., 1999). The advantages of CT examination must be carefully weighed against the risk to the client of being transported for the study.

Collaborative Management

Despite numerous studies, no effective therapy for treating ARDS at the pathophysiologic level is available. Identification of the precipitating event is a priority and treatment is focused on resolving the symptoms of the disease process, which include impaired gas exchange, inadequate tissue perfusion, and excess fluid volume (Gal & Shaffer, 2002).

Mechanical Ventilation in Acute Lung Injury/Acute Respiratory Distress Syndrome

Intubation and provision of ventilatory support provides the foundation for medical therapy of ALI/ARDS, and the goals of this therapy are to ensure sufficient oxygenation to protect organ function (Moss & Ingram, 2001). Researchers continue to develop new understandings and manipulate the various components of mechanical ventilation to improve outcomes in ARDS.

Oxygenation

Clients with ARDS are suffering from inability to exchange gas. Mechanical ventilation provides additional O_2 to support the failing lungs; however, supplemental O_2 alone will not enhance gas exchange. The nurse should anticipate early intubation and PEEP to reduce intrapulmonary shunting (Conrad, 2005). The prevalent atelectasis in ARDS results from decreased functional surfactant experience. The addition of PEEP will provide

TABLE 3-11

Ventilator Management Goals in ARDS

GOAL	PURPOSE
Tidal volume between 4 and 8 mL/kg	Protects lungs from VILI
Plateau pressure ≤ 30 cm H_2O	Protects lungs from VILI
Keep FiO_2 ≤ 60%	Minimize O_2 toxicity
Utilize PEEP at 5–15 cm H_2O	Recruit alveoli
Permissive hypercapnea ($PaCO_2$ 60–100)	Protects lungs from VILI
Maintain SaO_2 between 88% and 95%	Support tissue oxygenation

Source: Adapted from Kane, C., & Galanes, S. (2004). Adult respiratory distress syndrome. *Critical Care Nursing Quarterly 27*, 325–335.

additional surface area in the alveoli to enhance gas exchange, thus increasing the FRC and may allow the health care team to decrease FiO_2 while maintaining an acceptable SaO_2. Amato et al. (1995) found that setting PEEP at levels between 14 and 16 cm H_2O could return collapsed alveoli to a functional status; however, there is no method for predicting the optimal level of PEEP (Burns, 2005).

Ventilation

Possibly the most daunting challenge of providing adequate ventilation to clients with ARDS is how to achieve that goal without causing injury from the high pressures or large volumes required to inflate the noncompliant lungs, such as stress fractures in the ACM. Prevention of ventilator-induced lung injury (VILI) is a major focus of research at present. The goals of mechanical ventilation during ALI/ARDS are found in Table 3–11.

Lower Tidal Volumes and Permissive Hypercapnea. The ARDS network study (2000) examined the use of lower V_{Ts} to prevent VILI in clients with ARDS and found that V_{Ts} of 4 to 6 mL/kg of body weight reduced mortality as well as decreased days on the ventilator. The lower V_{Ts} result in alveolar hypoventilation, resulting in a rise in serum CO_2 levels. Therefore, hypercapnea is an expected outcome of using lower V_{Ts} or pressures, and permissive hypercapnea is a deliberate exchange to protect lungs from VILI as opposed to maintaining normal $PaCO_2$ levels. However, CO_2 levels must be allowed to rise slowly and the pH maintained with bicarbonate administration (Stacy, 2006b). Hypercapnea has been associated with alterations in neurological status, alterations in cardiac and vascular status, and some studies have linked hypercapnea to impaired gas exchange (Feihl et al., 2000) and the distribution of blood flow (Hickling & Joyce, 1995). However, one study in rats found that early induction of hypercapneic acidosis actually protected the lungs against endotoxin-induced injury (Laffey et al., 2004). Hypercapnea is contraindicated in clients with increased intracranial pressure and hypoxia that is not corrected, and it should be used with caution in clients with renal impairment or metabolic acidosis. Despite conflicting results from these studies, Burns (2005) identifies low-volume ventilation as a preferred protective lung strategy.

Another lung protective strategy considered for use is **inverse ratio ventilation (IRV)**. Normally, inspiration takes less time in one breath than does expiration, and the normal inspiration:expiration ratio is 1:1–1:2. In IRV, this ratio is reversed so that inspiration takes more time than expiration. Conceptually, this should allow the lungs more time to adapt to the increasing airway pressure required for the breath, thus protecting the lungs. Conflicting study results led Marini (2006) to conclude that IRV does not offer a benefit to clients over standard practice.

Alternative Modes of Ventilation

Pressure mode ventilation focuses on protecting the lungs from VILI by monitoring ventilatory pressures rather than volumes. Pressure ventilation is heavily affected by lung compliance (Burns, 2005) and instinctually seems very attractive in protecting the lungs from injurious levels of pressure. The obvious downside is that if pressures are restricted by the ventilator, V_{Ts} will be sacrificed to maintain pressure limits, may change unpredictably, and may be widely variable. However, insufficient studies are available to determine if this mode is appropriate for ARDS patients (Burns, 2005).

Another mode of ventilatory support researched for use is **high-frequency oscillation** (HFO). HFO uses very small V_{Ts}, allowing the lungs to retain higher volumes at end expiration. Burns (2005) explains that the oscillator scatters the oxygen into the lung via "augmented dispersion" at high frequency, creating a vibration in the chest. HFO also oscillates the mean airway pressure at a higher mean than conventional ventilation is able (Derdak et al., 2002). One randomized clinical trial found a nonsignificant decrease in mortality in clients with ARDS receiving HFO after 30 days (Derdak et al., 2002) but other lung protective strategies were not used. Mentzelopoulos et al. (2007) recently reported HFO in conjunction with tracheal gas insufflation, which Epstein (2002) defines as continuous flow of O_2 throughout the ventilatory cycle, and found that oxygenation could be improved. However, nurses must be aware that clients generally require significant sedative and paralytic agents to allow them to tolerate the intervention (Burns, 2005). Further, this mode alters lung sounds, making assessment for nurses challenging.

Partial liquid ventilation (PLV) is another mode being studied to determine efficacy in ARDS. In this mode, the lungs are filled with 5 to 30 mL/kg of perfluorocarbon, which is a clear, odorless liquid with very low surface tension. When inserted, the perfluorocarbon goes to the dependent portion of the lungs, thus redistributing air into more adequately perfused alveoli while also recruiting the alveoli in the dependent areas of the lung (Seetharamaiah, Tredici, & Hirschl, 2006). One study found no significant difference in mortality between PLV and control groups (Hirschl et al., 2002). Kacmarek et al. (2006) found that adult experimental groups with PLV had higher mortality, more pneumothoraces, and more hypotensive episodes than control, and they concluded that evidence does not support PLV in adults with ARDS.

Pharmacological Support

A number of trials are in progress to test pharmacological intervention for clients with ARDS. These include anti-inflammatories, vasodilators, agents to decrease alveolar surface tension, and inhibition of inflammatory cytokines.

Anti-inflammatories

The anti-inflammatory properties of corticosteroids seemed a logical solution to the cytokine-mediated inflammatory response in ARDS, and studies investigating corticosteroids have been ongoing since the 1980s. Sadly, the most recent results from the Late Steroid Rescue Study do not support the use of methylprednisolone in late ARDS (Steinberg et al., 2006). Prostaglandin seemed to be another logical agent as it also combats inflammation; however, a randomized multicenter study was unable to document efficacy from this agent, and, further, the clients suffered from hypotension. Studies have not been able to provide evidence of survival benefit or decreased ventilator time.

Vasodilators

One of the vasodilators investigated in ARDS is inhaled nitric oxide. Nitric oxide is produced in the lungs and relaxes pulmonary vascular smooth muscle, therefore playing a role in ventilation perfusion ratios. Rossaint et al. (1993) demonstrated that inhaled nitric oxide reduced pulmonary artery pressures and improved oxygenation without concurrent hypotension. Despite several studies, the most recent by Gerlach et al. in 2003, no improvement in survival has been documented. Unfavorable effects of inhaled nitric oxide include increases in pulmonary edema and methemoglobinemia (Jain & DalNogare, 2006).

Surfactant and β-Agonists

Surfactant therapy is delivered in one of three ways: via the endotracheal tube, bronchial installation during bronchoscopy, or aerosolized via the ventilator circuit (Stacy, 2006b). Although the use of exogenous surfactant is supported in neonates, benefit to adult clients has not been supported (Anzueto, 2002). Better results have been obtained in the β-Agonist Lung Injury Trial (BALTI). Intravenous salbutamol was infused into clients with ARDS over 7 days, and the experimental group had significantly lower plateau airway pressures as well as less lung water (Perkins, McAuley, Thickett, & Gao, 2006). However, it must be noted that the experimental group also had more supraventricular arrhythmias.

Cytokine Inhibitors

Lisofylline is a xanthine derivative known to inhibit release of cell-mediated free fatty acids (Jain & DalNogare, 2006). It is these free fatty acids that convert into proinflammatory mediators. Lisofylline seemed to be a good choice for limiting cytokines, but the ARDS Network study on lisofylline was stopped after 28 days as designated outcomes were not being met, and there was increased mortality in the experimental group (ARDS Clinical Trials Network, 2002). The ARDS Network also investigated ketoconazole, which inhibits thromboxane. Thromboxane is known to increase capillary permeability and platelet aggregation, providing reasonable belief that the agent could contribute to positive outcomes in ARDS. However, the study showed no difference in gas exchange, number of days on the ventilator, or mortality (ARDS Network, 2000).

Fluid Management

Managing fluids in the ARDS patient remains an area of controversy as well. The conundrum revolves around maintaining sufficient preload to maintain tissue perfusion as opposed to drying out pulmonary tissue to reduce interstitial and alveolar edema (Taylor, 2005). An ARDS Network study (2006) found that while mortality remained the same between groups, conservative fluid management improved lung function and decreased days on the ventilator and in ICU (NHLBI ARDS Clinical Trials Network, 2006). For fluid resuscitation, no difference between crystalloids and colloids was documented relative to mortality, length of stay, or organ failure (SAFE Study Investigators, 2004). Therefore, fluids should be managed conservatively as research continues.

Nursing Management

Nursing care of clients with ALI/ARDS is supportive of the medical goals of maintaining tissue perfusion and protecting the lungs from injury. Vollman (2007) suggests the six Ps of ARDS treatment: prevention, PEEP, pump, pipes, paralysis, and position. Pump and pipes (i.e., fluid management) and PEEP are discussed in the previous section.

Prevention

As always, prevention is the ideal treatment method for any syndrome. Fundamental nursing actions such as hand washing play a pivotal role in preventing the spread of pathogens (Potter & Perry, 2005). Attention to line care and oral care and keeping the head of the bed in the proper position all contribute to prevention of nosocomial infections. VAP is a major risk occurring in 22.8%

TABLE 3–12

Activities That Increase Oxygen Consumption

ACTIVITY	PERCENT INCREASE IN VO$_2$
Dressing change	10
Physical exam	20
Bath	23
Chest x-ray	25
Suctioning	27
Increased work of breathing	40
Position change	31
Linen change—occupied bed	22

Source: Adapted from Vollman, K. M. (2007, May). *ARDS care: Prevention, PEEP, pipes, pump, paralysis, & position.*

of mechanically ventilated patients (Safdar, Dezfulian, Collard, & Saint, 2005), and VAP comprises 80% of nosocomial pneumonias (Richards, Edwards, Culver, & Gaynes, 1999). A more detailed discussion of VAP can be found in Chapter 17. ∞

Paralysis

The purpose of paralysis or sedation in the client with ARDS is to minimize O$_2$ demand, thereby minimizing O$_2$ debt. Table 3–12 lists the impact of various activities on O$_2$ consumption.

To minimize these effects, sedation is a standard of care. Commonly used agents include propofol, fentanyl, and midazolam. A more detailed discussion of sedation can be found in Chapter 2. ∞ However, the negative effects of paralysis, such as continued neuromuscular weakness, have been linked to both increased ventilator time and length of stay (LOS). Overall, Amato and Marini (2006) suggested that deep sedation combined with short-acting sedatives is superior to paralysis. The importance of daily sedation vacations is also documented, not only for neurological assessment, but researchers found a decrease in length of time on the ventilator as well as decreases in length of stay (Kress, Pohlman, O'Connor, & Hall, 2000). It is worth noting that a sedation protocol managed by nurses can reduce the length of time on the ventilator as well (Brook et al., 1999).

Positioning

Prone positioning in ARDS patients is a case study in the lag between evidence production and practice implementation. The first publication supporting prone positioning came out in 1976 (Piehl & Brown, 1976), but implementation remains limited (Essat, 2005) as studies are still not considered definitive (Broccard, 2003). The theory behind the intervention is that the majority of alveolar-capillary units are positioned posteriorly and dependently.

Placing the patient face down assists with redistributing blood flow to less damaged areas of the lung, improving O_2 delivery (Breiburg, Aitken, Reaby, Clancy, & Pierce, 2000). Prone positioning is most effective when utilized early in the disorder (Rance, 2005). Patients must be evaluated carefully prior to implementation as this position is contraindicated in clients with large abdomens (including pregnant women), head injuries, seizures, open abdominal wounds, and hemodynamic instability (Essat, 2005).

Practically, the procedure is deemed a success if the client's PaO_2 rises 10 mm Hg within 30 minutes of being turned. The ideal length of time for the position is not yet established. Before turning, the client's eyes are lubricated and secured, and great attention is given to the security of all lines and drains. A team is required to implement the protocol to ensure client safety (Stacy, 2006c). Figure 3-14 displays a ventilated patient in the prone position.

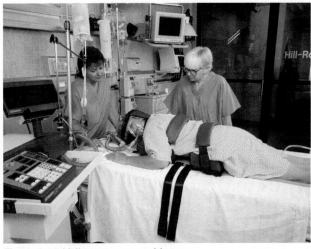

Figure 3-14 Vollman prone positioner.
(Copyright 2008 Hill-Rom Services, Inc.)

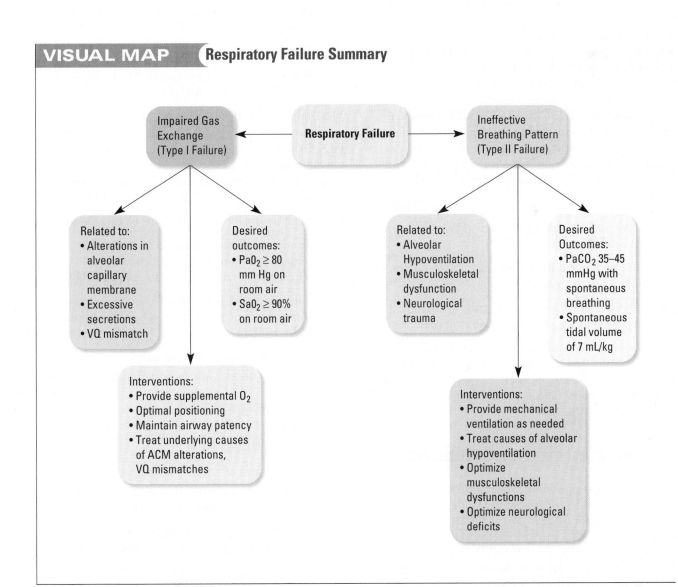

VISUAL MAP **Respiratory Failure Summary**

Impaired Gas Exchange (Type I Failure) ← Respiratory Failure → Ineffective Breathing Pattern (Type II Failure)

Related to:
• Alterations in alveolar capillary membrane
• Excessive secretions
• VQ mismatch

Desired outcomes:
• $PaO_2 \geq 80$ mm Hg on room air
• $SaO_2 \geq 90\%$ on room air

Interventions:
• Provide supplemental O_2
• Optimal positioning
• Maintain airway patency
• Treat underlying causes of ACM alterations, VQ mismatches

Related to:
• Alveolar Hypoventilation
• Musculoskeletal dysfunction
• Neurological trauma

Desired Outcomes:
• $PaCO_2$ 35–45 mmHg with spontaneous breathing
• Spontaneous tidal volume of 7 mL/kg

Interventions:
• Provide mechanical ventilation as needed
• Treat causes of alveolar hypoventilation
• Optimize musculoskeletal dysfunctions
• Optimize neurological deficits

RESPIRATORY FAILURE SUMMARY

Caring for clients with ALI provides a significant challenge for the health care team. The paucity of effective medical or nursing treatment for ALI is frustrating to the team and families of the client. However, the array of supportive modalities, such as mechanical ventilation, requires skilled nursing care and the constant application of critical thinking. Health care researchers, including nurses, continue to research interventions that will optimize the care of clients with ALI. The needs of these clients and their families require the entire health care team, including spiritual caregivers. The nurse functions as the coordinator for this team and ensures the provision of holistic, optimal care to clients with ALI. The care these patients require is summarized in the concept map.

CASE STUDY

Mark Donnelly is a 54-year-old patient admitted 2 days ago in severe DTs. Immediately prior to his admission, he vomited, had a seizure, and probably aspirated. His previous medical history includes: hypertension, COPD, and an MI treated with angioplasty and a stent. According to his wife, he was taking Toprol and Lipitor regularly prior to admission and has smoked a pack a day for the past 30 years. He had been drinking a fifth of vodka daily until 3 days prior to admission when he stopped completely. He was 5' 11" and weighed approximately 180 pounds. On arrival in the ED, his blood pressure was 193/124 with a heart rate of 150. He was tremulous, nauseated, and agitated. Lorazepam was started according to CIWA protocol but he began to vomit and had several seizures. He was sedated with propofol and Zemuron, emergently intubated, ventilated, and transferred to the ICU. On arrival in the ICU, his blood pressure was 80/52.

1. What probably caused his blood pressure to drop?

2. What strategies should the nurse institute immediately to prevent VAP?

3. Will his current BP impact the implementation of any of the strategies?

4. Would his DTs and mental status impact the implementation of any of these strategies?

During the initial assessment on his second day of hospitalization, his ET tube was noted to be 24 cm at the lips. His nurse heard crackles and rhonchi in the bases, especially on the right. His chest x-ray showed that his ET tube was approximately 5 cm above the carina. He had infiltrates and a consolidation on the right with an elevated diaphragm. The nurse suctioned him for copious amounts of very pale yellow secretions.

5. What, if any inferences can the nurse draw from these assessment findings and the results of the chest x-ray?

6. What should the nurse do about these?

7. What factors could predispose Mr. Donnelly to the development of ARDS?

Mr. Donnelly was being mechanically ventilated. On ventilator settings of SIMV rate 14, tidal volume 600, FiO_2 50%, PEEP 8, his respiratory rate was 15, he was maintaining an oxygen saturation of 94%, and his peak inspiratory pressures were 22 to 28. His ABGs revealed pH 7.42, PaO_2 96, $PaCO_2$ 48, and HCO_3 29.

8. What information, if any, do his blood gases reveal?

9. Are the ventilator settings in line with recommendations for patients who might potentially develop or have developed ARDS?

10. If his ventilator is set for 14 breaths per minute with a mode of SIMV, how is he able to breathe at a rate of 15?

11. Why is this useful for a patient?

See answers to Case Studies in the Answer Section at the back of the book.

CRITICAL THINKING QUESTIONS

1. What conditions may cause ALI/ARDS? Why can so many different conditions result in the development of ALI/ARDS?

2. How does ALI/ARDS progress?

3. What are the early manifestations of ALI/ARDS? What is the hallmark of ARDS?

4. What factors are associated with increased mortality for patients with ARDS?

5. What does the evidence suggest are the best ventilator settings for patients with ARDS? Why?

6. What are three nursing priorities when caring for the ventilated patient with ARDS?

7. Explain the following ventilator settings:
   a. Oxygen concentration (FiO_2)
   b. Tidal volume
   c. Rate
   d. Inspiratory:expiratory ratio
   e. High-pressure limit

f. Pressure support
g. Positive end-expiratory pressure (PEEP)

See answers to Critical Thinking Questions in the Answer Section at the back of the book.

EXPLORE MEDIALINK
http://www.prenhall.com/perrin

Additional interactive resources for this chapter can be found on the Web site at http://www.prenhall.com/perrin. Click on "Chapter 3" to select activities for this chapter.

Case Study: ARDS

Nursing Care Plan

NCLEX Review Questions

MediaLinks:
- American Family Physician: Acute Respiratory Distress Syndrome
- American Journal of Respiratory and Critical Care Medicine: Acute Respiratory Distress Syndrome: A historical perspective
- American Lung Association: Adult (Acute) Respiratory Distress Syndrome Fact Sheet

- Clinical Trials for ARDS
- Critical Care Medicine Tutorials: Mechanical Ventilation in Critical Care
- National Heart Lung and Blood Institute: Diseases and Conditions Index: ARDS
- NHLBI ARDS Network
- VentWorld: What Is a Ventilator?

MediaLink Applications

REFERENCES

AHCPR. (1996). *Hospital inpatient statistics.* Healthcare Cost and Utilization Project HCUP Research Note, Publication No. 99-0034. Rockville, MD: Author.

Akgul, S., & Akyolcu, N. (2002). Effects of normal saline on endotracheal suctioning. *Journal of Clinical Nursing, 11,* 826–830.

Amanullah, S., Golbin, J. M., Theodoris, A. C., Lowenstein, S. J., Rogers, M. R., & Lessnan, K. D. (2003). The alveolar-arterial O_2 gradient as perceived by hospital-based health care professionals: A survey of 100 individuals. *Chest, 124,* 86S.

Amato, M. B. P., Basbas, C. S. V., Medeiros, D. M., Schettino, G. P., Lorenzi, F. G., Kairalla, R. A., et al. (1995). Beneficial effects of the "open lung approach" with low distending pressures in acute respiratory distress syndrome. *American Journal of Respiratory and Critical Care Medicine, 152,* 1835–1846.

Amato, M. B. P., & Marini, J. J. (2006). Pressure-controlled and inverse-ratio ventilation. In M. J. Tobin (Ed.), *Principles and practice of mechanical ventilation* (2nd ed.). New York: McGraw-Hill.

Ambrosino, N. (1996). Noninvasive mechanical ventilation in acute respiratory failure. *European Respiratory Journal, 9,* 795–807.

Anzueto, A. (2002). Surfactant supplementation in the lung. *Respiratory Care Clinics of North America, 8,* 211–236.

ARDS Clinical Trials Network, National Heart, Lung, and Blood Institute, National Institutes of Health. (2002). Randomized, placebo-controlled trial of lisofylline for early treatment of acute lung injury and acute respiratory distress syndrome. *Critical Care Medicine, 30,* 1–6.

ARDS Network. (2000). Ketoconazole for the early treatment of acute lung injury and acute respiratory distress syndrome. *Journal of the American Medical Association, 283,* 1995–2002.

Augustyn, B. (2007). Ventilator-associated pneumonia: Risk factors and prevention. *Critical Care Nurse, 27*(4), 32–39.

Bergbom-Engberg, I., & Haljamae, H. (1989). Assessment of patients' experience of discomforts during respirator therapy. *Critical Care Medicine, 17,* 1068–1072.

Blackwood, B. (1999). Normal saline installation with endotracheal suctioning: Primum non nocere (first do no harm). *Journal of Advanced Nursing, 29,* 928–934.

Breiburg, A. N., Aitken, L., Reaby, L., Clancy, R. L., & Pierce, J. D. (2000). Efficacy and safety of prone positioning for patients with acute respiratory distress

syndrome. *Journal of Advanced Nursing, 32,* 922–929.

Broccard, A. (2003). Prone position in ARDS: Are we looking at a half-empty or half-full glass? *Chest, 123,* 1334–1336.

Brook, A. D., Ahrens, T. S., Schaiff, R., Prentice, D., Sherman, G., Shannon, W., et al. (1999). Effect of a nursing-implemented sedation protocol on the duration of mechanical ventilation. *Critical Care Medicine, 27,* 2609–2615.

Burns, S. M. (2005). Mechanical ventilation of patients with acute respiratory distress syndrome and patients requiring weaning. *Critical Care Nurse, 25*(4), 14–23.

Byrd, R. P., Eggleston, D. L., Takubo, T., & Roy, T. M. (2006). *Ventilation, mechanical.* Retrieved July 16, 2007, from http://www.emedicine.com/med/topic3370.htm

Charlebois, D. L., Earven, S. S., Fisher, C. A., Lewis, R., & Merrel, P. K. (2005). Patient management: Respiratory system. In P. G. Morton, D. Fontaine, C. M. Hudak, & B. M. Gallo (Eds.), *Critical care nursing: A holistic approach* (8th ed.). Philadelphia: Lippincott, Williams & Wilkins.

Chatila, W. M., & Criner, G. J. (2002). Complications of long-term mechanical ventilation. *Respiratory Care Clinics of North America, 8,* 631–647.

Christie, H. A., & Goldstein, L. S. (2003). *Respiratory failure and the need for ventilatory support.* In R. L. Wilkins, J. K. Stoller, & C. L. Scanlan (Eds.), *Egan's fundamentals of respiratory care* (8th ed.). St. Louis, MO: Mosby.

Conrad, S. A. (2005). *Respiratory distress syndrome, adult.* Retrieved September 15, 2007, from http://www.emedicine.com/EMERG/topic503.htm

Demir, F., & Dramali, A. (2005). Requirement for 1005 oxygen before and after closed suction. *Journal of Advanced Nursing, 51,* 245–251.

Derdak, S., Mehta, S., Stewart, T. E., Smith, T., Rogers, M., Buchman, T. G., et al. and the Multicenter Oscillatory Ventilations for Acute Respiratory Distress Syndrome Trial (MOAT) Study investigators. (2002). High-frequency oscillatory ventilation for acute respiratory distress syndrome in adults: A randomized, controlled trial. *American Journal of Respiratory and Critical Care Medicine, 166,* 801–808.

Des Jardin, T., & Burton, G. (2002). *Clinical manifestations and assessment of respiratory disease* (4th ed.). St. Louis, MO: Mosby.

Dodek, P., Keenan, S., Cook, D., Heyland, D., Jacka, M., Hand, L., et al. (2004). Evidence-based clinical practice guideline for the prevention of ventilator-associated pneumonia. *Annals of Internal Medicine, 141,* 305–313.

Drummond, J. (2004). Non-invasive mechanical ventilation (NIMV) for exacerbation of COPD. *Canadian Journal of Respiratory Therapy, 1,* 22–25.

Epstein, S. K. (2002). TGIF: Tracheal gas insufflation: For whom? *Chest, 122,* 1515–1517.

Essat, Z. (2005). Prone positioning in patients with acute respiratory distress syndrome. *Nursing Standards, 20,* 52–55.

Feihl, F., Eckert, P., Brimioulle, S., Jacobs, O., Schaller, M., Melot, C. H., et al. (2000). Permissive hypercapnea impairs pulmonary gas exchange in the acute respiratory distress syndrome. *American Journal of Respiratory and Critical Care Medicine, 162,* 209–215.

Fein, A. M., & Clallang-Colucci, M. G. (2000). Acute lung injury and acute respiratory distress syndrome in sepsis and septic shock. *Critical Care Clinics, 16,* 289–317.

Fenstermacher, D., & Hong, D. (2004). Mechanical ventilation: What have we learned? *Critical Care Nursing Quarterly, 27,* 258–294.

Gal, P., & Shaffer, C. L. (2002). Acute respiratory distress syndrome. In J. T. DiPiro, R. L. Talbert, G. C. Yee, G. R. Matzke, B. G. Wells, & L. M. Posey (Eds.), *Pharmacotherapy: A pathophysiologic approach* (5th ed., p. 539). New York: McGraw-Hill.

Garpestad, E., & Hill, N. (2005). Noninvasive ventilation for acute respiratory failure: But how severe? *Chest, 128,* 3790–3791.

Gerlach, H., Keh, D., Semmerow, A., Busch, T., Lewandowski, K., Pappert, D. M., et al. (2003). Dose-response characteristics during long-term inhalation of nitric oxide in patients with severe acute respiratory distress syndrome: A prospective, randomized controlled study. *American Journal of Respiratory and Critical Care Medicine, 167,* 1008–1015.

Goodman, L. R., Fumagalli, R., Tagliabue, P., Tagliabue, M., Ferrario, M., Gattinoni, L., et al. (1999). Adult respiratory distress syndrome due to pulmonary and extrapulmonary causes: CT, clinical and functional correlations. *Radiology, 213,* 545–552.

Guyton, A. C., & Hall, J. E. (2000). *Textbook of medical physiology* (10th ed.). Philadelphia: W. B. Saunders.

Heffner, J. E. (2003). Tracheotomy application and timing. *Clinics in Chest Medicine, 24,* 389–398.

Hess, D. R. (1999). Indications for translaryngeal intubation. *Respiratory Care, 44,* 604–609.

Hickling, K. G., & Joyce, C. (1995). Permissive hypercapnea in ARDS and its effect on tissue oxygenation. *Acta Anaesthesiologica Scandinavica, 107,* 201–208.

Hirschl, R. B., Croce, M., Gore, D., Wiedemann, H., Davis, K., Zwischenberger, J., et al. (2002). Prospective, randomized controlled pilot study of partial liquid ventilation in adult acute respiratory syndrome. *American Journal of Respiratory and Critical Care Medicine, 165,* 781–787.

Hudson, L., Milberg, J., Anardi, D., & Maunder, R. (1995). Clinical risks for development of the acute respiratory distress syndrome. *American Journal of Respiratory and Critical Care Medicine, 151,* 293–301.

Jain, R., & DalNogare, A. (2006). Pharmacological therapy for acute respiratory distress syndrome. *Mayo Clinic Proceedings, 81,* 205–212.

Kacmarek, R. M., Wiedemann, H. P., Lavin, P. T., Wedel, M. K., Tutuncu, A. S., & Slutsky, A. S. (2006). Partial liquid ventilation in adult patients with acute respiratory distress syndrome. *American Journal of Respiratory and Critical Care Medicine, 173,* 882–889.

Kane, C., & Galanes, S. (2004). Adult respiratory distress syndrome. *Critical Care Nursing Quarterly 27,* 325–335.

Kaplan, J. D., Calandrino, F. S., & Schuster, D. P. (1991). A positron emission tomographic comparison of pulmonary vascular permeability during the adult respiratory distress syndrome and pneumonia. *American Review of Respiratory Diseases, 143,* 150–154.

Khadaroo, R. G., & Marshall, J. C. (2002). ARDS and the multiple organ dysfunction syndrome. Common mechanisms of a common systemic process. *Critical Care Clinics, 18,* 127–141.

Kress, J. P., Pohlman, A. S., O'Connor, M. F., & Hall, J. B. (2000). Daily interruption of sedative infusions in critically ill patients undergoing mechanical ventilation. *New England Journal of Medicine, 342,* 1471–1476.

Kwok, H., McCormack, J., Cece, R., Houtchens, J., & Hill, N. S. (2003). Controlled trial of oronasal versus nasal mask ventilation in the treatment of acute respiratory failure. *Critical Care Medicine, 31,* 468–473.

Laffey, J., Honan, D., Hopkins, N., Hyvelin, J., Boylan, J. F., & McLoughlin, P. (2004). Hypercapneic acidosis attenuates endotoxin-induced acute lung injury. *American Journal of Respiratory and Critical Care Medicine, 169,* 46–56.

Levitan, R., & Ochroch, E. A. (2000). Airway management and direct laryngoscopy: A review and update. *Critical Care Clinics, 16,* 373–388.

Liesching, T., Kwok, H., & Hill, N. S. (2003). Acute applications of noninvasive positive-pressure ventilation. *Chest, 124,* 669–713.

MacCallum, N. S., & Evans, T. W. (2005). Epidemiology of acute lung injury. *Current Opinion in Critical Care, 11*(1), 43–49.

Manno, M. S. (2005). Managing mechanical ventilation. *Nursing 2005, 35,* 36–41.

Marini, J. J. (2006). Mechanical ventilation in the acute respiratory distress syndrome. In M. J. Tobin (Ed.), *Principles and practice of mechanical ventilation* (2nd ed.). New York: McGraw-Hill.

Marshak, A. B., & Scanlan, C. L. (1999). Emergency life support. In R. L. Wilkins, J. K. Stoller, & C. L. Scanlan (Eds.), *Egan's fundamentals of respiratory care* (8th ed.). St. Louis, MO: Mosby.

Matthay, M., Zimmerman, G., Esman, C., Bhattacharya, J., Coller, B., Doerschuk, C. M., et al. (2003). Future research directions in acute lung injury: Summary of a National Heart, Lung, and Blood Institute working group. *American Journal of Respiratory and Critical Care Medicine, 167,* 1027–1035.

Mentzelopoulos, S. D., Roussos, C., Koutsoukou, A., Sourlas, S., Malachias, S., Lachana, A., et al. (2007). Acute effects of combined high-frequency oscillation and tracheal gas insufflation in severe acute respiratory distress syndrome. *Critical Care Medicine, 35,* 1500–1508.

Moss, M., & Ingram, R. H. (Eds.). (2001). Acute respiratory distress syndrome. In *Harrison's Principles of Internal Medicine* (15th ed.). New York: McGraw-Hill.

National Heart, Lung, and Blood Institute Acute Respiratory Distress Syndrome (ARDS) Clinical Trials Network. (2006). Comparison of two fluid-management strategies in acute lung injury. *New England Journal of Medicine, 354,* 2564–2575.

Neff, M. J. (2003). The epidemiology and definition of the acute respiratory distress syndrome. *Respiratory Care Clinics of North America, 20,* 273–282.

Newmarch, C. (2006). Caring for the mechanically ventilated patient: Part one. *Nursing Standard, 20*(17), 55–64.

Perkins, G. D., McAuley, D. F., Thickett, D. R., & Gao, F. (2006). The β-agonist lung injury trial (BALTI): A randomized placebo-controlled clinical trial. *American Journal of Respiratory and Critical Care Medicine, 173,* 281–287.

Piehl, M.A., & Brown, R.S. (1976). Use of extreme position changes in acute respiratory failure. *Critical Care Medicine, 4,* 13–14.

Potter, P. A., & Perry, A. G. (2005). *Fundamentals of nursing* (6th ed.). St. Louis, MO: Mosby.

Rance, M. (2005). Kinetic therapy positively influences oxygenation in patients with ALI/ARDS. *Nursing in Critical Care, 10,* 35–41.

Raper, S., & Maynard, N. (1992). Feeding the critically ill patient. *British Journal of Nursing, 1,* 273–280.

Richards, M. J., Edwards, J. R., Culver, D. H., & Gaynes, R. P. (1999). Nosocomial infections in medical intensive care units in the United States. *Critical Care Medicine, 27,* 887–892.

Rocco, T. R., Reinert, S. E., Cioffi, W., Harrington, D., Buczko, G., & Simms, H. H. (2001). A 9-year, single-institution, retrospective review of death rate and prognostic factors in adult respiratory distress syndrome. *Annals of Surgery, 233,* 414–422.

Rossaint, R., Falke, K. J., Lopez, F., Slama, K., Pison, U., & Zapol, W. M. (1993). Inhaled nitric oxide for the adult respiratory distress syndrome. *New England Journal of Medicine, 328,* 399–405.

Safdar, N., Dezfulian, C., Collard, H. R., & Saint, S. (2005). Clinical and economic consequences of ventilator-associated pneumonia: A systematic review. *American Journal of Respiratory and Critical Care Medicine, 33,* 2184–2193.

SAFE Study Investigators. (2004). A comparison of albumin and saline for fluid resuscitation in the intensive care unit. *New England Journal of Medicine, 350,* 2247–2256.

Schuster, D. P. (1995). What is acute lung injury? What is ARDS? *Chest, 107,* 1721–1726.

Seetharamaiah, R., Tredici, S., & Hirschl, R. B. (2006). Liquid ventilation. In M. J. Tobin (Ed.), *Principles and practice of mechanical ventilation* (2nd ed.). New York: McGraw-Hill.

Smith, S. F., Duell, D. J., & Martin, B. C. (2008). *Clinical nursing skills: Basic to advanced skills* (8th ed.). Upper Saddle River, NJ: Pearson Prentice Hall.

Springhouse. (2007). Respiratory care. In *Best practices: Evidence-based nursing procedures*. Philadelphia: Lippincott, Williams & Wilkins.

Stacy, K. M. (2006a). Pulmonary anatomy and physiology. In L. Urden, K. Stacey, & M. Lough (Eds.), *Thelan's critical care nursing*. St. Louis, MO: Mosby.

Stacy, K. M. (2006b). Pulmonary disorders. In L. Urden, K. Stacey & M. Lough (Eds.), *Thelan's critical care nursing*. St. Louis, MO: Mosby.

Stacy, K. M. (2006c). Pulmonary therapeutic management. In L. Urden, K. Stacey, & M. Lough (Eds.), *Thelan's critical care nursing*. St. Louis, MO: Mosby.

Steinberg, K. P., Hudson, L. D., Goodman, R. B., Hough, C. L., Lanken, P. N., Hyzy, R., et al. (2006). Efficacy and safety of corticosteroids for persistent acute respiratory distress syndrome. *New England Journal of Medicine, 354,* 1671–1684.

Taylor, M. M. (2005). ARDS diagnosis and management: Implications for the critical care nurse. *Dimensions of Critical Care Nursing, 24*(5), 197–207.

The Acute Respiratory Distress Network. (2000). Ventilation with lower tidal volumes as compared with traditional tidal volumes for acute lung injury and the acute respiratory distress syndrome. *New England Journal of Medicine, 342,* 1301–1308.

Tobin, M. J. (2001). Advances in mechanical ventilation. *New England Journal of Medicine, 344,* 1986–1996.

Van Soeren, M. H. (2005). Acute respiratory distress syndrome. In P. G. Morton, D. K. Fontaine, C. M. Hudak, & B. M. Gallo (Eds.), *Critical care nursing: A holistic approach* (8th ed.). Philadelphia: Lippincott, Williams & Wilkins.

Vollman, K. M. (2007, May). ARDS care: Prevention, PEEP, pipes, pump, paralysis, & position. Paper presented at the National Teaching Institute and Critical Care Exposition of the American Association of Critical Care Nurses in Atlanta, GA.

Vollman, K. M., & Aulbach, R. K. (1998). Acute respiratory distress syndrome. In *AACN clinical reference for critical care nursing* (4th ed., pp. 529–564). Philadelphia: Mosby.

Zeitoun, S. S., de Barros, A. L., & Dicini, S. (2003). A prospective, randomized study of ventilator-associated pneumonia in patients using a closed vs. open suction system. *Journal of Clinical Nursing, 12*(4), 484–489.

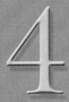

Interpretation and Management of Basic Dysrhythmias

Catherine Fogg PhD(c), RN, ARNP-FNP

Learning Outcomes

Upon completion of this chapter, the learner will be able to:

1. List and briefly describe the four properties of cardiac cells.

2. Explain the normal cardiac conduction system, beginning with the sinus node and ending with the Purkinje fibers.

3. Draw a normal cardiac cycle as seen in normal sinus rhythm and identify the waveforms, intervals, and complexes.

4. List the seven steps of interpreting an ECG rhythm strip.

5. Identify sinus tachycardia and sinus bradycardia on ECG rhythm strips.

6. Identify atrial fibrillation (AF) on an ECG rhythm strip and list some of the treatment measures for AF.

7. Distinguish between second-degree AV block, type I, and second-degree AV block, type II, and complete heart block on an ECG rhythm strip.

8. Discuss three antidysrhythmic medications that can be used for ventricular dysrhythmias.

9. Explain the difference between defibrillation and synchronized cardioversion.

10. Describe the four malfunctions of pacemakers.

Abbreviations

ACLS	Advanced Cardiac Life Support
CHF	Congestive Heart Failure
CPR	Cardiopulmonary Resuscitation
CRT	Cardiac Resynchronization Therapy
ECG, EKG	Electrocardiogram
ICD	Implantable Cardioverter-Defibrillator
RFCA	Radiofrequency Catheter Ablation
TEE	Transesophageal Echocardiogram

MEDIALINK
http://www.prenhall.com/perrin
See the Companion Website for chapter-specific resources at www.prenhall.com/perrin.

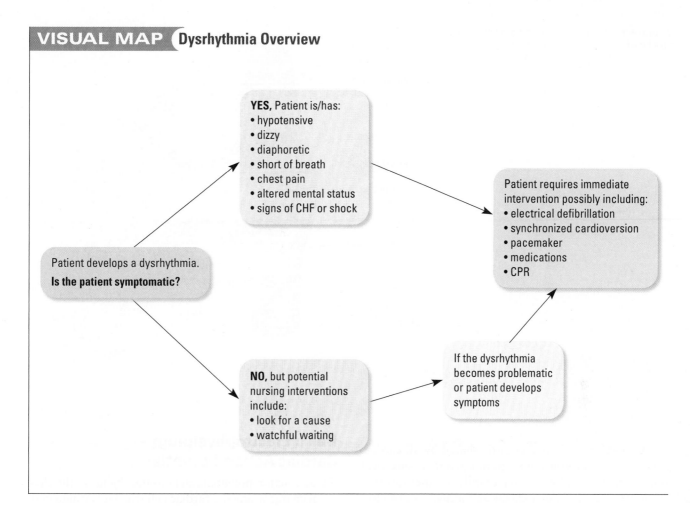

VISUAL MAP Dysrhythmia Overview

Patient develops a dysrhythmia. **Is the patient symptomatic?**

YES, Patient is/has:
• hypotensive
• dizzy
• diaphoretic
• short of breath
• chest pain
• altered mental status
• signs of CHF or shock

NO, but potential nursing interventions include:
• look for a cause
• watchful waiting

If the dysrhythmia becomes problematic or patient develops symptoms

Patient requires immediate intervention possibly including:
• electrical defibrillation
• synchronized cardioversion
• pacemaker
• medications
• CPR

To understand basic cardiac dysrhythmias, an understanding of the electrical activity of the heart and the normal heart rhythm is needed. The cardiac rhythm is usually determined by recording and examining an electrocardiogram, or ECG, strip. Another common abbreviation for electrocardiogram is EKG, which comes from the German word "elektrokardiogramm." A normal heart rhythm, referred to as normal sinus rhythm, is seen on the ECG when an electrical impulse begins at the heart's primary pacemaker, the sinus node or sinoatrial (SA) node, and travels through the heart's electrical conduction system unimpaired at a normal rate and rhythm. If there are disturbances of the cardiac electrical impulse formation or conduction, or both, an abnormal rhythm, or cardiac dysrhythmia, results. The terms "dysrhythmia" and "arrhythmia" are used interchangeably; however, some people prefer to use arrhythmia to refer to the loss of rhythm, as the prefix "a" means "without." Dysrhythmias may be life threatening, markedly altering the cardiac output and causing deterioration in vital signs, or they may be benign, or somewhere in between. To interpret and manage basic dysrhythmias, an understanding of basic cardiac electrophysiology is necessary, including the special properties of cardiac cells, the conduction system, and the electrocardiogram.

Basic Electrophysiology

Cardiac electrophysiology is the study of the electrical properties of the cardiac muscle. These properties ensure that electricity flows through the heart in a regular, measured pattern and results in contraction of the cardiac muscle.

Properties of Cardiac Cells

Specialized cardiac cells have unique characteristics that allow them to regulate heart rate and rhythm. These characteristics include automaticity, excitability, conductivity, and contractility.

Automaticity is the pacing function or ability of cardiac pacemaker cells to spontaneously initiate an electrical impulse. Normally only the primary pacemaker cells, the sinoatrial SA node, the atrioventricular (AV) junction, and the Purkinje fibers possess the characteristic of automaticity. Figure 4-1 depicts the electrical conduction system of the heart.

Under certain conditions, however, such as myocardial infarction (MI), electrolyte imbalances, hypoxia, and drug toxicity, any cardiac cell may exhibit this characteristic and initiate electrical impulses, generating dysrhythmias.

Figure 4-1 The electrical conduction system of the heart.

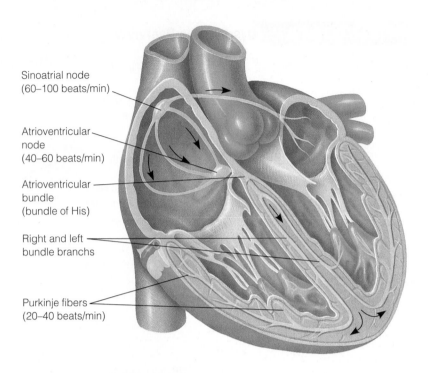

Sinoatrial node
(60–100 beats/min)

Atrioventricular node
(40–60 beats/min)

Atrioventricular bundle
(bundle of His)

Right and left bundle branchs

Purkinje fibers
(20–40 beats/min)

Excitability is a characteristic shared by all cardiac cells that refers to the ability to respond to an electrical impulse generated by pacemaker cells or other external stimulus, such as from a chemical, mechanical, or electrical source, and to depolarize. Depolarization occurs when the cells become electrically excited due to an ionic imbalance across the membrane of the cells.

Conductivity is the ability of the cardiac cells to transmit the electrical impulse to adjacent cardiac cells. This allows an electrical impulse in any part of the myocardium to spread throughout the heart as excitable cells depolarize in rapid succession. The resultant wave of depolarization creates the deflections seen on the ECG. Disturbances in conduction can result in electrical impulses that travel too fast or too slow, that are blocked, or that follow abnormal electrical pathways, generating dysrhythmias.

Contractility is the ability of the cardiac cells to shorten in response to electrical stimulation. Contractility is a mechanical event rather than an electrical event. The wave of depolarization initiates the contraction of the cardiac cells, creating the mechanical activity of the heart and propelling the blood forward. Certain medications, such as digoxin, dopamine, and epinephrine, can help to enhance the contractility of the heart. Conductivity without contractility is a medical emergency known as pulseless electrical activity (PEA) and happens when the electrical activity of the heart can be seen on the ECG; however, the patient does not have a pulse because there is no mechanical activity in response to the electrical stimuli.

Basic Electrophysiology— Cardiac Action Potential

Cardiac action potential refers to the change in the electrical charge inside the cardiac cell when it is stimulated. This electrical change is caused by the flow of specific ions, or electrically charged particles, into and out of the cardiac cell. This electrical change creates a series of events to occur known as polarization, depolarization, and repolarization. Figure 4-2 depicts the action potential of the cardiac cell.

Polarization is the electrical state that exists at the cardiac cell membrane when the cell is at rest. In this state no electrical activity is occurring and the ECG displays a flat, isoelectric line. When the cardiac cell is polarized, the inside of the cell is more negative than the outside of the cell because of the ions found inside it. During the resting state, potassium ions leak out of the cell, leaving the negatively charged ions inside.

Depolarization is the opposite of polarization and occurs when there is a reversal of the electrical charges at the cell membrane. The inside of the cell becomes more positive due to the rapid influx of sodium ions into the cell. On the ECG, the P wave represents atrial depolarization and the QRS complex represents ventricular depolarization. Depolarization is the electrical event that results in a contraction of the cardiac muscle, a mechanical event.

Repolarization is the restoration of the polarized state at the cell membrane. Repolarization can be thought of as the recovery of the cell to its original po-

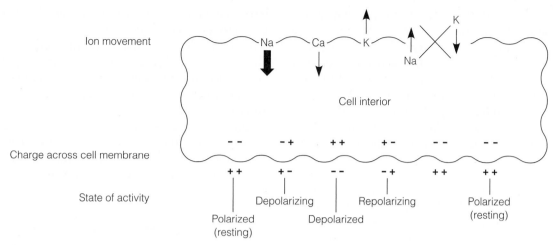

Figure 4-2 The action potential of a cardiac cell.

larized state. After the cell depolarizes, the diffusion of sodium ions into it stops and potassium ions diffuse out, leaving mostly negatively charged ions inside the cell. On the ECG, the ST segment and the T wave represent ventricular repolarization.

Refractory Periods

Refractory is a term that refers to the resistance of the cell membrane to respond to a stimulus. The refractory period extends beyond the length of the cardiac contraction and protects the cardiac muscle from spasm or tetany. There are three refractory periods: the absolute refractory period, the relative refractory period, and the supernormal period. Figure 4-3 depicts where the refractory periods fall in the cardiac cycle.

The **absolute refractory period** is the brief period during depolarization when the cells will not respond to further stimulation, no matter how strong the stimulus. This period corresponds with the onset of the QRS complex to the peak of the T wave.

The **relative refractory period** is also known as the vulnerable period. During this period some cardiac cells have repolarized and if they receive a stronger than normal stimulus they may respond. This response is known as the "R-on-T phenomenon," because it occurs when a stimulus, causing Q"R"S depolarization, lands on the vulnerable downslope of the "T" wave. This phenomenon may cause a life-threatening dysrhythmia known as ventricular fibrillation.

The **supernormal period** comes after the relative refractory period. During this period a weaker than normal stimulus can cause depolarization of cardiac cells. On the ECG, this period corresponds to the end of the T wave. Cardiac dysrhythmias may also occur during this period.

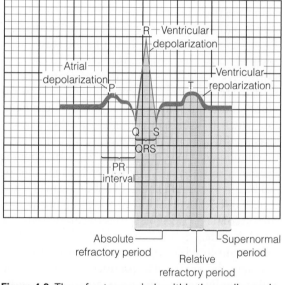

Figure 4-3 The refractory periods within the cardiac cycle.

The Cardiac Conduction System

The cardiac conduction system is composed of the SA node, the AV node, the bundle of His, the left and right branch bundles, and the Purkinje fibers. This system of specialized cardiac cells is responsible for the generation and conduction of electrical impulses that cause atrial and ventricular depolarization (refer to Figure 4-1).

The **sinoatrial (SA) node**, also referred to as the sinus node, is the heart's dominant pacemaker and is located in the upper-posterior wall of the right atrium. The SA node generates stimuli at regular intervals that result in a wave of depolarization. This electrical activity is recognized on the ECG monitor as "Sinus Rhythm." The SA node possesses the greatest degree of automaticity of the cardiac cells and spontaneously generates electrical impulses at a rate of 60 to 100 beats a minute. The wave of depolarization disperses away from the SA node, via slow and fast conduction pathways, in all directions throughout both atria, causing them to contract. The waves of depolarization are created by movement of the positively charged sodium ions into the cardiac cells. This positive charge is seen on the ECG monitor as an upward wave, which represents atrial depolarization. This upward wave is called the P wave. The depolarization of the atria should lead to atrial contraction. This atrial contraction forces blood through the atrioventricular valves (mitral and tricuspid) located between the atria and ventricles.

When the wave of atrial depolarization enters the atrioventricular junction area, the AV node, conduction markedly slows down. The **atrioventricular (AV) node** is located on the posterior wall of the right atrium just behind the tricuspid valve and is the only electrical conduction pathway between the atria and ventricles. The slowed conduction is attributed to the slow-moving calcium ions that carry the electrical stimuli through the AV node. This slowed conduction allows time for the atria to contract and the ventricles to fill with blood and creates an electrical pause on the ECG monitor, which is seen as a flat line after the P wave known as the PR interval. The AV junction, if not electrically stimulated from the SA node, can spontaneously generate electrical impulses at a usual rate of 40 to 60 beats per minute and act as the pacemaker for the heart. This is known as an "escape mechanism" because this secondary pacemaker tries to compensate for the failed SA node.

Conduction speeds up again as the wave of depolarization enters the ventricular conduction system. The ventricular conduction system originates at the **bundle of His**, which penetrates the AV valves, and then bifurcates into the right and left bundle branches to the terminal filaments of the **Purkinje fibers**. The entire ventricular conduction system is composed of Purkinje fibers, which use fast-moving sodium ions for the conduction of depolarization. This allows for rapid depolarization of the ventricles, which is recorded on the ECG monitor as the QRS complex. Ventricular depolarization causes ventricular contraction, sending the blood out of the ventricles into the aorta and pulmonary artery. Occasionally, some of the cells that make up the Purkinje fibers will demonstrate automaticity, initiating an electrical impulse and causing ventricular beats or rhythms. These cells can generate electrical impulses at a rate of 20 to 40 beats a minute. If there are no electrical impulses being generated from the SA or AV nodes, the Purkinje fibers may try to compensate by acting as a tertiary pacemaker.

The Electrocardiogram

The electrocardiogram (ECG) provides a graphic picture of the electrical activity of the heart. The electrical waves of depolarization and repolarization are weakly transmitted to the body surface, where they are picked up by the conductive gel within the electrode pads and transmitted to the ECG machine. Besides monitoring a client's heart rate, the ECG can provide information related to conduction disturbances, electrical impulse disturbances, the presence of myocardial ischemia, and electrical effects of medications and electrolyte imbalances.

The Leads

Most cardiac monitors will show one or two leads, or views, of the heart's electrical activity. The standard ECG provides 12 leads, or separate views of the same myocardial electrical activity. The lead is a graphic picture of the electrical current flowing between two electrodes. The 12 leads are divided into two main types: six limb leads and six chest leads. The limb leads are identified as Leads I, II, III, and $_aV_r$, $_aV_l$, and aV_f. The chest leads are identified by V_1 through V_6. Figure 4-4 shows the leads of the 12-lead ECG.

The limb leads provide a view of the frontal plane of the heart, or the heart viewed from the front of the body. The chest leads provide a view of the horizontal plane of the heart, or the heart viewed in a cross-sectional slice, as if it were sliced in half horizontally. All of the leads are recording the same electrical activity, but the ECG tracing looks different in each lead because the electrical activity is viewed from different positions. The placement of the

Figure 4-4 Leads of the 12-lead ECG.

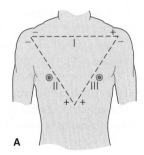

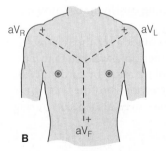

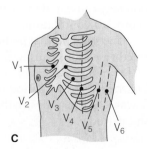

TABLE 4-1

Position of Lead and Heart Surface Viewed

LEAD	POSITION OF POSITIVE ELECTRODE	HEART SURFACE VIEWED
Limb Lead 1	Left arm or under the left clavicle	Lateral
Limb Lead 2	Left leg or lowest rib, left midclavicular line	Inferior
Limb Lead 3	Left leg or lowest rib, left midclavicular line	Inferior
Limb Lead aV_R	Right arm or under the right clavicle	None
Limb Lead aV_L	Left arm or under the left clavicle	Lateral
Limb Lead aV_F	Left leg or lowest rib, left midclavicular line	Inferior
Chest Lead V_1	Right side of sternum, fourth intercostal space	Septum
Chest Lead V_2	Left side of sternum, fourth intercostal space	Septum
Chest Lead V_3	Midway between V_2 and V_4	Anterior
Chest Lead V_4	Left midclavicular line, fifth intercostal space	Anterior
Chest Lead V_5	Left anterior axillary line, horizontal to V_4	Lateral
Chest Lead V_6	Left midaxillary line, horizontal to V_4	Lateral

positive electrode determines the portion of the heart viewed by that lead; in other words, it acts as the camera. Table 4–1 describes where the positive electrode for each lead is placed on the body, and which aspect of the heart is electrically visualized by that lead.

Each lead also has a negative and a grounding electrode, but to emphasize the relationship between the positive electrode and the aspect of the heart that is visualized, only the positive lead is shown in the table.

The ECG Paper

The electrical activity that is viewed from the various leads is recorded on ECG paper. The paper is graph paper made up of small and large boxes, with each small box measuring 1 mm high and 1 mm wide. Each large box has the width and height of 5 mm as shown in Figure 4-5.

The horizontal axis of the paper represents time. ECG monitors all record at a standard speed of 25 mm/sec. At this speed, each small horizontal box represents 0.04 second (25 mm/sec × 0.04 sec = 1 mm). Each large box contains five small boxes, which is equivalent to 0.20 second (5 × 0.04 sec = 0.20 sec). Following this same logic, five large boxes represent 1 second (5 × 0.20 sec = 1 sec). Vertical lines, or hash marks, at the top or bottom of the ECG strip denote 15 large block segments, representing 3-second strips. This information is useful when ECG strips are analyzed to determine the cardiac rate.

The vertical axis of the ECG paper represents voltage or amplitude of the waveforms. The height and depth of a waveform is measured vertically from the baseline in millimeters (mm). The waveform is a deflection either upward or downward from the baseline of the ECG recording. When a wave of depolarization (positive charges) moves toward a positive electrode, this produces a posi-

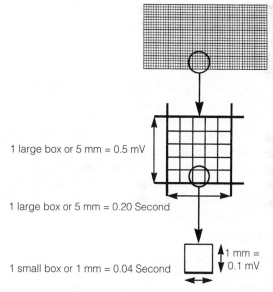

1 large box or 5 mm = 0.5 mV

1 large box or 5 mm = 0.20 Second

1 small box or 1 mm = 0.04 Second

1 mm = 0.1 mV

Figure 4-5 Time and voltage measurements on ECG paper recording at a speed of 25 mm/second.

tive or upward deflection on the ECG. This is a measurement of the wave's voltage. Conversely, when a wave of depolarization moves away from a positive electrode, this produces a negative or downward deflection on the ECG.

ECG Waveforms

A full cardiac cycle of depolarization and repolarization creates particular waveforms on the ECG. The cardiac cycle is composed of waveforms, segments, intervals,

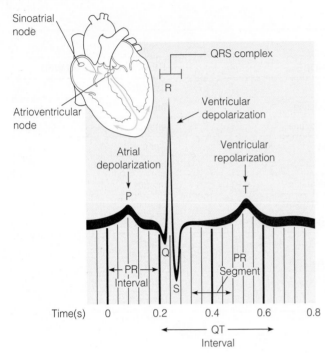

Figure 4-6 The normal cardiac cycle with ECG waveforms, segments, and intervals.

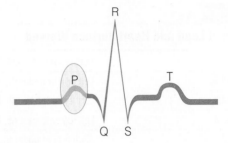

Figure 4-7 P wave.

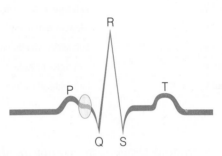

Figure 4-8 PR segment.

and complexes. Figure 4-6 depicts a normal cardiac cycle. As discussed earlier, a waveform is a deflection either upward or downward from the ECG baseline, such as the P wave or T wave. A segment is a line between waveforms that usually falls on the ECG baseline, such as the PR segment and the ST segment. An interval is a waveform and an adjoining segment, such as the PR interval and the QT interval. A complex is made up of multiple deflections, such as the QRS complex.

The P Wave

The cardiac cycle starts with the P wave. The P wave results from electrical firing of the SA node, and the resulting atrial depolarization. P waves are usually round and smooth, positive deflections on the ECG. However, in certain leads, the P waves may be negative or biphasic deflections. For the sake of this chapter, however, Lead II is referred to in the examples and discussions of wave deflections because this lead is quite commonly used and normally has a positively deflected P wave, QRS complex, and T wave. When all of the P waves originate from the SA node, they all have the same configuration, so they all look the same. If an ectopic pacemaker, or different cardiac cell, fires and stimulates atrial depolarization, the P wave will have a different configuration from the other P waves. See Figure 4-7.

The PR Segment

After the P wave, there is a short segment that usually falls on the isoelectric line (or ECG baseline). This results from the short pause in electrical conduction as the wave

of depolarization slows down while traveling through the AV junction. The duration of the PR segment depends on the length of time it takes for the electrical impulse to conduct through the AV junction. See Figure 4-8.

The PR Interval

The entire P wave and PR segment make up the PR interval. Electrically speaking, the PR interval reflects depolarization of the right and left atria (P wave) and the impulse delay through the AV junction (PR segment). This interval measures from the beginning of the P wave to the beginning of the QRS complex. It normally measures 0.12 to 0.20 second, or three to five small boxes on the ECG paper. A PR interval longer than 0.20 second usually indicates a delay in impulse conduction through the atria or AV junction. A PR interval shorter than 0.12 second may indicate that the impulse originated from an ectopic pacemaker in the atria, rather than the SA node, that was located closer to the AV node. See Figure 4-9.

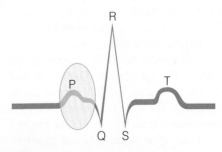

Figure 4-9 PR interval.

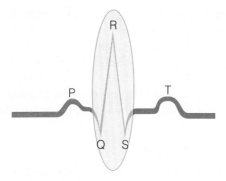

Figure 4-10 QRS complex.

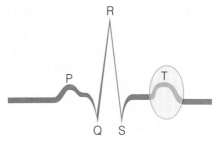

Figure 4-12 T wave.

The QRS Complex

The QRS complex is made up of three waveforms. Not all three waveforms are visualized in all leads, so the QRS complex may actually have one, two, or three waveforms. The Q wave is the first downward deflection after the P wave. The R wave is the first upward deflection in the QRS complex. The S wave is the downward deflection following the R wave. The QRS complex represents the depolarization of both ventricles. The QRS is larger than the P wave because the ventricles have a much larger muscle mass to depolarize than the atria. The QRS complex is measured from the point where the first waveform of the complex deviates from baseline to the point where the last waveform begins to level out. The QRS complex normally measures less than 0.12 second, or less than three small boxes. A QRS complex that is larger than 0.12 second usually is the result of an electrical impulse originating from an ectopic pacemaker in the ventricles. An abnormally large Q wave may indicate cardiac cell necrosis from a previous myocardial infarction. See Figure 4-10.

The ST Segment

The ST segment is usually an isoelectric line between the QRS complex and the T wave. It begins at the end of the QRS complex and ends at the beginning of the T wave. The ST segment represents early repolarization of the ventricles. The ST segment is considered elevated if it deviates above the isoelectric line, and it is considered depressed if it deviates below the isoelectric line by more than about 1 mm, or one small box. ST segment elevation may be indicative of myocardial injury and may occur during an MI. See Figure 4-11.

T Wave

The T wave follows the ST segment and represents ventricular repolarization. The T wave is usually rounded and deflected in the same direction as the preceding QRS complex. A negative T wave following a positive QRS complex is suggestive of myocardial ischemia. Tall and peaked T waves may be suggestive of hyperkalemia. If an ectopic stimulus excites the ventricles during the downward slope of the T wave, the vulnerable period, it may cause ventricular irritability and a resulting lethal dysrhythmia. This is known as the R-on-T phenomenon. See Figure 4-12.

The QT Interval

The entire QRS complex, ST segment, and T wave make up the QT interval. The QT interval represents the total time required for ventricular depolarization to repolarization. It is measured from the beginning of the QRS complex to the end of the T wave. The length of the QT interval varies with the client's age, gender, and heart rate but, typically, it is 0.38 to 0.42 second. The interval becomes shorter with faster heart rates, and longer with slower heart rates; therefore, the corrected QT (QTc) is usually calculated taking into account the patient's heart rate. Most cardiac monitors will calculate the QTc. A prolonged QT interval may be congenital or as a result of certain medications and electrolyte imbalances such as some antidysrhythmic drugs and low levels of potassium, calcium, or magnesium. A prolonged QT interval may develop into fatal dysrhythmias such as ventricular tachycardia or ventricular fibrillation. See Figure 4-13.

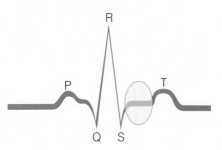

Figure 4-11 ST segment.

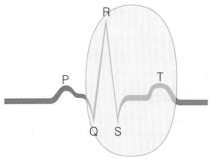

Figure 4-13 QT interval.

Interpreting the Electrocardiogram

Until the nurse has gained experience at reading ECG rhythm strips, it is important to approach reading them in a step-by-step manner. The six steps leading up to the interpretation of a rhythm are:

1) Determine the heart rhythm.
2) Measure the heart rate.
3) Examine the P waves.
4) Examine the P to QRS ratio.
5) Measure the PR interval.
6) Examine the QRS complex.
7) Interpret the rhythm.

Step One: Determine the Heart Rhythm

The first step is to determine whether the cardiac rhythm is regular or irregular. Irregular rhythms can be regularly irregular, mostly regular with some irregularity, or totally irregular. The SA node generates impulses at regular intervals, producing waves of depolarization in regularly repeating cycles. If the ventricular rhythm is regular, the R to R interval will be relatively the same for all of the cardiac cycles. If the atrial rhythm is regular, the P to P interval will be relatively similar for all of the cardiac cycles. A dysrhythmia that does not have a regular rhythm may be caused by the firing of ectopic pacemakers, resulting in a rhythm that is mostly regular with some irregularity. Atrial fibrillation is a common dysrhythmia that usually causes a totally irregular cardiac rhythm. Once the rhythm has been determined, then it is time to calculate the heart rate. For a regular heart rhythm, any of the three methods discussed next can be used to calculate the rate. For irregular rhythms, only the first method (the 6-second method) will be accurate.

Step Two: Measure the Heart Rate

As mentioned earlier, in adults the SA node generates electrical impulses at a rate of 60 to 100 beats a minute; therefore, the normal heart rate is 60 to 100 beats a minute. A rate that is less that 60 beats per minute is considered bradycardic, and a rate that is greater than 100 is considered tachycardic. Both the atrial and ventricular rates should be the same if there are no problems with the conduction and impulse generation. There are many different ways to calculate the cardiac rate. Following are some of the most common methods.

Six-Second Method

Most ECG paper is printed with a 3-second hash mark at the top or bottom of the rhythm strip. The fastest way to determine the cardiac rate is to count the number of R waves (usually the most prominent deflection of the QRS complex) in a 6-second period and multiply it by 10 to find the ventricular heart rate in 1 minute. For example, in Figure 4-8 there are eight R waves in the 6-second ECG strip; multiply 8 by 10 and the result is a ventricular rate of about 80. This method gives a quick average of the cardiac rate and is most appropriate for irregular cardiac rhythms. For regular rhythms the large box method may also be used.

Large-Box Method

This method is appropriate for regular cardiac rhythms, but it would not be appropriate for irregular heart rhythms. To determine the atrial rate, the number of large boxes between two consecutive P waves is counted. To determine the ventricular rate, the number of large boxes between two consecutive R waves is counted. The number of large boxes between the waveforms is then divided by 300, because there are 300 large boxes in 1 minute. For example, if there are two large boxes between two consecutive R waves, the ventricular rate would be 150 (300/2 = 150). This method is similar to the memory method.

Memory Method

To determine the ventricular rate, the nurse should find an R wave that falls on one of the dark lines of a large box. Then, with the first dark line that the R wave falls on being 0, the nurse should recite the following numbers while counting each large box line after that R wave until the second R wave is reached: 300, 150, 100, 75, 60, 50, 43, 38, 33, and 30. This method is the same as the large-box method, except that the math is already figured out if both of the R waves fall on dark lines; however, if the second R wave does not fall on a dark line, the nurse can make a guesstimate of the difference between the two or calculate a more exact heart rate. The calculation is done by taking the difference of the two memorized numbers between which the second R wave falls and dividing it by 5. This number is used as the value of each little box that lies between the second R wave and the last dark line that immediately precedes it. From that last dark line, the number of small boxes is counted between it and the second R wave. That value is added to the memorized number above to get the heart rate. For example, if the second R wave lies between the memorized numbers of 60 and 50, the nurse would calculate the difference, 60 − 50 = 10, then divide 10 by 5 to determine the value of each small box, which would be 2. If the second R wave lies two small boxes beyond the dark line that represented 60, the value of 2 would be added for each of the two boxes to 60; therefore, the heart rate would be 64.

Step Three: Examine the P Waves

As the SA node initiates the wave of depolarization in the atria, the P wave is produced. If all of the P waves are similar in size and shape, and occurring regularly, it can be assumed that they are all originating from the SA node. If there are differently shaped P waves, it can be assumed that they are originating from an irritable foci in the atria. If the P waves are negatively deflected or absent, the rhythm may be originating from the AV junction, or the ventricles. Premature atrial contractions (PACs) are an example of a dysrhythmia that may cause irregularly shaped P waves.

Step Four: Examine the P to QRS Ratio

Each P wave should be followed by a QRS complex, signifying that the wave of depolarization has successfully moved from the atria to the ventricles. If there are more P waves than QRS complexes, it can be assumed that a dysrhythmia exists.

Step Five: Measure the PR Interval

The PR intervals should be the same for all cardiac cycles on the monitor strip, measuring approximately 0.12 to 0.20 second. AV blocks are an example of dysrhythmias in which the PR interval may be longer than normal.

Step Six: Examine the QRS Complex

The QRS complexes, like the P waves, should all be similar in shape and size and should occur with regularity across the ECG strip. The QRS complexes should all measure approximately less than 0.12 second. A wide QRS complex measuring greater than 0.12 second probably originated in the ventricles. An example of this would be a premature ventricular contraction (PVC). A narrow QRS complex measuring less than 0.12 second probably originated above the ventricles, for example, in the SA node or AV node.

Step Seven: Interpret the Rhythm and Evaluate the Patient's Reaction

The final step is to interpret the cardiac rhythm and the assumed pacemaker site of origin. For example, "the monitor pattern reads sinus tachycardia at a rate of 120 beats per minute." However, when interpreting the cardiac monitor always remember to examine and treat the patient, not the monitor! The nurse needs to determine how the patient is tolerating the cardiac rate and rhythm. The patient in sinus tachycardia at 120 beats per minute may be symptom-free and not require any treatment at all, aside from determining the cause of this tachycardia and resolving the cause. On the other hand, the patient may be showing signs of distress in this tachycardic rhythm and may need immediate interventions to decrease the cardiac rate. With any dysrhythmia, treatment will depend on the patient's reaction to the rhythm, which ultimately is determined by the patient's underlying health, length of time in the dysrhythmia, and amount of hemodynamic compromise being caused by the dysrhythmia.

Hemodynamic Consequences of Dysrhythmias

Hemodynamics refers to the study of the forces that aid in circulating blood throughout the body. If any of these forces are compromised, the cardiovascular system is affected. The hemodynamic status of a patient is monitored by frequently assessing the blood pressure, pulse, mental status, urinary output, and cardiac output. A deviation from the patient's normal values may indicate hemodynamic compromise. With both tachydysrhythmias and bradydysrhythmias, a patient may experience hemodynamic compromise because the cardiac output may be affected. Cardiac output is a product of stroke volume and heart rate. A decrease in either stroke volume or heart rate will decrease the cardiac output. In tachydysrhythmias, the rate may be too fast to enable the ventricles to fill completely, causing a shortened diastole and thereby decreasing stroke volume. As a result, after an initial increase, cardiac output and blood pressure will begin to decrease. In bradydysrhythmias, the rate may be too slow to provide adequate blood pressure and cardiac output. In both cases, coronary perfusion may be compromised.

There are many symptoms that may indicate a compromised hemodynamic status. These symptoms include, but are not limited to, hypotension, chest pain, congestive heart failure, decreased urine output, altered mental status, and other signs of shock. Symptoms may also include dizziness, diaphoresis, palpitations, shortness of breath, and syncope. After interpreting the rhythm, it is important to evaluate the clinical significance of the rhythm by determining the patient's reaction to the cardiac rhythm. With many dysrhythmias, the intervention will be dependent on the patient's reaction to the cardiac rhythm. As the following dysrhythmias are discussed, when reference is made to patients being symptomatic, it is important to refer to the above-mentioned symptoms. Also, it is important to remember that dysrhythmias may look somewhat different from patient to patient so following the steps of interpreting ECGs will be important as the heart rhythms are read.

Sinus Rhythms and Dysrhythmias

Sinus rhythms and dysrhythmias refer to rhythms that result from electrical impulses generated from the SA node. These rhythms typically have similarly shaped P waves because they all originate from the SA node. See Figure 4-14. A QRS complex follows each P wave, and the QRS complexes are usually narrow, or less than 0.12 second. The most common rhythms in this category include normal sinus rhythm, sinus arrhythmia, sinus bradycardia, and sinus tachycardia.

Figure 4-14 Origination of sinus rhythms.

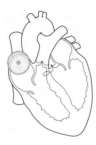

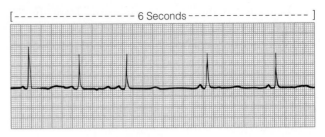

Figure 4-16 Sinus arrhythmia.

Sinus Rhythm

Sinus rhythm (SR), also referred to as normal sinus rhythm (NSR), is the rhythm that originates at the SA node. The SA node typically initiates electrical impulses at a rate of 60 to 100 beats per minute; therefore, the atrial and ventricular rate for SR is 60 to 100. The P to P intervals and R to R intervals are regular. The P waves are uniform and upright, with one P wave preceding each QRS complex. The PR interval is between 0.12 and 0.20 second and remains constant throughout the monitor strip. The QRS complexes are less than 0.12 second and are uniform and upright. Figure 4-15 shows an example of sinus rhythm. In the 6-second strip there are eight QRS complexes; multiply this by 10 seconds and the result is a rate of 80. The PR interval measures approximately three small boxes, and each small box is 0.04 second. Using the calculation of 3 × 0.04 = 0.12 second, the PR interval is found to be within normal parameters. The QRS complex is about two small boxes, so using the calculation of 2 × 0.04 = 0.08 second, the QRS complex is also within normal limits.

Evaluation

In summary, for NSR the ECG interpretation will be as follows:

1) Heart rhythm—regular
2) Heart rate—60 to 100 beats per minute
3) P waves—uniform and upright
4) P to QRS ratio—one to one
5) PR interval—0.12 to 0.20 second
6) QRS complex—narrow, less than 0.12 second

Sinus Arrhythmia

Sinus arrhythmia is a variation of normal sinus rhythm and not a true arrhythmia in the sense that arrhythmia means "without rhythm." Sinus arrhythmia is also referred to as respiratory sinus arrhythmia because it occurs with respiration. The heart rate increases during inspiration and decreases during expiration. The rhythm still originates at the SA node but is irregular with a repetitive variation in cycle length. The difference between the shortest and longest R to R interval is usually more than 0.12 second. The rate is usually 60 to 100 beats per minute but may be slightly faster or slower with inspiration and expiration. For example, Figure 4-16 shows sinus arrhythmia with a slower than normal rate of 50 beats a minute. The PR interval and the QRS duration are normal and consistent.

Evaluation

In general, for sinus arrhythmia the ECG interpretation will be as follows:

1) Heart rhythm—irregular, heart rate increases gradually with inspiration and decreases with expiration
2) Heart rate—60 to 100 beats per minute
3) P waves—uniform and upright
4) P to QRS ratio—one to one
5) PR interval—0.12 to 0.20 second
6) QRS complex—narrow, less than 0.12 second

Etiology

This normal phenomenon may be a result of reflex enhancement of sympathetic tone during inspiration and parasympathetic tone with expiration. Sinus arrhythmia is commonly seen in healthy children but may be seen in any age group. Occasionally sinus arrhythmia may be due to nonrespiratory causes as a result of medications such as digitalis and morphine.

Collaborative Management

Sinus arrhythmia usually does not require any treatment because it seldom produces symptoms. If it is accompanied by a bradycardic heart rate that causes hemody-

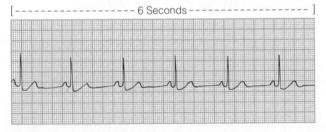

Figure 4-15 Normal sinus rhythm.

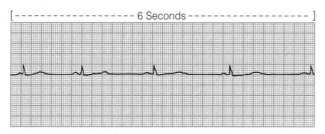

Figure 4-17 Sinus bradycardia.

namic compromise, it can be treated as symptomatic sinus bradycardia as described in the next section.

Sinus Bradycardia

In sinus bradycardia (SB), the rhythm still originates at the SA node but at a decreased rate of less than 60 beats per minute for both the atria and ventricles. The P to P intervals and R to R intervals are regular. The P waves are uniform and upright, with one P wave preceding each QRS complex. The PR interval is between 0.12 and 0.20 second and remains constant throughout the strip. The QRS complexes are less than 0.12 second and are uniform and upright. Figure 4-17 shows an example of SB that has a rate of 50 beats per minute.

Evaluation

In summary, for SB the ECG interpretation will be as follows:

1) Heart rhythm—regular
2) Heart rate—less than 60 beats per minute
3) P waves—uniform and upright
4) P to QRS ratio—one to one
5) PR interval—0.12 to 0.20 second
6) QRS complex—narrow, less than 0.12 second

Etiology

SB may be normal during sleep and in well-trained athletes. It also results from excessive vagal or parasympathetic stimulation. Excessive vagal stimulation may be caused by vomiting, carotid sinus massage, suctioning, and Valsalva maneuvers such as bearing down for a bowel movement, choking, or gagging. SB may also result from an acute myocardial infarction, hypoxia, and medications such as digitalis, beta blockers, and calcium channel blockers.

Nursing Management

Treatment of SB is only needed if the patient is exhibiting signs of hemodynamic compromise. If any of these symptoms exist (as discussed earlier under Hemodynamic Consequences of Dysrhythmias), immediate intervention should be provided. All patients should receive oxygen, IV access, and continuous monitoring. The unstable patient should be immediately prepared for temporary external pacing (see the discussion of selected technologies later in this chapter). The drugs to consider while awaiting the temporary pacemaker include atropine (see Commonly Used Medication, page 90) and epinephrine or dopamine (American Heart Association [AHA], 2005).

Sinus Tachycardia

In sinus tachycardia (ST), the rhythm still originates at the SA node but at an increased rate of greater than 100 beats per minute for both the atria and ventricles. The heart rate is usually between 100 and 180 beats per minute. The P to P intervals and R to R intervals are regular. The P waves are uniform and upright, with one P wave preceding each QRS complex. The PR interval is between 0.12 and 0.20 second and remains constant throughout the strip. The QRS complexes are less than 0.12 second and are uniform and upright. In Figure 4-18 there are 15 QRS complexes in the 6-second strip; multiplied by 10, this gives a rate of 150 beats per minute. The PR intervals are equal to three small boxes, or $3 \times 0.04 = 0.12$ second. The QRS complexes measure approximately two small boxes or $2 \times 0.04 = 0.08$ second. This strip is an example of sinus tachycardia.

Evaluation

In summary, for ST the ECG interpretation will be as follows:

1) Heart rhythm—regular
2) Heart rate—greater than 100 beats per minute
3) P waves—uniform and upright
4) P to QRS ratio—one to one
5) PR interval—0.12 to 0.20 second
6) QRS complex—narrow, less than 0.12 second

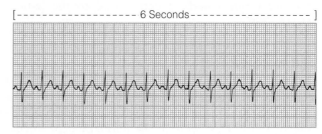

Figure 4-18 Sinus tachycardia.

COMMONLY USED MEDICATIONS

ATROPINE

INTRODUCTION Atropine is the first-line drug of choice for symptomatic bradycardia of any origin.

Desired Effect: Atropine is an anticholinergic drug that blocks the cholinergic and parasympathetic stimulation of the heart, resulting in an increased heart rate. This effect should be seen within 1 to 2 minutes of the IV bolus administration.

Nursing Responsibilities:
- Administration of the therapeutic dose. The usual dose of atropine is 0.5 mg IV boluses repeated every 3 to 5 minutes to a total dose of 3 mg (AHA, 2005). Atropine may be given down an endotracheal tube or intraosseous cannulation (into a long bone) if IV access is unobtainable.
- Atropine administration should not delay the implementation of temporary external pacing for patients with poor perfusion.
- Assessment of cardiac rhythm for increase in heart rate.

Side and/or Toxic Effects: Because of the parasympathetic-blocking effect, side effects of atropine can include mouth dryness, urinary retention, blurred vision, and increased intraocular tension. Doses of less than 0.5 mg boluses may further slow the heart rate and should be avoided.

Etiology

ST is usually the result of a normal physiological response to physical exercise, fever, anxiety, pain, hypoxia, congestive heart failure (CHF), acute MI, infection, sympathetic stimulation, anemia, or other stressors that may increase the body's requirement for increased oxygen. Certain medications such as epinephrine, atropine, and dopamine may cause sinus tachycardia. Caffeine, nicotine (a catecholamine), and cocaine may also cause ST.

Collaborative Management

Treatment of Sinus Tachycardia is directed toward identifying and correcting the underlying cause. Interventions may include decreasing the fever, anxiety, or pain; treating the infection, CHF, or MI; or removing the offending medication or substance. According to the AHA (2005), no emergent drug treatment is needed for ST, and in patients where cardiac function is poor, the cardiac output may be dependent on a compensatory tachycardia. In this case, normalizing the heart rate could be detrimental to the patient (AHA, 2005).

Sick Sinus Syndrome

Sick sinus syndrome (SSS) is actually a combination of a few different dysrhythmias caused by an unhealthy sinus node. SSS is most commonly identified by SB with periods of sinus arrest without the normal escape mechanisms of atrial and junctional foci, which are also dysfunctional. Sinus arrest, also called sinus pause, occurs when the sinus node fails to pace for at least one complete cycle.

Etiology

SSS most often occurs in elderly patients with heart disease. The SB is usually a result of excessive parasympathetic activity, which innervates the SA node and depresses the pacing rate of the node. The atrial and junctional foci are depressed as well and fail to fire as an escape mechanism when sinus arrest occurs. Periods of asystole result. Depending on the degree of SB and the sinus arrest episodes, the patient may experience hemodynamic compromise.

Collaborative Management

If hemodynamic compromise is present, IV atropine 0.5 mg may be given. If the episodes of sinus arrest are frequent and lasting longer than a few seconds, insertion of a permanent pacemaker may be required.

Atrial Dysrhythmias

Atrial dysrhythmias refer to those dysrhythmias or complexes that originate in the atria but outside the SA node. See Figure 4-19. The P wave configuration will be upright but shaped differently from the P waves originating in the SA node, as the electrical conduction will follow a different pathway to the AV node. The common dysrhythmias in this category include premature atrial complexes, atrial tachycardia, atrial flutter, and atrial fibrillation. The term "supraventricular tachycardia (SVT)" is often used interchangeably with atrial tachycardia (AT); however, it is actually a general term to describe tachydysrhythmias that originate above the ventricles, either of atrial or junctional origin, or of uncertain origin but with a rapid ventricular rate and narrow QRS complexes.

Premature Atrial Complexes

Premature atrial complexes (PAC) are early beats that most often originate from an irritable focus in the atria.

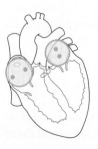

Figure 4-19 Atrial dysrhythmia.

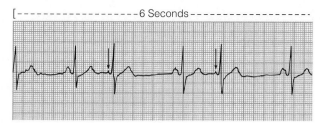

Figure 4-20 Premature atrial complex (PAC).
(From Jacobs, S. H. [1976]. *Intensive coronary care multimedia learning system: ECG exercises.* Van Nuys, CA: Sutherland Learning; Dubin, D. [2000]. *Rapid interpretation of EKG's* [6th ed.]. Hong Kong: Cover; Kinney, M. R., & Packa, D. R. *Andreoli's comprehensive cardiac care* [8th ed.]. Boston: Mosby.)

PACs are single early beats within an underlying rhythm rather than an abnormal rhythm in and of itself. The rhythm is regular except for the premature beats occurring earlier than would otherwise be expected. There is a P wave before each QRS; however, as shown in Figure 4-20, the P wave with the early beat may have a different configuration because it is not initiated in the SA node. The P wave may also be hidden in the preceding T wave; therefore, if no P wave is identified, the T wave should be examined for changes in size and shape compared with the other T waves. The PR interval of the PAC may be normal or prolonged. QRS complexes are usually narrow and similar in both the PAC beats and normal beats as they are all conducted through the AV node; however, occasionally the PAC may have a wide (aberrant) QRS complex or no QRS complex. The wide QRS complex may occur if the PAC is conducted abnormally down one of the bundle branches first and down the second bundle branch afterward. This would be called an aberrantly conducted PAC and the QRS would look wider than the QRSs from the normal beats. Occasionally a QRS complex does not follow the premature P wave because it occurred so early that the AV junction was still in the refractory period and was unable to conduct the impulse to the ventricles. This is referred to as a nonconducted PAC and will appear as a P wave on the monitor that is not followed by a QRS complex. A pause usually occurs following the PAC and represents the time delay during which the SA node resets its rhythm for the next beat. There are two types of pauses following premature complexes: compensatory, meaning complete; or noncompensatory, meaning incomplete. Noncompensatory pauses usually follow a premature atrial complex and compensatory pauses usually follow a premature ventricular complex (PVC). When a PAC is wide due to aberrant conduction, examining the pause may help identify the origin of the premature beat. To distinguish between the two types of pauses, the distance between three normal beats is measured and that measurement is compared with the distance between three beats that includes the premature complex. If the premature beat has a noncompensatory pause then the measurement of the three complexes that includes the premature complex will be less than the measurement containing the three normal beats. If the premature beat has a compensatory pause, the two measurements will be the same.

Evaluation

In summary, for PACs the ECG interpretation will be as follows:

1) Heart rhythm—regular except for the premature beats
2) Heart rate—usually within normal range
3) P waves—the P waves of the early beat may be upright, flattened, notched, or lost in the preceding T wave
4) P to QRS ratio—one to one
5) PR interval—0.12 to 0.20 second or prolonged in the PAC
6) QRS complex—narrow, less than 0.12 second

Etiology

PACs can be caused by emotional stress, anxiety, fatigue, infection, or lack of sleep or from substances such as nicotine, caffeine, alcohol, and stimulants. PACs may also be caused by medications, CHF, electrolyte imbalances, and myocardial ischemia. Patients may have no symptoms, or they may complain of palpitations, feelings of skipped beats, or an unpleasant awareness of their heart beating. PACs do not usually cause hemodynamic compromise.

Nursing Management

Usually no treatment for Premature Atrial Complexes is necessary other than treating the cause, such as stress reduction, rest, avoidance of substances known to cause atrial irritability, correcting electrolyte imbalances, or treating CHF.

Supraventricular Tachycardia

SVT is a rapid dysrhythmia that originates above the ventricles in either the atria or the AV junction. When the origin of the rhythm is clearly in the atria it may be referred to as atrial tachycardia (AT). It is referred to as paroxysmal atrial tachycardia (PAT) or paroxysmal supraventricular tachycardia (PSVT) when its abrupt onset or cessation is observed via cardiac monitoring. The rhythm in SVT is usually very regular. SVT has an atrial and ventricular rate of more than 120 beats per minute, typically 150 to 250 beats per minute. The P waves are hidden in the

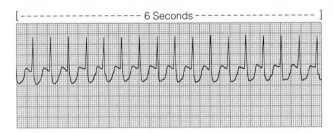

[- - - - - - - - - - - - - - - - 6 Seconds - - - - - - - - - - - - - - - - -]

Figure 4-21 Atrial tachycardia or superventricular tachycardia (SVT).

preceding T waves because of the rapid rate; therefore, the PR interval is usually not measurable. The QRS interval is usually narrow, less than 0.12 second. Figure 4-21 shows an example of SVT; it has a rate of 170 beats per minute.

Evaluation

In general, for supraventricular tachycardia the ECG interpretation will be as follows:

1) Heart rhythm—regular

2) Heart rate—150 to 250 beats per minute

3) P waves—may differ in shape from sinus P waves; may be hidden in preceding T wave

4) P to QRS ratio—one to one

5) PR interval—may be difficult to measure

6) QRS complex—narrow, less than 0.12 second

Etiology

AT is often initiated by PACs so the factors that cause PACs can also cause AT. Runs of AT are common in young, healthy people with no evidence of cardiac disease, as well as in people with hypertension or atherosclerosis.

Collaborative Management

The intervention for a Supraventricular Tachycardia depends on the patient's reaction to the dysrhythmia. Stable patients can be treated with oxygen, IV access, cardiac monitoring, and vagal maneuvers. Vagal maneuvers may successfully terminate SVT in about 20% to 25% of the patients (AHA, 2005). These maneuvers include gagging, bearing down, and carotid sinus massage. Carotid massage should be performed only by the physician.

If the vagal maneuvers are unsuccessful or give only transient relief from SVT, adenosine is the first-line drug of choice.

Atrial Flutter

In atrial flutter, the atrial rhythm is usually regular and the ventricular rhythm can be regular or irregular de-

COMMONLY USED MEDICATIONS

ADENOSINE

Desired Effect: Adenosine is an antiarrhythmic drug. When administered intravenously, adenosine causes a transitory block at the AV node. This blockade results in a short run of asystole when the patient has no heart rhythm. An effect from adenosine should be seen within 1 to 2 minutes.

Nursing Responsibilities:
- Administration of a therapeutic dose. The dosage of adenosine is 6 mg rapid IV push, followed by a second bolus of 12 mg within 2 minutes if the dysrhythmia does not convert back to normal sinus rhythm. A third bolus of 12 mg may follow in another 2 minutes if the SVT continues.
- Adenosine has a very short half-life; therefore, it must be given rapidly over 1 to 3 seconds through an IV in the antecubital vein followed by a 20 mL saline flush and elevation of the arm; a lower dose may be used if it is given through a central line.
- HR, BP, and cardiac rhythm pattern should be monitored constantly while administering adenosine; the nurse should be prepared for a code situation by having a code cart, oxygen, suction, and defibrillator readily available.

Side and/or Toxic Effects: Many individuals experience facial flushing, diaphoresis, lightheadedness, chest pain, and a sense of doom after administration of adenosine. These symptoms usually last less than 1 minute. If the dysrhythmia returns or does not convert with adenosine, a longer-acting AV node blocking agent, such as a calcium channel blocker or beta blocker, is the second-line drug of choice (AHA, 2005).

COMMONLY USED MEDICATIONS

CALCIUM CHANNEL BLOCKER (DILTIAZEM OR VERAPAMIL)

Desired Effect: Diltiazem and verapamil are both calcium channel blockers and work by slowing the conduction of electrical activity of the heart and increasing the refractory period of the AV node. The slowing of conduction through the AV node causes a decrease in the heart rate and may terminate the AT/SVT, which depends on the AV node for its depolarization circuit.

Nursing Responsibilities:
- Ensuring appropriate dosage: Diltiazem is given by slow IV push at a dose of 15 to 20 mg. A repeat bolus of 20 to 25 mg may be given after 15 minutes if needed. An IV infusion dose of 5 to 15 mg/hr may also be started and titrated to the desired heart rate. Verapamil is also given slow IV push at a dose of 2.5 to 5 mg. If there is no response to the verapamil, repeat doses of 5 to 10 mg may be given every 15 to 30 minutes to a total dose of 20 mg.
- Each single dose of diltiazem or verapamil is administered slow IV push over at least 2 minutes.
- Cardiac rhythm, HR, and BP should be monitored during administration.

Side and/or Toxic Effects: Diltiazem and verapamil may cause hypotension, bradycardia, AV heart block, flushing, burning or itching at the injection site, and CHF.

pending on the AV conduction. Atrial flutter is usually initiated by an irritable focus in the atria, which causes rapid depolarization at an atrial rate of about 250 to 350 beats per minute. The ventricular rate will be slower due to a protective mechanism in the AV node, which does not allow all of the atrial impulses to be

BETA BLOCKERS (METOPROLOL, ATENOLOL, LABETALOL, AND PROPRANOLOL)

Desired Effect: Beta blocker is an abbreviated name for "beta-adrenergic blocking agent." Beta blockers decrease the heart rate and blood pressure by reducing the effects of circulating catecholamines. Beta blockers also have cardioprotective effects for MI patients.

Nursing Responsibilities:
- Administration and dosage depend on the beta blocker being administered; however, beta blockers are administered via slow IV push and the dose is often checked with another nurse prior to administration.
- Continuous monitoring of HR, BP, and cardiac rhythm is mandatory during IV administration.
- Beta blockers should not be administered to patients with heart rate of less than 50 or those with second- or third-degree AV block.

Side and/or Toxic Effects: Side effects include bradycardia, hypotension, AV conduction delays, AV heart block, or heart failure.
   Synchronized cardioversion (see the discussion of selected technologies later in this chapter) may be needed if the above-mentioned medications do not successfully convert the patient back to sinus rhythm, or if the patient is not tolerating the dysrhythmia due to hemodynamic compromise.

conducted to the ventricles. There are usually no identifiable P waves; instead there are "flutter" waves that have a saw-toothed, or picket fence top, appearance. The rhythm is often described in terms of the number of flutter waves for each QRS complex, for example, a 3 to 1 flutter would refer to a pattern with three flutter waves for every one QRS complex. The PR interval is usually hard to measure. The QRS duration is usually narrow. In Figure 4-22, the ventricular rate is about 90; however, the atrial rate is approximately 250. There are two to three flutter waves for each QRS complex.

Evaluation

In general, for atrial flutter the ECG interpretation will be as follows:

1) Heart rhythm—atrial regular, ventricular may be regular or irregular

2) Heart rate—atrial rate 250 to 350 beats per minute; ventricular rate is usually slower

3) P waves—flutter waves that look like the top of a picket fence

4) P to QRS ratio—more flutter waves than QRSs

5) PR interval—not measurable

6) QRS complex—normal unless flutter waves are buried in the QRS, which would make the QRS appear wider

Etiology

Atrial flutter is usually seen in the presence of heart disease, CHF, cardiac valvular disease, and following car-

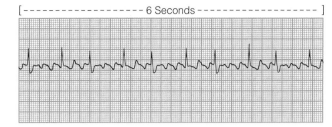

[- - - - - - - - - - - - - - - - - 6 Seconds - - - - - - - - - - - - - - - - -]

Figure 4-22 Atrial flutter.

diac surgery. The rhythm may be paroxysmal, suddenly converting back to NSR or to atrial fibrillation either spontaneously or with treatment. Expert consultation may be needed because the dysrhythmia may be difficult to distinguish from other SVTs.

Collaborative Management

The treatment for atrial flutter depends on the patient's condition. The patient is usually asymptomatic; however, the more rapid the ventricular rate, the more likely the patient is to be symptomatic. The goal with rapid ventricular response to atrial flutter is to slow down the ventricular rate. To decrease the heart rate, medications such as calcium channel blockers or beta blockers (as described under Supraventricular Tachycardia) may be used. Antiarrhythmic medications such as amiodarone or synchronized cardioversion may be attempted to convert the rhythm back to normal sinus.

Atrial Fibrillation

Atrial fibrillation (AF, Afib) occurs from the rapid firing of multiple irritable foci in the atria, resulting in no effective atrial contraction because there is no uniform wave of depolarization. The loss of an effective atrial contraction results in the loss of the "atrial kick" and a subsequent decrease in cardiac output. Atrial kick refers to the blood that is pushed out of the atria into the ventricles after they depolarize and contract together. The loss of the atrial kick can result in a 20% to 30% reduction in cardiac output. The rapid and erratic fibrillation of the atria also results in a risk for an embolic event due to the pooling and clotting of blood in the atria. The atrial rate is around 350 to 600 beats per minute. There are no consistently identifiable P waves; instead there are fibrillatory waves causing an erratic and wavy baseline. The ventricular rate is variable and has an irregular rhythm. In an untreated or uncontrolled AF, the ventricular rate may be between 100 and 160 beats per minute; this is referred to as a rapid ventricular response. When the ventricular rate is less than 100, the dysrhythmia is usually referred to as controlled atrial fibrillation. There

SAFETY INITIATIVES Prevent Harm from High-Alert Medication: Warfarin

PURPOSE: To prevent harm from high-alert medications by implementing the changes in care recommended in the Institute for Healthcare Improvement (IHI) guide. High-alert (or high-hazard) medications are medications that are likely to cause significant harm to the patient, even when used as intended.

RATIONALE: Warfarin (Coumadin) has a very narrow therapeutic index, making appropriate dosing and monitoring critical. Patients and their families are usually involved in administration; therefore, they must understand how to take the medication, avoid specific medications, and recognize symptoms that indicate likely problems. The IHI recommends changes in three areas to decrease adverse events. These areas for change are standardization of dosing, ensuring adequate monitoring, and ensuring partnering with patients and their families.

HIGHLIGHTS OF RECOMMENDATIONS:

THE IHI RECOMMENDS: Changes designed to ensure standardization such as standardizing protocols and dosing of warfarin but also vitamin K dosing guidelines.

Changes designed to ensure adequate monitoring such as making lab results available on the unit within 2 hours and plotting the INR results and dose changes on a chart.

Changes designed to ensure better partnering with patients and families such as developing appropriate educational programs that include self-monitoring and how to avoid drug and food interactions and carrying an accurate list of medications.

Source: Institute for Healthcare Improvement Available: http://www.ihi.org/IHI/Programs/Campaign/HighAlertMedications.htm

VISUAL MAP Narrow Complex Dysrhythmia

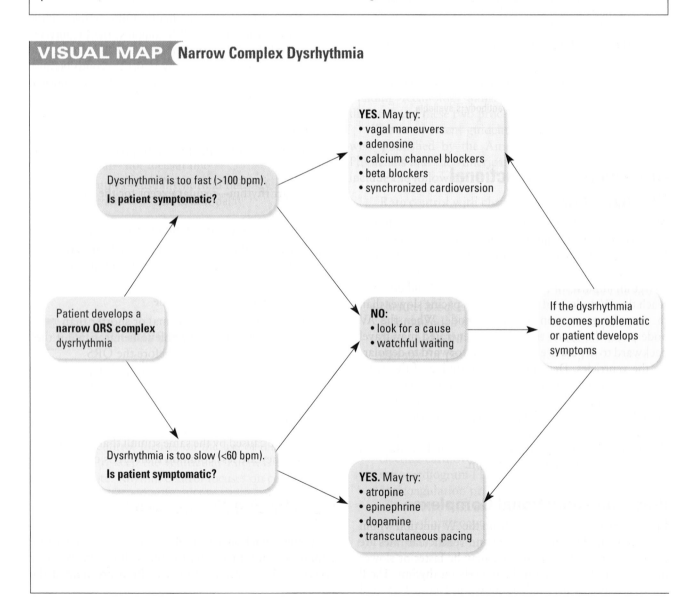

Junctional Escape Rhythm

Junctional escape rhythm occurs because the SA node has failed to pace the heart, or the impulse has failed to reach the AV node. The atrial and ventricular rate is 40 to 60 beats per minute as that is the rate of automaticity of the nodal cells at the AV junction. The rhythm is regular. The P wave is usually inverted and may occur before, during, or after the QRS complex. In Figure 4-26, the junctional escape rhythm has a rate of 50 and the P wave looks like an inverted notch and occurs immediately after the QRS complex. If the P wave occurs before the QRS, the PR interval will probably be shorter than normal. The QRS complex will be normal and narrow.

Evaluation

In summary, for junctional escape rhythm the ECG interpretation will be as follows:

1) Heart rhythm—regular

2) Heart rate—40 to 60 beats per minute

3) P waves—may occur before, during, or after the QRS, and may be inverted

4) P to QRS ratio—one to one

5) PR interval—usually normal or shorter than normal, or may not be able to be measured if the P wave does not appear before the QRS

6) QRS complex—usually narrow, less than 0.12 second, unless there is a conduction delay

Etiology

Junctional escape rhythm may be seen in acute MI, valvular disease, SA node disease, and postcardiac surgery, and in patients taking certain medicines such as digitalis, beta blockers, and calcium channel blockers. The junctional rhythm may serve as a safety mechanism if the primary pacemaker fails to pace the heart.

Collaborative Management

The treatment for junctional escape rhythm depends on the patient's symptoms and the underlying cause of the dysrhythmia. If the dysrhythmia is due to a medication, such as digitalis toxicity, the medication should be held. If the patient is hemodynamically unstable because of the slow heart rate, the same intervention as for sinus bradycardia may be used.

Atrioventricular Blocks

Up to this point the dysrhythmias involved problems with automaticity, or the pacing function of the heart; in discussing AV blocks, the focus shifts to conductivity problems of the heart. An AV block exists when the electrical conduction through the AV node or bundle of His is delayed or blocked. See Figure 4-27. The blocks are differentiated by their level of severity or degree of block, becoming more acute with each additional degree: first-degree AV block; second-degree AV block, type I and type II; and third-degree AV block, or complete heart block.

First-Degree Atrioventricular Block

First-degree AV block is really a conduction delay rather than a block. Every impulse is conducted to the ventricles but just in a delayed manner. The rate is usually within normal limits but depends on the underlying rhythm; for example, the underlying rhythm may be sinus bradycardia with first-degree AV block. The rhythm is regular. The P waves are normal configuration with one P wave preceding each QRS complex, and the QRS duration is usually narrow. The distinguishing feature of first-degree AV block is that the PR interval is greater than 0.20 second due to the conduction delay. All PR intervals are consistent in that they all measure roughly the same length. Figure 4-28 gives an example of sinus rhythm with a first-degree AV block where the PR interval is approximately six small boxes, or 0.24 second.

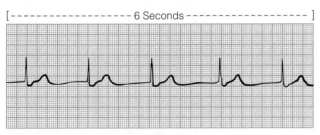

[- - - - - - - - - - - - - - - 6 Seconds - - - - - - - - - - - - - - -]

Figure 4-26 Junctional escape rhythm.

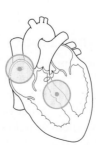

Figure 4-27 Atrioventricular (AV) blocks.

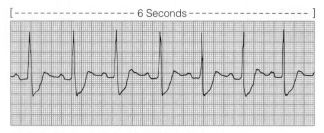

Figure 4-28 Sinus rhythm with first-degree AV block.

Evaluation

In summary, for first-degree AV block the ECG interpretation will be as follows:

1) Heart rhythm—regular

2) Heart rate—usually normal, but depends on the underlying rhythm

3) P waves—normal in size and shape

4) P to QRS ratio—one to one

5) PR interval—consistently prolonged from cycle to cycle, greater than 0.20 second

6) QRS complex—usually narrow, less than 0.12 second, unless there is a conduction delay

Etiology

First-degree AV block may be a normal finding for some individuals, or it may be due to a diseased heart. Some causes of first-degree block include AV nodal ischemia, which may occur from an inferior MI; digitalis toxicity or toxicity to other medications such as beta blockers, calcium channel blockers, and narcotics; excessive vagal stimulation; or postcardiac surgery due to edema in the AV junction.

◀ Collaborative Management

Generally, first-degree atrioventricular block does not cause hemodynamic compromise, so the patient remains without symptoms. If the dysrhythmia is due to a medication, the drug should be stopped or the dosage decreased. If the dysrhythmia is due to an acute MI, the patient should be monitored closely for progression to a more severe AV block.

Second-Degree Atrioventricular Blocks

In a second-degree block, not all of the impulses from the atria are conducted to the ventricles. The SA node is firing at regular intervals, but some of the impulses are blocked at the AV junction. There are two types of second-degree AV blocks: type I, also called Wenckebach, and type II, which is more serious than type I. Just as the PR interval was the distinguishing factor in first-degree block, the PR interval is the distinguishing factor differentiating type I from type II second-degree block.

Second-Degree Atrioventricular Block, Type I (Wenckebach)

The rhythm appears irregular due to the nonconducted P waves, or P waves that are not followed by a QRS complex. The atrial rate is greater than the ventricular rate due to the nonconducted P waves. The P waves are normal, but some P waves are not followed by a QRS complex. The QRS duration is narrow. The PR interval lengthens with each consecutive cardiac cycle until a P wave is not followed by a QRS complex. The pattern of progressively longer PR intervals and a dropped QRS repeats itself. The impulses from the SA node take an increasingly longer time to conduct through the AV node until one is unable to conduct to the ventricles. The conduction pause then allows the AV node time to recover so that the next impulse starts the cycle over again with an initial shorter conduction time. Figure 4-29 shows an example of second-degree AV block, type I. After the first QRS in the strip, there is a P wave that is not conducted into the ventricles and, therefore, is not followed by a QRS. The PR interval of the second cardiac cycle is 0.24 second, the PR interval of the third cardiac cycle is 0.28 second, the PR interval of the fourth cardiac cycle is 0.36 second, and then a nonconducted P wave is seen again.

Evaluation

In summary, for second-degree AV block, type I, the ECG interpretation will be as follows:

1) Heart rhythm—regularly irregular due to repeating patterns with a dropped QRS complex

2) Heart rate—the atrial rate is greater than the ventricular rate due to the dropped QRS complex

3) P waves—normal in size and shape

4) P to QRS ratio—some P waves are not followed by a QRS complex

5) PR interval—lengthens with each cycle until a P wave is not followed by a QRS complex

6) QRS complex—usually narrow, less than 0.12 second

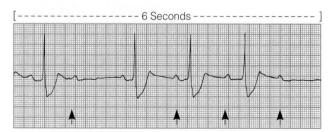

Figure 4-29 Second-degree AV block, type I (Wenckebach).

Etiology

The conduction delay through the AV node is thought to be caused by AV nodal ischemia from occlusion to the right coronary artery, or from acute inferior wall MI, or from increased parasympathetic stimulation. It is usually transient and rarely progresses to second-degree AV block, type II, or third-degree AV block.

◄ Collaborative Management

This dysrhythmia is usually asymptomatic as the cardiac output is not significantly affected. If the patient does become symptomatic and the rhythm is slow, treatment will follow that for sinus bradycardia, using atropine as the first-line drug of choice, and temporary pacing should be considered depending on the patient's symptoms.

Second-Degree Atrioventricular Block, Type II

Second-degree AV block, type II, is less common than type I. It is more serious than type I because it may suddenly progress to a third-degree AV block and because it is usually bradycardic in nature. The block occurs below the bundle of His in the bundle branches of the conduction system. The atrial and ventricular rhythms are usually regular. The atrial rate is greater than the ventricle rate because of the nonconducted P waves. The ventricular rate is often slow. If the nonconducted P waves are blocked in a random pattern, the ventricular rate will be irregular. When the P waves are blocked at regular intervals, such as in a 2 to 1 block (two P waves for every one QRS), the ventricular rate will be regular. The P waves are normal in size and shape. Unlike type I block, the PR interval is constant for the conducted beats. The QRS duration is usually wider than normal (>0.12 second) because of the delay in conduction below the bundle of His. Figure 4-30 shows an example of a second-degree AV block, type II. Notice that there is a nonconducted P wave and a conducted P wave before each QRS complex.

Evaluation

In summary, for second-degree AV block, type II, the ECG interpretation will be as follows:

1) Heart rhythm—usually regular, but may be irregular for the ventricular rhythm

2) Heart rate—the atrial rate is greater than the ventricular rate due to the dropped QRS complexes

3) P waves—normal in size and shape

4) P to QRS ratio—some P waves are not followed by a QRS complex

5) PR interval—normal or slightly prolonged and constant for the conducted P waves

6) QRS complex—usually narrow, less than 0.12 second

Etiology

Second-degree AV block, type II, may occur in patients with left coronary artery disease, such as an anterior wall MI, because the bundle branches receive their blood supply from the left coronary artery. Type II block may also result from other forms of heart disease. The patient may experience hemodynamic compromise if there are frequently dropped P waves, resulting in a slow ventricular rate and inadequate cardiac output.

◄ Collaborative Management

The treatment for unstable patients with second-degree AV block, type II, is immediate temporary pacing. Atropine 0.5 mg may be considered while waiting for the pacer, but its administration should not delay temporary pacing. If temporary pacing is ineffective, preparations should be made for a permanent pacemaker and expert consultation should be obtained. (See the section on pacemakers under Building Technology Skills.)

Third-Degree Atrioventricular Block (Complete Heart Block)

Second-degree AV blocks are incomplete blocks because some of the impulses are conducted through the AV junction to the ventricles and some of the impulses are blocked. Third-degree AV block is referred to as complete heart block because none of the impulses from the atria are conducted through the AV junction to the ventricles. The atria and ventricles beat independently of each other. Both the atrial and ventricular rhythms are usually regular, but they have no relationship to each other. The atrial rate is greater than the ventricular rate. The ventricular rate is determined by the site of the ventricular pacemaker. The atria may be paced by the SA node or by an ectopic focus in the atria; the ventricles may be paced by the AV node, the bundle of His, or the Purkinje fibers. The P waves are normal in shape and size and are equal distances from each other. The QRS complexes may be narrow or wide depending on the location of the escape pacemaker. Narrow QRS complexes are indicative of an escape pacemaker at the AV junction

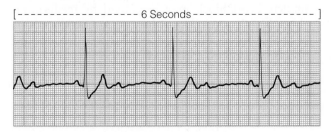

[------------------- 6 Seconds -------------------]

Figure 4-30 Second-degree AV block, type II.

COMMONLY USED MEDICATIONS

EPINEPHRINE

INTRODUCTION According to the AHA (2005), an epinephrine infusion should be used for patients with symptomatic bradycardia or hypotension after atropine or pacing has failed.

Desired Effect: Epinephrine is a catecholamine and as such causes vasoconstriction, thereby increasing the heart rate. Epinephrine is also a potent cardiac stimulant, strengthening myocardial contraction and increasing heart rate.

Nursing Responsibilities:
- An infusion may need to be prepared according to hospital policy (usually 1 mg of 1:1,000 concentration in 500 mL NS) and hung on an infusion pump at a rate of 1 to 5 mL/min to equal 2 to 10 mcg/min (Gahart & Nazareno, 2007); most drug books provide drug calculation charts to help calculate the drug dosage.
- Epinephrine is rapidly destroyed in alkaline solutions, so alkaline medications such as sodium bicarbonate should be administered through a separate IV line.
- The patient's response to the medication should be assessed by monitoring the ECG, BP, and HR every 5 minutes.
- The epinephrine label must be checked because the medication comes in a 1:1,000 solution and a 1:10,000 solution.

Side and/or Toxic Effects: Many side effects are transitory and can include anxiety, dizziness, dyspnea, and palpitations. Overdose can include bradycardia, tachycardia, cerebrovascular hemorrhage, fibrillation, pulmonary edema, renal failure, and death (Gahart & Nazareno, 2007).

COMMONLY USED MEDICATIONS

DOPAMINE

INTRODUCTION According to the AHA (2005), dopamine infusion may be used with epinephrine or administered alone as a second drug of choice after atropine.

Desired Effect: Dopamine is a catecholamine agent, a cardiac stimulant, and a vasopressor. Dopamine causes an increase in heart rate and blood pressure in similar fashion as epinephrine, and it also increases contractility of the heart and cardiac output. An effect should be seen in less than 5 minutes.

Nursing Responsibilities:
- A dopamine infusion should be started at 2 to 10 mcg/kg/min and titrated to the patient's response. Drug calculation charts for dopamine are available in most drug books.
- An infusion may need to be prepared according to hospital policy (a 400-mg or 800-mg ampule must be diluted in 250 to 500 mL of IV solution).
- The slowest possible rate should be used to maintain adequate heart rate and blood pressure.
- Blood pressure and heart rate should be checked every 5 minutes to avoid hypertension.
- A central line is preferred for infusion as infiltration into the tissues can cause necrosis and sloughing of the tissue.

Side and/or Toxic Effects: Side effects may include bradycardia, dyspnea, ectopic beats, hypertension, hypotension, palpitations, tachycardia, and widened QRS complex (Gahart & Nazareno, 2007).

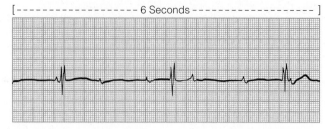

[- - - - - - - - - - - - - - - - - - 6 Seconds - - - - - - - - - - - - - - - - - -]

Figure 4-31 Third-degree AV block (complete heart block).

and will usually have a rate of 40 to 60 beats per minute, as in the junctional escape rhythm. Wide QRS complexes are indicative of an escape pacemaker in the ventricles and will usually have a rate of less than 40 beats per minute. The QRS complexes are equal distances apart, but there is no relationship between the P waves and the QRS complexes. There is no consistent PR interval, as the atria and ventricles are beating independently of each other, so the PR intervals are all different. Complete heart block may deteriorate into a fatal dysrhythmia such as ventricular asystole, ventricular tachycardia, or ventricular fibrillation. Figure 4-31 shows an example of complete heart block. Notice how the P waves march out independently of the QRS complexes. The atrial rate is 60, whereas the ventricular rate is 30.

Evaluation

In summary, for third-degree AV block the ECG interpretation will be as follows:

1) Heart rhythm—the atrial and ventricular are regular, but there is no relationship between the two rhythms
2) Heart rate—the atrial rate is greater than the ventricular rate
3) P waves—normal in size and shape
4) P to QRS ratio—there are usually more P waves than QRS complexes
5) PR interval—none, as the atria and ventricles beat independently of each other
6) QRS complex—narrow or wide depending on the location of the escape pacemaker; narrow indicates a junctional pacemaker, whereas wide indicates a ventricular pacemaker

Etiology

Complete heart block may be caused by medications such as digitalis toxicity and by degenerative heart disease. It may also be caused by acute MI and myocarditis.

Collaborative Management

The nurse should prepare for emergent temporary pacing in patients with symptomatic third-degree AV block.

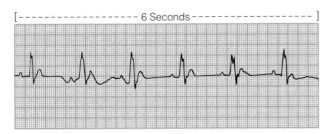

[- - - - - - - - - - - - - - - 6 Seconds - - - - - - - - - - - - - - - -]

Figure 4-32 Normal sinus rhythm with a bundle branch block.

Atropine 0.5 mg IV may be given, while awaiting the pacemaker, to a total of 3 mg. Epinephrine or dopamine infusing may also be considered while awaiting the pacemaker or if the pacing is ineffective (AHA, 2005). If temporary pacing is ineffective, the nurse should prepare for permanent pacemaker insertion. Third-degree AV block with a narrow QRS is usually better tolerated than third-degree block with a wide QRS.

Bundle Branch Block

Bundle branch block (BBB) is a type of intraventricular conduction block. After the AV node, the electrical impulse enters the bundle of His, which bifurcates into the right and left bundle branches. BBB is a conduction delay or block in one of the two main bundle branches. Instead of both ventricles being depolarized simultaneously, the unblocked bundle branch conducts normally, and then the wave of depolarization is spread from the first ventricle, cell by cell, to the second ventricle. The electrical impulses spread much slower through the cardiac cells than through the specialized bundle branch cells. This slowed depolarization prolongs the QRS duration to 0.12 second or longer. Its appearance varies depending on the affected bundle branch. See Figure 4-32.

Evaluation

In general, for BBB the ECG interpretation will be as follows:

1) Heart rhythm—depends on the underlying rhythm, usually sinus in origin
2) Heart rate—depends on the underlying rhythm
3) P waves—not affected by the BBB, usually normal
4) P to QRS ratio—not affected by the BBB, usually one to one
5) PR interval—not affected by the BBB
6) QRS complex—usually 0.12 second or wider; usually appears notched with an R and R prime wave or as a widened QRS with two peaks. The second notch, or peak, represents the delay in ventricular depolarization

Etiology

BBB may be a temporary or permanent conduction disorder. A temporary BBB may occur after acute conditions such as MI or heart failure. A permanent BBB may occur with congenital heart disease, rheumatic heart disease, cardiomyopathy, severe aortic stenosis, or other cardiac diseases that may cause scarring of the conduction system. Typically, the patient with a BBB is asymptomatic.

Nursing Management

BBBs do not usually require intervention; however, a new block should be reported to the health care provider, and the patient should be assessed for signs of hemodynamic compromise.

Ventricular Dysrhythmias

Ventricular dysrhythmias are those dysrhythmias that originate in the ventricles. See Figure 4-33. The ventricles may take over as the primary pacemaker of the heart if the SA node fails to discharge an impulse, or the impulse is blocked and does not reach the ventricles, or if the SA node and AV node are pacing slower than the impulse generation of the ventricles, or if an irritable site in one of the ventricles produces a rapid rhythm. When one of the ventricles paces the heart, the impulse generated must first spread a wave of depolarization through one ventricle and then depolarize the other ventricle. This creates a QRS complex that is wide (>0.12 second) and abnormally shaped. The impulse is usually blocked in the AV junction and does not depolarize the atria. Tachycardic rhythms that have narrow QRS complexes (<0.12 second) usually originate above the ventricles, whereas tachycardic rhythms that have wide QRS complexes (>0.12 second) usually originate in the ventricles. Some common ventricular dysrhythmias include PVCs, ventricular escape rhythm, ventricular tachycardia (VT), ventricular fibrillation (VF), ventricular asystole, and PEA.

Premature Ventricular Complexes

PVCs are early beats within an underlying rhythm that are initiated by an irritable focus in one of the ventricles. There is no PR interval with the PVC because the beat originated in the ventricles and does not have a P wave. The QRS duration is wide (> 0.12 second) and bizarre. The T wave is usually deflected in the opposite direction of the QRS complex. A pause usually occurs following

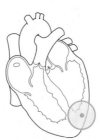

Figure 4-33 Ventricular dysrhythmias.

the PVC. As discussed in the section on PACs, there are two types of pauses following premature complexes: compensatory, meaning complete, and noncompensatory, meaning incomplete. Noncompensatory pauses usually follow a PAC, and compensatory pauses usually follow a PVC. When a PAC is wide due to aberrant conduction, examining the pause may help identify the origin of the premature beat. Figure 4-34A shows an example of a PVC with an irregular underlying rhythm of AF. Multiple PVCs may be described as unifocal or multifocal. Unifocal PVCs mean they look the same and originate from the same irritable focus in the ventricles. Multifocal PVCs mean they look different and may originate from different irritable foci in the ventricles. When the rate is fast, PVCs may occur in pairs, called couplets. A run of three of more PVCs at a fast rate is known as VT. PVCs may also appear in repetitive patterns known as bigeminy or trigeminy. Bigeminy refers to a repetitive pattern in which every other beat is a PVC. Trigeminy refers to a repetitive pattern in which every third beat is a PVC. Figure 4-34B shows an example of bigeminy.

Evaluation

In general, for PVCs the ECG interpretation will be as follows:

1) Heart rhythm—depends on the underlying rhythm, essentially regular with premature beats

2) Heart rate—depends on the underlying rhythm

3) P waves—usually absent

4) P to QRS ratio—the PVC does not have a P wave preceding it

5) PR interval—none with the PVC

6) QRS complex—greater than 0.12 second, wide and bizarre, with T waves in the opposite direction as the QRS complex

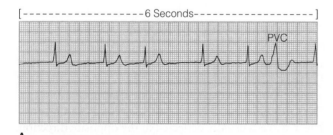

A

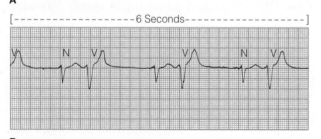

B

Figure 4-34 *A*, A premature ventricular complex (PVC) with an underlying rhythm of atrial fibrillation. *B*, Ventricular bigeminy.

Etiology

PVCs can occur in healthy patients, and the incidence of PVCs increases with age. PVCs may produce no symptoms or may cause a feeling of skipped beats, racing heart, or chest and neck discomfort. PVCs may or may not produce a palpable pulse. PVCs may be caused by hypoxia; myocardial ischemia or infarction; CHF; stress; medications such as digitalis, epinephrine, and dopamine; or electrolyte imbalances such as hypokalemia or hypomagnesemia. PVCs may also be caused by ingestion of caffeine, alcohol, and tobacco, and by an increase in catecholamines. PVCs may also be caused by successful fibrinolytic therapy.

Collaborative Management

Occasional PVCs in otherwise healthy patients do not need intervention, except to eliminate contributing factors such as medications or caffeine. Treatment of post-MI patients with frequent PVCs includes correction of hypoxia, pain relief, and correction of electrolyte imbalances and heart failure. Occasionally an antiarrhythmic medication, such as amiodarone or lidocaine, may be needed. However, due to the potential adverse effects of many antiarrhythmic medications, the health care practitioner needs to weigh the costs and benefits of each particular patient in treating PVCs with medications.

COMMONLY USED MEDICATIONS

AMIODARONE

Desired Effect: Amiodarone is an antiarrhythmic agent. It has actions similar to calcium channel blockers on slowing conduction and prolonging refractoriness at the AV node. Amiodarone also prolongs the duration of cardiac action potential via the sodium and potassium channels, raising the threshold for SVT and ventricular fibrillation, and may prevent its recurrence (Gahart & Nazareno, 2007).

Nursing Responsibilities:
- Ensuring administration of therapeutic dose. Amiodarone 150 mg IV (diluted in 100 mL D₅W) is administered over 10 minutes and repeated as needed to a maximum dose of 2.2 grams in 24 hours. If the amiodarone is effective in converting the tachydysrhythmias back to NSR, the patient is maintained on an IV infusion of amiodarone. Amiodarone infusion is dosed at 1 mg/min over 6 hours, followed by 0.5 mg/min maintenance infusion over 18 hours (AHA, 2005).
- The preferred route of administration is through a central venous line due to risk of vein phlebitis; use of a 0.2 micron in-line filter is recommended, along with a glass bottle for infusions that will take over 2 hours to infuse, because amiodarone may leach out chemicals in plastics (Gahart & Nazareno, 2007).
- Continuous monitoring of HR, BP, and cardiac rhythm pattern is essential during IV administration.

Side and/or Toxic Effects: Side effects include hypotension, bradycardia, or QT interval prolongation; amiodarone may cause torsades de pointes, a type of ventricular tachycardia. Amiodarone has a long half-life; therefore, side effects to the drug may continue even after the drug has been discontinued.

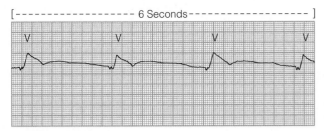

Figure 4-35 Ventricular escape rhythm (idioventricular rhythm).

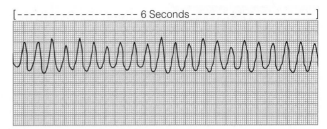

Figure 4-36 Ventricular tachycardia.

Ventricular Escape Rhythm (Idioventricular Rhythm)

Ventricular escape rhythm is also called idioventricular rhythm because it occurs in the ventricles without any association with the atria. This rhythm may exist when both the SA and AV nodes fail to pace the heart, or when their impulses are blocked. The ventricular rate is 20 to 40 beats per minute, and the ventricular rhythm is usually regular. P waves are usually absent. The QRS duration is greater than 0.12 second and the T wave is deflected opposite the QRS complex. Figure 4-35 shows an example of ventricular escape rhythm with a rate of 40 beats per minute.

Evaluation

In general, for ventricular escape rhythm the ECG interpretation will be as follows:

1) Heart rhythm—usually regular
2) Heart rate—20 to 40 beats per minute
3) P waves—usually absent
4) P to QRS ratio—the PVC does not have a P wave preceding it
5) PR interval—none
6) QRS complex—greater than 0.12 second; T waves are frequently in the opposite direction as the QRS complex

Etiology

Ventricular escape rhythm indicates significant slowing of the supraventricular pacemakers and is often seen in the dying heart. The rhythm is typically too slow to provide adequate perfusion.

▌ Collaborative Management

Ventricular escape rhythm usually requires immediate resuscitation efforts, including cardiopulmonary resuscitation (CPR) and advanced cardiac life support (ACLS) measures. If there is no pulse with the rhythm, it is treated as PEA and the interventions for PEA are followed. If there is a pulse, the patient should be treated for symptomatic bradycardia with immediate temporary pacing, and the use of atropine, epinephrine, and dopamine should be considered.

Ventricular Tachycardia

Ventricular tachycardia (VT or VTach) is a run of three or more PVCs in rapid succession. The ventricular rate is usually between 110 and 250 beats per minute and the rhythm is usually regular. The P waves are usually absent, or hidden in the QRS complexes. The QRS duration is greater than 0.12 second. The rhythm is referred to as nonsustained VT if it lasts less than 30 seconds, and sustained VT if it persists for more than 30 seconds. Figure 4-36 shows an example of ventricular tachycardia.

Evaluation

In general, for VT the ECG interpretation will be as follows:

1) Heart rhythm—usually regular
2) Heart rate—110 to 250 beats per minute
3) P waves—usually absent
4) P to QRS ratio—the PVC does not have a P wave preceding it
5) PR interval—none
6) QRS complex—greater than 0.12 second; the shape, width, and amplitude of QRS complexes are all similar; T waves are often difficult to distinguish from QRS complexes

Etiology

VT is usually indicative of significant cardiac disease. VT can be seen in patients with acute MI, coronary artery disease, cardiomyopathy, heart failure, and valvular heart disease. It may also be seen in electrolyte imbalance such as hypokalemia or hypomagnesemia. This rhythm can be mimicked by artifact, such as by scratching or tapping the electrodes, or by shivering. When a dysrhythmia is seen on the monitor, the nurse should always assess the patient, not just the monitor, before initiating treatment! Disconnected monitor leads, loose electrode patches, and patient shivering can all mimic dysrhythmias.

▌ Collaborative Management

Patients in VT may present with a pulse and in a relatively stable condition, or without a pulse and in significant hemodynamic compromise. The treatment will depend on the patient's presentation. A stable patient in sustained VT

VISUAL MAP Wide Complex Dysrhythmia

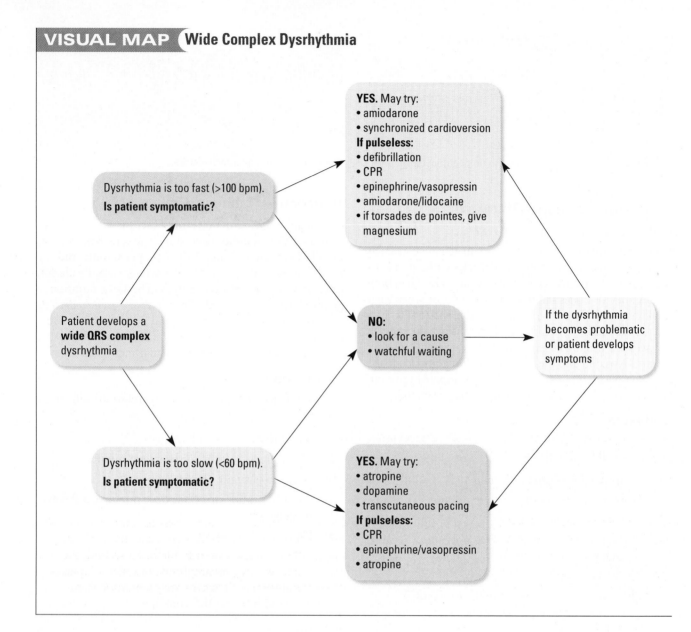

COMMONLY USED MEDICATIONS

LIDOCAINE

Desired Effect: Lidocaine is an antiarrhythmic drug that blocks the sodium channels, decreasing cardiac automaticity and depolarization. It is similar in action to procainamide, but more potent.

Nursing Responsibilities:
- The initial dose is 1 to 1.5 mg/kg IV. If ventricular ectopy persists, repeat doses of 0.5 to 0.75 mg/kg IV may be given at 5- to 10-minute intervals to a maximum dose of 3 mg/kg (AHA, 2005). A maintenance IV infusion of 1 to 4 mg/min is usually hung if the bolus was able to terminate the ventricular dysrhythmia.
- The nurse should continuously monitor the ECG.

Side and/or Toxic Effects: Many side effects are transient because of the short duration of action of lidocaine; these include confusion, dizziness, numbness of tongue and lips, hallucinations, and vomiting. Major side effects include anaphylaxis, bradycardia, seizures, cardiac arrest, hypotension, respiratory depression, and cardiovascular collapse.

COMMONLY USED MEDICATIONS

MAGNESIUM

Desired Effects: Magnesium is an electrolyte replenisher and a central nervous system (CNS) depressant and cardiac muscle depressant. It acts as an anticonvulsant and antidysrhythmic. It can reverse VT or VF caused by hypomagnesemia. Its onset of action is immediate and it is effective for about 30 minutes.

Nursing Responsibilities:
- Ensuring accurate dosage: 1 to 2 grams is administered diluted in 10 mL D_5W over 5 to 20 minutes slow IV push.
- The nurse should continuously monitor the ECG and the magnesium level.

Side and/or Toxic Effects: Side effects usually result from magnesium intoxication and include CNS depression, respiratory depression, hypotension, complete heart block, circulatory collapse, and cardiac arrest (Gahart & Nazareno, 2007).

COMMONLY USED MEDICATIONS

PROCAINAMIDE

Desired Effect: Procainamide is an antiarrhythmic agent that blocks sodium channels and prolongs the cardiac action potential. This results in slowed conduction of both atrial and ventricular dysrhythmias and a reduction in myocardial irritability. An effect from the medication should occur in 2 to 3 minutes.

Nursing Responsibilities:
* According to the AHA (2005), procainamide is given via IV infusion as a loading dose at 20 mg/min until the arrhythmia is suppressed, hypotension ensues, the QRS complex widens by 50%, or a total of 17 mg/kg of the drug has been given. A maintenance dose is started after the dysrhythmia is suppressed or a maximum dose is reached at 1 to 4 mg/min.
* For the loading dose, 1 gram of procainamide can be diluted in 50 mL D_5W to yield 20 mg/mL. This is administered via an infusion pump at 1 mL/min to get the desired dose of 20 mg/min. A total loading dose for a patient weighing 70 kg at 17 mg/kg would be 1190 mg, or the entire 1 gram, unless the loading dose needs to be discontinued due to hypotension, widened QRS complex, or suppression of the dysrhythmia. Gahart and Nazareno (2007) suggest the use of dopamine to correct hypotension.
* The nurse should continuously monitor the ECG and BP, assessing for widened QRS and hypotension.

Side and/or Toxic Effects: Side effects include blood dyscrasias, hypotension, PR interval prolongation, QRS complex widening, QT interval prolongation, and ventricular asystole (Gahart & Nazareno, 2007).

    If the patient becomes unstable during the administration of an antiarrythmic drug, immediate synchronized cardioversion is performed. If the rhythm progresses to a pulseless VT at any time, the rhythm is treated as ventricular fibrillation, and the patient is immediately defibrillated with an unsynchronized shock.

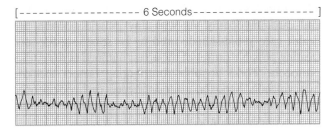

Figure 4-37 Torsades de pointes.

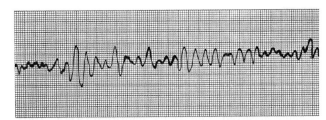

Figure 4-38A Ventricular fibrillation.

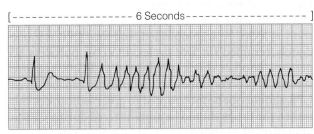

Figure 4-38B Sinus rhythm that deteriorated into a few beats of ventricular tachycardia, and then into ventricular fibrillation.

may be successfully treated with an antiarrythmic drug such as amiodarone. According to the AHA (2005), amiodarone is the first drug of choice in ventricular tachycardia. It should be given while synchronized cardioversion is being prepared as a backup measure. An alternative drug for patients in stable VT is procainamide (AHA, 2005).

Magnesium may be effective in terminating a particular type of VT called torsades de pointes. "Torsades de pointes" is a French term that means "twisting of the points." It is a polymorphic VT characterized by long QT intervals and QRS complexes that change shape, width, and amplitude. The strip in Figure 4-37 shows the changing of the amplitude in torsades de pointes as the complexes gradually increase and then gradually decrease, giving the tracing a wavy appearance. It may be caused by certain medications, hypomagnesemia, and other conditions that prolong the QT interval. Magnesium can be considered when VT is associated with torsades de pointes.

Ventricular Fibrillation

VF represents severe electrical chaos in the ventricles. Multiple irritable foci fire in an erratic and disorganized manner, resulting in no organized depolarization of the ventricles and, therefore, no ventricular contraction, resulting in no cerebral, myocardial, or systemic perfusion. Without successful termination of this dysrhythmia, death will follow within minutes. The ventricular rate cannot be determined as there are no discernible waveforms. The rhythm is rapid and chaotic and is described as coarse or fine VF depending on the amplitude of the irregular undulations. Figure 4-38A shows an example of VF. Figure 4-38B shows an example of a sinus rhythm that deteriorated into a few beats of VT and then into coarse VF, maybe due to the R-on-T phenomena.

Evaluation

In general, for VF the ECG interpretation will be as follows:

1) Heart rhythm—regular or irregular
2) Heart rate—unable to determine, no identifiable wave patterns
3) P waves—undetectable
4) P to QRS ratio—none
5) PR interval—none
6) QRS complex—undetectable

Etiology

The patient in VF rapidly loses consciousness and becomes pulseless and apneic. Respiratory and metabolic acidosis develops. Death rapidly follows if the VF is not converted to an organized rhythm that can sustain a cardiac output.

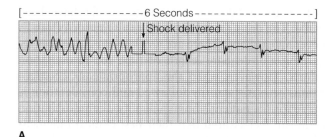

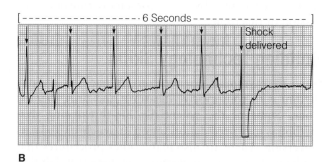

Figure 4-40 *A,* Pulseless ventricular tachycardia/ventricular fibrillation defibrillated into a sinus rhythm. *B,* Atrial fibrillation cardioverted into a sinus rhythm.

CPR is resumed. Figure 4-40A gives an example of a pulseless ventricular fibrillation that was successfully defibrillated into a sinus rhythm.

Synchronized **cardioversion** is a shock that is synchronized with the QRS complex. The "synchronize" button on the defibrillator must be pressed to put the defibrillator in the synchronized mode. In this mode, the defibrillator will recognize the QRS complexes and shock on an R wave, thus avoiding discharging during the vulnerable period of the T wave, which could cause VF. Synchronized cardioversion is indicated for unstable SVT, AF, atrial flutter, and VT with a pulse. The procedure should be explained to the patient and the consent signed, unless the cardioversion is an emergency because the patient is hemodynamically unstable. The patient should be premedicated with sedation and pain medication. Figure 4-40B shows an example of AF that was successfully cardioverted into a sinus rhythm.

Pacemakers

A pacemaker is a medical device designed to assist in stimulating the heart when the natural pacemaker is too slow or its impulses are blocked from reaching the ventricles. There are two different methods of pacing: temporary and permanent. There are also two different modes of pacing: fixed-rate and demand pacing. There are pacemaker codes that are used to describe the functions of the pacemaker and there are malfunctions of pacers. This section discusses these areas. The two major methods of pacing include temporary and permanent pacemakers.

Temporary Pacemaker

A temporary pacemaker can be internal or external.

External Temporary Pacemaker. An external temporary pacemaker is the type that is commonly used in emergency situations for patients with unstable bradycardia, including unstable second-degree type II block or third-degree block. It is the least invasive type of pacing, and it is quick and effective until a more permanent pacemaker can be inserted. The external temporary pacemaker is also referred to as transcutaneous pacing because it is performed through the skin by placing two self-adhesive pacing pads on the chest wall. The anterior (negative) pad is placed to the left of the sternum and the posterior (positive) electrode on the left side of the thoracic spine, opposite the anterior pad, or along the left axilla near the bottom of the rib cage. Most emergency defibrillators can also function as external pacemakers, using the same pads to monitor the heart rhythm, defibrillate, and/or pace the patient. The pacer rate is set as ordered and the threshold is set by finding the lowest current that achieves electrical and mechanical capture. Electrical capture indicates that the electrical impulse from the pacemaker successfully caused depolarization so that on the ECG (1) the pacer spike is followed by a QRS complex, (2) the QRS complex is wide, and (3) the T wave is deflected in the opposite deflection of the QRS complex. Mechanical capture is determined by the presence of pulse, indicating cardiac output. The electrical current from the pacemaker travels from one pacer pad to the other through the chest wall and heart, electrically stimulating the muscles in its path. The chest wall will contract with each paced beat. If the patient is conscious, the stimulation of the chest wall muscles may be uncomfortable. Analgesics or sedatives should be given as prescribed to provide comfort.

Internal Temporary Pacemaker. The other type of temporary pacemaker is the internal temporary pacemaker, also called transvenous pacing. Figure 4-41 shows a picture of the temporary pacemaker. If the external pacing is ineffective, or if the patient will need tempo-

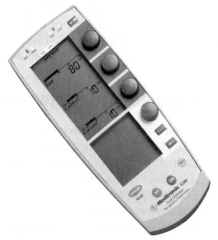

Figure 4-41 Temporary transvenous pacemaker.
(Reproduced with permission of Medtronic, Inc.)

rary pacing for any length of time (more than 24 hours), transvenous pacing should be initiated. Transvenous pacing usually involves insertion of a pacing wire into either the right atrium or right ventricle via a central venous catheter. The other end of the pacer wires are attached to an external, battery-operated pulse generator. The electrical impulses, at the set rate and current, are emitted from the generator and flow through the lead wire and hopefully depolarize the cardiac cells. The electricity is sent to the cells, but the cells must be capable of conducting the electricity. Transvenous pacing is not as uncomfortable as transcutaneous pacing; however, if the patient does experience some discomfort, it is usually alleviated by decreasing the pacer current. The QRS complex often is wide due to the fact that one ventricle is being depolarized at a time.

Permanent Pacemaker.
The permanent pacemaker is used to resolve dysrhythmias that are not temporary, such as third-degree heart block, or SSS (the malfunctioning of the SA node). A permanent pacemaker involves placing one or more wires into the heart chambers. One end of each wire is attached to the heart muscle in the atria and/or ventricles, and the other end is attached to the pacemaker generator. The generator is usually inserted below the subcutaneous fat of the chest wall, usually in the subclavicular space.

Modes of Pacing

The two basic modes of pacing are demand (synchronous) pacing and fixed-rate (asynchronous) pacing.

Demand Pacemaker.
A demand pacemaker is synchronized with the patient's heart rate, in that it only fires (delivers an electrical stimulus) when the patient's rate drops below a preset amount. The temporary pacemakers often use the demand mode. Figure 4-42 is an example of ventricular demand pacing. It should be noted that there are no pacing spikes before the patient's natural cardiac beats

Fixed-Rate Pacemaker.
Fixed-rate pacing is asynchronized with the patient's heart rate in that it continually fires at a preset rate regardless of the patient's intrinsic heart rate. This pacing mode is not used often because if the patient's heart rate increases above the pacer set rate, competition will occur. VF may result if the pacer fires an impulse during the vulnerable period

of repolarization, causing the pacer spike to fall on the T wave. If the nurse observes pacer competition, the pacemaker should be changed to the demand mode. This mode may be used in a severely bradycardic patient.

Codes in Pacing

The functions of a pacemaker have been coded into three to five letter codes to describe the main features of the pacemaker. The pacemaker codes have been used since 1974, and have been updated and expanded most recently by the North American Society for Pacing and Electrophysiology (NASPE) and the British Pacing and Electrophysiology Group (BPEG). The first letter in the code identifies the heart chambers that are paced, and the second letter identifies the heart chambers that are sensed by the pacemaker. The codes for these first two letters are: *A* means *atrium*, *V* means *ventricles*, *D* means *dual* chambers (both atrium and ventricles), and *O* means *no* chambers. The third letter in the code identifies the mode of response of the pacemaker. The codes for the third letter are: *I* means the pacer can be *inhibited* by the patient's heart rate, *T* means the pacer can be *triggered* by the patient's heart rate, *D* means the pacer can be atrial *triggered* and ventricular *inhibited*, and *O* means *no* response of the pacer to the patient's heart rate. Therefore, an *O* in the third letter of the code would mean a fixed-rate or asynchronous pacer, whereas any of the other codes would be a demand or synchronous pacer. The fourth and fifth letters of the code describe the pacemaker's programmable functions and antitachycardia functions. To understand how the codes are used, assume a patient has a DDD pacer. This would mean the pacemaker can pace both chambers, can sense both chambers, and is a demand pacer with a dual mode of response. This is also known as a dual-chamber pacemaker. Figure 4-43 is an example of DDD pacing, or dual-chamber pacing. The atria are paced first and then the ventricles; therefore, this is also referred to as AV sequential pacing.

A new type of pacemaker is the biventricular pacemaker (BVP). This pacer paces both the left and right ventricles and is also known as cardiac resynchronization therapy (CRT). By pacing both ventricles, the pacemaker can resynchronize the heart to depolarize the ventricles at the same time. This improves the functional ability of the heart for patients with moderate to severe heart failure.

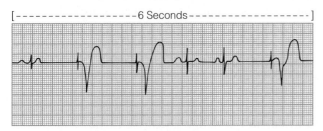

Figure 4-42 Ventricular demand pacing.

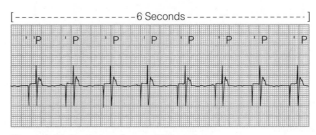

Figure 4-43 Dual-chamber or DDD pacing.

Malfunctions of Pacemakers

The four types of pacemaker malfunctions that the nurse can check for while reading the rhythm strip include: failure to pace, failure to capture, failure to sense (undersensing), and oversensing. Figures 4-44A, B, and C give examples of some of these pacemaker malfunctions.

Failure to Pace. Failure to pace occurs when the pacemaker fails to deliver an electrical stimulus (fire) when it should have fired. This can be seen on the ECG as an absence of pacer spikes when the patient's heart

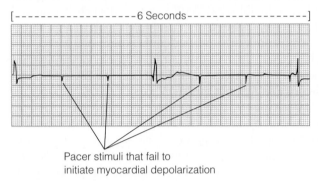

Pacer stimuli that fail to initiate myocardial depolarization

Figure 4-44A Pacemaker malfunction: Failure to capture (noncapture). Notice the pacemaker spikes that are not followed by QRS complexes.

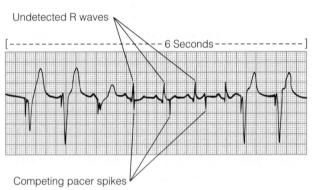

Undetected R waves

Competing pacer spikes

Figure 4-44B Pacemaker malfunction: Failure to sense (undersensing). Notice the pacemaker spikes immediately following two of the patient's own cardiac beats.

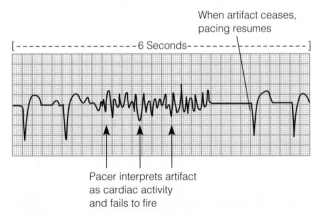

When artifact ceases, pacing resumes

Pacer interprets artifact as cardiac activity and fails to fire

Figure 4-44C Pacemaker malfunction: Oversensing. Notice that there are no QRS complexes during the artifact because the pacemaker interprets this activity as the patient's own cardiac beats.

rate is less than the demand pacer rate is set, indicating that the pacemaker did not fire. The patient may become bradycardic and hypotensive, and hemodynamically compromised. Causes of failure to pace may include a loose connection between the pacer wire and the generator, a broken pacing wire, or battery failure. The health care provider should be notified because the patient will probably need to return to the EP lab for a pacemaker check.

Failure to Capture (Noncapture). Failure to capture occurs when the pacemaker fires, but the chamber that is being paced (atria or ventricles, or both) does not depolarize. This is seen on the ECG strip as a pacer spike that is not followed by a P wave or QRS complex. Again, the patient may become bradycardic and hypotensive. Common causes of failure to capture include displacement of the pacing wire or the energy level set too low. The patient may need to be repositioned or the energy level may need to be slowly increased until capture occurs. Failure to capture can also be seen when the patient expires and has an asystolic rhythm with the pacemaker still on.

Failure to Sense (Undersensing). Failure to sense occurs when the pacer fails to recognize, or sense, the heart's natural electrical activity. This is seen on the ECG as pacer spikes that occur too closely behind the patient's QRS complex. This can result in a pacemaker spike that falls in the vulnerable period of the T wave and cause an R-on-T phenomenon. Causes of failure to sense include the same problems as noted in the malfunctions above; however, the most common cause is displacement of the electrode tip, or fibrosis at the electrode tip. Treatment may include increasing the sensitivity or replacing the pacing lead.

Oversensing. Oversensing occurs when the pacer senses extraneous electrical stimuli, or artifact, for actual atrial or ventricular depolarization and therefore fails to fire. This is seen on the ECG as pacemaker spikes that are at a slower rate than the pacemaker's preset rate or no paced beats, even though the patient's heart rate is slower than the pacer's preset rate. The patient should be taught to avoid strong electromagnetic fields, such as magnetic resonance imaging (MRI) machines, and arc welding equipment because electromagnetic interference (EMI) may affect the pacemaker settings. EMI is caused by devices that work on radiofrequency waves of 50 to 60 Hz. This includes such common devices as cellular phones and iPods; and less common devices such as arc welders, antitheft devices, HAM radios, and airport radar. In the hospital the devices that can cause EMI include electrocautery, defibrillation, radiation, radiofrequency ablation, and MRI. These devices can affect the pacemaker in many ways, including: oversensing, undersensing, inappropriate reprogramming, mode changes, and pacing rate changes. To avoid EMI with the pacemaker, iPods and cellular phones should not be carried in a shirt pocket over an implanted pacemaker; the ear on the opposite side of the pacemaker should be used when talking on the cellular phone; pacer pads for cardioversion or defibrillation should be placed at least 4 to 6 inches away from the implanted pacemaker. To avoid EMI from airport radar, the patient should inform airport security workers about the pacemaker and have an individual security check performed. If any of these devices are used on a patient with a pacemaker in the hospital setting, the pacemaker can be interrogated or checked to verify correct pacemaker settings after the procedure.

Implantable Cardioverter-Defibrillator

The implantable cardioverter-defibrillator (ICD) is a device similar in size to a pacemaker, and implanted in a patient similar to a pacemaker. It is used in patients who are at risk of sudden cardiac death due to VF and those patients who have experienced one or more episodes of VT or VF unrelated to an MI. An ICD constantly monitors the patient's heart rate and rhythm and is multiprogrammable to deliver pacing, cardioversion, and/or defibrillation according to the patient's needs. The ICD is programmed to deliver an electric shock if the patient goes into VF. Most are also programmed to provide overdrive pacing, or fast pacing, if the patient declines into VT in an attempt to break the tachycardia before it progresses to VF. The ICD may also be programmed to pace the heart if severe bradycardia develops.

Radiofrequency Catheter Ablation

Radiofrequency catheter ablation (RFCA) is useful in the treatment of many tachydysrhythmias. RFCA is a high-frequency form of electrical current that creates small necrotic lesions in the heart by means of thermal injury. The necrotic lesions are approximately 5 to 7 mm in diameter (Greenberg & Chandrakantan, 2005). The high-frequency energy is delivered through a catheter and the tip of the catheter delivers the current to the site of the dysrhythmia origin. RFCA has successfully treated SVT, atrial flutter, and AF. RFCA has also successfully treated VT in patients who have ICDs that frequently discharge in response to a VT rhythm. RFCA is performed in the EP lab under IV conscious sedation. Cardiac medications, such as beta blockers, calcium channel blockers, digoxin, and coumadin, are often held prior to the procedure so that an assessment of the best response of the heart can be detected. In the procedure, two to five electrode catheters are inserted via the femoral or internal jugular veins and positioned in the right and left side of the heart. For left heart catheterization, the catheter may be placed retrograde across the aortic valve, or transseptally via the interatrial septum. Multiple catheters are used prior to the ablation to map the various tachydysrhythmia pathways. Anticoagulation with IV heparin is used during the procedure to reduce the risk of thromboembolism.

Major complications occur in approximately 3% of patients who have an ablation procedure. These complications include death in less than 0.3% of all procedures; cardiac complications, such as AV block, cardiac tamponade, and pericarditis; vascular complications, such as bleeding, hematoma, thrombolemboism, and stroke; and pulmonary complications, such as pneumothorax (Greenberg & Chandrakantan, 2005).

Some common forms of SVT, such as AT and atrial flutter, have successful cure rates of about 90% with one or two ablation procedures. Cure rates for AF are about 70% to 80% for paroxysmal AF without structural heart disease, and about 50% for persistent AF with structural heart disease. VT that occurs spontaneously and without heart disease has a cure rate of about 80%, whereas VT with structural heart disease has a cure rate of less than 50% (Greenberg & Chandrakantan, 2005).

Maze Procedure

The maze procedure is the precursor to RFCA therapy and was developed in the 1980s to eliminate AF. The procedure was originally performed as an open heart procedure and has developed into a minimally invasive procedure using endoscopy and radiofrequency ablation. The maze procedure is done by making a series of incisions arranged in a maze-like pattern in the atria. It is hoped that the incisional scars block the electrical impulses that cause AF. The maze procedure is still employed for patients in chronic AF who are scheduled for an open heart procedure for other cardiac problems such as valve repair or coronary artery bypass, thereby eliminating the need for the RFCA procedure.

Cardiac Mapping

To diagnose and treat cardiac dysrhythmias, cardiac mapping may be utilized. Cardiac mapping is also referred to as electrophysiologic mapping and is performed in the EP lab. To determine the origin or origins of a dysrhythmia, multiple flexible wires, called electrode catheters, are threaded into the heart. These catheters can track and stimulate the heart's electrical impulses, allowing the physician to identify the dysrhythmia foci. Other types of catheters may be used to create three-dimensional pictures of the heart. These catheters have multiple miniature electrodes on them that act as radio antennae; they receive signals from all around the heart chamber and relay the signals to a computer. The computer processes the signals into a three-dimensional picture of the heart chamber. By determining the cause of the dysrhythmia, the physician is able to determine if the patient would be best treated by medication, an ICD, a pacemaker, or an ablation procedure. If an ICD or pacemaker is to be inserted or if ablation procedure is to be preformed, it can usually be done at the time of the mapping and with the guidance of the mapping graphics. Complications of cardiac mapping are similar to those of catheter ablation.

CASE STUDY

As you enter the ICU for your oncoming shift, you are told to go immediately to your assigned room because your patient, a 55-year-old male, is in full cardiac arrest. You quickly learn that your patient had open heart surgery 2 days ago for a coronary bypass graft and mitral valve repair. He is on the ventilator and has a central line for IV medications. You enter the cardiac room and find the code team performing CPR and charging the monitor for another defibrillation. You see ventricular tachycardia on the monitor; however, the patient has no pulse and no blood pressure. The team leader tells you that this is the second shock and

no medications have been given yet. The team leader asks you to be the medication nurse for the code.

1. What medication do you assume will be given first?

2. What is the implication of giving this/these medication(s)? After the second shock, continued CPR, and the administration of epinephrine and vasopressin, the team prepares for another shock. The "all clear" sign is given and you watch the monitor as the shock is delivered. To the left is the rhythm that you see.

3. How would you interpret what you see on the monitor and what should be done next?

4. What medication(s) should be given next?

5. What might have caused this ventricular dysrhythmia and what labs might be drawn to help determine the cause of this dysrhythmia?

See answers to Case Studies in the Answer Section at the back of the book.

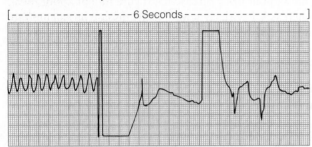

[- - - - - - - - - - - - - - - - - - 6 Seconds - - - - - - - - - - - - - - - - - -]

CRITICAL THINKING QUESTIONS

1. What are the four properties of cardiac cells?

2. Why is the development of atrial fibrillation significant for a patient?

3. Why is anti-coagulation important for the patient in af?

4. What are the common treatment modalities for af?

5. What are the characteristics of third degree heart block?

6. What are four ways in which pacemakers can malfunction?

See answers to Critical Thinking Questions in the Answer Section at the back of the book.

EXPLORE MEDIALINK
http://www.prenhall.com/perrin

Additional interactive resources for this chapter can be found on the Web site at http://www.prenhall.com/perrin. Click on "Chapter 4" to select activities for this chapter.

Case Study: Interpretation and Management of Basic Dysrhythmias

Nursing Care Plan

NCLEX Review Questions

MediaLinks:
- Ambulance Technology Study
- Heart Rhythm Society

MediaLink Applications

REFERENCES

American Heart Association. (2005). Guidelines for cardiopulmonary resuscitation and emergency cardiovascular care, part 2: Ethical issues. *Circulation, 112*(Suppl. IV). Also see http://www.americanheart.org.

Andrews, M., & Nelson, B. (2006). Atrial fibrillation. *The Mount Sinai Journal of Medicine, 73*(1).

Cummings, R. O. (Ed.). (2001). *ACLS provider manual*. Dallas, TX: American Heart Association.

Fang, M. C., Chen, J., & Rich, M. W. (2007). Atrial fibrillation in the elderly. *American Journal of Medicine, 120*(6).

Gahart, B. L., & Nazareno, A. R. (2007). *Intravenous medication* (23rd ed.). St. Louis, MO: Mosby.

Greenberg, M., & Chandrakantan, A. (2005). *Radiofrequency catheter ablation*. Retrieved September 24, 2006, from http://www.emedicine.com/med/topic2957.htm

Cardiodynamics and Hemodynamics Regulation

Shirley Jackson, MS, RN, CCRN, CCNS

Learning Outcomes

Upon completion of this chapter, the learner will be able to:

1. Explain how preload, afterload, and contractility determine cardiac output.

2. Describe how oxygen supply and demand can be evaluated.

3. Evaluate the accuracy of a pressure monitoring system.

4. Explain nursing responsibilities in the care of the patient with invasive pressure monitoring systems, including arterial, central venous, and pulmonary artery pressure lines.

Abbreviations

CI	Cardiac Index
CO	Cardiac Output
CVP	Central Venous Pressure
ECG	Electrocardiogram
L/min/m²	Liters/Minute/Square Meters
MAP	Mean Arterial Pressure
PA	Pulmonary Artery
PAWP	Pulmonary Artery Wedge Pressure
PVR	Pulmonary Vascular Resistance
RA	Right Atrial
RAP	Right Atrial Pressure
RV	Right Ventricle; Right Ventricular
SaO₂	Oxygen Saturation
ScvO₂	Central Venous Oxygen Saturation
SV	Stroke Volume
SvO₂	Oxygen Saturation of Venous Blood
SVR	Systemic Vascular Resistance

Cardiodynamics and Hemodynamic Regulation

Cardiodynamics and hemodynamic regulation deal with the forces the heart must develop to circulate blood through the cardiovascular system. These hemodynamic forces demonstrate themselves as blood pressure and blood flow. This chapter concentrates on systemic hemodynamics—the blood pressure and blood flow at the output of the left heart. Chapter 6 ∞ utilizes this information on cardiodynamics and hemodynamic regulation to review the pathophysiology, manifestations, and management of hypotension and heart failure.

Heart Anatomy and the Cardiac Cycle

The heart consists of four chambers: the right and left atrium and the right and left ventricles. Major vessels lead into and out of the chambers, moving blood within the systemic and pulmonary systems. Deoxygenated blood returns from the body via the inferior and superior vena cavae into the right atrium. Blood then moves over the tricuspid valve into the right ventricle. The right ventricle, structurally thinner than the left ventricle, moves blood over the pulmonary valve into the

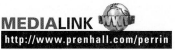

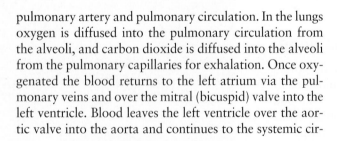

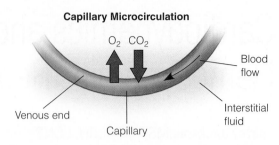

Figure 5-1 Cardiopulmonary circulation: *A*, The deoxygenated blood (blue in color) returns to the right side of the heart, exiting through the pulmonary artery into the pulmonary circulation where carbon dioxide is released into the alveoli and oxygen diffuses into the pulmonary circulation. The oxygenated blood (red in color) returns to the left side of the heart and exits through the aorta. *B*, In the capillaries, the oxygen is released to the tissues.

culation. Once in the systemic circulation, blood travels to the capillaries where the oxygen and carbon dioxide are exchanged at the tissue level (Figure 5-1). One of the important functions of the cardiopulmonary circulation is tissue perfusion.

The Cardiac Cycle: Diastole and Systole

The **cardiac cycle** is the sequence of events related to the flow of blood from the beginning of one heartbeat to the beginning of the next. It is divided into two phases: diastole and systole (Figure 5-2). The diastolic phase is further divided into the passive phase and the active phase. During the passive phase, when the heart is at rest, blood returning to the right and left atria create a pressure exceeding that in the ventricles. At this point the tricuspid and mitral valve open, allowing blood to passively fill the right and left ventricles. Immediately following this passive filling is the active phase. During this phase the atria contract, emptying the atria and fully filling the ventricles. This atrial con-

pulmonary artery and pulmonary circulation. In the lungs oxygen is diffused into the pulmonary circulation from the alveoli, and carbon dioxide is diffused into the alveoli from the pulmonary capillaries for exhalation. Once oxygenated the blood returns to the left atrium via the pulmonary veins and over the mitral (bicuspid) valve into the left ventricle. Blood leaves the left ventricle over the aortic valve into the aorta and continues to the systemic cir-

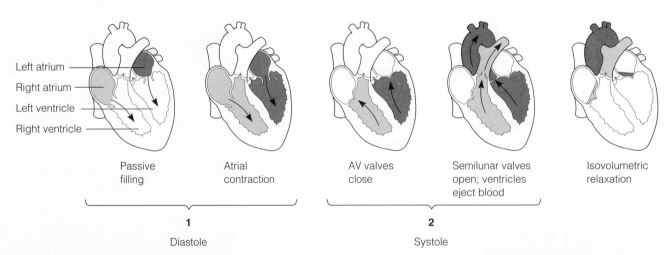

Figure 5-2 The cardiac cycle. The cardiac cycle is divided into diastole and systole. During diastole there is passive flow of blood from the atria to the ventricles followed by an active phase of atrial contraction. Once the ventricles are fully filled blood is ejected into the aorta and pulmonary circulation.

traction makes up 20% to 30% of the cardiac output and is an important contribution to the ventricle filling. The atrial contraction is stimulated by the electrical impulse originating in the sinoatrial node or atria and traveling through the atrial conduction pathways. This electrical impulse is seen on the electrocardiogram as the P wave (see Chapter 4 ∞ for discussion of ECG waveform). The nurse should be aware that if the patient is in a rhythm that does not have a P wave (i.e., atrial fibrillation) or a P wave positioned normally before the QRS (i.e., junctional rhythms), the patient may exhibit signs of decreased cardiac output.

Once the ventricles are fully filled and the pressure in the ventricle exceeds the pressure in the atria, the tricuspid and mitral valves close. Pressure builds up in the ventricles, opening the pulmonic and aortic valves. Blood is ejected into the pulmonary circulation from the right ventricle and into the systemic circulation from the left ventricle. This is the systolic phase.

Concepts in Basic Hemodynamics

In order to understand basic hemodynamics, it is essential to understand basic cardiac anatomy, the cardiac cycle, blood pressure, cardiac output, preload, afterload, and contractility.

Blood Pressure

The blood pressure is determined by the flow through the vessels and the vessel resistance. The peak pressure is known as the systolic pressure and the lowest point of the pressure is known as the diastolic pressure. The difference between the systolic and diastolic pressure is known as the **pulse pressure**. The **mean arterial pressure** (MAP) is the average pressure over one cardiac cycle. The MAP is thought to be a very good estimate of the perfusion seen by the organs. In many situations, the MAP is a better indicator of overall perfusion than the systolic pressure. A MAP of greater than 60 mm Hg indicates adequate perfusion. Most patient monitoring systems (noninvasive and invasive) automatically calculate the MAP. The formula for calculating the MAP reflects (at

normal heart rates) the extended time the heart is in diastole during the cardiac cycle.

$$MAP = \frac{(\text{systolic pressure}) + (\text{diastolic pressure} \times 2)}{3}$$

Cardiac Output

The **cardiac output** (CO) is the volume of blood ejected by the left ventricle every minute. The normal value is 4 to 8 L/min. The **cardiac index** (CI) is the CO divided by the body surface area and is the preferred value because it reflects the CO related to patient size. The normal CI is 2.8 to 4.2 L/min/m². Most bedside monitors automatically calculate the CI once height and weight are entered.

Determinants of Cardiac Output

CO is determined by the heart rate (HR) × stroke volume (SV). HR affects the CO when it is either too slow or too fast. Tachycardic rhythms shorten the time in diastole when the heart fills, therefore reducing the amount of blood available for ejection, thus lowering CO. Patients who are bradycardic have a reduced CO simply due to reduced ejection time. **Stroke volume** is the volume of blood ejected from each ventricle with each heartbeat. The right and left ventricles eject about the same amount, which normally is between 60 and 100 mL per heartbeat (Table 5–1). The primary factors that determine stroke volume are preload, afterload, and contractility.

Preload

Preload is the stretch on the ventricular myocardium at end diastole. Preload is determined by volume left in the ventricles. Pressures are used to evaluate volume at the end of diastole; these are also known as the "filling pressures" of the ventricles. The volume of blood at end diastole is determined by the circulating blood volume and the atrial contraction. Patients who have a reduced circulating volume (i.e., trauma or gastrointestinal [GI] bleed) or who are in an electrocardiogram (ECG) rhythm that does not have an effective atrial contraction (i.e., atrial fibrillation) may present with a reduced preload. Additionally, end-diastolic volume is also determined by the

TABLE 5–1

Hemodynamic Calculations

PARAMETER	CALCULATIONS	NORMAL VALUES
Pulse pressure	Systolic pressure – diastolic pressure	–
Mean arterial pressure (MAP)	$MAP = \frac{(\text{systolic pressure}) + (\text{diastolic pressure} \times 2)}{3}$	70–105 mm Hg
Cardiac output	Heart rate × stroke volume	4–8 L/min
Cardiac index	Cardiac output ÷ body surface area	2.8–4.2 L/min/m²
Stroke volume	Cardiac output × 1000 ÷ heart rate	60–100 mL/beat

TABLE 5–2

Causes of Elevated and Decreased Preload

	RIGHT VENTRICLE	LEFT VENTRICLE
Elevated preload	• Fluid overload • Tricuspid stenosis • Tricuspid insufficiency • Pulmonary stenosis • Pulmonary insufficiency • Pericardial tamponade • Constrictive pericarditis • Right ventricular infarction • Pulmonary hypertension	• Left-sided heart failure • Volume overload • Mitral stenosis • Mitral insufficiency • Cardiomyopathy • Myocarditis • Pericardial tamponade • Constrictive pericarditis
Decreased preload	• Hypovolemia • Venodilation	• Hypovolemia

TABLE 5–3

Causes of Elevated and Decreased Afterload

	ELEVATED	DECREASED
Systemic vascular resistance (SVR)	• Hypertension • Vasopressor use • Aortic stenosis • Hypothermia	• Septic shock • Anaphylactic shock • Neurogenic shock • Use of vasodilators • Side effects of some medications
Pulmonary vascular resistance (PVR)	• Pulmonary hypertension • Hypoxia • Pulmonary embolism • Pulmonary stenosis	• Use of vasodilators • Side effects of some medications

distribution of blood volume. Increases in intrathoracic pressure and venodilation, perhaps as a side effect of medications like nitroglycerin, can reduce the volume of blood returning to the heart and therefore reduce the preload. Preload exists for the right and left ventricles. Both the right and left preload are decreased in states of reduced circulating blood volume (e.g., trauma or GI bleed). As the preload decreases, the CO/CI may be reduced. Right heart preload is elevated in patients with fluid overload, tricuspid stenosis or insufficiency, pulmonary stenosis or insufficiency, pulmonary hypertension, and right ventricular infarction. Left heart preload is elevated in left-sided heart failure, volume overload, and mitral stenosis. Both right and left preload are elevated in conditions that cause increases in pericardial pressures like pericardial tamponade or constrictive pericarditis (Table 5–2).

Afterload

Afterload is the pressure (resistance) against which the right or left ventricle has to pump to eject the blood. The right ventricular resistance is the pulmonary vascular resistance (PVR). Elevations in PVR occur in pulmonary hypertension, hypoxia, pulmonary embolism, and pulmonary stenosis. The left ventricular resistance is the systemic vascular resistance (SVR). Elevations in SVR occur in hypertension, vasopressor use, aortic stenosis, and hypothermia. Decreased afterload may occur in cases of septic shock, anaphylactic or neurogenic shock, use of vasodilators, and side effects to some medications (e.g., narcotics) (Table 5–3). If the PVR is elevated less blood is available to the left ventricle, potentially decreasing the CO/CI. If the SVR is elevated less blood is able to be ejected from the left ventricle and may decrease the CO/CI.

Contractility

Contractility is the ability of the myocardium to shorten the muscle fibers. Contractility of the heart is influenced by electrolyte abnormalities (potassium and calcium), acid-base abnormalities, or myocardial oxygen supply/demand

abnormalities. Decreased contractility may be found in patients with hyperkalemia, hypocalcemia, myocardial ischemia, administration of negative **inotropic** medications, hypercapnea, hypoxia, and acidosis. Increased contractility may be found in patients with hypercalcemia, administration of positive inotropic medications, or sympathetic stimulation (Table 5–4).

A relationship known as the Frank Starling law of the heart exists between end-diastolic volume and contractility. As the end-diastolic volume increases, the myocardial fibers stretch, thus increasing the force of contractions. In some situations the end-diastolic volume is so large that it causes overstretching of the myocardial fibers, leading to heart failure. Adequate CO is dependent on adequate end-diastolic volume to optimize the contractility.

Tissue Oxygen Supply and Demand

The primary goal of the cardiopulmonary system is to maintain a balance between oxygen supply to the tissues and oxygen demand of the tissues at any given time. An imbalance of oxygen supply and demand can lead to tissue hypoxia and eventual organ failure and cellular death.

Determinants of Oxygen Supply to the Tissues

Oxygen supply to the tissues is dependent on how much oxygen is in the arterial bloodstream (**oxygen content**)

TABLE 5–4

Causes of Elevated and Decreased Contractility

ELEVATED	DECREASED
• Hypercalcemia • Administration of positive inotropic medications • Sympathetic stimulation	• Hyperkalemia • Hypocalcemia • Myocardial ischemia • Administration of negative inotropic medications • Hypercapnea • Hypoxia • Acidosis

and how effectively that oxygen content is being delivered to the tissues.

Oxygen Content

The two determinants of oxygen content in the arterial blood are the oxygen saturation (SaO_2) of the hemoglobin and the oxygen dissolved in the blood (pO_2). The majority of oxygen in the blood is in the form of oxygen bound to hemoglobin. An adequate amount of hemoglobin is required for effective oxygen-carrying capacity. The SaO_2 value indicates what percentage of available hemoglobin is saturated. The nurse must always evaluate the patient's hemoglobin level when assessing oxygen supply. If a patient has a low hemoglobin level, the SaO_2 may appear adequate but the overall oxygen-carrying capacity will be reduced due to the low hemoglobin level. A small percent of oxygen is dissolved in the blood and is indicated by the pO_2 value. At the bedside the arterial oxygen saturation can be estimated by pulse oximetry or measured via an arterial blood gas analysis. The pO_2 is measured as part of an arterial blood gas analysis. Oxygen content may also be calculated on an arterial blood gas report.

Cardiac Output

The oxygen content is delivered to the tissues by the CO. An adequate oxygen supply to the tissues is dependent on a normal CO.

Oxygen Demand

Oxygen demand is the tissue's need for oxygen. Oxygen demand is increased when the patient's metabolic rate is increased such as in infection, hyperthyroidism, shivering, or seizure activity. Stressful states can also increase oxygen demand such as with surgery, pain, and trauma. Oxygen demand cannot be assessed directly; therefore, the nurse must utilize measures to assess the balance of oxygen supply and demand.

Evaluating the Balance of Oxygen Supply and Demand

Tissue oxygenation is adequate if the oxygen supply and demand is balanced (Figure 5-3). An imbalance can occur with the following conditions: decreased arterial oxygen saturation, decreased cardiac output, decreased hemoglobin, or increased cellular demand (over the supply). Commonly used methods to determine an imbalance of supply and demand are laboratory measurements of lactic acid and measurement of mixed venous oxygen saturation.

Lactate

Under normal conditions when oxygen is available to the tissues, glucose is metabolized into carbon dioxide (CO_2) and water. When the cells experience an oxygen debt, anaerobic metabolism of glucose occurs, resulting in lactate formation instead of CO_2 and water. If the liver is also hypoxic, clearance of the lactate is delayed further

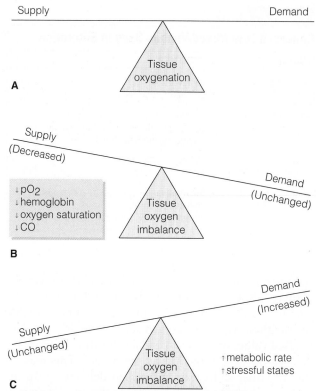

Figure 5-3 Tissue oxygenation supply and demand. *A,* Balanced supply and demand. *B,* A decreased supply compared to demand, creating an imbalance of tissue oxygenation. *C,* An increased demand with an unchanged supply creates an imbalance of tissue oxygenation.

(Kee, 2005). Lactate accumulates in the blood during conditions of tissue hypoxia; therefore, elevated levels of lactate (serum lactate greater than 4 mmol/L) are a reliable indicator of tissue hypoxia.

Mixed Venous Oxygen Saturation

The oxygen saturation returning from the tissues to the venous system is a reflection of the oxygen supply and demand. The oxygen saturation of venous blood (SvO_2) or the central venous oxygen saturation ($ScvO_2$) is influenced by the concentration of hemoglobin and the oxygen saturation of the hemoglobin, CO, and the amount of oxygen extracted and utilized by the tissues. The percentage of saturation in the venous system is normally lower than the arterial system due to consumption at the tissue level and the hemoglobin giving up the oxygen at the tissue level. The SvO_2 is normally 60% to 75%. It can be continuously monitored by the nurse using a specialized (fiberoptic) catheter that is positioned in the pulmonary artery, or it can be intermittently evaluated by drawing a sample from a similar pulmonary artery catheter. The $ScvO_2$ levels are generally 3% to 11% higher than the SvO_2 levels and are obtained by continuously or intermittently sampling the saturation from a catheter positioned near the right atrium (Reinhart, Kuhn, Hartog, & Bredle, 2004). The advantage of the $ScvO_2$ measurement is that it can be

TABLE 5-5

Causes of Low Mixed Venous Oxygen Saturation

CAUSE	CONDITION
Low CO/CI	• Hypovolemia • Left ventricular failure
Low hemoglobin	• Bleeding • Dyshemoglobinemia (carbon monoxide poisoning, methmeglobinemia)
Low SaO$_2$	• Pulmonary disease • Low inspired oxygen
High O$_2$ demand	• Elevated metabolic rate (fever, hyperthyroidism, shivering, or seizure activity) • Stressful states (surgery, pain, and trauma)

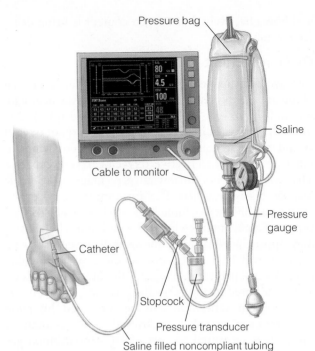

Figure 5-4 Pressure monitoring system. The system consists of a flush system, transducer, and monitor. The flush system is attached to solution in a pressure bag and connected to the patient using noncompliant tubing. The transducer is connected to a monitor via a cable.

obtained from a simple device such as a central venous catheter. Regardless of which method is used, the trending of the information can give the nurse valuable information regarding oxygen supply and demand. Decreased values of venous oxygen saturation indicate increased oxygen extraction by the tissues. This may be due to either a decrease in oxygen delivery or an increase in tissue oxygen demands. As the arterial oxygen saturation or hemoglobin level is reduced or the cardiac output decreases, less oxygen returns to the venous system after tissue extraction. This in turn reduces the SvO$_2$ or ScvO$_2$. If the hemoglobin, arterial oxygen saturation, and CO remain the same but the tissue demand increases, this will also reduce the SvO$_2$ and ScvO$_2$ (Table 5–5). Occasionally, the oxygen supply exceeds the demand of the tissues or the tissue extraction is dysfunctional as in late sepsis. In this case the SvO$_2$ and ScvO$_2$ may be elevated.

Technology

The technologies covered in this section assist the nurse in determining the hemodynamic status of the patient. Like with many technologies utilized in health care, interpretation of the values must be done in context with the patient's condition and the nurse's physical assessment. Many of the invasive technologies used to assess hemodynamic status rely on pressure monitoring systems to display the data.

Overview of Pressure Monitoring Systems

The basic components of any invasive hemodynamic pressure monitoring system are the flush system, transducer, and monitor. The catheter is attached to the fluid-filled flush system. The mechanical pressure through the catheter is communicated to the transducer. The transducer converts the mechanical pressure into an electrical signal. The monitor converts the electrical sig-

nal to a waveform and digital number for the nurse to see (Figure 5-4). The tubing from the catheter to the transducer must be noncompliant to accurately display the pressures. The flush system is attached to a flush solution of normal saline commonly containing heparin. Some institutions do not use heparinized saline. Data are unclear as to the need for heparinized solutions to maintain catheter patency (Preuss & Wiegand, 2005). Use of heparinized flush solution is contraindicated in any coagulopathy or history of heparin-induced thrombocytopenia. The solution is placed in a pressure bag that is inflated to 300 mm Hg. At this pressure, the flush system continuously delivers a small amount of solution (e.g., 3 mL/hr) through the catheter, thus maintaining patency.

Zero and Level the Pressure Monitoring System

In order to obtain accurate readings, the pressure monitoring systems must be zeroed and leveled periodically. The pressure monitoring system must be leveled from the air-fluid interface to the patient's left atrium. Leveling the transducer to the location of the left atrium corrects for changes in the readings due to hydrostatic pressure above and below the heart. The level of the left atrium, in the supine position, is the fourth intercostal space halfway between the anterior-posterior diameter of the chest. This is known as the **phlebostatic axis**. The nurse should mark this site on the chest wall and use a commercial level to properly level the transducer air-fluid interface to the phlebostatic axis. The air-fluid interface on the pressure monitoring system is at the level of the stopcock closest to the transducer (Figure 5-5). Releveling is done anytime the patient's position is changed. In some settings, the flush/transducer system is attached directly to the patient at the phlebostatic axis, preventing a need to relevel upon patient position change. As long as the patient is supine, studies have found that measurements are accurate when the head of the bed is elevated between 0 and 60 degrees (AACN, 2004).

Once the system is leveled it can now be zeroed. Zeroing is the process of negating the influence of atmospheric air. The zeroing procedure is done by turning the stopcock on the pressure monitoring system off to the patient and open to air. The nurse then activates the zero button on the monitor (Figure 5-6). Zeroing must be done for each pressure monitoring system used. It is done initially during setup, when the monitoring cable is disconnected from the flush system (Ahrens, Penick, & Tucker, 1995). Zeroing is also customarily done at the beginning of each shift and when the values do not fit the clinical picture.

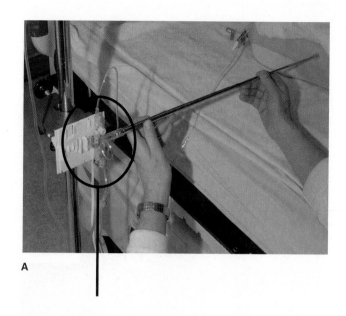

A

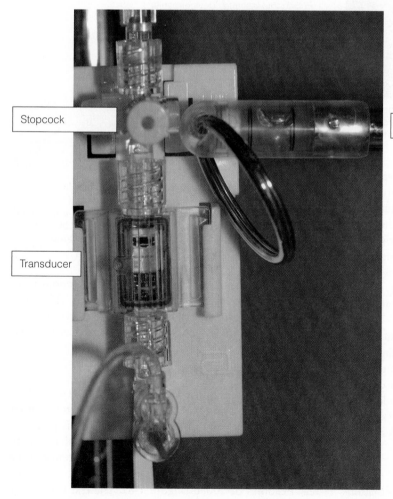

Stopcock

Transducer

Commercial Level

Figure 5-5 Leveling procedure. *A,* The nurse levels the transducer to the phlebostatic axis on the patient and the air-fluid interface. *B,* The air-fluid interface on the pressure monitoring system is at the level of the stopcock closest to the transducer.
(Courtesy Elliot Hospital, Manchester, NH)

B

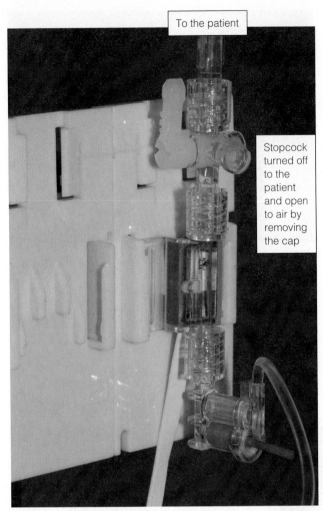

Figure 5-6 Zeroing procedure. To zero the system the stopcock is turned off to the patient and open to air by removing the stopcock cap. The nurse then activates the zero button on the monitor. (Courtesy Elliot Hospital, Manchester, NH)

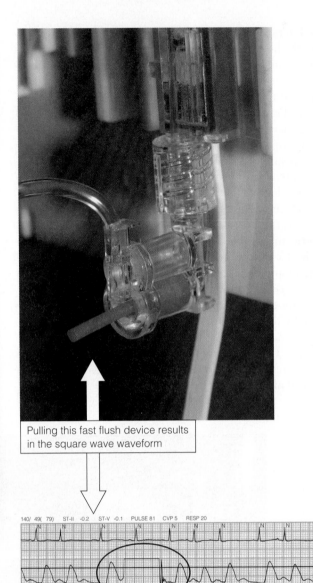

Figure 5-7 Square wave test. By activating the fast flush device, a square wave is displayed on the monitor. The waveform should have a sharp upstroke, a plateau, and a rapid downstroke extending below the baseline followed by one or two small waveforms lasting no more than 0.12 second. (Courtesy Elliot Hospital, Manchester, NH)

The Square Wave Test. The **square wave test** allows the nurse to test the ability of the pressure monitoring system to accurately reflect pressure values. The test is accomplished by activating the fast flush device on the pressure monitoring system and observing the monitor for the resultant pressure waveform (Figure 5-7). The nurse should perform the square wave test on the initial system setup, on every shift, after opening the system (i.e., when drawing blood), and when the values are suspected to be inaccurate (AACN, 2004).

Inaccurate values in pressure monitoring systems can be a result of an overdamped (pressures are underestimated) or underdamped (pressures are overestimated) system. Factors that can cause overdamped values are catheter patency, air bubbles or blood in the tubing, and kinks in the tubing. Factors that can cause underdamped values are excessive tubing length and use of multiple stopcocks.

Arterial Pressure Monitoring

Invasive arterial pressure monitoring is used in situations where blood pressure must be continuously monitored as in

unstable patients or in patients receiving intravenous medications such as vasopressors or vasodilators. The placement of an arterial line also provides the opportunity to easily sample arterial blood for arterial blood gas analysis.

Insertion and Measurement

The arterial catheter insertion can be placed in several arteries. The most common site is the radial artery. Other sites include the femoral, brachial, and doralis pedis arteries. Prior to inserting a catheter in the radial artery, an Allen's test should be performed to test the patency of the radial and ulnar arteries in the event that the radial artery becomes occluded (Figure 5-8). The test is done by having the patient open and close the fist while the radial

TABLE 5-6

Troubleshooting Overdamped and Underdamped Pressure Monitoring Systems

	CAUSE	NURSE CORRECTIVE ACTION
Overdamped waveforms	Reduced catheter patency	• Ensure that the pressure bag is inflated to 300 mm Hg to maintain continuous flow of saline solution through the catheter. • Ensure that there is adequate saline solution in the flush bag. • Inspect for kinks in the tubing preventing the flush solution from reaching the catheter. • Heparinize the solution per institution policy.
	Air bubbles	• Ensure that air is removed from the flush system on intial setup.
	Blood in the tubing	• Ensure that the pressure bag is inflated to 300 mm Hg because a reduction in inflated pressure can cause blood to back up in the tubing. • Ensure that there is adequate saline solution in the flush bag. • Fully clear the pressure system after blood is drawn from the line.
	Kinks in the tubing	• Inspect the tubing periodically to ensure that no kinks are present.
	Incorrect pressure scale on the monitor	• Use of a pressure scale on the monitor significantly higher than the actual monitored pressure can cause the waveform to appear overdamped.
Underdamped waveforms	Excessive tubing length	• Do not add tubing to the premanufactured flush system.
	Use of multiple stopcocks	• Utilize stopcocks available with the premanufactured flush system. Reduce the number added to the system.

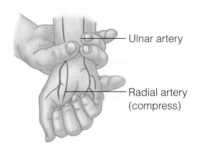

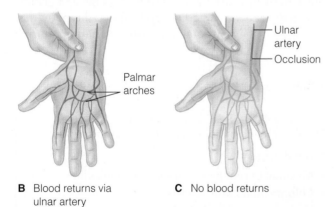

A Open and close fist

B Blood returns via ulnar artery

C No blood returns

Figure 5-8 Allen's test. *A,* Compress both the radial and ulnar arteries and have the patient open and close the fist. *B,* Release the ulnar artery compression and blood should return to the hand. *C,* Ulnar artery compression is released and no blood returns. Occlusion in the ulnar artery. Do not use this radial artery for arterial line insertion.

and ulnar arteries are compressed. Once the hand is open it will appear blanched. When the ulnar compression is released the color should return in 5 seconds. If it does not, the ulnar artery cannot provide collateral flow in the

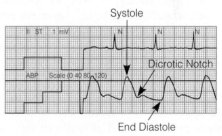

Figure 5-9 Arterial waveform.
(Courtesy of Elliot Hospital, Manchester, NH)

event that the radial artery becomes occluded from the catheter or a thrombus. Another site for the arterial catheter placement should be chosen.

Once the catheter is placed and attached to a pressure monitoring system a waveform and digital value will be displayed on a monitor.

Waveform Interpretation

The arterial waveform has a rapid upstroke as ventricular ejection occurs and the aortic pressure rises (Figure 5-9). The peak of the waveform is the systolic pressure. The ventricular pressure then falls to a point below the aortic pressure and the aortic valve closes. This point is called the **dicrotic notch**. The dicrotic notch signals the end of systole. The pressure continues to fall to the lowest pressure on the waveform, which is the diastolic pressure.

The average pressure during the entire cardiac cycle is the MAP. Identification of the dicrotic notch is one indication that the waveform is accurate. As the waveform becomes overdamped, the dicrotic notch is lost. A waveform that appears overdamped can be a

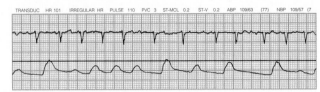

Figure 5-10 Effect of atrial fibrillation on the arterial waveform. Note the varying arterial pressures due to erratic cardiac filling and rhythm irregularity.
(Courtesy of Elliot Hospital, Manchester, NH)

pressure monitor system problem or a hypotensive episode in the patient. The nurse should immediately evaluate the arterial system for accuracy and perform a square wave test. The nurse can easily identify the effects of dysrhythmias on blood pressure by observing the simultaneous invasive arterial pressure waveforms (Figure 5-10).

Nursing Management

The arterial system should be routinely checked to ensure that the connections are tight, that sterile nonvented caps are present on the flush system, that the pressure bag is at 300 mm Hg, and that there is an adequate volume of solution in the flush system. The nurse should perform a neurovascular assessment in the cannulated extremity immediately after insertion and periodically according to institution protocol. The monitor pressure alarm should be activated at all times to alert the nurse of changes in hemodynamic stability or unintentional dislodgment. The nurse should observe the insertion site for signs of infection. Periodic dressing changes and flush tubing and solution changes per institution protocol prevent infection.

Complications

Complications of arterial pressure monitoring include:

- Hemorrhage from the site of insertion
- Thrombosis in the cannula
- Tissue ischemia in the cannulated extremity
- Infection

Central Venous Pressure Monitoring

The **central venous pressure** (CVP) or the **right atrial pressure** (RAP) measures the right-sided preload also known as the right filling pressures. The CVP values are helpful in determining volume status, pulmonary status (i.e., pulmonary hypertension or pulmonary embolism), right-sided cardiac function, and medication effects, particularly those that decrease preload such as nitroglycerin.

Insertion and Measurement

A central venous catheter is placed within a central vein near the right atrium. Once the catheter is connected to a monitoring device a CVP value is obtained. If a pulmonary artery (PA) catheter is in place the RAP is obtained from the proximal port of the catheter (see discussion of PA catheters). The CVP value can be obtained through a pressure monitoring system or through a manometer. The value obtained from a pressure monitoring system is more common and provides the nurse with a pressure value as well as a waveform.

Waveform Interpretation

After ensuring that the system is leveled and zeroed, the nurse must measure the CVP or RAP at the end expiration in the patient's breathing cycle. It is at this point that the effects of intrathoracic pressure variations during

---

SAFETY INITIATIVES   Prevent Central Line Infections

PURPOSE: To prevent catheter-related bloodstream infections by implementing the five components of care called the "central line bundle"

RATIONALE: Central lines (lines that terminate in great vessels) are being used with increasing frequency in hospitalized patients. In fact, nearly half of all intensive care unit (ICU) patients have central lines. The majority of catheter-related bloodstream infections occur in patients with central lines. These infections are particularly dangerous because they may cause hemodynamic changes, organ dysfunction, and, possibly, even death. It is estimated that between 14,000 and 28,000 deaths occur annually due to central line infections. Therefore, instituting a group of best practices, known as a central line bundle, to prevent central line infections is recommended.

HIGHLIGHTS OF RECOMMENDATIONS:
The central line bundle has five key components:

- Hand hygiene
- Maximal barrier precautions on line insertion
- Chlorhexidine skin asepsis
- Utilization of the subclavian vein when possible for nontunneled catheters
- Daily review of line necessity with prompt removal of unnecessary lines

Source: Institute for Healthcare Improvement Available: http://www.ihi.org/IHI/Programs/Campaign/CentralLineInfection.htm

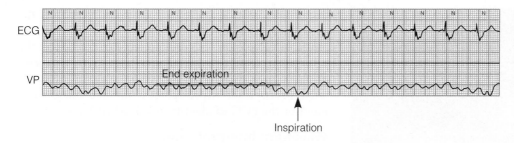

ECG

VP

End expiration

Inspiration

Figure 5-11 CVP tracing in a patient who is spontaneously breathing. Read the CVP value at end exhalation. (Courtesy of Elliot Hospital, Manchester, NH)

respiration are minimized. Because the digital readouts on the monitor reflect pressures throughout respiration, a graphic tracing will allow more accurate identification of end-expiration pressures. The location of end expiration on the graphic tracing is different depending on whether the patient is spontaneously breathing or receiving positive-pressure ventilation from a mechanical ventilator. In the spontaneously breathing patient, the pressures at end expiration are higher (Figure 5-11).

In the patient receiving ventilator breaths, pressures at end expiration are lower than the positive-pressure inspiration breaths. Normal CVP/RAP are 2 to 6 mm Hg (mean). CVP/RAP that are lower than normal usually indicate fluid volume deficit. Conditions causing elevation of the CVP/RAP include:

- Fluid volume excess
- Right ventricular failure
- Pulmonary hypertension
- Tricuspid stenosis or insufficiency
- Pulmonic stenosis or insufficiency
- Pulmonary embolism

Nursing Management

The nurse should record the CVP/RAP values hourly or more frequently based on patient condition. As with all hemodynamic values the trending of the values over time is most valuable. The CVP system should be routinely checked to ensure that the connections are tight, that sterile nonvented caps are present on the flush system, that the pressure bag is at 300 mm Hg, and that there is an adequate volume of solution in the flush system. The monitor pressure alarm should be activated at all times to alert the nurse of changes in hemodynamic stability or unintentional dislodgment. The nurse should observe the insertion site for signs of infection. Periodic dressing changes and flush tubing and solution changes per institution protocol prevent infection. The nurse participates in the multidisciplinary daily review of line necessity to reduce central line catheter-related bloodstream infections (Institute for Healthcare Improvement, 2005).

Complications

Complications for the CVP/RAP measurements are primarily related to central line placement:

- Pneumothorax/hemothorax
- Laceration of major vessels
- Catheter malposition possibly leading to dysrhythmias
- Thrombus formation occurring at the tip of the catheter

Pulmonary Artery Pressure Monitoring

The PA catheter is used to:

- Establish a diagnosis during hemodynamic instability such as determining heart failure
- Guide therapy such as volume repletion, or medication effects such as vasopressors or vasodilators
- Monitor cardiac function for cardiac surgery or in high-risk patients while undergoing vascular procedures such as abdominal aneurysm repair
- Assess the determinants of oxygen delivery such as cardiac output or assess the balance of oxygen supply and demand such as with SvO_2

Catheters

The standard catheter is 7.5 Fr and 110 cm long. The standard catheter has four ports, and when inserted into the heart it has an opening in the right atrium that corresponds to the proximal port, an opening in the pulmonary artery that corresponds to the distal port, a port for inflating a balloon at the distal tip, and a thermistor port for obtaining a cardiac output (Figure 5-12). Additional ports are available in some catheters to provide supplemental volume or medication administration.

Insertion

Prior to PA catheter insertion, an introducer is placed through the internal jugular, subclavian, or femoral vein by a physician or advanced practice nurse. The PA catheter is then threaded through the introducer and into the right atrium. At this point the balloon at the

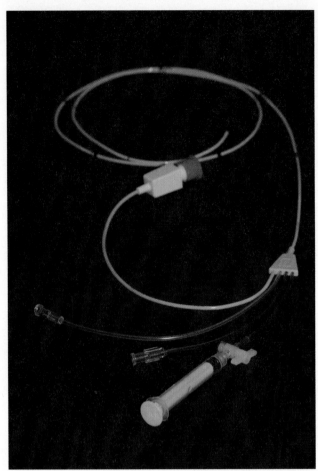

Figure 5-12 Pulmonary artery catheter with four ports.
(Courtesy of Elliot Hospital, Manchester, NH)

distal tip is inflated and the catheter advanced over the tricuspid valve into the right ventricle then over the pulmonary valve into the pulmonary artery. Here the catheter sits for the routine monitoring of PA waveforms and pressures (Figure 5-13). During insertion the ECG must be continuously displayed and the nurse must monitor the ECG to identify any dysrhythmias.

Waveform Interpretation

The following pressures and waveforms can be obtained from the PA catheter: right atrial (RA), PA systolic, PA diastolic, PA mean, and **pulmonary artery wedge pressure (PAWP)**. After ensuring that the system is leveled and zeroed, the measurement of the PA pressures must be done at end expiration in the patient's breathing cycle as described in the section on CVP/RAP.

Waveform Interpretation During Pulmonary Artery Catheter Insertion

Insertion of the PA catheter is guided and placement is validated by waveform analysis (Figure 5-14).

As the catheter is advanced from the central vessel into the right atrium the balloon is inflated to facilitate movement through the heart. In the right atrium, the RAP is obtained. The normal RA value is 2 to 6 mm Hg. Conditions causing elevated or decreased RAPs are found under the CVP/RAP section.

As the catheter is advanced over the tricuspid valve there is a marked increase in systolic pressure. The nurse must pay close attention to the ECG monitor during the

Figure 5-13 Pulmonary artery catheter positioned in the heart. The proximal port communicates with an opening in the right atrium for RA pressures. The distal port communicates with an opening at the end of the catheter for pulmonary artery pressure. The balloon at the end of the catheter is inflated for PAWPs.

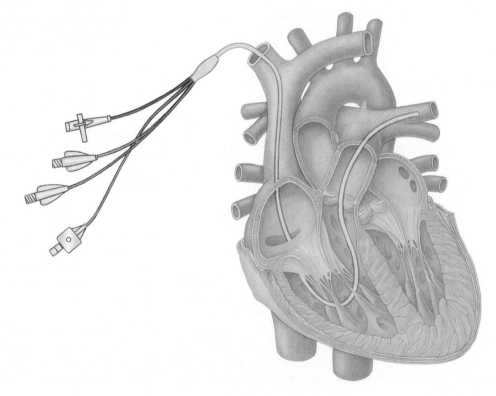

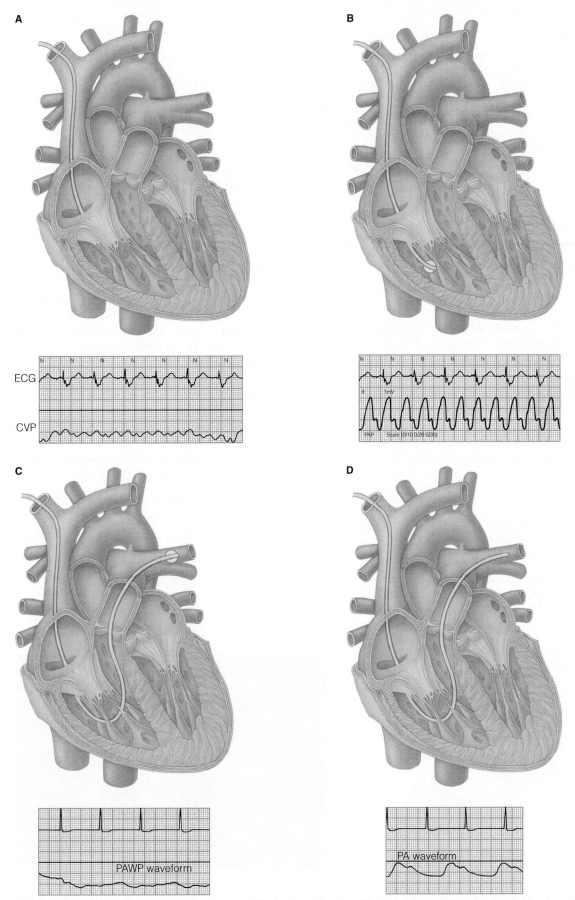

Figure 5-14 Insertion of the pulmonary artery catheter. *A,* During insertion the catheter is first positioned in the right atrium, displaying an RA pressure tracing. *B,* The distal balloon is inflated and the catheter is advanced into the right ventricle, displaying the RV pressure tracing. Note the elevation in systolic pressure. *C,* The catheter is advanced into the pulmonary artery where the distal balloon is wedged in a capillary, displaying the PAWP tracing. *D,* The balloon is deflated, displaying the PA tracing. Note the dicrotic notch.

passing of the catheter through the right ventricle (RV) as ventricular dysrhythmias such as premature ventricular contractions or ventricular tachycardia can occur. Normal RV pressure value is 15 to 25 mm Hg (systolic) and 0 to 8 mm Hg (diastolic). The right ventricular pressure is usually only obtained during insertion of the catheter. The RV pressure that is lower than normal usually indicates fluid volume deficit. Conditions causing elevation of RV pressures include:

- Pulmonary hypertension
- Pulmonic valve stenosis
- Increased pulmonary vascular resistance
- Fluid volume excess
- Cardiac tamponade
- Right heart failure

Once the catheter leaves the RV it is advanced across the pulmonary valve to the PA. The PA waveform has a dicrotic notch that identifies the closure of the pulmonary valve. The systolic pressure is fairly consistent with the RV systolic pressure; however, the diastolic pressure increases once the catheter is in the PA. Normal PA pressure value is: 15 to 25 mm Hg (systolic), 8 to 15 mm Hg (diastolic), 10 to 20 mm Hg (mean). Conditions causing elevation of PA pressures include:

- Increased pulmonary vascular resistance
- Pulmonary hypertension
- Mitral stenosis or insufficiency
- Left heart failure

Conditions causing decreased PA pressure include:

- Fluid volume deficit
- Pulmonic stenosis
- Tricuspid stenosis

Pulmonary Artery Wedge Pressure

During insertion, the catheter is advanced further into the PA until the PAWP is obtained. With the balloon inflated, the catheter floats into, or "wedges," in a smaller pulmonary arteriole or capillary and temporarily stops forward blood flow in that area. When the balloon is inflated the opening at the end of the catheter looks through the pulmonary circulation into the pulmonary veins and into the left atrium (Figure 5-15).

The waveform obtained when the balloon is inflated is the PAWP. This pressure reflects the left atrial pressure. During diastole when the normal mitral valve is open, the PAWP also reflects the left ventricular end-diastolic pressure. Thus, the PAWP gives the nurse an estimate of the preload of the left ventricle. During insertion, once the PAWP is obtained, the position of the catheter is confirmed by deflating the balloon and observing a PA tracing. Normal PAWP value is: 8 to 12 mm Hg (mean). The PAWP that is lower than normal usually indicates fluid volume deficit. Conditions causing elevation of PAWP pressures include:

- Fluid volume excess
- Left ventricular failure
- Mitral stenosis or insufficiency
- Aortic stenosis or insufficiency

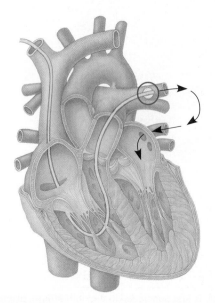
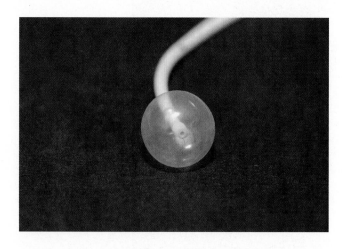

Figure 5-15 When the distal balloon is inflated the catheter is wedged in a small pulmonary capillary, stopping forward flow. The opening at the distal tip (see insert) "looks" forward through the pulmonary circulation and the pulmonary veins and into the left atrium. If the mitral valve is normal, left ventricular end-diastolic pressures can be obtained.
(Balloon insert photo: Courtesy of Elliot Hospital, Manchester, NH)

TABLE 5-7

Pulmonary Artery Catheter Pressures— Normal Values

PRESSURE	NORMAL VALUE
RA	2–6 mm Hg
RV systolic/diastolic	15–25 mm Hg/0–8 mm Hg
PA systolic/diastolic PA mean	15–25 mm Hg/8–15 mm Hg 10–20 mm Hg
PAWP	8–12 mm Hg

See Table 5–7 for normal values of the PA catheter pressures.

Routine Waveform Interpretation and Monitoring

The RAP is obtained from the proximal port of the PA catheter. Per institution policy, the waveform and pressure may be continuously monitored or monitored periodically.

The right ventricular (RV) pressure is not routinely monitored. It is important for the nurse to know the features of the RV waveform because, occasionally, the catheter can slip from the PA back to the RV. The hallmarks of the RV pressure are the lack of dicrotic notch and the low diastolic pressure. Prompt identification of that pressure is important to reduce the time the catheter spends in the RV. The position of the catheter in the RV can potentially cause ventricular dysrhythmia. The procedure for advancement of the catheter back into the PA depends on institution policy. In many institutions, the nurse must notify the physician or advanced practice nurse to advance the catheter back to the PA. Some institutions allow the bedside nurse to inflate the balloon, utilizing the blood flow within the heart to float the catheter back into the PA.

The PA pressures are obtained from the distal port of the PA catheter. The PA systolic, PA diastolic, and mean are routinely documented.

The PAWP is obtained by inflating the balloon at intervals per institution policy or at a frequency ordered by the physician or advanced practice nurse. The balloon should be inflated with the syringe that is provided by the manufacturer. This unique syringe has a stop on it, preventing inflation of more than 1.5 mL of air. Overinflation of the PA balloon can lead to pulmonary capillary rupture and/or inaccurate values. The nurse should slowly inflate the balloon with the air until the PA waveform changes to a PAWP (Figure 5-16). The nurse uses only the volume of air necessary to obtain a waveform change. The balloon is kept inflated for no more than 15 seconds because longer inflation times may lead to pulmonary infarction and rupture. The nurse lets the air passively escape from the balloon then disconnects the syringe and removes the air. Lastly, the nurse places the syringe back on the inflation port and closes the stopcock on the balloon inflation valve. This prevents inadvertent inflation of the balloon.

Occasionally, the PA catheter cannot be wedged. Despite inflation of the balloon the waveform does not change from PA to PAWP. The nurse should ensure that resistance is felt with balloon inflation. If it is not, the balloon may be ruptured. If balloon rupture is suspected, the nurse should (1) tape the balloon inflation port closed, (2) label the port to identify that the port should not be used, and (3) notify the physician or advanced practice nurse. If resistance is felt, the nurse should try repositioning the patient. If that does not work, the physician or advanced practice nurse should be notified because the catheter may need to be advanced.

In the event that the catheter independently migrates to the PAWP position, the nurse must identify the continuously wedged waveform and act quickly. The nurse must ensure that all the air is out of the syringe. Then the nurse should try repositioning the patient. The PA catheter should never be flushed when the catheter is stuck in wedge because this can lead to PA rupture. The physician or advanced practice nurse should be notified to reposition the catheter back into the PA. Some institutions have policies that allow the bedside nurse to withdraw the PA catheter until the PA waveform appears.

Nursing Management

During insertion, the nurse assists the physician or advanced nurse practitioner by priming the pressure monitoring tubing, preparing the insertion kits, connecting the system to appropriate solutions and pressure cables, leveling and zeroing the system, placing a sterile occlusive dressing on the insertion site, documenting the waveforms and values, and setting the appropriate alarms. The nurse should ensure that a chest x-ray has been done to verify catheter placement.

The nurse should record the RA, PA systolic, PA diastolic, and PA mean values hourly or more frequently based on patient condition. As with all hemodynamic

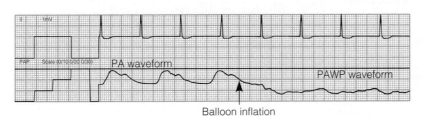

Balloon inflation

Figure 5-16 Pulmonary artery pressure to PAWP pressure with balloon inflation. (Courtesy of Elliot Hospital, Manchester, NH)

values, the trending of the values is most valuable. The PA system should be routinely checked to ensure that the connections are tight, that sterile nonvented caps are present on the flush system, that the pressure bag is at 300 mm HG, and that there is solution in the flush system. The PA pressure alarms should be activated at all times to alert the nurse of changes in hemodynamic stability or unintentional dislodgment. Periodic dressing changes and flush tubing and solution changes (per hospital protocol) prevent infection. The PA pressures should be continuously displayed on the monitor (bedside and central). The nurse monitors the PA waveform to ensure that it does not migrate into the PAWP position.

Complications

The nurse should be aware of complications from the insertion or use of the PA catheter, including:

- Ventricular dysrhythmias
- Pulmonary capillary rupture, pulmonary infarction
- Pneumothorax/hemothorax
- Infection
- Hematoma
- Valvular damage
- PA catheter knotting

Cardiac Output Measurement

Cardiac output measurements are used to assess the hemodynamic function of the patient. They are also used to guide therapy and evaluate patient responses to pharmacological interventions and mechanical ventilation.

Cardiac Output Measurement— Thermodilution Method

The thermodilution method of obtaining cardiac output measurements relies on a volume of normal saline (usually 5 to 10 mL) being injected through the proximal port of the PA catheter. That volume undergoes a temperature change as it moves through the RV and into the PA. This temperature change is picked up by the thermistor on the end of the PA catheter and is converted to a temperature-time curve on the monitor (Figure 5-17). The monitor calculates a CO from that curve. The CO measurement can have significant variations depending on the rate and smoothness of the saline injection. Therefore, between three and five injections are necessary to reliably select several values to average for the CO. Room temperature injectates can be used in most situations because research has proven that they reliably measure CO (Albert, 2005).

Cardiac Output Curve Interpretation

The CO curve should have a smooth upstroke followed by a gradual downslope to the baseline. Common errors

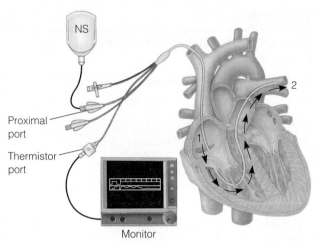

Figure 5-17 Thermodilution cardiac output. 5 to 10 mL of room temperature normal saline is injected through the proximal port. As the solution moves through the heart it changes temperature. This temperature change is picked up by the thermistor on the end of the PA catheter and is converted to a temperature-time curve on the monitor.

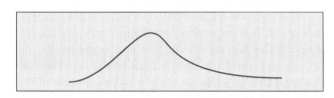

A

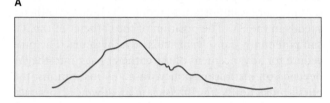

B

Figure 5-18 Thermodilution cardiac output curves. *A*, Normal curves showing a smooth injection technique. *B*, An abnormal curve caused by erratic injection.

with the curve are uneven upstrokes and long injection times (Figure 5-18).

Derived Hemodynamic Values

Once the CO value is obtained, several other derived hemodynamic values can be calculated. The CI and SV are commonly calculated. Indicators of afterload such as SVR and PVR as well as indicators of contractility such as stroke work index can also be calculated. Commonly, the bedside monitor system performs these calculations.

Nursing Management

Prior to the beginning of the procedure, the nurse must ensure that the computation constant is appropriate for the catheter size and volume of injectate. Any discrepancy in this value can lead to inaccurate readings. The nurse should inject at end expiration to limit variability in CO measurements related to respiratory cycle. Injections should be done smoothly and as fast as possible over less than 4 seconds. It is important to maintain the patency of the proximal port through a continuous infusion, because a clotted proximal port renders the catheter of no use for thermodilution CO measurement. Toward that end, at the completion of the CO procedure, the nurse should return the stopcock of the proximal port to its original position and ensure that infusions are flowing through the proximal port.

Alternatives to Thermodilution Cardiac Output Monitoring

The searches for less-invasive or noninvasive methods in obtaining CO and hemodynamic measurement have identified several techniques. Each one of these methods differs in how the information is derived. The nurse must review the research on each of these technologies to ensure that it is as accurate as the invasive CO techniques via a PA catheter.

Arterial Pressure-Based Cardiac Output Monitoring

In this system a sensor is attached to the patient's existing arterial pressure system. One branch of the cable goes to the monitor to display the arterial waveform and the other goes to a specialized monitor to analyze the wave-

form. The CO is determined from an algorithm, utilizing the arterial pulse waveform and pulse pressures. Studies have shown that the technology is comparable to existing invasive methods of CO determination (Headley, 2006).

Noninvasive Hemodynamic Monitoring Measurement

Noninvasive measuring of hemodynamic monitoring can be accomplished using impedance cardiography and esophageal Doppler monitoring (Prentice & Sona, 2006). Impedance cardiography measures resistance to transmission of small electrical currents either throughout the body or in one area such as the chest. These changes are associated with changes in the blood and plasma. During systole impedance is increased and during diastole the impedance returns to baseline. Through obtaining measured parameters such as HR, ejection time, and fluid content, calculated parameters such as SV, CO/CI SVR, and left cardiac work index can be obtained. The hemodynamic data are not directly equivalent to the conventional invasive PA catheter parameters; however, impedance cardiography can be a valuable adjunct to other monitoring devices (Albert, 2005).

In esophageal Doppler monitoring, a transducer probe is placed into the esophagus. This probe transmits and receives a signal that picks up the velocity and distance of the blood flow in the descending aorta. This device can provide an estimation of CO, preload, and contractility.

CARDIODYNAMIC SUMMARY

Understanding cardiodynamics and hemodynamic regulation helps the nurse and other members of the health care team to determine the status of the patient. The technologies described in this section must be utilized

carefully. The values they supply should be interpreted in conjunction with an accurate and thorough assessment of the patient.

CRITICAL THINKING QUESTIONS

1. What factors affect the tissue oxygen supply and demand?

2. What are the four determinants of cardiac output? What is the relationship between preload and contractility?

3. Upon entering a patient's room the nurse notices blood backing up in the tubing leading from the arterial catheter to the flush/transducer system.
   a. What are the nursing actions to correct this?
   b. Will this cause the arterial waveform to be overdamped or underdamped?

4. What patients would be candidates for a pulmonary artery catheter?

5. What conditions would cause an increase in RA pressure?

6. A patient has a PA catheter in place. The nurse notices that the waveform on the monitor has independently changed from a pulmonary artery tracing to a PAWP tracing.
   a. What are the potential complications of this change?
   b. What are the nursing actions to correct this?

See answers to Critical Thinking Questions in the Answer Section at the back of the book.

EXPLORE MEDIALINK
http://www.prenhall.com/perrin

Additional interactive resources for this chapter can be found on the Web site at
http://www.prenhall.com/perrin. Click on "Chapter 5" to select activities for this chapter.

Nursing Care Plan

NCLEX Review Questions

MediaLinks:
- Animation of Thermodilution Cardiac Output
- Animation of PA Catheter Placement
- Auscultation Assistant
- Medtronic
- Cardiac Cycle
- Spencer S. Eccles Health Sciences Library
- Thinkwell's Cardiac Cycle

- Interactive Physiology
- Central Venous Pressure Monitoring
- Central Venous Pressure Waveforms
- The Patient is Hypotensive: Is it Due to Hypovolemia?
- Hemodynamic Monitoring: Arterial Pressure Monitoring
- Monitoring Arterial Blood Pressure: What You May Not Know
- Pulmonary Artery Pressure Monitoring
- Pulmonary Artery Catheter Education Project

MediaLink Applications

REFERENCES

Ahrens, T., Penick, J. C., & Tucker, M. K. (1995). Frequency requirements for zeroing transducers in hemodynamic monitoring. *American Journal of Critical Care, 4*(6), 466–471.

Albert, N. (2005). Cardiac output measurement techniques (invasive). In D. J. Wiegand & K. K. Carlson (Eds.), *AACN procedure manual* (5th ed.). St. Louis, MO: Elsevier Saunders.

American Association of Critical-Care Nurses (AACN). (2004, May). *Pulmonary artery pressure measurement.* Retrieved April 26, 2007, from http://www.aacn.org/AACN/practiceAlert.nsf/Files/PAPM%20PDF/$file/PAP%20Measurement%2005-2004.pdf

Headley, J. (2006). Arterial pressure based technologies: A new trend in cardiac output monitoring. *Critical Care Nursing Clinics of North America, 18,* 179–187.

Institute for Healthcare Improvement. (2005). *Getting started kit: Prevent central line infections.* Retrieved April 26, 2007, from http://www.ihi.org/NR/rdonlyres/BF4CC102-C564-4436-AC3A-0C57B1202872/0/CentralLinesHowtoGuideFINAL720.pdf

Kee, J. L. (Ed.). (2005). *Laboratory and diagnostic tests with nursing implications* (7th ed.). Upper Saddle River, NJ: Pearson/Prentice Hall.

Prentice, D., & Sona, C. (2006). Esophageal Doppler monitoring for hemodynamic assessment. *Critical Care Nursing Clinics of North America, 18,* 189–193.

Preuss, T., & Weigand, D. (2005). Pulmonary artery catheter insertion (assist) and pressure monitoring. In D. J. Weigand & K. K. Carlson (Eds.), *AACN procedure manual* (5th ed.). St. Louis, MO: Elsevier Saunders.

Reinhart, K., Kuhn, H. J., Hartog, C., & Bredle, D. L. (2004). Continuous central venous and pulmonary artery oxygen saturation monitoring in the critically ill. *Intensive Care Medicine, 30,* 1572–1578.

Care of the Patient Experiencing Shock or Heart Failure

Shirley Jackson, MS, RN, CCRN, CCNS

Learning Outcomes

Upon completion of this chapter, the learner will be able to:

1. Recognize the manifestations of hypovolemia.

2. Describe hemodynamic findings indicative of hypovolemia.

3. Discuss volume replacement for the patient with hypovolemia.

4. Explain the pathophysiologic and neurohormonal mechanisms of heart failure.

5. Compare and contrast systolic and diastolic dysfunction.

6. Recognize the manifestations of heart failure.

7. Describe the hemodynamic findings indicative of heart failure.

8. Differentiate between the hemodynamic findings of hypovolemia and heart failure.

9. Explain collaborative management of the patient with heart failure.

10. Recognize the patient with acutely decompensated heart failure.

11. Describe collaborative management strategies appropriate for the patient with acutely decompensated heart failure.

Abbreviations

ACE	Angiotensin-Converting Enzymes
AHA	American Heart Association
ARBs	Angiotensin II Receptor Blockers
BiPAP	Bilevel Positive Airway Pressure
BNP	B-Type Natriuretic Peptide
CHF	Congestive Heart Failure
CPAP	Continuous Positive Airway Pressure
CRT	Cardiac Resynchronization Therapy
ICD	Implantable Cardioverter Defibrillator
LVEF	Left Ventricular Ejection Fraction
MAP	Mean Arterial Pressure
NYHA	New York Heart Association
SV	Stroke Volume
SVR	Systemic Vascular Resistance

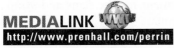

MEDIALINK
http://www.prenhall.com/perrin

See the Companion Website for chapter-specific resources at www.prenhall.com/perrin.

VISUAL MAP Heart Failure Overview

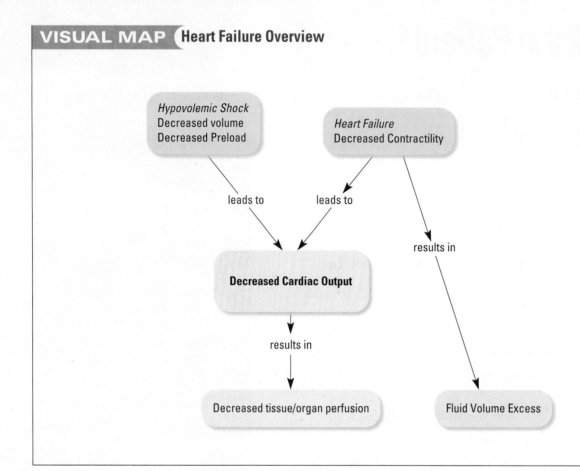

Shock

Shock is a condition in which a systemic decrease in perfusion to tissues and organs leads to poor gas and nutrient exchange. The nurse must be able to recognize the impending shock state and administer treatment in a timely fashion. Delays in recognition and treatment can lead to irreversible shock and multisystem organ failure.

Hypovolemic Shock

Hypovolemic shock results from a decreased circulating volume. Loss of approximately 15% to 30% or more of the normal blood volume can produce hypovolemic shock.

Etiology

The etiology of hypovolemic shock can be divided into two categories: hemorrhage and fluid loss. Causes of hemorrhage include GI bleeding, trauma, surgery, or ruptured aneurysm. Fluid loss may occur from vomiting or diarrhea, burns, or loss of fluids internally in cavities (e.g., ascites). In some situations the intravascular fluid is redistributed into the interstitial space (third spacing), resulting in a deficit in intravascular volume such as occurs in sepsis. Failure of mechanisms regulating water balance can lead to a fluid volume deficit. Diabetes insipidus (DI) results from a deficiency in antidiuretic hormone (ADH) release from the posterior lobe of the pituitary gland. Trauma or surgery to the pituitary gland can lead to de-

creased ADH. This deficiency in ADH leads to excessive urine output and, if left unchecked, hypovolemic shock.

Pathophysiology

A thorough understanding of the pathophysiology of hypovolemic shock can help identify the signs and symptoms of shock. Baroreceptors in the arch of the aorta and in the carotid arteries react to a drop in circulating volume and reduction in blood pressure by increasing the heart rate and vascular resistance. As the vasoconstriction occurs, blood is shunted away from the skin, kidneys, and gut to the major organs like the brain, heart, and lungs. The reduced blood flow to the kidneys stimulates the renin-angiotensin aldosterone system, leading to more vasoconstriction and conservation of water and sodium, maximizing the intravascular volume but further reducing the urine output. These compensatory mechanisms can keep the blood pressure and cardiac output normalized for a short period; however, as circulating volume is further reduced the compensatory mechanism fails.

Focused Assessment of the Patient

The nurse assesses the patient for the signs and symptoms indicating hypovolemia:

*   Hypotension
*   Orthostatic hypotension

VISUAL MAP Hypovolemia

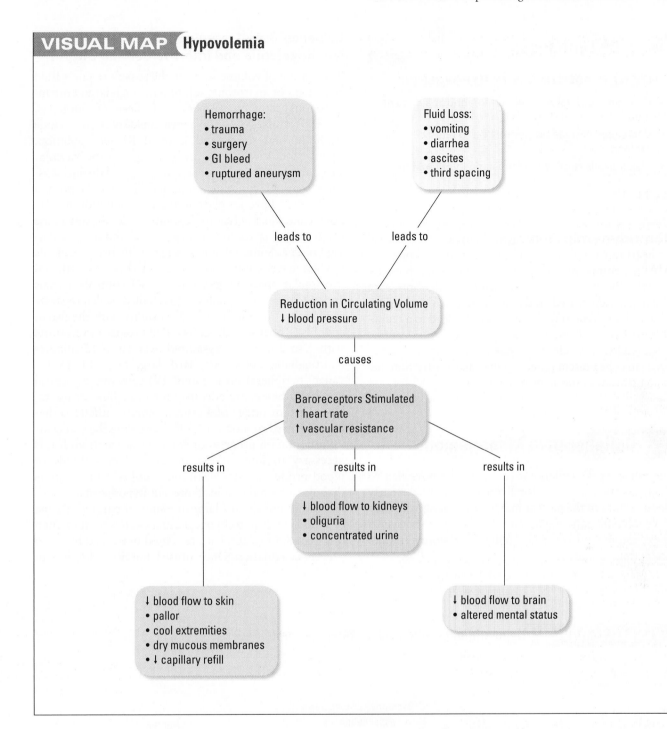

- Tachycardia
- Reduced capillary refill
- Dry mucous membranes
- Poor skin turgor
- Thirst
- Weight loss
- Oliguria
- Concentrated urine
- Altered mental status

Diagnostic Criteria

The nurse reviews laboratory studies for:

- Hypernatremia (serum levels above 145 mEq/L)
- Increased hematocrit (Hct) due to hemoconcentration (if patient is actively bleeding, Hct may drop)
- Arterial blood gases: metabolic acidosis
- Elevated serum lactate (serum lactate greater than 4 mmol/L)
- Reduced mixed venous oxygen saturation (SvO_2 less than 60%; $ScvO_2$ less than 70%)

Nursing Diagnoses

PATIENT PRESENTING WITH HYPOVOLEMIA

- Deficient fluid volume related to abnormal loss of fluid
- Decreased cardiac output related to altered preload
- Risk for falls related to orthostatic hypotension

Hemodynamic Findings. In hypovolemic shock the heart rate is increased and the mean arterial pressure (MAP), central venous pressure/right atrial pressure (CVP/RAP), and pulmonary artery wedge pressure (PAWP) are decreased, reflecting a reduced preload. A reduction in circulating volume may also lead to a reduction in stroke volume (SV) and cardiac output/cardiac index (CO/CI). An elevated systemic vascular resistance (SVR) may be present reflecting the vasoconstriction due to compensatory mechanisms.

Collaborative Management

The nurse works collaboratively with the physician to identify patients at risk for hypovolemic shock. Early identification of the patient in hypovolemic shock is key to a successful patient outcome. The goal of treatment is to expand the intravascular volume to restore a normal circulating volume.

Evidence-Based Interventions to Restore Normovolemia and Improve Cardiac Output

Restoration of volume status in the patient requires fluid challenges of an isotonic solution through large-bore intravenous catheters (American College of Surgeons, 2004). Examples of isotonic **crystalloid** solutions include 0.9% normal saline and lactated Ringer's solution. These isotonic solutions are infused into the vascular space and stay there long enough to expand the intravascular space. Hypotonic solutions, like 0.45% normal saline (NS), have no place in fluid resuscitation for hypovolemic shock. Hypotonic solutions do not stay in the intravascular space long enough to expand the circulating volume. Some references suggest the use of **colloids** in volume resuscitation. Even though they stay in the intravascular space longer, randomized controlled trials and extensive meta-analyses have failed to demonstrate a difference in morbidity and mortality with the use of colloids (Roberts et al., 2004). Fluid resuscitation starts with 1 to 2 liters of crystalloid over 10 to 15 minutes (Cottingham, 2006). Standard, large (e.g., 14- to 16-gauge) peripheral intravenous (IV) catheters or central venous catheters are adequate for most fluid resuscitation. The advantage of a central venous catheter is that it can be used to monitor CVP, thus giving the clinicians information on progress of volume resuscitation. If it is necessary to infuse large amounts of crystalloids or blood products, some institutions utilize rapid infusers that also warm the fluid to prevent hypothermia.

Rapid infusion of large amounts of citrated plasma or blood can lead to hypocalcemia (serum total calcium less than 8.5 mg/dL). Citrate is used in banked blood to prevent coagulation. Once infused, the citrate binds with

VISUAL MAP Hypovolemia Collaborative Management

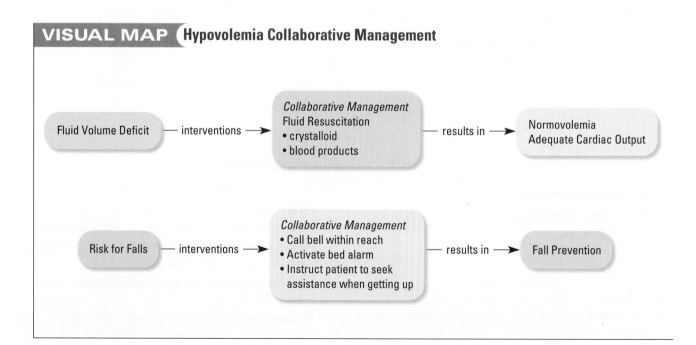

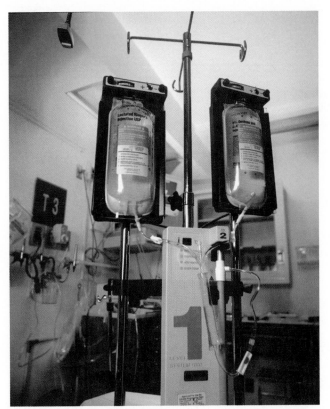

Figure 6-1 Rapid fluid infuser. Note the two solutions that can be infused together. The solutions are warmed by the blue heating cylinder.
(Courtesy Elliot Hospital, Manchester, NH)

the calcium in the patient's blood, leading to low serum calcium levels. A discussion of hypocalcemia, including manifestations and treatment, is found in Chapter 14, Care of the Patient with Acute Renal Failure. ∞ A positive response to fluid therapy would be indicated by an increasing CVP to a normal range, MAP of at least 60 mm Hg, and urine output greater than 0.5 to 1 mL/kg/hr (Merck Manual Online Medical Library, 2005). If the patient is in hypovolemic shock from hemorrhage, the nurse should anticipate orders for packed red blood cells (RBCs). The loss of RBCs diminishes oxygen (O_2)-carrying capacity and cannot be corrected by crystalloids alone. The nurse must assess the patient closely during fluid resuscitation for signs of respiratory compromise from pulmonary congestion. Signs and symptoms indicating pulmonary congestion and inadequate oxygenation include tachypnea, crackles on auscultation, and decreased oxygen saturation.

Evidence-Based Interventions to Prevent Falls

The patient who is experiencing a reduction in fluid volume will be at risk of falling. The presence of orthostatic hypotension may lead to dizziness, lightheadedness, and syncope when sitting up or ambulating. The nurse should remind the patient to seek assistance when getting up. The call bell should be placed within easy reach and the patient should be instructed to get up slowly.

The bed alarm should be activated to alert the nurse if the patient gets up independently.

Treatment of Specific Causative Disorder

Volume resuscitation in hypovolemic shock is only a temporary measure until the etiology can be identified and corrected. In the case of hypovolemia caused by trauma, GI bleeding, or ruptured aneurysm definitive surgery or other intervention is needed to correct the hemorrhaging. In the case of burns, fluid resuscitation must be continued until the patient is hemodynamically stable and the burn area is stable. In DI, administration of replacement ADH may be indicated to reduce the excessive urinary output.

Prevention and Detection of Common or Life-Threatening Complications

Renal insufficiency, cerebral ischemia, and irreversible shock are the primary concerns for complications. Renal insufficiency or renal failure due to the prerenal etiology of hypovolemia is a serious complication. Prevention strategies, early detection, and management can be found in Chapter 14. ∞

The brain is a major organ that depends on adequate perfusion for oxygenation and essential nutrients. Early identification and correction of the fluid volume deficit in hypovolemic shock is necessary to prevent cerebral ischemia. As the brain receives less blood flow as a result of hypovolemia, the reduction in end-organ perfusion leads to mental status changes. Mental status changes appear along a continuum from agitation and confusion to lethargy and coma. Identification of the early signs of cerebral ischemia can alert the nurse to the need for immediate volume resuscitation.

Authorities believe that irreversible shock leads to pooling of blood in the capillaries—the result of reduced vasomotor tone and reduced flow through capillaries due to a complex mechanism such as plugging by neutrophils and impaired vasomotor regulation (Rose & Mandel, 2005). Regardless of the mechanism, any administered fluid is sequestered in the capillary circulation. This elevation in the capillary hydrostatic pressure results in the movement of fluid out of the vascular space into the interstitium, further reducing tissue perfusion. Early identification and correction of the fluid volume deficit in hypovolemic shock is necessary to prevent the reduced tissue perfusion from becoming irreversible.

Heart Failure

Heart failure (HF) is a major health care concern. Over five million patients in the United States have heart failure and over 500,000 patients are newly diagnosed each year (Hunt, 2005). The incidence of heart failure among the elderly is higher than that among the younger population. As the population ages it is thought that the

VISUAL MAP Heart Failure

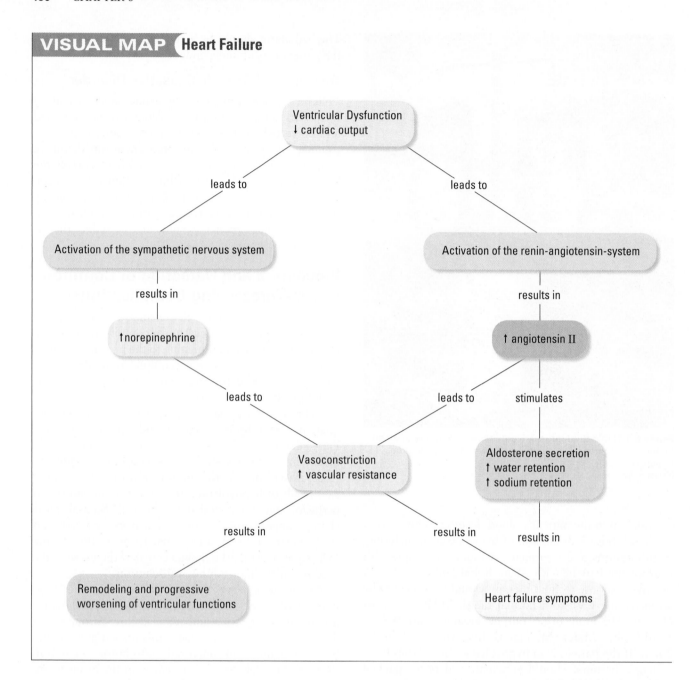

incidence of heart failure will increase. Heart failure is a clinical syndrome in which the ventricle is unable to fill or to eject blood. This abnormality of cardiac function results in an inability of the heart to deliver adequate volumes of blood to tissues at rest or during normal activity. As a result, tissues are inadequately perfused, leading to cellular hypoxia and disorders in metabolism. Heart failure may be acute or chronic.

Pathophysiology

Heart failure starts with some injury or stress to the myocardium and progresses over time. As the heart function fails and the CO decreases, compensatory mechanisms such as the sympathetic nervous system and renin-angiotensin-

aldosterone system are activated. The role of these compensatory mechanisms is to maintain perfusion to the vital organs. While these compensatory mechanisms are beneficial in the short term, long-term activation of these mechanisms can be deleterious, leading to increased afterload, pulmonary and peripheral edema, and eventual chamber dilation and/or hypertrophy—a process called **remodeling**. This remodeling leads to progressive worsening of ventricular dysfunction. The understanding of the role of these neurohormonal factors in the development of heart failure has improved in the past several years. The nurse must comprehend the pathophysiology of heart failure to understand the rationales for both pharmacological and nonpharmacological treatment.

TABLE 6–1

Etiologies of Heart Failure

- Ischemia to the heart
- Hypertension
- Myocarditis
- Valvular heart disease
- Dysrhythmias, particularly tachycardias
- Lupus erythematosus
- Alcohol abuse
- Cocaine abuse
- Peripartum cardiomyopathy
- Hyperthyroidism
- Obstructive sleep apnea
- Sarcoidosis
- Idiopathic

Neurohormonal Mechanisms

The primary neurohormonal mechanisms involved in response to heart failure are the sympathetic nervous system and the renin-angiotensin-aldosterone system. In response to a decreased CO, activation of the sympathetic nervous system releases norepinephrine, causing increases in vasoconstriction, heart rate, and contractility. Activation of the renin-angiotensin-aldosterone system further increases vasoconstriction through the activation of angiotensin II, a potent vasoconstrictor. Activation of the renin-angiotensin-aldosterone system also stimulates aldosterone, expanding fluid volume through sodium reabsorption.

Etiologies

The etiologies of heart failure are varied from direct insults to the myocardium to failure of the myocardium in specific systemic diseases. See Table 6–1.

The two most common etiologies of HF are ischemia to the heart and hypertension. Ischemic heart disease is a major cause of HF. Damage to the heart can be due either to damage from prior myocardial infarctions or chronic ischemia that is potentially reversible through myocardial revascularization. Hypertension is also the cause of heart failure in many patients. Chronic hypertension increases the load on the left ventricle, eventually causing failure.

Other cardiovascular causes of heart failure include myocarditis, valvular heart disease, and dysrhythmias. Damage to the myocardium can occur as a result of inflammation (viral) or when systemic disorders such as lupus erythematosus cause inflammation of the myocardium. Valve dysfunction such as aortic stenosis can increase the left ventricular load, leading to further cardiac injury. Dysrhythmias, particularly those that are tachycardic, can increase work on the heart, leading to failure. Alcohol consumption in large quantities has a toxic effect on heart muscle cells leading to alcoholic cardiomyopathy. Habitual abuse of alcohol results in a dilated heart that is too inefficient to pump adequately. The adrenergic stimulation and vasoconstrictive action

Gerontological Considerations

More than 80% of the people in the United States with heart failure are older than 65 years of age, with the majority of people being older than 75.

Heart failure is the leading diagnosis at hospital discharge for patients over the age of 65.

The leading causes of heart failure in older adults are hypertension and coronary artery disease. Most older adults with heart failure have other illnesses as well.

There is evidence that a significant number of older adults with heart failure do not receive evidence-based, AHA recommended care including angiotensin-converting enzymes (ACE) inhibitors and beta blockers.

Some studies indicate that older heart failure patients' knowledge of appropriate diet and medication management is poor. Pharmacy records indicate that prescriptions are not promptly refilled. Patient records indicate that daily weights are not consistently obtained.

The development of heart failure is associated with significant cognitive impairment in the older adult and mental performance may be at least partly related to ejection fraction.

Older patients with heart failure are more likely to be depressed and the presence of depression worsens patient outcomes.

of cocaine appear to be important factors leading to cocaine cardiomyopathy. Peripartum cardiomyopathy is the rare development of a dilated heart leading to heart failure within the last month of pregnancy or within 5 months after delivery. The exact etiology of peripartum cardiomyopathy is unknown. Patients with hyperthyroidism can develop hyperthyroid cardiomyopathy. This rate-related form of heart failure is thought to develop as a result of persistant sinus tachycardia or atrial fibrillation with an uncontrolled heart rate. Studies have suggested that obstructive sleep apnea may contribute to the progression of heart failure by causing recurrent myocardial hypoxemia, sympathetic activation, and an increased oxygen demand. The development of infiltrative granulomas called sarcoidosis can cause restrictive cardiomyopathy. Lastly, the cause can be idiopathic.

Classification

The classifications of heart failure are organized into a structural classification, systolic vs. diastolic dysfunction, and a functional classification or how well the patient can function with the disease.

Systolic Versus Diastolic Heart Failure

Systolic dysfunction is impaired left ventricular contractility with a reduced **ejection fraction**. The ejection fraction is the percentage of blood ejected from the left ventricle with each contraction—normal is 55% to 75%. This impaired contractility leads to a reduction in CO. Diastolic dysfunction appears when the ventricle is normal size but hypertrophied, leading to loss of left ventricular diastolic relaxation and distensibility. This preserves the normal ejection fraction but impairs filling, leading to elevated filling pressures and PAWPs.

Classifications

Traditionally the patients were classified according to the New York Heart Association (NYHA) by degree of symptoms. The patients are assigned to one of four categories according to the degree of exertion needed to elicit symptoms. The difficulty with this classification is that it is variable depending on what medications the patients are on or off and the degree of patient compliance with the medications and diet. In 2001, the American College of Cardiology/American Heart Association (ACC/AHA) developed a classification system that emphasized the development and progression of heart failure, concentrating on risk factors and structural abnormalities. It is categorized into four stages from high risk for development to refractory end-stage heart failure (Hunt, 2005). See Table 6–2 for a comparison between the NYHA and ACC/AHA classifications (Caboral, 2006).

Focused Assessment of the Patient

The assessment of the acutely ill patient with heart failure will exhibit signs, symptoms, and laboratory alterations from the effects of basically two major dysfunctions: decreased CO leading to volume overload and end-organ hypoperfusion.

Volume overload leads to:

- Dyspnea on exertion
- Orthopnea
- **Paroxysmal nocturnal dyspnea** (PND)
- Peripheral edema
- Abdominal pain and distention
- Weight gain
- Crackles on pulmonary auscultation

- Elevation of venous pressures (CVP, PAWP)
- Presence of S_3 or S_4 upon cardiac auscultation

End-organ hypoperfusion is manifested by:

- Decreased exercise tolerance
- Fatigue
- Dizziness
- Syncope or near syncope
- Palpitations
- Hypotension
- Tachycardia
- Cool extremities
- Delayed capillary refill
- Decreased urinary output

The nurse looks for evidence of worsening of the heart failure, including increasing dyspnea, tachypnea, tachycardia, fatigue, and exercise intolerance. Dysrhythmias such as ventricular ectopy or atrial fibrillation may exist in the presence of worsening disease. A dropping oxygen saturation, usually less than 90%, may indicate deteriorating pulmonary status due to pulmonary edema.

Diagnostic Criteria

In the labs of a heart failure patient, hyponatremia may indicate volume overload. Elevated BUN and serum creatinine may identify renal insufficiency due to low CO. Disorders of potassium may be present as a result of medication side effects. The nurse should be aware that most diuretics cause hypokalemia. Hyperkalemia may be present in patients taking ACE inhibitors or aldosterone inhibitors. Cardiac enzymes may be elevated if ischemia is the cause of the heart failure. Thyroid function tests may identify hyperthyroidism as a cause of heart failure or associated dysrhythmias. **B-type natriuretic peptide** (BNP) is released in response to increased ventricular filling pressures. In the patient who presents with increasing dyspnea, an elevated BNP suggests heart failure as a cause of the dyspnea.

TABLE 6–2

New York Heart Association (NYHA) and American College of Cardiology/American Heart Association (ACC/AHA) Classifications

ACC/AHA	NYHA
Stage A (at high risk for HF)	
Stage B (structural heart disease, asymptomatic)	I (no limitation on physical activity)
Stage C (structural heart disease, with symptoms)	II–III (limitations on physical activity)
Stage D (refractory end-stage HF)	IV (symptoms at rest)

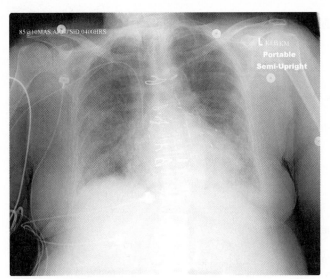

Figure 6-2 Chest x-ray showing infiltrates suggestive of pulmonary edema.
(Courtesy Elliot Hospital, Manchester, NH)

Chest X-Ray

A chest x-ray will be done looking for enlarged heart, enlarged pulmonary vessels, and/or pulmonary edema (Figure 6-2). The nurse works collaboratively with the physician or advanced practice nurse to review the chest x-ray reports.

Electrocardiogram

The nurse reviews the electrocardiogram (ECG) for dysrhythmias that may occur in patients with heart failure. Common dysrhythmias include sinus tachycardia at rest, atrial fibrillation, and ventricular ectopy such as premature ventricular complexes. Cardiac ischemia may appear as ST segment and T wave abnormalities.

Noninvasive Cardiac Testing

An echocardiogram is performed in most patients presenting with heart failure. Through this test, the function of the ventricles is assessed, including left ventricular (LV) size and wall thickness. Assessment of the heart valve function is also done looking for any valve stenosis or insufficiency. An estimate of the left ventricular ejection fraction (LVEF) is also done. Many patients with heart failure have a reduced ejection fraction (less than 40%); however, a normal LVEF does not exclude heart failure because diastolic dysfunction, ischemia, or valvular disease may all cause HF with normal LVEF.

Invasive Cardiac Testing

The patient may undergo a cardiac catheterization to further assess the patient's volume status, evaluate cardiac ischemia, measure CO, and/or assess pulmonary artery pressures.

Nursing Diagnoses

PATIENT PRESENTING WITH HEART FAILURE

- Excess fluid volume
- Impaired gas exchange (acute decompensated heart failure)
- Decreased cardiac output related to decreased myocardial contractility
- Fatigue related to decreased cardiac output
- Activity intolerance related to imbalance between oxygen supply and demand

Hemodynamic Findings

If the patient has a central line or a pulmonary artery (PA) catheter in place, the nurse monitors the hemodynamic values for trends indicating volume overload or cardiac decompensation. Elevated filling pressures may be present in heart failure. Elevations in right filling pressures (RA/CVP) can cause systemic venous pressure elevations, leading to peripheral edema and ascites. Elevations in left filling pressures (PAWP) can cause pulmonary capillary pressure elevations, leading to pulmonary edema. The CO may be normal due to adequate physiological compensation or reduced due to failure of those mechanisms. Elevation in systemic and pulmonary vascular resistance may be present, caused by the neurohormonal imbalances, which lead to vasoconstriction in an effort to preserve blood flow to the critical organs.

Collaborative Management

The nurse works collaboratively with the physician to manage the symptoms of heart failure, reduce the progression of the disease, and prolong survival. The management of the patient involves both pharmacological and nonpharmacological measures. Lifestyle modifications are important in all patients with heart failure. These include smoking cessation, restriction of alcohol consumption, salt restriction, weight reduction in obese patients, and cardiac rehabilitation in stable patients. One of the mainstays of treatment for the heart failure patient are medications directed at the neurohormonal activation of the sympathetic nervous system and the renin-angiotensin-aldosterone system. By blocking the neurohormonal activation, symptoms of heart failure are reduced and progression of the disease is slowed. Leading drug categories in this process are beta blockers, ACE inhibitors, and angiotensin II receptor blockers (ARBs). In some patients the use of aldosterone antagonists will also be beneficial.

VISUAL MAP **Heart Failure Collaborative Management**

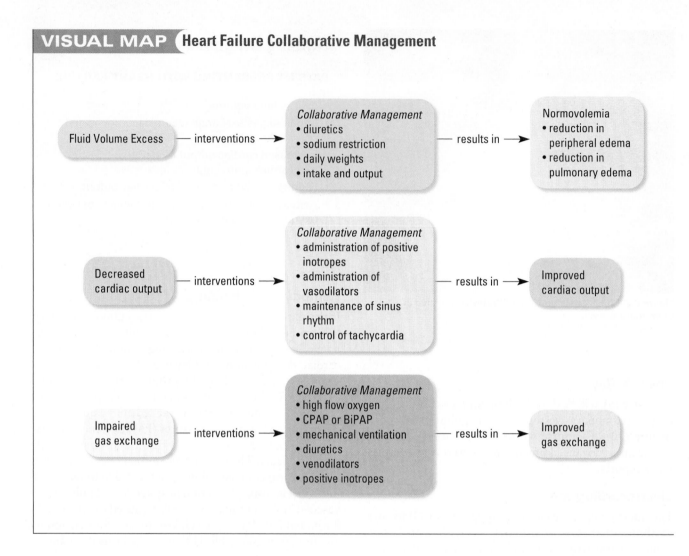

The blockade of the renin-angiotensin-aldosterone system takes place at different physiological points (Figure 6-3). The ACE inhibitors block the conversion of angiotensin I to angiotensin II, thus preventing vasoconstriction. The ARBs block the attachment of angiotensin II to the receptor, also preventing vasoconstriction. Examples of ACE inhibitors and ARBs are found in Table 6–3.

Nursing Management

The nurse should expect that patients with heart failure due to systolic dysfunction will be on ACE inhibitors unless they are contraindicated. Contraindication to ACE inhibitors are renal failure (serum creatinine greater than 3 mg/dL, hyperkalemia (greater than 5.5 mmol/L), **angioedema**, or very low systolic pressure, usually less than 80 mm-Hg. Patients with diastolic dysfunction may not be on these medications because the resultant hypotension can exacerbate the slow diastolic filling.

When administering any ACE inhibitor or ARB the nurse should:

- Assess for side effects; the two most common are dizziness and hypotension. Prior to administering either medication, the nurse should evaluate the patient's blood pressure ensuring that it is adequate before administration. Occasionally ARBs and ACE inhibitors are used together. If the patient is receiving both medications, the nurse must use particular caution to evaluate the patient's blood pressure prior to administration because both drugs can cause hypotension.

- Periodically review the lab values, looking for hyperkalemia and worsening renal function. ARBs can be used in patients who are unable to tolerate ACE inhibitors due to side effects.

- Assess for concomitant administration of nonsteroidal anti-inflammatory drugs (NSAIDs). NSAIDs may reduce the vasodilation and unloading effects of ACE inhibitors.

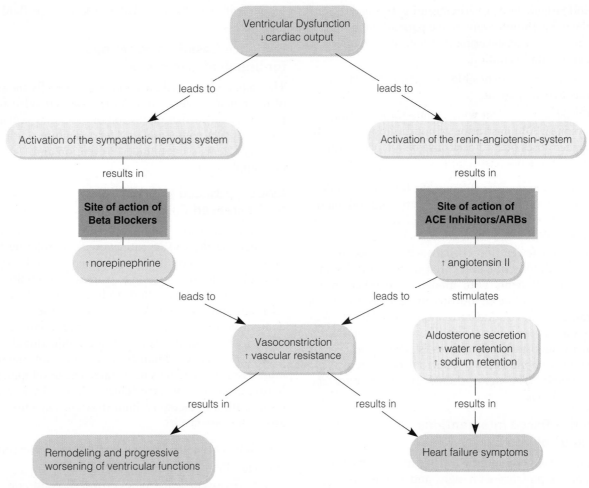

Figure 6-3 Beta blockers block the sympathetic nervous system and the ACE inhibitors and ARBs block the renin-angiotensin-aldosterone system.

TABLE 6–3

Medications Used to Block Neurohormonal Process

ACE INHIBITOR	ARBS	BETA BLOCKERS	ALDOSTERONE INHIBITORS
captopril (Capoten)	candesartan (Atacand)	carvedilol (Coreg)	spironolactone (Aldactone)
enalapril (Vasotec)	valsartan (Diovan)	metoprolol (Toprol XL)	eplerenone (Inspra)
fosinopril (Monopril)		bisoprolol (Zebeta)	
lisinopril (Prinivil) (Zestril)			
quinapril (Accupril)			
ramipril (Altace)			

Beta blockade inhibits the effects of the sympathetic nervous system stimulation in heart failure. Beta blockers can block the vasconstriction, reduce cardiac hypertrophy, and reduce dysrhythmias and tachycardia leading to heart failure. Beta blockers are indicated for all patients with stable heart failure and reduced ejection fraction. The earlier they are prescribed, the more positive effects they will have on the disease progression. Three common beta blockers are used in the treatment of heart failure (refer to Table 6–3). When administering the beta blockers the nurse should:

- Assess for the common side effects of hypotension, bradycardia, new atrioventricular blocks, dizziness, and fatigue. Prior to administering the medication, the nurse should evaluate the patient's blood pressure and pulse, ensuring that they are adequate before administration.

- Monitor the patient's blood sugar, particularly in the diabetic patient.
- Observe the patient with asthma for increasing dyspnea. Administration of noncardioselective and higher doses of cardioselective beta blockers can cause bronchoconstriction.

Aldosterone antagonists enhance the lowering of aldosterone in the serum, thus reducing water and sodium retention (refer to Table 6–3). Eplerenone (Inspra) selectively blocks the mineralocorticoid receptor and therefore has fewer side effects such as gynecomastia and sexual dysfunction compared with spironolactone (Aldactone). Patients with moderate to severe heart failure should be on an aldosterone antagonist unless contraindicated. As aldosterone inhibitors, these medications are potassium sparing. Therefore, a contraindication for aldosterone inhibitors is renal insufficiency. All patients on aldosterone antagonists are at risk for hyperkalemia. The nurse should closely monitor the potassium levels.

Evidence-Based Interventions for Fluid Volume Excess

Sodium and water retention lead to fluid volume excess. The patient presents with signs and symptoms of peripheral and pulmonary edema. Typically a loop diuretic like furosemide (Lasix) is used to control the pulmonary and peripheral edema. Usual starting doses are 20 to 40 mg. The expected response would be an increase in urine output and reduction in peripheral edema. If the patient was experiencing pulmonary edema, the expected response after diuretic administration would be less dyspnea, improving oxygen saturations, and a reduction in crackles upon auscultation. The nurse should assess for:

- Side effects of diuretics, including:
  - Hypokalemia (less than 3.5 mmol/L)
  - Hypomagnesemia (less than 1.5 mg/dL)
  - Metabolic alkalosis
- Signs of excessive diuresis, which will lead to volume contraction resulting in hypotension and renal insufficiency.
- Concomitant administration of NSAIDs, which may blunt the renal effects of diuretics.

Diuretics are usually combined with moderate sodium restriction (3 to 4 g daily) (Hunt, 2005). The nurse should weigh the patient daily to detect fluid accumulation. An increase in more than 3 lb in 1 day suggests fluid volume excess. Careful assessment of intake and output will identify an imbalance leading to fluid volume excess.

Evidence-Based Interventions for Impaired Gas Exchange

The impaired gas exchange in HF is generally the result of pulmonary edema from elevation of left-sided filling pressures. See further discussion of pulmonary edema in the Acute Decompensated Heart Failure with Pulmonary Edema section under Prevention and Detection of Complications.

Evidence-Based Interventions for Decreased Cardiac Output

A combination of vasodilators and positive inotropes can increase the CO in patients with systolic dysfunction. Orally, digoxin is given to patients with heart failure and systolic dysfunction to increase contractility and CO in patients who continue to be symptomatic despite ACE inhibitor, beta blocker, and diuretic use. The usual daily dose is 0.125 mg up to a maximum daily dose of 0.25 mg. Digoxin also decreases the conduction through the heart. Prior to administration of digoxin, the nurse must assess the patient's heart rate. The development of bradycardia or new atrioventricular blocks is a contraindication to digoxin administration. The nurse must assess the patient for:

- Bradycardia (less than 60 beats per minute [bpm])
- Development of dysrhythmias
  - Atrioventricular blocks (first-, second-, or third-degree heart block)
  - Accelerated junctional rhythms
- Blurred or yellow vision indicating digoxin toxicity
- Hypokalemia
- Elevated digoxin level (normal is 0.5–0.8 ng/mL)

Digoxin is not indicated to increase cardiac output for acute decompensated HF (see section under Prevention and Detection of Complications). Maintenance of sinus rhythm in HF is important in optimizing CO. Supraventricular dysrhythmias like atrial fibrillation can exacerbate HF by reducing CO through the absence of the "atrial kick" and, if the ventricular rate is tachycardic, ventricular filling may decrease during diastole. Both of these developments are particularly concerning in the patient with diastolic dysfunction who relies on an adequate filling volume to maintain CO. Conversion to sinus rhythm for atrial dysrhythmias may be accomplished through cardioversion or through medications such as amiodarone. See discussion of treatment for atrial dysrhythmias in Chapter 4. ∞ Cardiac resynchronization therapy (CRT) may improve ventricular contraction and enhance CO (see discussion in Building Technology Skills).

PURPOSE: To significantly improve care and reduce readmissions for patients with congestive heart failure (CHF) by implementing the components of care recommended by the Institute for Healthcare Improvement (IHI) and the American Heart Association (AHA)

RATIONALE: Heart failure results in a significant human toll because patients with CHF are often unable to function normally in their daily lives. "Yet, because of inadequate treatment, discharge guidance, and follow-up, many patients with CHF are caught in a 'revolving door' process that ultimately culminates in deterioration and rehospitalization. This is reflected in the following readmission rates among 616,000 Medicare discharges in 2005: 27% within 30 days, 39% within 60 days, and nearly 50% within 90 days of hospital discharge" (IHI Web site).

However, the human toll is not the only burden imposed by CHF. It also imposes a "substantial economic burden" (IHI). It has been estimated that direct and indirect costs of CHF approached $29.6 billion in the United States in 2006 due partially to high rehospitalization rates. Optimum management of heart failure through evidence-based approaches can reduce mortality and rehospitalization rates for patients with CHF.

HIGHLIGHTS OF RECOMMENDATIONS:
Numerous studies have established a firm evidence base indicating that specific components of CHF care reduce morbidity and mortality. Although care must

be tailored to the individual patient, the following seven key components of care should be provided to all CHF patients as long as there are no contraindications:

- Assessment of left ventricular systolic (LVS) function
- Provision of an ACE-inhibitor or angiotensin receptor blockers (ARB) at discharge for CHF patients with systolic dysfunction (LVEF less than 40%)
- Anticoagulant at discharge for CHF patients with chronic or recurrent atrial fibrillation (AF)
- Smoking cessation advice and counseling
- Discharge instructions that address all of the following: activity level, diet, discharge medications, follow-up appointment, weight monitoring, and what to do if symptoms worsen
- Influenza immunization (seasonal)
- Pneumococcal immunization

The campaign also strongly recommends consideration of one additional evidence-based intervention:

Beta-blocker therapy at discharge for stabilized patients with LVS dysfunction, without contraindications.

Source: Institute for Healthcare Improvement AHA/ACC 2005 Guideline Update for the Diagnosis and Management of Chronic Heart Failure in the Adult Available: http://www.ihi.org/IHI/Programs/Campaign/CHF.htm

Prevention and Detection of Complications

Many patients with heart failure have ventricular dysrhythmias, including ventricular premature beats and nonsustained and sustained ventricular tachycardia. Mortality is high with patients exhibiting these dysrhythmias. The nurse must continuously monitor the patient's rhythm for these types of dysrhythmias. The development of pulseless ventricular tachycardia or ventricular fibrillation must be promptly defibrillated. Most antiarrhythmic drugs are proarrythmic, cause an increase in arrhythmia, and have a negative inotropic effect, making them ineffective and dangerous for heart failure patients. Amiodarone is considered the exception and can be safely administered to treat symptomatic ventricular arrhythmia (see discussion of treatment for ventricular dysrhythmia in Chapter 4). ∞ Implantation of an implantable cardioverter defibrillator can immediately treat these ventricular dysrhythmias and prevent the development of sudden cardiac death (see the discussion in this chapter under the Building Technology Skills heading).

Acute Decompensated Heart Failure with Pulmonary Edema (Cardiogenic Shock)

Prevention of the development of acute decompensated heart failure is linked to the early identification and management of stable heart failure. Patient compliance with lifestyle modifications and appropriate pharmacological therapies may decrease the progression of heart failure and prevent the development of acute decompensation. The nurse assesses the patient for signs of deterioration, including:

- Dyspnea at rest
- Tachycardia
- Reduced oxygen saturation
- Crackles on lung auscultation
- Hypotension
- Worsening cough
- New dysrhythmias
- Elevation of PAWP
- Reduction in CO/CI

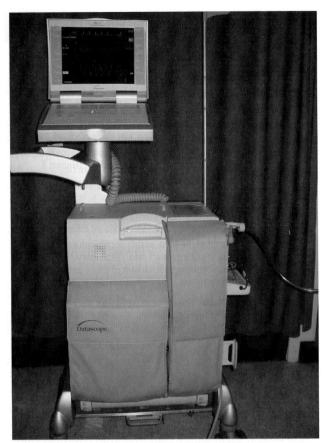

Figure 6-5 Intra-aortic balloon pump console.
(Courtesy Elliot Hospital, Manchester, NH)

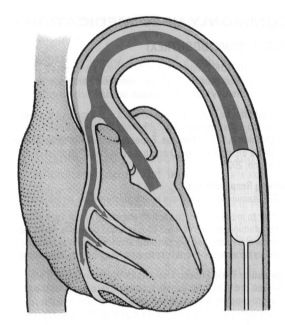

IAB Inflation

Figure 6-6A Inflation of the intra-aortic balloon. The blood in the aorta is pushed toward the coronary arteries, improving the oxygen supply to the myocardium.

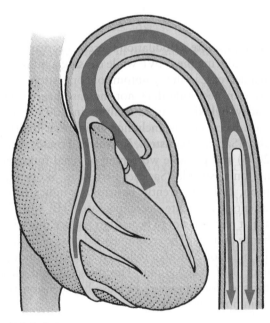

IAB Deflation

Figure 6-6B Deflation of the intra-aortic balloon. The heart pumps against the reduced resistance left by the balloon deflation, thus decreasing afterload and demand on the heart.

coronary arteries (Figure 6-5). The expected effects of IABP therapy are to improve CO/CI, improve MAP, and reduce PAWPs and pulmonary edema.

Access and Technological Requirements

A balloon catheter is inserted in the femoral artery and advanced into the aorta with the tip of the catheter just distal to the left subclavian artery and just above the renal arteries. The patient's ECG and arterial waveform are continuously monitored on the IABP console. Using the ECG as a trigger and the dicrotic notch as the timing indicator, the balloon is inflated during diastole and deflated during systole. During inflation, the blood in the aorta is pushed toward the coronary arteries, improving the oxygen supply to the myocardium. During deflation, the heart pumps against the reduced resistance left by the balloon deflation, thus decreasing afterload and demand on the heart (Figures 6-6A and B).

Nursing Responsibilities

Nursing responsibilities include:

- Assessing balloon timing within the cardiac cycle by evaluation of the arterial pressure values and tracings
- Maintaining stability of the balloon catheter
- Assessing for movement of the balloon catheter by evaluating the left radial pulse and the patient's urinary output
- Assessing perfusion of the legs by evaluating circulation, sensation, and movement
- Maintaining the head of the bed less than 30 degrees to avoid hip flexion and possible puncture of the femoral artery with the catheter

Implantable Cardioverter Defibrillator

The ICD is a generator implanted beneath the skin of the chest with wires leading to the atria and ventricle of the heart. Most of the newer ICDs are implanted in the same location as conventional pacemakers. The ICD detects dysrhythmias such as ventricular fibrillation and ventricular tachycardia and automatically delivers a shock to the heart. The shock may be in the form of cardioversion or defibrillation depending on the rhythm detected. Many ICDs also are able to perform antitachycardia pacing. This feature delivers bursts of pacing pulses at a rate faster than the ventricular tachycardia and can successfully terminate the tachycardic rhythms. If the rhythm becomes too slow, a pacemaker feature can restore the normal heart rate. ICDs have become useful in preventing sudden cardiac death. The 2005 ACC/AHA Heart Failure Guidelines recommend ICD implantation in patients who are at a II–III on the NYHA classification on optimal medical therapy with an LVEF less than or equal to 30%. A more detailed discussion of pacemakers and ICDs is available in Chapter 4. ∞

Nursing responsibilities in the acute setting include:

- Continuous monitoring of the ECG
- Identification of the active features and current settings
- Utilization of external defibrillation if the ICD fails to fire
- Knowledge of policies and resources for temporarily suspending function in the event that the device is misfiring

Cardiac Resynchronization Therapy

In heart failure there is a delay in atrioventricular synchrony with a reduced atrial systole, a delay in ventricular conduction causing disorganized ventricular contraction, and a decreasing pumping efficiency. CRT, also called biventricular pacing, is thought to improve the synchrony by coordinating atrial systole and simultaneously pacing the ventricles. The 2005 ACC/AHA Heart Failure Guidelines recommend implantation of CRT in patients who are at an NYHA III–IV, an ejection fraction (EF) less than or equal to 35%, and a QRS greater than 120 msec (0.12 second). The goal is to optimize the atrioventricular (AV) delay through consistent timing of the AV interval and simultaneously pace the ventricles 100% of the time. Optimizing the AV delay

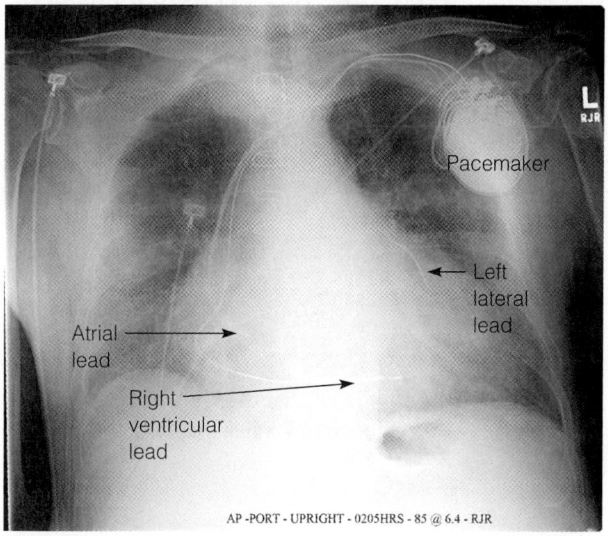

Figure 6-7 Biventricular pacemaker showing the atrial lead, right ventricular lead, and the left lead advanced through the coronary sinus to the lateral wall of the left ventricle. (Courtesy Elliot Hospital, Manchester, NH)

decreases mitral regurgitation and increases diastolic filling time. Simultaneous activation of the septum and LV lateral wall improves LV contraction, leading to increased CO and increased ejection fraction. Additional outcomes are improved quality of life, exercise tolerance, and survival.

Technological Requirements

The biventricular pacing system consists of one atrial lead, one right ventricular lead activating the septum, and activation of the lateral wall of the left ventricle via a lead placed in the coronary sinus and advanced to the lateral cardiac vein. Simultaneous pacing in the ventricles displays only one ventricular pacing spike for each ECG complex (Figure 6-7).

Nursing Responsibilities

Nursing responsibilities in the acute setting include:

- Continuous monitoring of the ECG.
- Measurement of the QRS duration. Widening of the QRS duration from the baseline may indicate a loss of ventricular synchronization.
- Identification of the active features and current settings (Boser & Ailing, 2006).

HEART FAILURE SUMMARY

The nurse caring for a patient with decreased tissue/organ perfusion must recognize that it may be caused by either hypovolemic shock or heart failure. The nurse will therefore need to carefully assess the patient for indications of fluid volume deficit or excess and collaborate with other members of the health care team to provide the appropriate therapies.

VISUAL MAP **Heart Failure Summary**

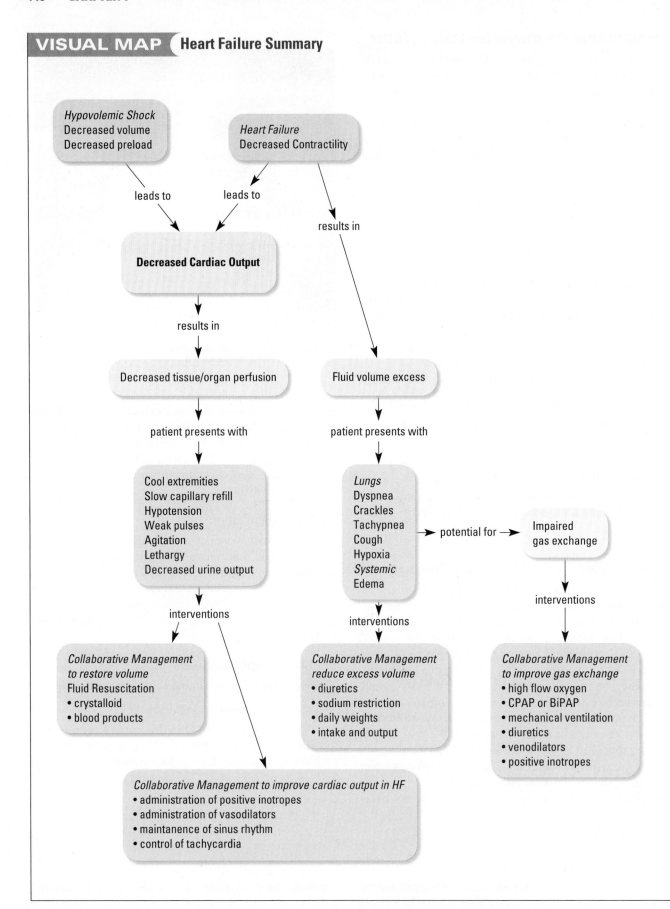

Hypovolemic Shock
Decreased volume
Decreased preload

Heart Failure
Decreased Contractility

leads to   leads to

results in

Decreased Cardiac Output

results in

Decreased tissue/organ perfusion

Fluid volume excess

patient presents with

patient presents with

Cool extremities
Slow capillary refill
Hypotension
Weak pulses
Agitation
Lethargy
Decreased urine output

Lungs
Dyspnea
Crackles
Tachypnea
Cough
Hypoxia
Systemic
Edema

potential for →

Impaired
gas exchange

interventions

interventions

interventions

*Collaborative Management
to restore volume*
Fluid Resuscitation
• crystalloid
• blood products

*Collaborative Management
reduce excess volume*
• diuretics
• sodium restriction
• daily weights
• intake and output

*Collaborative Management
to improve gas exchange*
• high flow oxygen
• CPAP or BiPAP
• mechanical ventilation
• diuretics
• venodilators
• positive inotropes

Collaborative Management to improve cardiac output in HF
• administration of positive inotropes
• administration of vasodilators
• maintanence of sinus rhythm
• control of tachycardia

CASE STUDY

An 84-year-old male was found at home unresponsive but breathing after vomiting large amounts of blood. He was transported by EMS to the emergency department with a massive GI bleed. Treatment by EMS en route included placement of two large-bore 16-gauge intravenous catheters and 100% oxygen via a nonrebreather mask. His vital signs on admission were HR 120 regular, BP 40/30, RR 12, pulse oximetry 96%. He appeared pale and slightly diaphoretic. He has delayed capillary refill and absent peripheral pulses but still has a carotid pulse. Lungs are clear to auscultation and his abdomen is distended. The patient has a remote history of excessive drinking but according to his wife he has not had a drink in 25 years. Past medical history includes: hypertension, depression, esophageal varices, cirrhosis, question of esophageal cancer, and abdominal aortic aneurysm repair 4 years ago. On admission labs revealed: sodium 150, potassium 3.9, BUN 30, creatinine 1, glucose 178, hemoglobin 5.6, hematocrit 25, INR 2.28, PT 22, PTT 35.

1. What signs and symptoms indicate hypovolemia in this patient?

2. What lab tests indicate hypovolemia?

3. Explain the relationship between the patient's hypotension, tachycardia, and peripheral vasoconstriction.

4. The patient's pulse oximetry is 96%. Further evaluate the saturation, considering his hemoglobin is 5.6.

5. What are the likely factors contributing to this massive GI bleed?

6. What are immediate priorities in the collaborative management of this patient?

7. What type of fluids should be administered to this patient in hypovolemic shock?

See answers to Case Studies in the Answer Section at the back of the book.

CRITICAL THINKING QUESTIONS

1. How would a patient most likely manifest hypovolemia?

2. What BP, CVP, and PA pressure would be indicative of hypovolemia?

3. How would a nurse recognize that a hypovolemic patient had received adequate volume replacement?

4. How do neurohormonal mechanisms contribute to the development of heart failure?

5. What are the differences between systolic and diastolic heart failure?

6. How do patients usually manifest heart failure (HF)? How do older adults manifest heart failure?

7. What BP, PA pressure, and CVP are indicative of heart failure?

8. What are the essential collaborative interventions for a patient with heart failure?

9. What are the indications that a patient with chronic heart failure is experiencing an acute decompensation with pulmonary edema?

10. What are the essential collaborative interventions for the patient with acutely decompensated heart failure?

11. What are the nursing priorities for the patient with acutely decompensated heart failure?

12. Why are isotonic solutions like 0.9% normal saline the preferred crystalloid in fluid resuscitation?

See answers to Critical Thinking Questions in the Answer Section at the back of the book.

EXPLORE MEDIALINK
http://www.prenhall.com/perrin

Additional interactive resources for this chapter can be found on the Web site at http://www.prenhall.com/perrin. Click on "Chapter 6" to select activities for this chapter.

Case Study: Hypervolemic Shock

Nursing Care Plan

NCLEX Review Questions

MediaLinks:
- Review of Lung Sounds
- Information of Catheter Placement for CRT. Animation of Placement at:

- Cardiac Cycle Animations at:
- American Heart Association
- American College of Cardiology

MediaLink Applications

REFERENCES

Albert, N. (2006). Evidence-based nursing care for patients with heart failure. *AACN Advanced Critical Care, 1*(2), 170–183.

American College of Surgeons. (2004). *Advanced trauma life support (ATLS) student manual*. Chicago: Author.

Bosen, D. M., & Ailing, E. (2006). Back on the beat: Cardiac resynchronization therapy. *Nursing 2006, 36*(3).

Caboral, M. (2006). Putting the 2005 American College of Cardiology/ American Heart Association heart failure guidelines into clinical practice; advice for advanced practice nurses. *Topics in Advanced Practice Nursing, 6*(2). Retrieved March 22, 2007, from http:// www.medscape.com/viewarticle/ 533626_print

Cottingham, C. (2006). Resuscitation of traumatic shock: A hemodynamic review. *AACN Advanced Critical Care, 17*(3), 317–326.

Gahart, B., & Nazareno, A. (2007). *2007 intravenous medications*. St. Louis, MO: Elsevier.

Hunt, S. (2005). *ACC/AHA 2005 guidelines update for the diagnosis and management of chronic heart failure in the adult*. Retrieved April 7, 2007, from http://www. acc.org/qualityandscience/clinical/ guidelines/failure/update/index.pdf

Merck Manual Online Medical Library. (2005). *Intravenous fluid resuscitation*. Retrieved April 15, 2007, from http:// www.merck.com/mmpe/sec06/ch067/ ch067c.html

Roberts, I., Alderson, P., Bunn, F., Chinnock, P., Ker, K., & Schierhout, G. (2004). Colloids versus crystalloids for fluid resuscitation in critically ill patients. *Cochrane Database of Systematic Reviews 2004*, Issue 4. Retrieved April 26, 2007, from http://www. mrw.interscience.wiley.com/cochrane/ clsysrev/articles/CD000567/frame.html

Rose, B., & Mandel, J. (2005). *Pathogenesis of irreversible shock*. Retrieved March 30, 2007, from http://www.utdol.com/utd/ content/topic.do?topicKey[equals]fldlytes/ 33374&view[equals]text

Sackner-Bernstein, J. D., Kowalski, M., Fox, M., & Aaronson, K. (2005). Short term risk of death after treatment with nesiritide for decompensated heart failure: A pooled analysis of randomized controlled trials. *JAMA, 293*(11), 1900–1905.

Sackner-Bernstein, J. D., Skopicki, H. A., & Aaronson, K. D. (2005). Risk of worsening renal function with nesiritide in patients with acutely decompensated heart failure. *Circulation, 111*(12), 1487–1489.

Stoltzfus, S. (2006). The role of noninvasive ventilation CPAP and BiPAP in the treatment of congestive heart failure. *Dimensions of Critical Care Nursing, 25*(2), 66–70.

Care of the Patient with Acute Coronary Syndrome

Susan A. Moore, PhD, RN

Learning Outcomes

Upon completion of this chapter, the learner will be able to:

1. Explain acute coronary syndrome.

2. Differentiate among different types of acute coronary syndrome.

3. Describe emergent assessment and collaborative management of the person with chest discomfort.

4. Evaluate various laboratory tests used to determine if a person is experiencing an acute coronary event.

5. Compare and contrast fibrinolysis and angioplasty for emergent reperfusion of the cardiac patient.

6. Describe nursing management of the patient post angioplasty with stent placement.

7. Discuss care of the patient following coronary artery bypass surgery.

8. Prioritize discharge teaching for the patient who has had an acute coronary event.

Abbreviations

ACS	Acute Coronary Syndrome
AHA	American Heart Association
ASA	Aspirin
BMI	Body Mass Index
CABG	Coronary Artery Bypass Graft
CAD	Coronary Artery Disease
CHD	Coronary Heart Disease
CK	Creatinine Phosphokinase
COPD	Chronic Obstructive Pulmonary Disease
CRP	C-Reactive Protein
DASH	Dietary Approaches to Stop Hypertension
ECG	Electrocardiogram
HDL	High-Density Lipoproteins
HRT	Hormone Replacement Therapy
LAD	Left Anterior Descending
Lcx	Left Circumflex
LDL	Low-Density Lipoprotein
LIMA	Left Internal Mammary Artery
MI	Myocardial Infarction
MIDCAB	Minimally Invasive Direct Coronary Artery Bypass
NCEP	National Cholesterol Education Program
NSTE	Non-ST-Segment Elevation
NSTEMI	Non-ST-Segment Elevation Myocardial Infarction
NTG	Nitroglycerin
PCI	Percutaneous Transluminal Intervention
RCA	Right Coronary Artery
STEMI	ST-Segment Elevation Myocardial Infarction
TC	Total Cholesterol
tPA	Tissue Plasminogen Activator

Acute coronary syndrome (ACS) is an inclusive term for conditions that cause chest pain due to insufficient blood supply to the heart muscle. ACS thus covers the spectrum of clinical conditions ranging from ST-segment elevation myocardial infarction (STEMI), non-ST-segment elevation (NSTE) ACS, which includes the diagnosis of unstable angina and NSTE myocardial infarction (NSTEMI). These life-threatening disorders are a major cause of emergency medical care and hospitalization in the United States. Coronary heart disease is the leading cause of death in the United States. Nearly 1.7 million Americans with ACS were discharged from hospitals in 2002, according to

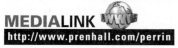

MEDIALINK
http://www.prenhall.com/perrin

See the Companion Website for chapter-specific resources at www.prenhall.com/perrin.

VISUAL MAP Coronary Artery Disease Overview

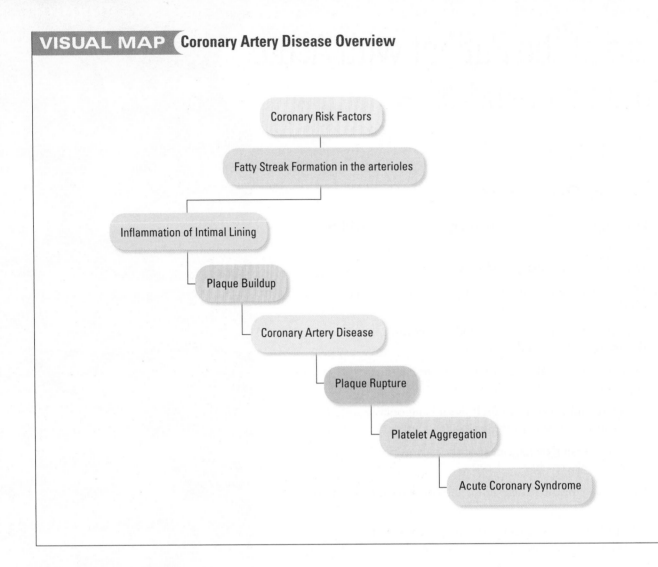

the American Heart Association (American Heart Association, 2006). This includes ACS as both primary and secondary discharge diagnoses.

Acute Coronary Syndrome

Acute coronary syndrome (ACS) is an all-inclusive term that often describes a progression of coronary events. The patient will have stable chest pain and can progress to unstable chest pain and eventually the infarction or death of the myocardial tissue. According to the AHA up to one third of the patients who are diagnosed with unstable angina will progress to a myocardial infarction (MI) in 1 year (2006).

Pathophysiology

ACS is the clinical manifestation of coronary heart disease, which includes the development of fatty plaques in the coronary arteries. The growth of the atherosclerotic

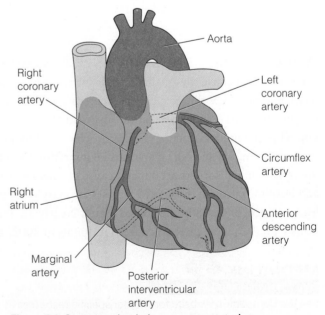

Figure 7-1 Coronary circulation, coronary arteries.

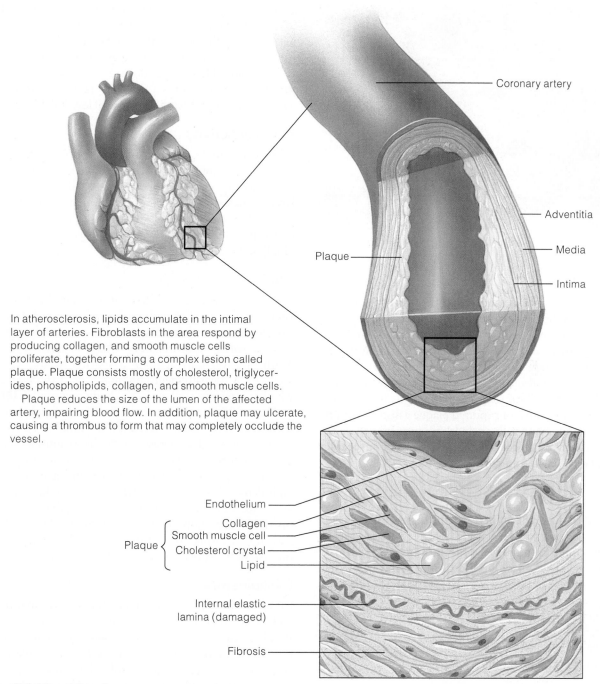

In atherosclerosis, lipids accumulate in the intimal layer of arteries. Fibroblasts in the area respond by producing collagen, and smooth muscle cells proliferate, together forming a complex lesion called plaque. Plaque consists mostly of cholesterol, triglycerides, phospholipids, collagen, and smooth muscle cells.

Plaque reduces the size of the lumen of the affected artery, impairing blood flow. In addition, plaque may ulcerate, causing a thrombus to form that may completely occlude the vessel.

Figure 7-2 Atherosclerosis.

plaques narrows the vasculature, which then limits the blood flow and delivery of oxygen to the coronary muscle (Figures 7-1 and 7-2). This buildup of plaque in the coronary arteries results in a less serious condition known as **stable angina**. A more serious condition exists when the plaque ruptures or becomes unstable in the vasculature (see Figure 7-3). The unstable plaque is characteristically composed of a large lipid core, large number of lipid-laden macrophages, and a thin fibrous cap.

Rupture of this cap exposes the thrombogenic contents of the plaque into a patient's circulation. This evolution of foreign material causes circulating platelets to adhere to the subendocardial collagen, thus causing more platelets to activate and aggregate at the site of injury (Mc Cance & Huether, 2005).

The formation of platelet-rich thrombi is the underlying cause of adverse ischemic events across the full spectrum of ACS. At first, the growth of the platelet-rich

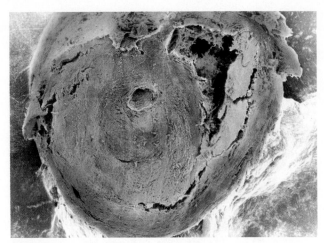

Figure 7-3 Ruptured plaque.

thrombi causes an occlusion, which leads to myocardial ischemia and the diagnosis of **unstable angina** (Figure 7-3). As the platelets continue to aggregate, they can cause blockage to smaller blood vessels resulting in an non-ST segment elevation myocardial infarction (**NSTEMI**). The plaque rupture also induces the formation of thrombin, which converts fibrinogen into fibrin. This formation of fibrin along the area of ruptured plaque assists the thrombus to stabilize and fully occlude the coronary vessel. The result of this full occlusion is a **ST elevated myocardial infarction STEMI** (Antman et al., 2004).

Risk Factors

The AHA has determined several factors that place a patient at risk for developing coronary artery disease, which could eventually evolve into an acute coronary syndrome. These have been determined through extensive research and statistical studies. Some of these risk factors can be modified, treated, or controlled, and others cannot. The more risk factors a person has, the greater the chance of developing an ACS sometime in the person's lifetime. The following section presents risk factors that can be modified.

Tobacco Smoke

Smoker's risk of coronary heart disease is two to four times that of nonsmokers. Cigarette smoking has been linked to sudden cardiac death as well as ACS. People who smoke cigars and pipes also have a high risk of dying from **coronary heart disease** (CHD) but it is still less than that of cigarette smokers. Exposure to secondhand smoke for nonsmokers also increases the risk of having an ACS event (Attebring et al., 2004).

Hypertension

Hypertension increases the heart's workload, causing increased stress and oxygen consumption to the myocardial muscle. There is a definite correlation between the degree of blood pressure (BP) elevation and CHD risk. The 20 mm Hg average increase in systolic BP that comes with age increases the occurrence of CHD two to three times for individuals between the ages of 30 and 65 years (Householder-Hughes, 2006). AHA strongly recommends people maintain a systolic pressure of less than 120 mm Hg and a diastolic pressure of less than 80 mm Hg.

Physical Activity

Sedentary lifestyles are a strong risk factor for heart disease. Regular, moderate to vigorous physical activity has been shown to prevent heart and blood vessel disease. Exercise has also been demonstrated to assist in controlling or eliminating other risk factors such as hypertension, hyperlipidemia, diabetes, and obesity (Householder-Hughes, 2006).

Obesity

People who have excess body fat are more likely to develop CHD even if they do not have other risk factors. **Obesity** has been defined as an excess of weight at least 20% above the ideal weight corresponding to the lowest death rate for individuals of a specific height, gender, and age. A measurement commonly used to determine whether a person is obese is the **body mass index (BMI)**. A BMI of 25.9 to 29.9 is considered overweight, and a BMI of over 30 is considered obese (Table 7–1). Excess weight causes added stress on the heart muscle, which increases coronary workload. An excess of weight has also been linked to hyperlipidemia and a decrease in high-density lipoproteins (HDL). It has also been associated with an increased risk of developing diabetes mellitus (DM), especially the type 2 prototype. Studies have shown that losing 10% of one's body weight can lower the risk of heart disease (Householder-Hughes, 2006).

Dyslipidemia

Cholesterol is the fatty substance found in animal tissue and is an important component of body functioning. Problems can occur if a person ingests too much animal protein or the body manufactures too much cholesterol. An overabundance of cholesterol is known as hyperlipidemia or hypercholesterolemia. Hypercholesterolemia is highly associated with the formation of atherosclerotic plaque, the precursor to ACS. High blood cholesterol can

TABLE 7–1
Body Mass Index
To determine: Weight × 703/Height in inches² Significant values: Below 25.9—Normal 25.9–29.9—Overweight 30–above—Obese

Source: From Longe, Jacqueline L. (editor). *The Gale Encyclopedia of Medicine,* 3E. Copyright 2006 Gale, a part of Cengage Learning Inc. Reproduced by permission. www.cengage.com/permissions.

TABLE 7–2

Lipid Levels

	TOTAL	LDL	HDL	TC/HDL
Optimal	< 160 mg/dL	< 100 mg/dL		
Desirable	160–199 mg/dL	100–129 mg/dL	> 45 mg/dL	< 3
Borderline	200–239 mg/dL	130–159 mg/dL	30–45 mg/dL	3–4
High Risk	> 240 mg/dL	> 160 mg/dL	< 35 mg/dL	> 4

Source: From Longe, Jacqueline L. (editor). *The Gale Encyclopedia of Medicine,* 3E. Copyright 2006 Gale, a part of Cengage Learning Inc. Reproduced by permission. www.cengage.com/permissions.

be the result of familial and/or nonfamilial forms. The nonfamilial form is exacerbated by foods containing excessive trans fat, saturated fats, and cholesterol. Familial hypercholesterolemia is an autosomal dominant disorder that causes marked elevation of total cholesterol (TC) and low-density lipoprotein (LDL) due to the absence or reduced number of LDL receptors. High-density lipoproteins (HDL) are often called good cholesterol because they remove excess cholesterol from blood vessels and transport it to the liver for metabolism. The ratio between the TC and HDL is referred to as the cardiac risk index. A cardiac risk index of less than 3 is desirable as shown in Table 7–2.

Risk Factors That Cannot Be Modified

- *Age* Over 83% of people who die of CHD are over the age of 65. As women get older, they experience more fatal heart attacks than men (Dulak, 2004).
- *Gender* Men have a greater risk of MIs than women, and they tend to experience them earlier in life.
- *Heredity* Children of parents with heart disease are at greater risk for developing it themselves. African Americans, due to the comorbidity of hypertension, have a higher risk than Caucasians. Due to the obesity factor, it has been found that Mexican Americans, American Indians, and some Asian Americans are also at increased risk for developing a heart disease-related syndrome (AHA, 2006).

Other Contributing Risk Factors

- *Diabetes Mellitus* Diabetes has been demonstrated to be a serious factor in the development of cardiovascular disease. This is particularly true in patients who do not have good glycemic control. More than 65% of people with diabetes die from some form of cardiovascular disease (American Diabetes Association).
- *Stress* People who are under extreme stress tend to participate in other unhealthy activities. This includes lack of exercise, overeating, and smoking. Stress also increases the workload on the cardiovascular system. Stress has the tendency to increase BP and heart rate (HR) and also contributes to the bloods ability to form clots, putting the patient at increased risk for a coronary event (Klieman, Hyde, & Berra, 2006).
- *Alcohol Consumption* Alcohol, when taken in large quantities, has been attributed to increasing a person's BP. It also contributes to an increase in triglycerides, an important component in the development of CHD (Klieman, Hyde, & Berra, 2006).
- *Hormone Replacement Therapy (HRT)* It was thought for a time that HRT after menopause had a protective factor against the formation of coronary artery disease (CAD). Evidence from the Women's Health Initiative released in 2002 and 2003 shows that HRT is a risk factor for CAD in postmenopausal women with existing CAD (Moriarity, 2004).

Table 7–3 provides a synopsis of the different risk factors and interventions to alleviate the cardiac risk from the main risk factors.

Angina Pectoris

Angina pectoris literally means "strangling of the chest." It is a general medical term used to define types of chest pain caused by myocardial ischemia.

Pathophysiology

The coronary arteries supply blood and oxygen to the myocardium. Due to plaque buildup and atherosclerosis, the myocardium can become deprived of blood and oxygen. Thrombus formation and further plaque formation eventually narrow the coronary arteries, causing ischemia and death of myocardial tissue. Ischemia occurs if the demand for oxygen exceeds its supply. Demand for myocardial oxygen increases with exercise, stress, and sympathetic nervous system stimulation.

Classification

Angina can be classified into three different phases: stable, unstable, and variant. The angina that is of more concern to the development of ACS is the unstable angina prototype. The stable and variant types are included to assist in the differentiation of the major anginal prototypes. Many factors can precipitate anginal pain (Table 7–4).

Stable Angina

Stable angina is chest pain that occurs predictably on exertion. This type of angina is associated with stable plaque buildup in the coronary arteries. The stenotic coronary vessel reduces coronary artery blood flow to a critical level. Symptoms of stable angina, although caused by decreased myocardial oxygen, can change from time to time depending on stress, oxygen consumption, and

TABLE 7-3

Secondary Prevention Guidelines for Risk Factors

RISK FACTOR	INTERVENTION
Smoking	• Ask about tobacco status. • Advise to quit if still smoking. • Assess willingness to quit. • Assist in developing a plan for quitting. • Arrange for a smoking cessation class. • Avoid environmental exposure.
Blood Pressure Control Goal: <140/90 mm Hg or <130/80 mm Hg if patient has diabetes or chronic kidney disease	• Initiate lifestyle modification, including weight control; increased physical activity; alcohol moderation; sodium restriction. • Include a diet of fresh fruits and vegetables and low-fat dairy products. • If blood pressure is elevated, control with medication—beta blockers and/or ACE inhibitors and diuretics.
Lipid Management	• Start dietary therapy. Reduce intake of saturated fats to < 7% of total calories. • Add fiber to the diet. • Encourage consumption of omega-3 fatty acids. • Initiate lipid-lowering medication if fasting lipid levels are abnormal.
Physical Activity Goal: 30 minutes, 7 days per week	• Assess risk with physical activity history and/or exercise test. • Encourage 30–60 minutes of activity every day. • Encourage resistance training 2 days per week. • Encourage cardiac rehabilitation program for people at high risk.
Weight Management Goal: BMI 18.5–24.9 kg/m² Waist circumference: men < 40 inches; women < 35 inches	• Assess measurements at each visit and encourage weight management through physical activity, caloric intake, and behavioral programs. • The initial goal of weight loss is to achieve a 10% reduction from baseline.
Diabetes Management Goal: HbA$_{1c}$ < 7%	• Initiate lifestyle and pharmacotherapy to achieve a normal HbA$_{1c}$. • Lifestyle changes as indicated in other risk factors. • Coordinate care between other medical providers.

Source: From Smith, S., et al. (2006). AHA/ACC secondary prevention for patients with coronary artery disease. *Circulation, 113*, 2363–2372.

VISUAL MAP Relationship Among Types of Angina

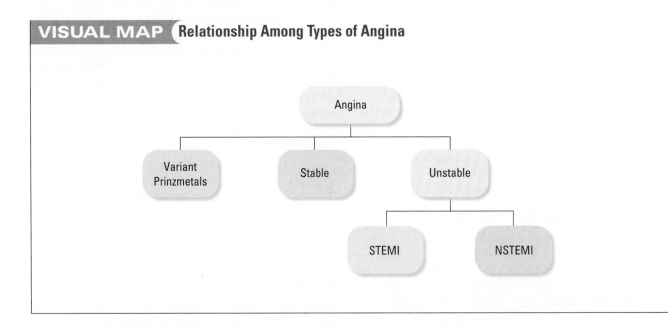

temperature extremes. Stable angina is often treated with nitroglycerin preparations and rest. Some patients are also placed on calcium channel blockers and beta adrenergic blockers (Reigle, 2005).

Variant (Prinzmetal's) Angina

Variant angina is a less common form of angina. It is characterized by episodes of chest pain that occur at rest. Unlike stable and unstable angina, variant angina is caused

TABLE 7-4

Precipitating Causes of Anginal Pain

Physical exertion
Temperature extremes
Emotions (stress and anger)
Consumption of a large meal
Tobacco use
Sexual activity
Stimulants (caffeine, cocaine, amphetamines)
Circadian rhythm patterns

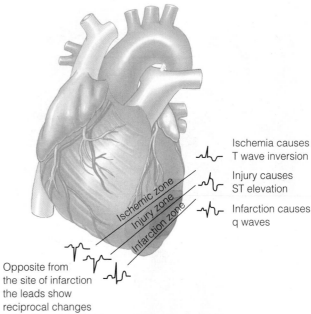

Ischemia causes T wave inversion

Injury causes ST elevation

Infarction causes q waves

Opposite from the site of infarction the leads show reciprocal changes

Figure 7-4 The evolution changes in acute MI.

by coronary artery vasospasms, which can cause an increase in myocardial oxygen demand and a transient ST-segment elevation. This type of angina is often treated with calcium channel blockers (Reigle, 2005).

Unstable Angina

Unstable angina is pain that occurs more often and in unpredictable patterns. It can occur while the patient is at rest, as well as with minimal exertion, and often causes the patient to limit his activity. According to Metules and Bauer (2005), unstable angina is actually the beginning of a process that can lead to a NSTEMI (Table 7–5).

Myocardial Infarction

An MI occurs when the heart muscle is abruptly deprived of oxygen. When the heart is deprived of oxygen, it proceeds through several phases of tissue injury (Figure 7-4). The first phase is the area of **ischemia**. If treatment is not immediate the tissue damage will continue onto injury and then **necrosis.**

Pathophysiology

Coronary plaque ruptures to initiate the events of an acute MI. Myocardial cells become ischemic within 10 seconds of coronary occlusion. During ischemia, cells experience a temporary shortage of oxygen, hypoxia, and downgrade their activity to conserve energy. Several minutes after the loss of contractile ability, the myocardium is deprived of its glucose source necessary for aerobic metabolism. This causes anaerobic processes to take over, and a buildup of lactic acid ensues. During this period the cells of the myocardium do not fully polarize. If this buildup continues without restoration of aerobic processes, MI occurs. Because infracted cells cannot respond to electrical impulses, they cannot help

TABLE 7-5

Classification and Treatment of Anginal Prototypes

CLASSIFICATION	ETIOLOGY	SYMPTOMS	TREATMENT
Stable	Myocardial ischemia CAD	• Episodic pain lasting 5–15 minutes • Aggravated by exertion • Relieved by rest	• NTG • Beta adrenergic blockers • Calcium channel blockers • ACE inhibitors
Unstable	Ruptured or thickened plaque	• Angina of increasing intensity • Occurs at rest or with minimal activity • Pain unresponsive to NTG	• NTG • Heparin • Clopidogrel • Morphine • Aspirin
Variant	Coronary vasospasm	• Occurs at rest • Triggered by smoking • Occurs with or without the presence of CAD	• Calcium channel blockers

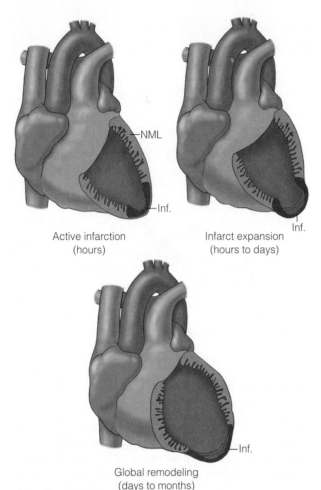

Active infarction
(hours)

Infarct expansion
(hours to days)

Global remodeling
(days to months)

Figure 7-5 Ventricular remodeling.

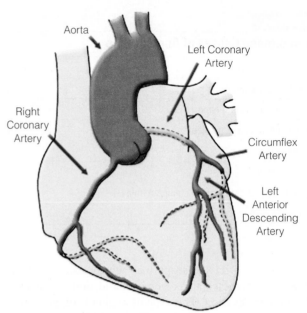

Figure 7-6 Coronary arteries with obstructions leading to various types of myocardial infarctions identified. (Courtesy Texas Heart Institute, www.texasheart.org)

the heart contract (McCance & Huether, 2005). The buildup of scar tissue from the ensuing necrotic heart tissue can lead to **ventricular remodeling**, which changes the shape and function of the heart muscle (Figure 7-5).

Location of Infarction

Myocardial injury and infarction occur mostly in the left ventricle, because it has the greatest oxygen demand and is more affected by occlusions of the coronary arteries. An MI is categorized by the wall of the left ventricle on which it occurs. This can be the anterior, lateral, septal, inferior, or posterior wall. The regions perfused by each of the coronary arteries are displayed in Figure 7-6.

An anterior wall MI is caused by occlusion of the left anterior descending artery (LAD). The higher or more proximal the occlusion, the more muscle damage ensues. Occlusion to the LAD can also cause an anterolateral or anteroseptal MI. Damage for this particular MI includes the anterior wall and anterior portion of the septal wall. Anterior wall MIs account for one fourth of the MIs and have the highest mortality rate (Householder-Hughes,

2006). These patients often suffer from the serious complications of ACS.

A lateral wall MI usually occurs with an occlusion of the circumflex artery or the diagonal branch of the LAD. Muscle damage occurs in the free, lateral wall of the left ventricle. Because the circumflex artery also supplies a portion of the sinoatrial (SA) node and atrioventricular (AV) node, clients often present with the complications of sinus dysrhythmias.

An inferior wall MI is most commonly due to an occlusion of the right coronary artery (RCA). The muscle damage is seen in the right ventricle and posterior and inferior left ventricle. More than half of all inferior wall MIs are associated with an occlusion of the proximal portion of the RCA, which can lead to significant damage to the right ventricle.

Myocardial injury to the posterior wall is uncommon due to the dual blood supply from the RCA and circumflex artery. If an infarction occurs in this portion of the heart muscle, it will also cause significant damage to the right ventricle (Householder-Hughes, 2006).

Q-Wave Versus Non-Q-Wave Myocardial Infarction

MIs can be classified as either a Q-wave or non-Q-wave MI. This depends on how deep the penetration of damage is in the heart muscle. A Q-wave MI, which is the most common, is usually transmural, where damage occurs to the full thickness of the myocardium. Electrocardiogram (ECG) changes result in ST-segment elevation, T-wave inversion, and pathologic T waves (see Figure 7-7).

Non-Q-wave MIs are considered subendocardial, where the damage is restricted to the innermost layer of

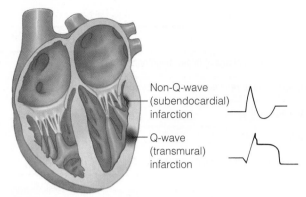

Figure 7-7 ECG and myocardial findings in Q-wave and non-Q-wave MIs.
(Courtesy Barbara Ritter, EdD, FNP-BS,CS)

the myocardium just beneath the epicardium. The most reliable diagnostic sign of a non-Q-wave MI is the presence of persistent, deep symmetrically inverted T waves (Desmarais & Cox, 2006). This is shown in Figure 7-7.

ST-Segment Elevation Myocardial Infarction (STEMI), Non-ST-Segment Elevation Myocardial Infarction (NSTEMI)

The most common cause of STEMI is reduced myocardial perfusion from an occlusive thrombus that developed on a ruptured portion of atherosclerotic plaque. This is associated with the term *acute coronary syndrome*. The STEMI is the newer term for a Q-wave MI. An NSTEMI is often associated with unstable angina.

Focused Assessment and Management

The classic sign and symptom a patient experiences during a cardiac event is pain. It is important for the nurse to differentiate the pain of an MI or angina attack from a multitude of other pain syndromes that can mimic a coronary event (Table 7–6). The pain during an MI is portrayed as a severe, crushing chest pain. This is often described by patients as a squeezing sensation. Patients often describe the pain as radiating down the left arm or up to the jaw. Similar to the discomfort of angina pectoris, the pain of an MI lasts for more than 20 minutes and it is not relieved by rest or nitroglycerin. A mnemonic device used for the evaluation of chest pain is the "APQRST" (Table 7–7). A history needs to be ascertained from the patient. This should include symptomatology of the anginal pain, history of CHD, and presence of CAD risk factors (DeVon & Ryan, 2005).

Nursing Management

Upon arrival to the emergency department (ED), the nurse needs to perform the following interventions to alleviate pain and anxiety and increase the myocardial oxygen level.

- The patient is placed in a semi-Fowler's position to allow for comfort and proper cardiovascular functioning.
- An intravenous line should be started to keep the vein open for immediate access for the administration of emergency drugs.
- Medications and treatments are then started in a standard progression.
- Aspirin is given first and consists of four "baby strength" aspirin or the equivalent of 325 mg. Baby aspirin is the treatment of choice because the patient can chew or have the medication dissolve in the mouth without a bitter taste. It is used to prevent platelet aggregation and the formation of blood clots in the coronary vasculature.
- Nitroglycerin—This is given if the patient's systolic blood pressure is above 90 mm Hg. It can be given in either the sublingual form, which will reduce the pain that is currently present, or the intravenous form to prevent future episodes.

TABLE 7–6

Noncardiovascular Causes of Chest Pain

PULMONARY	GASTROINTESTINAL	MUSCULOSKELETAL	PSYCHOGENIC	VASCULAR
Pulmonary Embolus	GERD	Costochondritis	Panic Disorder	Aortic Dissection
Pulmonary Hypertension	Esophageal Rupture	Rib Fracture		Aortic Aneurysm
Pneumothorax	Peptic Ulcer Disease	Cervical Disk		Mitral Valve Prolapse
Pleuritis	Pancreatitis			
Pneumonia	Biliary Disease			

Source: From Reigle, J. (2005). Evaluating the patient with chest pain. *Journal of Cardiovascular Nursing*, 227.

TABLE 7-7

"APQRST" Mnemonic for the Evaluation of Chest Pain

A = Associated symptoms	Dyspnea, nausea/vomiting, diaphoresis, palpitations, feelings of impending doom
P = Precipitating factors	Exertion; exposure to cold; following meals; movement; relieved by rest, nitroglycerin, or positional changes
Q = Quality	Heaviness; tightness; pressure; sharp, stabbing burning
R = Region, radiation, risk factors	Radiates to arm, jaw, back, below diaphragm Region is substernal, left lateral, right chest Risk factors include hypertension, diabetes, obesity, dyslipidemia, smoking
S = Severity	Pain scale of 0–10
T = Timing	Onset and duration: nocturnal, constant or intermittent

Source: Adapted from Reigle, J. (2005). Evaluating the patient with chest pain: The value of a comprehensive history. *Journal of Cardiovascular Nursing, 20*(4), 226–231.

- Supplemental oxygen—Oxygen is administered at 2 to 4 liters per nasal cannula to increase myocardial oxygenation. The oxygen saturation level of 92% is used as a guideline for the proper amount of oxygen to be administered.
- Morphine—Morphine sulfate is given in a dose of 2 to 5 mg intravenous every 5 to 30 minutes as needed. Morphine is used for both pain management and as an antianxiety medication. If this medication is given first it can mask the patient's perception of pain and mask the underlying cause of ischemia.
- Vital signs should be taken at frequent intervals.
- Electrocardiogram—This should be obtained within the first 10 minutes of arrival (see specifics of the ECG in the following topics).
- The patient will also be evaluated with a series of blood tests and cardiac markers, which are discussed in detail later in this chapter (American College of Cardiology, 2002).

Pain

Patients commonly describe the discomfort as crushing, oppressive, or constricting or as a pressure that may radiate to the left arm, neck, jaw, intrascapular area, or epigastric region. Transient symptoms that last less than 15 minutes and disappear at rest are classified as angina. The discomfort associated with an MI typically lasts more than 30 minutes, is not relieved by rest or nitroglycerin, and may or may not be severe. The patient is asked to evaluate the level of pain using the universal 0 to 10 scale, with 10 being the highest level of discomfort.

Additional signs and symptoms of an MI include nausea, vomiting, diaphoresis, palpitations, and dyspnea. The patient may have cool, clammy skin due to vasoconstriction and a low-grade fever caused by the systemic response to inflammation.

Special populations may cause a challenge to a correct assessment of MI. The elderly and patients with

TABLE 7-8

Differential Causes of Heart Disease in Special Populations

Women	Atypical signs and symptoms, nausea or vomiting, diaphoresis, palpitations, gastrointestinal problems
Diabetics	Atypical and silent signs and symptoms due to autonomic dysfunction
Elderly	Generalized weakness, stroke or cerebral vascular accident, syncope or change in mental status

Source: Adapted from ACC Guidelines 2002.

diabetes may not experience chest discomfort but may present with only dyspnea and palpitations. According to DeVon and Ryan (2005), women often arrive in the ED complaining of fatigue, jaw pain, back pain, nausea, vomiting, and dyspnea (Table 7–8).

Diagnostic Criteria

Diagnostic criteria are extremely important for the patient with an MI. It helps to determine the location of the muscle damage as well as the extent of the damage. Several diagnostic tests are included as the mainstay of MI or ACS diagnosis.

Electrocardiogram

The 12-lead **electrocardiogram (ECG)** is one of the most crucial diagnostic tools available for ACS. In a normal ECG, the ST segment is level with the tracing's isoelectric line. Any deviation of the ST segment from this isoelectric line will determine the amount of damage to the heart muscle. According to the 2002 American College of Cardiology/American Heart Association (ACC/AHA) guidelines, patients presenting to an ED with chest discomfort should have a 12-lead ECG performed within 10 minutes of arrival and should also be evaluated with telemetry monitoring. The presence of severe and prolonged elevation of the ST segment, or, less frequently, new Q waves, indicates that the patient is likely experiencing a STEMI. Patients with NSTE ACS may present with ST depression, T-wave inversion, transient ST-segment elevation, or with any ischemic ECG abnormalities.

Ischemia. Myocardial ischemia is the result of an imbalance between the myocardial oxygen supplies versus the myocardial oxygen demand. If this supply and demand scenario is not corrected in a timely fashion, cell death will occur. There are several key ECG changes that coincide with myocardial ischemia. The first is a T-wave inversion. Other ECG changes are a ST-segment depression of greater than 0.5 mm, an ST segment that remains on the baseline longer than 0.12 second, and inverted U waves.

Injury. Myocardial injury is most often indicated by ST-segment elevation of 1 mm or more above the baseline. The T wave may also become taller and pointed in configuration. There is also symmetric T-wave inversion.

Infarction. Infarction is suspected when the ECG shows either new Q waves, or a deepening of existing Q waves. Q waves appear within hours of pain onset and usually remain for the remainder of a patient's lifetime. A Q wave that is either 0.04 second wide or that has a depth of at least 25% of the size of the R wave is considered pathologic (Robinson, 2004). T-wave inversion occurs within hours of an infarction and can last for several months after the complete evolution of the MI.

Specific 12-Lead Changes

An anterior MI is correlated to ST elevation in leads V_2 through V_4. An MI caused by the occlusion of the left main artery is characterized by ST-segment elevation in leads V_1 through V_6. This represents a large amount of damage. An anterior lateral MI caused by an occlusion of the LAD shows ST-segment elevations in V_3 through V_6 and leads I and aVL. An anteroseptal MI shows ST elevations in leads V_1 through V_4 (Figure 7–8).

ST-segment changes in leads I and aVL indicate a high lateral wall infarct, whereas elevations in leads V_5 and V_6 reveal a lower lateral infarct. Inferior wall MI is shown with elevations in leads II, III, and aVF.

ECGs look primarily at the front of the heart; therefore, in order to assess damage to the posterior wall, a nurse needs to look for reciprocal changes in the pattern. As shown in Table 7–9, these changes include ST depression accompanied by tall, upright R waves and tall, symmetrical T waves in leads V_1 through V_3 (Goldich, 2006).

Laboratory Assessment

Within 10 minutes of arrival to the ED, the patient should have blood drawn to measure substances released when myocardial inflammation, injury, and necrosis are present.

Creatinine Kinase. Creatinine kinase (CK) may not be helpful in immediate diagnosis of an MI due to the 4 to 6 hours needed to see a significant rise. It is believed that the CK levels are more important in gauging the size and timing of an acute MI than the actual diagnosis. CK levels will peak in 12 to 24 hours and return to normal in 72 to 96 hours. The CK levels are further differentiated by bands, signifying the different muscles affected. The CK-MB is used for myocardial damage. These levels increase within 2 to 6 hours, peak at 18 hours, and return to normal within 24 hours. The CK-MB is considered positive when it is greater than 3% of the total CK.

- Reference Level:

Total CK	Women	40–150 U/L
	Men	60–400 U/L
CK-MB		<3% or 0–7.5 ng/mL

Troponin. Troponin T and troponin I assays are very useful in the diagnosis of an acute MI. These are highly sensitive tests that can determine myocardial damage at the bedside. Troponin I is the most accurate marker of myocardial injury. This marker appears in the bloodstream 4 to 12 hours after the onset of injury, peaks in 12 hours, and remains elevated for 4 to 10 days. Data has suggested that a troponin T concentration measured 72 hours after an acute MI may be predictive of MI size, independent of reperfusion. The guidelines consider values greater than 0.01 ng/mL as elevated and values of 0.1 ng/mL as markedly elevated and indicating a high risk of death. Cardiac troponins may not be released until 6 hours after symptoms begin; therefore, the ACC/AHA recommend that patients who have a negative troponin level within 6 hours of symptom onset be retested at 8 to 12 hours after onset.

- Reference Level:

Troponin I	<0.6 ng/mL
	>1.5 ng/mL consistent with MI
Troponin T	>0.1–0.2 ng/mL consistent with MI

Troponin T (bedside) can detect limits as low as 0.08 ng/mL.

Myoglobin. Damaged cardiac cells rapidly release myoglobin into the bloodstream. Peak levels occur between 1 and 4 hours, allowing for an early diagnosis of an acute MI. The levels return to normal in less than 24 hours. The drawback is that myoglobin lacks cardiac specificity; therefore, it needs to be used in conjunction with other definitive laboratory tests. A doubling of the myoglobin level in 2 hours strongly suggests MI, and a negative myoglobin within 4 to 8 hours after the onset of symptoms is used to rule out an MI.

- Reference Level: Myoglobin   50–120 ug/mL

C-Reactive Protein. C-reactive protein (CRP) is an acute-phase reactant produced by the liver in response to

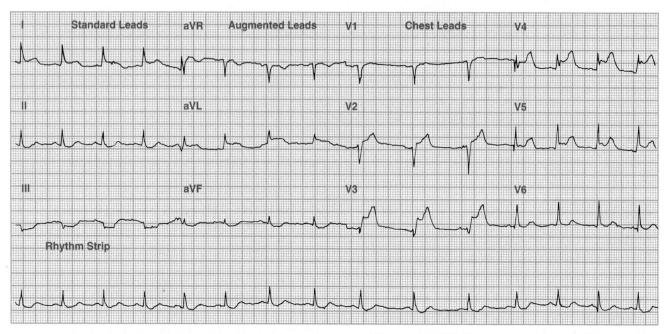

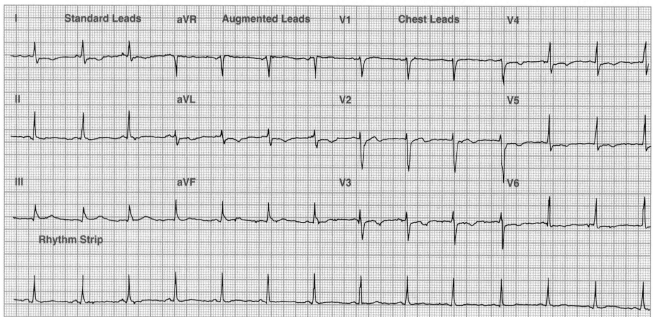

Figure 7-8 12-lead ECG of patient with an anterior MI before and after reperfusion.

inflammation. Recent scientific evidence strongly suggests that C-reactive protein levels should be used as an additive measure in performing a global risk assessment for CHD (Corbett, 2004).

- Reference Level:

CRP	Low	<0.7 mg/L
	Moderate	1.2–1.9 mg/L
	High	3.9–15.0 mg/L

Chest X-ray

A chest x-ray upon admission can be used to determine signs of impending heart failure. It can also be useful in ruling out pulmonary causes for chest pain and to evaluate for cardiomegaly.

Exercise Testing

Exercise testing with continuous electrocardiographic monitoring is a widely used and reliable method of evaluating patients who have or are at risk for developing an ACS (Table 7–10). This type of change can focus on the changes in the electrocardiograph tracing during exercise as well as give information about dysrhythmias, HR, BP, exercise perceived exertion rate, and exercise capacity. The ACC/AHA has selected categories for evidence-based classifications for patients who need to undergo exercise testing.

TABLE 7-9

ECG Changes in MI

SITE OF INFARCTION	CHANGES SEEN	POSSIBLE OCCLUSION	PICTURE ASSOCIATING ECG CHANGES
Large anterior wall	V_1–V_6: ST-segment elevation II, III, aVF: ST-segment depression	Left main coronary artery	
Anterior wall	V_2–V_4: ST-segment elevation II, III, aVF: ST-segment depression	Left anterior descending artery	
Anteroseptal	V_1–V_4: ST-segment elevation II, III, aVF: ST-segment depression	LAD and branches supplying blood to the septal wall	
Anterolateral	I, aVL, V_3–V_6: ST-segment elevation II, III, aVF: ST-segment depression	LAD and branches supplying blood to the lateral wall	
Lateral wall	V_5, V_6, I, aVL: Pathologic Q wave, ST-segment elevation, inverted T wave	Left circumflex (LCx) and/or LAD	
Inferior wall	II, III, aVF: Pathologic Q wave, ST-segment elevation, inverted T wave	RCA and/or LCx	
Posterior wall	V_1–V_3: ST-segment depression, tall, upright, symmetrical R wave, and tall, symmetrical T wave	RCA and/or LCx	

Source: Adapted from Robinson, S. (2005, May). Is it an MI? What the leads tell you. *RN, 67*(5), 48–54.

TABLE 7-10

Exercise Testing Recommendations in Patients with Acute Coronary Syndrome

Patients undergoing initial evaluation with suspected or known CAD, including those with complete right bundle branch block or less than 1 mm of resting ST depression

Patients with suspected or known CAD, previously evaluated, now presenting with significant change in clinical status

Low-risk patients with unstable angina 8–12 hours after presentation who have been free of active ischemic or heart failure symptoms

Intermediate-risk patients with unstable angina 2 or 3 days after presentation who have been free of active ischemic or heart failure symptoms

Intermediate-risk patients with unstable angina who have initial cardiac markers that are normal, repeat electrocardiography without significant change, and cardiac markers that are normal 6 to 12 hours after onset of symptoms and no other ischemia during observation

Source: From Gibbons, R., et al. (2002). ACC/AHA 2002 guideline update for exercise testing. *Circulation, 116*(14), 1883–1892.

The timing of the exercise stress test in patients with ACS depends on the specific risk. It is suggested that the patient be clinically stable before undergoing any type of exercise stress testing. Class 1 evidence is for patients who are undergoing an initial evaluation with suspected or known CAD, who have less than 1 mm of resting ST depression, or present with a significant change in clinical status. Low-risk patients with unstable angina 8 to 12 hours after presentation to an ED who have been free of ischemic or heart failure symptoms are also considered for testing. Intermediate-risk patients with unstable angina for 2 to 3 days post presentation who have been free of ischemic changes or signs of failure are also considered Class 1 evidence (Fletcher, Mills, & Taylor, 2006).

Class 2a evidence is the second category for exercise stress testing. These include immediate-risk patients with unstable angina whose initial cardiac markers are normal and now show other signs of ischemia during observation.

Diagnostic Imaging

Echocardiography is safe and easy to use as a diagnostic test. In patients with a suspected STEMI, the two-dimension echocardiography always reveals abnormalities in wall motion. It is also useful in determining left ventricular function, which assists the practitioner in determining the patient's prognosis.

Cardiac Catheterization

A cardiac catheterization is performed to determine the exact location of the myocardial injury and specific obstructions to the coronary vasculature. See specific care of patient undergoing percutaneous transluminal intervention (PCI) later in this chapter. The cardiac catheterization assists the physicians in determining whether a client would benefit from a PCI or a coronary artery bypass graft (CABG) surgery.

Collaborative Management

The immediate treatment goals for the patient with MI are to restore coronary artery blood flow, limit the infarction size, and balance myocardial oxygen supply and demand (Lackey, 2006). The nurse would use the following interventions to promote treatment of the patient with ACS.

Pharmacological Therapy

According to Wilson, Shannon, Shields, and Stang (2008), pharmacological therapy remains an important intervention for clients with ACS. There are many therapies involved including those that will decrease ischemia, assist in a decrease in platelet aggregation, and provide pain relief.

Anti-Ischemic Therapy

Anti-ischemic therapy is used to promote pain relief and increase myocardial blood perfusion. There are several drugs used for this type of therapy.

Antithrombotic Therapy

The primary effect of antithrombins is the prevention of thrombin-mediated fibrin deposition and stabilization of platelet-rich thrombi. Heparin is the most commonly used anticoagulant for a patient with ACS. It blocks thrombin formation by accelerating the action of circulating antithrombin, an enzyme that inactivates factors needed to produce thrombin. Drugs that prevent platelet aggregation are also included in this discussion.

Invasive Therapy/Interventions

NSTEMI patients who have definitive ischemic ECG changes and/or elevated cardiac markers are typically managed with an early invasive strategy. This strategy involves the use of diagnostic catheterization, followed by a PCI or CABG surgery as soon as possible. Procedural and nursing cares are similar to the PCI, so they are included in the discussion later.

COMMONLY USED MEDICATIONS

ANTI-ISCHEMIC THERAPY

NITROGLYCERIN

Nitroglycerin is an arterial and venous vasodilator. It increases coronary blood flow by dilating the coronary arteries. It is first given as a 0.4-mg sublingual tablet or spray. This initial dose is followed by an intravenous drip starting at 10 mcg/min.

Desired Effects: It reduces systolic, diastolic, and mean BP and has antianginal, anti-ischemic, and antihypertensive effects. When administered sublingually to a patient with angina, it usually results in a reduction in pain in 3 to 5 minutes.

Nursing Responsibilities:
- Ensuring administration of a therapeutic dose: Sublingual: 0.3 to 0.4 mg. q 3 to 5 min (maximum dose is three tablets in 15 minutes); Intravenous: Start infusion at 5 mcg/min and titrate every 3 to 5 minutes until the desired response is achieved.
- Ensuring use with extreme caution in patients with hypotension; monitoring for unresponsiveness and cardiac dysrhythmias.
- Checking blood pressure every 3 to 5 minutes if on intravenous dose, because this may cause a precipitous drop in systolic and diastolic blood pressure.
- If the patient's blood pressure does decrease, lowering the head of the bed, increasing the rate of IV fluids, or decreasing the dose of nitroglycerin temporarily should resolve the problem.
- Assessing the patient for a headache because 50% of patients develop this effect.

Side and/or Toxic Effects: Symptoms of overdose include hypotension; tachycardia; warm, flushed skin; headache; confusion, nausea; convulsions; and cardiovascular collapse. These symptoms may occur because ethanol is the diluent in IV nitroglycerin. When high doses of IV nitroglycerin are administered, the patient may experience ethanol intoxication (Wilson, 2008).

MORPHINE SULFATE

Morphine sulfate, an opioid analgesic, is used when chest discomfort is not relieved with nitroglycerin, when the patient becomes agitated, or when he or she is experiencing the complication of pulmonary congestion.

Desired Effects: Morphine helps to increase the coronary blood flow by dilating arteries and veins while it controls severe pain and anxiety. It also reduces preload, which, in effect, decreases the workload of the myocardial tissue.

Nursing Responsibilities:
- Providing a therapeutic dose, usually 2 to 10 mg IV in divided doses.
- Obtaining baseline respiratory rate, depth and rhythm, and size of pupils.
- Recording pain level and duration of analgesia.
- Continuing to monitor for respiratory depression.

BETA BLOCKERS

Blocking beta-1 receptors located primarily in the myocardium and beta-2 receptors in the vasculature and bronchial smooth muscle decrease myocardial contractility, slow heart rate, and decrease systolic BP. These in effect lower the cardiac oxygen demand. A slower heart rate will also assist in increasing the ventricular filling time and coronary artery blood flow, so more oxygen will reach the myocardial tissue. Receiving beta blockers within 24 hours of hospital arrival after an MI reduces mortality in the first week by 14%. Patients who were placed on intravenous doses of metropolol have been shown to have lower rates of reinfarction and recurrent ischemia (Roberts et al., 1991).

Beta-blocker therapy is contraindicated when the patient has a heart rate less than 60 beats per minute, systolic blood pressure less than 100 mm Hg, moderate or severe left ventricular failure, shock, PR interval on the electrocardiogram greater than 0.24 second, second- and third-degree heart block, and active asthma and/or reactive airway disease.

Desired Effects: Beta blockers block the cardiac effects of beta-adrenergic stimulation; as a result heart rate, myocardial irritability, and force of contraction decrease. They have also been associated with a decrease in platelet aggregability. When administered intravenously the effects occur within 1 to 2 minutes.

Nursing Responsibilities:
- Administering a therapeutic dose once the patient's hemodynamic condition has stabilized following an MI. AHA recommends an initial intravenous dose of 5 mg of metoprolol followed by two additional doses at 5-minute intervals for a total of 15 mg. The patient is converted to oral dosing if IV is tolerated.
- Observing monitor pattern, heart rate, respiration, blood pressure, and circulation closely during administration. Administration is stopped if bradycardia, heart block, or hypotension develop.
- Monitoring for signs and symptoms of heart failure.

Side and/or Toxic Effects: Bradycardia, hypotension, and heart blocks are serious side effects. Bronchospasm and dyspnea may also occur as may indications of poor perfusion such as syncope, confusion, or dizziness.

COMMONLY USED MEDICATIONS

ANTI-THROMBOTIC THERAPY

ASPIRIN

Giving aspirin as soon as possible inhibits platelet activity and interrupts platelet aggregation at the site of plaque rupture. Patients who receive aspirin in the acute phase have a 15% lower mortality rate than those who do not. Aspirin was shown to reduce the incidence of death or MI by approximately 50% in clinical trials with UA and has a Class IA recommendation in the 2002 ACC/AHA guidelines.

Desired Effects: It inhibits platelet aggregation, reducing the ability of blood to clot. It is used to prevent recurrence of MI and in prophylaxis against MI in patients with unstable angina.

Nursing Responsibilities:
- Administration of a therapeutic dose. If a patient does not take aspirin regularly the initial dose should be 160 to 325 mg. The patient should chew the dose in the acute phase to increase absorption. If a patient regularly takes an aspirin daily, check with the physician for orders on appropriate dosage.
- Monitoring prothrombin time and international ratio unit in patients with concurrent anticoagulant therapy.
- Using enteric-coated tablets to reduce gastrointestinal disturbances.

Side and/or Toxic Effects: The most common side effects are bleeding, GI discomfort, and tinnitus.

CLOPIDOGREL

Clopidogrel (Plavix) is a drug that inhibits platelet aggregation. It has recently been approved by the Food and Drug Administration (FDA) to prevent thrombotic events in patients who have had a myocardial infarction with acute ST-segment elevation. Clopidogrel should be administered with aspirin, unless a surgical intervention is planned.

Desired Effect: The desired effect is a prolongation of bleeding time and prevention of MI in patients with recent MI or unstable angina.

Nursing Responsibilities:
- Administration of a therapeutic dose: Often the initial dose is a loading dose of 300 mg, followed by 75 mg daily.
- Observing for bleeding episodes, especially GI bleeding.
- Reviewing periodic platelet count, bleeding time, and lipid profile.

Side and/or Toxic Effects: The most serious adverse effects include bleeding and purpura.

UNFRACTIONATED HEPARIN (UHF)

This is administered intravenously, but the anticoagulant is unpredictable and must be monitored with the frequent use of activated partial thromboplastin time (aPTT) blood testing.

Desired Effects: UHF inhibits formation of new clots but does not lyse already existing thrombi. It prevents thromboembolic complications during the acute stage of an MI.

Nursing Responsibilities:
- Administration of a therapeutic dose, usually 5,000 units subcutaneously every 8 to 12 hours. Doses are usually checked with a second person prior to administration.
- Monitoring aPTT levels closely: keeping INR between 1.5 and 2.5.
- Checking platelet count.
- Observing for signs and symptoms of internal and external bleeding.

Side and/or Toxic Effects: The most common problematic adverse effect is bleeding.

LOW MOLECULAR WEIGHT HEPARINS

Low molecular weight heparins (LMWH) have a relatively low degree of binding to plasma proteins and cells; they also have a more predictable anticoagulant effect, a longer half-life, and a lower incidence of thrombocytopenia than UHF. The low molecular weight heparin enoxaparin (Lovenox), given subcutaneously, is preferred. Enoxaparin has a longer half-life than heparin and provides more sustained and predictable anticoagulation. The 2002 ACC/AHA guidelines recommend the use of enoxaparin as the preferred antithrombin in patients with NSTEMI who will not undergo bypass surgery within 24 hours.

Contraindications for both forms include hypersensitivity to heparin, previous heparin-induced thrombocytopenia, uncontrollable active bleeding, and the inability to monitor platelet counts.

Desired Effects: As with UHF, enoxaparin inhibits the formation of new clots but does not lyse existing clots. Antithrombotic properties are due to its antifactor Xa and antithrombin (antifactor IIa) in coagulation activity.

Nursing Responsibilities:
- Administration of a therapeutic dose: usually 1 mg/kg every 12 hours for 2 to 8 days; given concurrently with aspirin 100 to 325 mg per day.
- Monitoring baseline coagulation studies.
- Watching platelet count closely and withholding the drug if the level of platelet count is less than 100.000 mm^3.
- Assessing for signs of unexplained bleeding.

Percutaneous Transluminal Intervention

PCI consists of coronary arteriography and percutaneous balloon angioplasty of the infarcted artery with stent placement to maintain vessel patency. To be most effective, this procedure should be performed within 90 minutes of the patient's arrival in the ED. The goal of treatment is to open the blockage in the coronary artery and reperfuse the myocardium, limiting the amount of damage. Percutaneous angioplasty alone increases the risk of restenoses; therefore, many physicians are opting to place stents in the coronary vessels to help maintain vessel patency. These stents can be mesh, tube coil, or ring in design to assist in the prevention of restenoses (Figure 7-9).

Procedure

During a PCI, for an angioplasty or stent placement, a catheter with a balloon is inserted into the femoral artery and guided to the desired site. The balloon is inflated, expanding the stent, which in turn squeezes the atherosclerotic plaque against the vessel wall and widens the arterial lumen (Figure 7-10). After the stent is in place, the balloon is deflated and removed. The stent remains

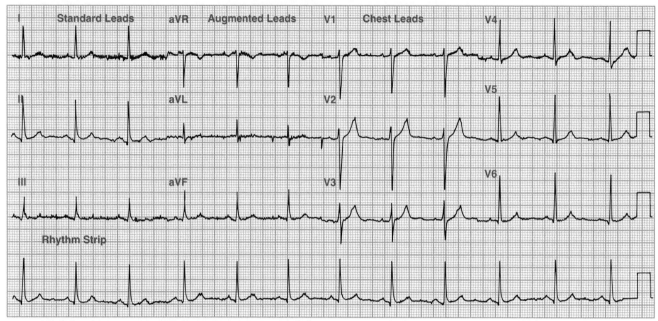

Figure 7-9 EKG of patient following percutaneous coronary intervention with stent placements.

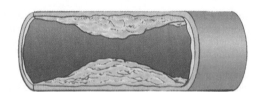

Artery is diseased.

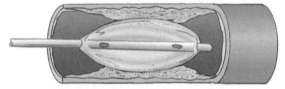

Inflated balloon presses plaque
against arterial wall.

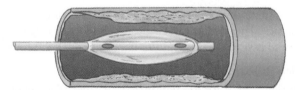

Balloon is deflated and
blood flow is reestablished.

Figure 7-10 Coronary angioplasty procedure.

in place, holding the plaque against the arterial walls and providing structural support (Figure 7-11).

The physician may also give the patient platelet GP IIb-IIIa inhibitors. These are new drugs in the regime of MI treatment. These drugs prevent platelet aggregation by keeping fibrinogen from binding to the GP IIb-IIIA receptors on the platelet surface. Studies have shown that administering this drug within 24 hours of admission for unstable angina without response to conventional therapy or NSTEMI significantly reduces the risk of death while hospitalized, but few patients receive the therapy. Initially, the patient needs to be assessed for any risk factors that might preclude the administration of these drugs (Table 7–11).

Other drugs that are considered for reperfusion therapy are the fibrinolytics. Fibrinolysis is achieved with the use of tissue plasminogen activator (tPA), to quickly lyse the thrombus. To be a candidate, the patient must have STEMI and have developed the symptoms within 12 hours of the therapy. tPA within the first 2 hours can occasionally abort an MI and dramatically reduce mortality. The ideal entrance to the ED for reperfusion would be within 30 minutes of arrival to the ED.

Contraindications to fibrinolytic therapy are displayed in Table 7–12.

Patients with stent placement usually require antiplatelet therapy with aspirin and clopidogrel for up to 6 months after stenting to reduce the risk of vessel thrombosis. During this time the endothelium grows over the stent, incorporating the device into the artery and reducing the tendency to clot (Figures 7-12 and 7-13).

Artery cross-section

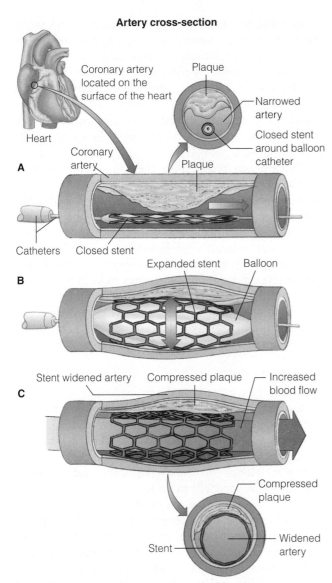

Figure 7-11 Stent placement following angioplasty.

PLATELET AGGREGATION INHIBITORS

INTRODUCTION

Three different agents fall into this category: eptifibatide (Integrelin) and tirofiban (Aggrastat), which are small molecular agents, and abciximab (ReoPro), which is a monoclonal antibody fragment. These drugs should be given as soon as possible and can be given prior to catheterization or PCI. The GP IIb-IIIa inhibitors are contraindicated for patients with bleeding diathesis, acute abnormal bleeding, or history of stroke within the last month. Renal dialysis, a history of major surgery within 6 weeks, or a platelet count of less than 100,000 mm[3] are also contraindications (Fesmire, Peterson, Roe, & Wojcik, 2003).

Desired Effects: The desired effect is inhibition of platelet aggregation, and effectiveness is indicated by minimizing thrombotic events during treatment of ACS.

Nursing Responsibilities:
- Administering the appropriate doses as prescribed: Abciximab (ReoPro)—Intravenous dose of 0.25 mg/kg bolus over 5 minutes followed by a continuous infusion of 0.125 mcg/kg/min for the next 12 hours; eptifibatide (Integrelin)—Intravenous infusion of 180 mcg/kg initial bolus followed by a 2 mcg/kg/min drip for up to 72 hours; tirofiban (Aggrastat)—Intravenous loading dose of 0.4 mcg/kg/min for 30 minutes followed by 0.1 mcg/kg/min for 12 to 24 hours.
- Monitoring platelet count, hemoglobin, and hematocrit prior to initiation of therapy and throughout treatment.
- Monitoring partial thromboplastin time (PTT) and international ratio (INR).
- Withholding the medication if thrombocytopenia is confirmed.
- Monitoring for signs and symptoms of internal and external bleeding at all invasive sites but especially at the sheath insertion site by observing the site and palpating the site and pulses distal to it.

Side and/or Toxic Effects: The most significant adverse effect is bleeding.

TABLE 7-11

Risk Factors for Contrast-Induced Acute Renal Failure

Creatinine level ≥1.5 mg/dL
Glomerulo-filtration rate (GFR) ≥60 mL/min
Diabetic nephropathy
Congestive heart failure
Hypovolemia
High-dose contrast medium

Source: From Marenzi, G., et al. (2006). N-Acetylcysteine and contrast induced nephropathy in primary angioplasty. *New England Journal of Medicine, 354*, 2773–2782.

TABLE 7-12

Contraindications for the Use of Fibrinolytic Therapy

Absolute Contraindications
Active internal bleeding
Known history of cerebral aneurysm or arteriovenous malformation (AVM)
Previous cerebral hemorrhage
Recent ischemic stroke
Suspected aortic dissection

Relative Contraindications
Active peptic ulcer disease
Current use of anticoagulants
Pregnancy
Prior ischemic stroke
Dementia
Recent surgery
Recent internal bleeding
Severe uncontrolled hypertension

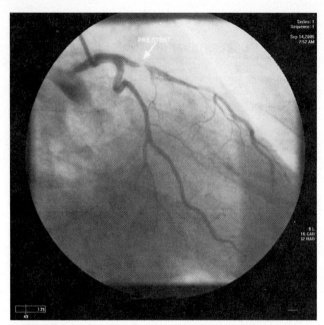

Figure 7-12 Coronary artery before angioplasty with stent insertion.
(Courtesy Elliot Hospital, Manchester, NH)

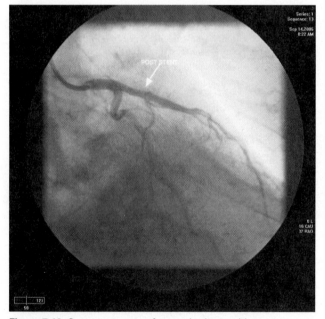

Figure 7-13 Coronary artery after angioplasty with stent insertion.
(Courtesy Elliot Hospital, Manchester, NH)

Nursing Care

The nurse prepares the patient for the procedure. The first step is to ascertain that the patient understands the procedure and that the consent form is signed. A medication history, and any allergic reactions, especially to radiographic contrast media, aspirin, or clopidogrel, needs to be obtained. The nurse must then check for lab work, especially a blood urea nitrogen and creatinine levels, due to the nephrotoxic effects of the contrast media, and report any abnormalities to the cardiac intra-

ventionalist (see Table 7-11). The drug N-acetylcystine is given to prevent contrast nephropathy because it is inexpensive, has a relatively low risk, and may have other antioxidant benefits. If risk factors for acute renal failure are ascertained, the patient will receive 600 mg twice daily for 2 days. This is usually started on the day before the procedure. In order to make the drug more palatable, the liquid should be mixed in a juice of the patient's choice.

Intravenous access must then be established with fluid at a keep-vein-open rate. The nurse must document arterial pulses in both legs, using a 0 to 4 scale. The pulses that need to be checked include the femoral, popliteal, dorsalis pedis, and posterior tibial.

The nurse should explain to the patient what to expect during the procedure. The patient will be awake but will receive analgesics and sedatives to keep him or her relaxed and comfortable. The patient should be notified that he or she might experience chest pain during balloon inflation. This may feel like a twitch rather than the severe pain of an MI (Householder-Hughes, 2006).

During the Procedure

Throughout the procedure, the patient's vital signs will be monitored as will the pulse oximetry. The patient needs to be assessed for chest pain and shortness of breath, signs and symptoms of bleeding, changes in cardiac rhythm, and presence of ST-segment or T-wave abnormalities. The nurse must also monitor for neurological status and peripheral vascular status, especially in the leg used for the procedure.

Vasovagal reactions can occur during sheath insertion and removal. If the patient's BP and HR drop and the patient starts to complain of dizziness, nausea, and possible vomiting, the nurse should administer IV fluids and atropine according to advanced cardiac life support guidelines until the HR and BP return to normal (Householder-Hughes, 2006).

Post Procedure

After the procedure the patient needs to be monitored for signs and symptoms of myocardial ischemia, thrombosis, and bleeding. Myocardial ischemia and possible thrombosis are assessed by chest pain; ST-segment changes, especially elevation on the telemetry; and shortness of breath. Changes in vital signs can include decreased oxygen saturation, a drop in BP, or a decrease or increase in HR.

Bleeding can include hematuria as well as bleeding from the catheterization site or other body orifices. The formation of a hematoma at the catheter insertion site can be a sign of internal bleeding. Vital signs can also indicate more serious internal bleeding problems. The patient's hemoglobin, hematocrit, and platelet levels should also be monitored. These can give indications for the tendency to bleed, especially if the patient has been given glycoprotein IIb/IIIa receptor inhibitors and/or tPA because these can cause thrombocytopenia. According to Householder-Hughes (2006), if the patient should start to

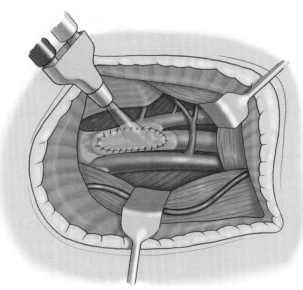

Figure 7-14 Collagen patch for arterial insertion site.

bleed from the insertion site, the nurse can either apply manual pressure to the site, or use a special clamp that can be placed over the insertion site to maintain appropriate pressure.

A newer device to maintain hemostasis after a PCI is the collagen sheath or patch (Figure 7-14). This method provides a secure method of achieving hemostasis following a femoral artery puncture. It allows the patient to achieve early ambulation and hospital discharge. The patient needs to be monitored for peripheral thrombosis and ischemia in the leg used for the procedure. Any change in pulses from the preprocedure assessment should be reported immediately to the intraventionalist (Abando & Hood, 2004).

Upon return to the unit, the patient needs to keep the catheterized leg straight and remain on bedrest for 4 to 6 hours until femoral artery hemostasis occurs. Early sheath removal reduces post procedure vascular complications (Table 7–13).

Discharge Teaching

The patient should report any signs or symptoms of an MI or angina to the physician. The patient also needs to notify the intraventionalist if any signs or symptoms of infection or bleeding occur. These can include fever, swelling, ooz-ing, or extension of bruising around the catheter insertion site. Pain, numbness, or tingling of the leg used for the procedure must also be reported.

The patient will be discharged on antiplatelet medication, either aspirin or clopidogrel, a statin to lower lipids, and a beta blocker to reduce the cardiac workload. (These medications are discussed later in the chapter.) Instructions on the proper administration of these drugs should be given to the patient. If the patient remains on antiplatelet medications, he or she must notify the physician of record, so adjustments in the medication regime can be made prior to any medical procedure.

For the first 2 weeks at home the patient should avoid excessive pressure on the puncture site or lifting items heavier than 10 pounds. The patient should not drive for 3 to 4 days or as directed. The patient can usually resume normal exercise, housework, and employment after a week.

Coronary Artery Bypass Grafting

CABG is a procedure in which the patient's diseased coronary arteries are bypassed with the patient's own venous (saphenous vein) or arterial (internal mammary artery) vessels.

CABG is indicated for patients with ACS to relieve symptoms, improve quality of life, and, it is hoped, prolong life. Proper preparation of the patient and significant others increase the likelihood of a positive outcome for the patient. CABG is indicated for the patient who:

- Has failed medical management
- Has more than two diseased coronary vessels with significant blockage
- May not be a candidate for PCI
- Has failed a PCI attempt with ongoing chest discomfort (Martin & Turkelson, 2006)

TABLE 7–13

Post-PCI/Catherization Nursing Care

Monitor for signs of myocardial ischemia, thrombosis, and bleeding from the catheterization or sheath site.
Monitor vital signs and the catheterization insertion site frequently. Report any significant changes to the intraventionalist.
Monitor the patient's hemoglobin, hematocrit, and platelet counts.
Monitor the extremity below the insertion site for pulses. Report any changes to the intraventionalist.
Maintain the patient on bedrest with the catheterized extremity straight for 4–6 hours as ordered.

Preoperative Phase

Research has shown that education of the patient prior to surgery assists with recovery, increases patient contentment, and decreases postoperative complications. Because open heart surgery is anxiety producing, it is important for the nurse to assess the individual for needs and provide the information in a timely manner to decrease that anxiety. The experienced professional nurse individualizes preoperative instruction to meet the specific needs of the client.

Information that may be included in preoperative teaching includes: sights and sounds that will be experienced, invasive lines that will be inserted, anticipated preoperative medications, and anticipated length of the operation. The nurse should also provide information on the expected postoperative course. Teaching should also include proper techniques to prevent respiratory complications, including the proper splinting of the incision for effective turning, coughing, and deep breathing.

Teaching about insertion of an endotracheal tube during surgery should be stressed. The patient needs to know that he will not be able to speak, but a nurse will be available close by to anticipate the patient's needs at that time.

Nursing interventions for the significant others should include how communication will be handled during the intraoperative period and about the patient's expected appearance once the surgery is completed (Martin & Turkelson, 2006). The patient may appear pale, cool, and edematous due to the cooling of the body during surgery and the blood loss. The nurse should also explain the equipment they will see during the intensive care and postoperative course, including chest tubes, ventilator, nasogastric tubes, urinary catheter, and multiple intravenous and other invasive lines (Table 7–14).

Intraoperative Phase

Prior to the initiation of anesthesia, cardiac surgical patients undergo the insertion of a large-bore peripheral in-

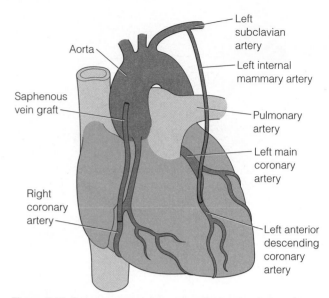

Figure 7-15 Coronary artery bypass graft showing internal mammary and saphenous vein graft.

travenous catheter, a triple lumen subclavian catheter, an arterial line, and a pulmonary artery catheter. These are needed for the monitoring and stabilization of fluid balance and hemodynamics.

The standard surgical approach is via a median sternotomy. Sources of grafts can be the internal mammary artery, the radial artery, and/or the saphenous vein (Figure 7-15).

Heparin is administered during surgery, and anticoagulation studies are performed at specific intervals to assess and guide the amount of heparin to be administered. The patient is placed on cardiopulmonary bypass, and cardioplegia is introduced. Cardioplegia is a cold solution that has a high concentration of potassium.

Rewarming of the body occurs after the surgery to offset the surgically induced hypothermia. The intrinsic heart rhythm is often spontaneously reestablished once the rewarming starts and the cross clamp is removed from the patient. Once the patient has a good return of BP and pulse, the cardiopulmonary bypass is removed and protomine sulfate is administered to reverse the effects of the intraoperative heparin. Epicardial atrial and ventricular pacing wires may be inserted at this time. Mediastinal and pleural chest tubes will also be inserted. The sternum is then wired and the incision is sutured and the patient is transported to the intensive care unit (Martin & Turkelson, 2006).

Collaborative Management

The patient must be monitored carefully because changes are subtle and occur rapidly during this period. It is

TABLE 7-14

Important Preoperative Teaching Points

Sights and sounds of the perioperative environment
Insertion of monitoring lines
Preoperative medications and anticipated sensations
Use of incentive spirometer
Length of the operation
Expectations of the postoperative environment
Postoperative pain management
Splinting of incision for pain control
Postoperative presence of an endotracheal tube
Communication issues
Postoperative activity
Preparation of significant others

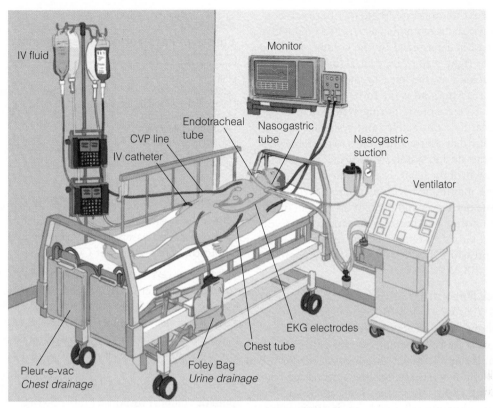

Figure 7-16 Patient returning from the OR following coronary artery bypass surgery.

important for the nurse to anticipate the possible complications so the proper interventions can be initiated in a timely manner to ensure a positive outcome for the patient. While the admitting nurse is doing an overall assessment of the patient and connecting the monitoring equipment, the operating room nurse and anesthesiologist report on the patient's condition to a receiving nurse (Figure 7-16).

Pulmonary Management

Pulmonary dysfunction is a common complication of CABG surgery. Patient history and intraoperative complications must be considered for proper management postoperatively.

Most patients will be intubated and mechanically ventilated when they first arrive in the intensive care unit. Early extubation, adequate ventilation, and oxygenation are the desired outcomes for the patient. Studies have shown that there is an increase in pulmonary complications if the patient is intubated for longer than 24 hours postoperatively. It is the goal to have the patient extubated within 12 hours after surgery.

Postoperative management includes accurate and frequent assessment, arterial blood gas analysis, and pulse oximetry, pulmonary care, including suctioning if intubated, and incentive spirometry after extubation. Early mobilization has also been shown to be important to decrease pulmonary complications postoperatively.

The nurse must assess for patient readiness for extubation. Extubation is considered when the patient is arousible, able to follow commands, hemodynamically stable, and initiating spontaneous ventilations without excessive respiratory effort. Specific hospital protocols and parameters must be followed for extubation. These can vary, but standard parameters include a blood gas analysis of a PO_2 greater than 80 mm Hg on a FiO_2 of 40% or less, a pCO_2 less than 45 mm Hg, a pH between 7.35 and 7.45, and an oxygen saturation of greater than 92%. During the weaning process the nurse should assess the patient for an increase in respiratory effort and HR, use of accessory muscles, fatigue, and color changes. These changes may indicate the patient is not ready for extubation (Martin & Turkelson, 2006).

Postoperative Management of Hemodynamics

Movement of the patient from the operating room to the intensive care unit can cause hemodynamic instability. Therefore, it is important to reconnect the patient to the monitoring equipment in a timely and orderly fashion. A manual BP should be obtained to correlate to the reading obtained on the arterial line.

The nurse needs to constantly assess for cardiac instability during the immediate postoperative period. The intensive care nurse must monitor the interrelationship between heart rhythm and rate, preload, afterload, contractility, and myocardial compliance to achieve a positive outcome. Preload is determined by the volume of blood returning to the right atrium as well as by myocardial compliance. Preload is the measurement of the end-diastolic pressure. Afterload is the force the left ventricle must overcome to eject blood during systole. It is determined by myocardial contractility and systemic vascular resistance. Myocardial contractility refers to the force generated by the heart during systole. Myocardial compliance is the ease with which the heart distends during diastole.

BP must be maintained within ordered parameters to provide tissue perfusion and prevent disruption of the surgical anastomosis. The nurse must monitor the volume in the circulatory system, which is reflected by the right arterial pressure (RAP) and pulmonary capillary wedge pressure (PCWP).

Low Blood Pressure. If the BP, cardiac output (CO), and RAP/PCWP are low, the patient will need replacement volume. Volume can be replaced by packed cells or a colloid solution depending on the cause of volume depletion. If the BP and CO are low but the PCWP is high, the patient may be experiencing a decreased contractility, and inotropic support with an agent such as dobutamine or dopamine should be instituted (see Chapter 6). ∞ If the BP is low and the CO is adequate or elevated, the systemic vascular resistance (SVR) may be low, and the patient may need a constrictive agent such as phenylephrine (see Chapter 17). ∞ Low pressure can be temporarily increased by turning off the positive end-expiratory pressure and by position changes to the Trendelenburg position.

High Blood Pressure. If the BP is too high, the surgical anastomosis can be disrupted. Nitroprusside, a vasodilator, is often administered to lower BP. Nitroglycerin may also be used to cause vasodilation as described previously in this chapter and to lower the BP. These medications need to be started slowly and carefully titrated according to patient response.

The nurse needs to rewarm the patient if hypothermia persists. The negative effects of hypothermia include ventricular dysrhythmias, vasoconstriction, and depression of clotting factors. Rewarming can be accomplished by the use of warm blankets, warm humidified oxygen, convective air mattresses, and other procedures as dictated by individual hospitals.

It is important to maintain effective CO after surgery to provide adequate tissue perfusion. The cardiac index (CI) can also be decreased with bradycardia or if the SVR is elevated. After the cause is determined proper management can be instituted. If the CO/CI is low and the PCWP is high, inotropic support is needed. If the CO/CI is low and the PCWP is low, volume is likely needed. If the SVR is elevated in the early postoperative period it can be due to hypothermia or lack of volume.

TABLE 7–15
Causes of Postoperative Dysrhythmias
Hypothermia
Inhaled anesthetics
Electrolyte disturbances (hypokalemia, hypomagnesium, hypocalcemia, and hypercalcemia)
Metabolic acidosis
Manual manipulation of the heart
Myocardial ischemia
Increased catecholamine levels

The nurse must also correlate pressure reading with clinical assessment. Peripheral perfusion assessment by neurovascular assessments can provide information about the effectiveness of CO.

Postoperative Dysrhythmias. Dysrhythmias are common after CABG surgery. The patient will be constantly monitored by telemetry monitor. Ventricular dysrhythmias are common the first 24 hours post-op, whereas supraventricular dysrhythmias are more likely 24 hours to 5 days postoperatively. There are many factors that can cause dysrhythmias post-op, and management depends on the type of dysrhythmia and the patient's clinical response (Table 7–15).

The nurse needs to treat the patient, not the monitor. Effectiveness of BP and CO should be considered when evaluating the dysrhythmia. Because surgeons place epicardial pacer wires during surgery, temporary pacing can be instituted to override an improper intrinsic rhythm so CI and BP can be maintained. The intensive care nurse needs to utilize the protocols of the individual institution as well as current advanced cardiac life support protocols.

Postoperative Management of Bleeding

Many factors need to be considered when assessing the patient's potential for bleeding. Patients who were on anticoagulants and antiplatelet agents prior to surgery may be at risk for postoperative bleeding.

The nurse should monitor the patient for signs of bleeding from the chest tubes and the surgical sites as well as clinical signs of hypovolemia due to blood loss. Hemoglobin and hematocrit should be monitored at regular intervals during the postoperative period according to physician orders and institutional protocol. Pharmacological intervention may include protomine sulfate to reverse heparin or antifibrinolytic agents such as aminocaproic acid or desmopressin (DDVP) may be ordered. Blood products such as fresh frozen plasma and platelets may also be ordered.

Because bleeding increases the risk for blood to accumulate in the pericardium the nurse needs to be cognizant to the signs and symptoms of pericardial tamponade. The clinical manifestations of tamponade include lack of chest tube drainage, decreased BP, narrowed pulse pressure, increased HR, jugular venous distention, elevated central venous pressure (CVP), and muffled heart tones.

The patient will need to have an emergent surgical procedure to reverse the cause of tamponade.

Postoperative Neurological Management

Patients post CABG are at risk for neurological complications. Cerebrovascular accidents (CVA) can be the cause of hypoprofusion or an embolic event during or after surgery. The risk of CVA is approximately 2.5%.

The nurse needs to routinely perform a complete neurological assessment of the patient. This should include pupil size and reactivity, the ability to follow commands, equality of strength of the extremities, and the ability to move all extremities. The patient should be assessed for orientation to time, place, and person.

Postoperative Renal Management

There is about an 8% risk for postoperative renal complications. Renal insufficiency can be caused by advanced age, hypertension, diabetes, decreased left ventricular function, and the length of time on cardiopulmonary bypass. Normal urinary output should be at least 0.5 mL/kg/hr. The urinary output should be monitored hourly for the first 24 to 48 hours postoperatively. The patient's potassium level should be measured every 4 to 6 hours during the first 24 hours, because potassium can be lost with diuresis. Intravenous potassium should be administered to keep levels within normal limits. Other laboratory tests that need to be monitored are the blood urea nitrogen and serum creatinine (Martin & Turkelson, 2006).

Postoperative Gastrointestinal Management

Complications can include peptic ulcer disease, perforated ulcer, pancreatitis, choleycystitis, and liver dysfunction. The risk factors for gastrointestinal (GI) dysfunction include age over 70, history of GI disease, history of alcohol abuse, emergent operation, prolonged cardiopulmonary bypass postoperative hemorrhage, use of vasopressors, and low postoperative CO.

The nurse should monitor the patient's bowel sounds, abdominal distention, and nausea and vomiting. The intubated patient will have a nasogastric tube in place so placement and assessment of the amount, color, and characteristics of drainage should be noted. After discontinuance of the nasogastric tube, the nurse should continue to assess for potential complications. The nurse can administer antiemetics and histamine-blocking agents as ordered by the physician.

Postoperative Pain Control

Poorly controlled pain can lead to cardiovascular consequences. The HR and BP can increase and the blood vessels constrict, causing an increase in cardiac workload and myocardial oxygen demand. Effective pain control is important for patient comfort and hemodynamic stability.

Pain control is achieved with intravenous or patient-controlled anesthesia (PCA) until the patient is able to tolerate and maintain control with oral narcotic agents.

The nurse must assess for respiratory depression when the patient is using narcotic pain relievers. In addition to opioid analgesics, a nonsteroidal anti-inflammatory agent, ketorolac, can be used as an adjunct and decrease the amount of narcotic pain relievers administered. The patient needs to be monitored for renal status while on ketorolac and discontinue use if the serum creatinine is too high.

Additional Postoperative Management

The nurse must monitor for signs and symptoms of infection. This source can be respiratory or from the incisions. These signs and symptoms can be increased temperature, drainage from incision, increased color in sputum, or redness at the incision site. The patient may be treated with antibiotics.

Minimally Invasive Direct Coronary Artery Bypass

If a patient presents with only lesions to the LAD, the patient may be referred for a minimally invasive direct coronary artery bypass (MIDCAB). This is also called off-pump bypass or beating heart surgery. This approach utilizes a thoracotomy approach, and cardiopulmonary bypass is not required during the procedure. During the procedure a 2-inch incision is made at the level of the fourth rib. This rib is then removed for access to the left internal mammary artery (LIMA). The LIMA is then dissected and anastomosed to the level below the lesion in the LAD while the heart is still beating. After the surgery the patient needs to be monitored for signs of acute graft closure, including a new presence of Q waves and ST-segment changes in leads V_2 through V_6. The cardiothoracic surgeon should be notified if the nurse ascertains these ECG changes.

The patient will need to have good pain management, because the incision is in the chest area and a chest tube has been inserted. The nurse also should encourage the use of the incentive spirometer and be certain that the patients turns, coughs, and deep breathes at least every two hours. The patient recovers faster from the MIDCAB, spending less time in intensive care and is often discharged from the hospital within 2 to 3 days.

Transmyocardial Laser Revascularization

A newer approach to cardiac surgery is the use of lasers. In this surgery a thoracotomy approach is used to visualize the heart. A laser beam is then utilized to create 20 or more long, narrow channels into the left ventricle. These will allow oxygenated blood to travel to the cardiac muscle during diastole. The patient is monitored in the intensive care unit after surgery to assess for reoccurrence of angina and bleeding. This procedure is still in the experimental stages.

Robotics

The use of robotics in cardiac surgery is another experimental and new procedure. This requires an endoscopic approach in which 8- to 10-mm incisions are made in the chest wall. The advantages are the ability to reach lesions that were considered inoperable in the past. The patient is in the hospital for a shorter time, there is less incisional pain, and the recovery period at home is shorter.

Nursing Care

The care of the patient with ACS not only includes the hospitalization, but many months of recuperation and rehabilitation. The patient will be monitored by the cardiologist and nursing staff, and the plan of care will include medications, anxiety control, exercise management, and nutrition management. As with any program that involves a lifestyle change, frequent contact with health care providers is highly suggested to provide time for evaluation and encouragement to continue with the promoted changes. The ACC/AHA has adapted the mnemonic ABCDE to assist with discharge and medical management of the ACS patient.

- A = Aspirin and antianginals
- B = Beta blockers and blood pressure
- C = Cholesterol and cigarettes
- D = Diet and diabetes
- E = Education and exercise (American College of Cardiology, 2002)

Pharmacological Therapies

The patient will be discharged from the hospital after an acute coronary event on multiple medications. These medications will include ones that control platelet adhesion, prevent the expenditure of myocardial oxygen, and prevent ventricular remodeling so that the complication of congestive heart failure is less likely to develop.

Risk Factor Modification

The strategy of changing lifestyle habits has been demonstrated to be successful in the patient with coronary syndromes (Jensen, 2003). Patients need interactions with health care providers in the form of personal contact, phone surveys, and support groups. Therapeutic lifestyle changes along with medications are found to be independent, but both contribute to the patient having successful outcomes.

Cardiac Rehabilitation Programs

The particular goal of a cardiac rehabilitation program is to promote lifestyle changes and secondary prevention of CHD. The programs strive to improve both the quantity and the quality of life by alleviating the psychological and physiological constraints in the form of reducing risks, managing symptoms, and having patients regain control of their lives. The programs consist of a monitored exercise program and an educational program on lifestyle changes. The length of the programs varies from program to program.

The monitored exercise program is usually supervised by a physiotherapist and a registered nurse who assesses the patient's HR, BP, ECG, and cardiac symptoms

---

SAFETY INITIATIVES | Improve Care for Acute Myocardial Infarction

PURPOSE: To reduce the gap between what is known to be effective management of the patient who has experienced an MI and the care delivered to MI patients in the United States

RATIONALE: Numerous studies have demonstrated that patients with acute myocardial infarction should receive specified components of care in order to reduce morbidity and mortality. Despite the fact that seven evidence-based care components should be included in the care of MI patients, many patients' medical records have no documentation that these care components were either provided or contraindicated. Delivery of all appropriate components could substantially improve patient outcomes following MI.

HIGHLIGHTS OF RECOMMENDATIONS:
Unless contraindicated, the patient experiencing an MI should receive:

- Early administration of aspirin
- Early administration of a beta blocker
- Timely initiation of reperfusion (thrombolysis or percutaneous intervention)
- Aspirin at discharge
- Beta blocker at discharge
- ACE-inhibitor or angiotensin receptor blockers (ARB) at discharge for patients with systolic dysfunction
- Smoking cessation counseling

Source: What Are the Key Components of Reliable, Evidence-Based AMI Care? Available: http://www.ihi.org/IHI/Programs/Campaign/AMI.htm

COMMONLY USED MEDICATIONS

AT DISCHARGE FOLLOWING AN ACUTE CORONARY EVENT

ASPIRIN

Long-term aspirin therapy significantly reduces the risk of MI, stroke, and vascular death among patients with CHD. Taking a maintenance dose of 75 to 325 mg/day significantly reduces the risk of reinfarction. Any STEMI patient without aspirin sensitivity should take a maintenance dosage indefinitely, unless contraindications are present.

Desired Effects: The therapeutic dose of 81 to 325 mg per day is intended to inhibit platelet aggregation and prevent reoccurrence of MI or ACS.

Nursing Responsibilities:
- Monitoring the INR, especially in patients with concurrent antithrombotic therapy.
- Monitoring the patient for signs and symptoms of bleeding.

BETA BLOCKERS

Continued beta blocker use post ACS reduces long-term mortality by 23%. The AHA, ACC, and American College of Physicians recommend that beta blockers be started and continued indefinitely in all patients after an MI and ACS. Drug selection is based on the desired mechanism for the patient. Beta blockers such as metoprolol and atenolol are cardioselective. Others, including labetalol, have both alpha- and beta-blocker properties and may be prescribed for concurrent management of such disorders as hypertension.

Desired Effects: See Commonly Used Medications Section 7-1. When effective, the patient has a slower heart rate, less cardiac irritability, and is able to be more active without chest discomfort.

Nursing Responsibilities:
- Administering the appropriate dose of the indicated medication such as carvedilol (Coreg) 25 mg once a day; atenolol (Tenormin) 25 to 100 mg per day; metoprolol tartrate (Topral XL; Lopressor) 50 to 100 mg twice a day; propranolol hydrochloride (Inderal) 180 to 240 mg per day in divided doses; labetolol 100 mg twice a day.
- Obtaining a history to rule out asthma and chronic obstructive pulmonary disease (COPD).
- Monitoring apical pulse, respiration, BP, and circulation to extremities closely during dose adjustment.
- Monitoring for signs and symptoms of heart failure.
- Instructing the patient not to fast for more than 12 hours because the drugs can cause hypoglycemic effects.

Side and/or Toxic Effects: Common long-term adverse effects are fatigue and weakness that, if accompanied by impotence, may cause a patient to stop complying with therapy. Bradycardia and heart failure potentially resulting in pulmonary edema are some of the most serious side effects. However, because beta blockers may mask the symptoms of hypoglycemia, it can be dangerous if it develops.

ACE INHIBITORS

By causing vasodilation, these drugs reduce afterload, the pressure against which the heart must pump, and thus its workload. ACE inhibitors help decrease ventricular remodeling after MI; thus, they may decrease the risk of heart failure. Long-term use also may improve the endothelial integrity in abnormal segments of the coronary arteries. These drugs have also been shown to be effective for BP control and stroke prevention.

Desired Effects: ACE inhibitors improve CO and exercise tolerance due to inhibition of ACE. They decrease peripheral resistance or afterload and pulmonary vascular resistance. Effectiveness may be noted by an improvement in blood pressure for a hypertensive patient, fewer symptoms of CHF, and survival following MI or ACS.

Nursing Responsibilities:
- Administering the appropriate dose such as Benazepril hydrochloride (Lotensin) 10 to 40 mg/day in divided doses; captopril (Capoten) 6.25 to 12.5 mg three times a day; enalapril maleate (Vasotec) 2.5 mg one to two times a day and may increase to 20 mg a day in divided doses; lisinopril (Prinivil, Zestril) 5 to 40 mg per day; ramipril (Altace) 2.5 to 5 mg per day.
- Watching for postural hypotension when initiating therapy.
- Monitoring blood pressure before dosing and holding per agency protocol if BP is too low.
- Monitoring for the development of hyponatremia and/or hypokalemia.

Side and/or Toxic Effects: The most common adverse effects are hypotension (which occurs most commonly in patients who are hyponatremic), an increase in serum potassium, and cough.

CHOLESTEROL-LOWERING MEDICATIONS

In 2004, the National Cholesterol Education Program (NCEP) Adult Treatment Panel (ATP III) guidelines recommended that the optimal level for LDL-C should be less than 100 mg/dL for all adults. Achieving this level produces reductions in recurrent MI, coronary death, stroke, and coronary artery procedures. The management of triglyceride elevation and a low HDL-C also deserves attention in the treatment regime. The goal for triglycerides should be less than 150 mg/dL. An HDL-C level of less than 40 is considered a major risk for CHD progression. Low HDL-C is often correlated to a high triglyceride level in adults (Metules & Bauer, 2005).

High triglycerides can be treated with lifestyle changes and "statin" therapy. The most common statins are Zocor (simvastatin), Crestor (rosuvastatin), and Lipitor (artorvastatin calcium). Fibrates, such as Lopid (gemfibrizol), and Niacin (nicotinic acid), may also be added to the regime if needed.

DRUG: HMG-COA REDUCTASE INHIBITORS (STATINS)

Desired Effects: These medications increase HDL cholesterol while decreasing LDL cholesterol and total cholesterol synthesis. They are used for patients with hypercholesterolemia, familial hypercholesterolemia; and when effective, they reduce the risks of coronary death and nonfatal MI.

Nursing Responsibilities:
- Administering the appropriate dose of the medication: Lovastatin (Mevacor) 20 mg daily, may increase to 40 to 80 mg daily; simvastatin (Zocor) 5 to 10 mg daily, may increase to 80 mg daily; atorvastatin (Lipitor) 10 mg daily, may increase to 80 mg daily; rosuvastatin (Crestor) 5 to 10 mg daily to start and increase to 20 mg daily for very high cholesterol levels.
- Obtaining baseline and periodic liver function tests.
- Monitor cholesterol levels.
- Monitoring INR: If the patient is on concurrent anticoagulants, the INR may be prolonged.
- Reporting unexplained muscle pain.
- Instructing the patient to not take the medication with grapefruit juice.

NICOTINIC ACID (NICOBID, NIASPAN)

Desired Effects: Nicotinic acid inhibits hepatic synthesis of very low density lipoproteins (VLDL), cholesterol, and triglyceride, and indirectly LDL. Large doses effectively reduce elevated serum cholesterol and total cholesterol in hypercholesterolemia. It is used as adjuvant therapy to patients with hyperlipidemia who do not respond to diet and weight loss.

(*continued*)

COMMONLY USED MEDICATIONS (*continued*)

Nursing Responsibilities:
- Ensuring administration of therapeutic dose 1.5 to 3 grams daily with a maximum dose of 6 grams daily.
- Monitoring for therapeutic effectiveness.
- Monitoring diabetics for increase in blood sugar.
- Telling patients they may feel warm and experience a flushed face within 2 hours after ingestion.

FIBRIC ACID DERIVATIVES (FIBRATES)
Desired Effect: Fibrates decrease VLDL and triglyceride synthesis, produce a moderate increase in HDL cholesterol levels, and reduce levels of total and LDL cholesterol and triglycerides. They are used for patients with high triglycerides who have not responded to diet restrictions.

Nursing Responsibilities:
- Ensuring administration of the therapeutic dose. The therapeutic doses are gemfibrozil (Lopid) 600 mg twice daily; fenofibrate (Tricor) 67 mg daily.
- Monitoring cholesterol and triglyceride levels.
- Notifying the physician if the patient presents with signs and symptoms of cholelithiasis or cholecystitis.

NITROGLYCERIN
Action and Expected Outcomes: Nitroglycerin is a vasodilator. It increases the coronary blood flow by dilating the coronary arteries.

Nitroglycerin has also been shown to potentiate the hypotensive effects of patients who take drugs for erectile dysfunction. These include sildenafil (Viagra), tadalafil (Cialis), or vardenafil (Levitra). Examples of nitrates are: Nitroglycerin (Nitro-Bid, Nitro-Dur, Nitrostat).

Desired Effects: Nitroglycerin reduces systolic, diastolic, and mean BP; produces antianginal, anti-ischemic, and antihypertensive effects. When effective, nitroglycerin prevents angina pectoris; controls CHF related to MI; and controls hypertension in the cardiac patient.

Nursing Responsibilities:
- Ensuring administration of a therapeutic dose: Sublingual: 0.3 to 0.4 mg q3–5 min (maximum dose three tablets in 15 minutes); Transdermal: Apply once every 24 hours (12 hours on–12 hours nitro free); Topical: 1 to 1½ inches of ointment every 4 to 6 hours.
  - Teaching the patient to sit or lie down before taking sublingual nitroglycerin and to keep sublingual tablets in a dark bottle with the top tightly sealed to prevent moisture from deactivating the medication.
  - Checking BP until the patient's response is known if the patient recently initiated treatment.

Side and/or Toxic Effects: The most common adverse effects are headache and hypotension.

---

during the exercise session. This is to provide data for compliance and exercise tolerance so complications can be avoided.

The programs consist of three phases. Phase 1 is provided on an inpatient basis. It is started a few days after the coronary event and ends at discharge. At this time the patient is referred to Phase 2, which is an outpatient exercise/educational program and can last for 8 to 12 weeks depending on the particular program. After completing the outpatient program, some patients elect to continue on to a Phase 3 or maintenance program. In this program the patients are in a controlled setting for exercise but are no longer monitored for ECG changes. If the patient does not elect to go onto a maintenance program in the hospital, a home exercise program is given to maintain the lifestyle change of physical activity.

Physical Activity. Physical activity provides a multitude of benefits for the cardiac patient. An exercise program can include aerobic and resistance training. Aerobic exercise has been found to positively affect lipid levels, hypertension, diabetes, weight, and obesity. Resistance training has a positive correlation with muscle mass, bone density, and functional capacity. Physical activity also has a positive correlation with psychological health.

The recommendation is for all adults to participate in a program of 30 minutes of moderate physical exercise for at least 5 days a week. The nurse or physical therapist can give the patient specific information about the type, intensity, frequency, and duration of the particular exercise session. Studies have shown that a program of moderate activity over 5 years significantly lowered the mortality rate of people who participated in the pro-

Gerontological Considerations

More than 80% of deaths in patients 65 years of age and older in the United States are from cardiovascular disease. This makes cardiovascular disease the leading cause of death in older adults. It is also one of the major causes of ED visits, hospitalization, morbidity, and disability in older adults.

Older adults, especially older women, may manifest acute coronary events differently than younger adults and men. Older women may be less likely to experience the classic chest discomfort and more likely to have nonspecific discomfort, dyspnea, diaphoresis, and fatigue.

Because age often excludes patients from clinical trials and research studies, there is not sufficient evidence to say whether cardiovascular disease ought to be managed differently in older adults than younger individuals.

However, secondary prevention strategies have been shown to be effective. When older adults participate in light to moderate physical activity and have hypertension managed aggressively, their outcomes are better.

Older adults are more likely to become depressed and isolated following a cardiovascular event.

gram as compared to sedentary individuals (Chan, Chau, & Chang, 2005).

Smoking Cessation. The patient with an ACS is often forced to quit smoking during hospitalization. Many patients can continue with the elimination of smoking post cardiac event, but it has been found that some patients relapse into the smoking habit after about 3 months at home. Studies have shown several predictive factors of success or failure of a smoking cessation program. These can include a previous medical event of a coronary nature, use of sedatives and antidepressants, nonparticipation in a cardiac rehabilitation program, and the level of cigarette consumption prior to the coronary event.

It is known that smoking cessation after a myocardial event enhances the patient's outcomes and rehabilitation. It has been found that the patient who has contemplated smoking cessation prior to the coronary event will be more successful after the event (Attebring et al., 2004). It was found that patients with a previous history of a coronary event were more likely to continue smoking than if they were newly diagnosed.

Patients who were being treated with antianxiety medications or antidepressives prior to admission also had trouble with a smoking cessation program. This correlates well with the fact that patients who have mental health issues often find it difficult to adhere to a smoking cessation program.

Patients who participate in a cardiac rehabilitation program have been reported to having a greater success at smoking cessation. This can be attributed to the patient's motivation to ensure a healthier lifestyle and peer support throughout the program.

Cigarette consumption per day is considered an indicator of nicotine dependency. It has been found that the higher average consumption was associated with a patient's continuing to smoke after a coronary event, whereas a patient who smokes a few cigarettes or is not as dependent on nicotine has a better chance of being successful in a smoking cessation program.

With short-term stay hospitalizations, it is often difficult for nurses to find time to broach the subject of smoking cessation with the patient. Literature supports that counseling by nurses and other health professionals during a patient's admission will increase the chances of the patient being successful at smoking cessation. Health care professionals need to invest more time and effort in assisting patients to stop smoking and provide the proper follow-up with the patient to ensure adherence to the program.

Nutrition

Nutrition and cardiovascular health have many facets to include. These include dietary changes to control lipids, hypertension, diabetes, and overall obesity. There are many diets on the market for a patient to follow, but ones recommended by the AHA and the American Diabetes Association appear to be the healthiest and easiest to meet the patient's particular needs (Table 7–16).

Dyslipidemia. LDL cholesterol lowering can be achieved by reducing saturated fats to less than 7% of total calories and consuming less than 200 mg of cholesterol. The National Cholesterol Educational Panel also recommends an intake of monounsaturated fatty acids

---

COMMONLY USED MEDICATIONS

MEDICATIONS USED FOR SMOKING CESSATION

NICOTINE
Desired Effect: To reduce withdrawal that accompanies smoking cessation. It is used in conjunction with a medically supervised behavior modification program and a temporary and alternate source of nicotine by the nicotine-dependent smoker who is withdrawing from cigarette smoking.

Nursing Responsibilities:
- Ensuring administration of the appropriate dose: Gum: Chew 1 piece of gum whenever there is an urge to smoke; do not exceed 20 pieces of gum per day; Intranasal: 1 dose = 2 sprays, 1 to 2 doses every hour with a maximum of 5 doses per hour (40 doses per day); Topical: Apply one patch every 24 hours in gradually decreasing strengths.
- Monitoring for skin reactions when using the transdermal approach.
- Reviewing with the patient the explicit instructions of drug use; gradually decreasing doses of all nicotine replacement forms.
- Instructing the patient to not smoke while using the transdermal approach.

BUPROPION HYDROCHLORIDE (WELLBUTRIN, ZYBAN)
Desired Effect: Bupropion is an antidepressive agent used for smoking cessation.

Nursing Responsibilities:
- Administering the drug as indicated: Start with 150 mg once daily for 3 days, then increase to 150 mg twice a day for 7 to 12 weeks.
- Monitoring for therapeutic effect; do not abruptly discontinue the drug.

VARENICLINE TARTRATE (CHANTIX)
Desired Effect: By binding to nicotinic acetylcholine receptor subtypes, it reduces the craving to smoke and nicotine withdrawal symptoms. If effective, the patient will be able to quit smoking.

Nursing Responsibilities:
- Administering the appropriate dose 0.5 mg once a day on days 1 to 3, followed by 0.5 mg twice a day in the morning and evening on days 4 to 7, then 1 mg twice a day from day 8 until the end of the 12-week course of treatment.
- Teaching the patient to start 1 week before he or she plans to stop smoking.
- Instructing the patient to take the drug with a full glass of water after eating (Aschenbrenner & Price, 2007).

---

of up to 20% of total calories. Carbohydrates have been shown to be effective when used to replace fats in the diet; however, they also tend to increase triglyceride levels and decrease HDL. Therefore, it is recommended that carbohydrate intake be limited to 60% of total calories. Fiber has also shown positive effects on lipid management and it is recommended that the patient receive a minimum of 5 to 25 grams of soluble fiber per day. Americans typically eat six or seven meals away from home each week so they must also be aware of how to eat reasonably when eating out (Table 7-17).

Hypertension. The Dietary Approaches to Stop Hypertension (DASH) study showed that a diet low in saturated fat, cholesterol, and total fat and one that emphasizes fruits, vegetables, and low-fat dairy products

TABLE (7-16

Dietary Recommendations

- Use up at least as many calories as you take in.
- Aim for at least 30 minutes of physical activity on most, if not all, days. To lose weight, do enough activity to use up more calories than you eat every day.
- Eat a diet rich in vegetables and fruits.
- Choose whole-grain, high-fiber foods.
- Eat fish at least twice a week.
- Limit how much saturated fat, trans fat, and cholesterol you eat.
- Select fat-free, 1 percent fat, and low-fat dairy products.
- Cut back on foods containing partially hydrogenated vegetable oils to reduce trans fat in your diet.
- Cut back on beverages and foods high in calories and low in nutrition, such as soft drinks and foods with added sugar.
- Choose and prepare foods with little or no salt.
- If you drink alcohol, drink in moderation.

Source: From American Heart Association.

TABLE (7-17

Dietary Recommendations for Eating Out

- To keep portions smaller, split an entrée with your dining partner or take half home when dining alone.
- Ask for sauces and dressing on the side to control the fats, sodium, and calories you eat.
- When ordering, choose foods that have been grilled, baked, steamed, or poached instead of fried, sautéed, smothered, or au gratin.
- Try ordering two or three appetizers instead of a full meal and add a salad (watch the dressing) or soup.
- If you choose a dessert, split it with your dining partners or ask for fresh fruit. Another alternative is a fat-free cappuccino or espresso beverage instead.

Source: From American Heart Association.

reduces BP. The DASH diet also provided information on sodium control in the diet. It was found that the largest reduction in BP is with a sodium intake of 1,500 mg per day. In order to adhere to these dietary constraints the patient needs to be taught how to read food labels, avoid processed food, and use an alternative seasoning to salt.

Diabetes. Because diabetic patients present with a higher risk for CAD, they should receive individualized attention on dietary management. Because they usually present with comorbidities of increased cholesterol, hypertension, and obesity, following the above recommendations plus management of glucose control will give these patients some control over their dietary habits. The diabetic patient must maintain tight glycemic control. The goal is to maintain a hemoglobin A_1C (HbA$_1$C) of less than 7%.

Weight Management

Obesity is a risk factor highly suggestive of second coronary events, especially in the older population. The obese patient presents with the comorbidities of hypertension, hypercholesterolemia, and diabetes. By controlling weight with a medically supervised weight loss program, the patient should also find success in controlling the comorbid conditions.

Anxiety/Depression

Depression has emerged as a risk factor for CAD. It has been estimated that up to 30% of patients experience depression after a coronary event (Arthur, 2006). Depression is associated with reduced participation in cardiac rehabilitation programs. The thoughts of a person who is depressed often accompany feelings of worthlessness, hopelessness, and even death. Anxiety often coexists with depression in a patient with CAD. Anxiety may present itself with feelings of tension and impending catastrophe as well as insecurity, inadequacy, and helplessness. In a recent study it was found that a primary depressive episode after an MI signals a considerably greater risk for a future coronary event.

It is important for the nurse to understand depression and anxiety in order to enhance patient recovery from the coronary event. Patients often feel that they are to blame for their health situation and that they have no control over what is going to happen over the course of rehabilitation.

Patients' anxiety and depression can be controlled by medications, but often they feel that having a nurse or medical team member keeping them informed of the situation gives them more control. Patients need to have an emphasis on psychoeducational programs, such as stress management and relaxation techniques, in the rehabilitation setting. It is important for the nurse to identify the patients' current coping strategies. The nurse can assist patients in attaining the appropriate coping mechanisms by keeping them informed and helping them sort out the important information they need to be successful in the rehabilitation process. Nurses also can assist patients to adapt and use the appropriate defense mechanisms for healthy control of depression and anxiety.

Medications commonly used to treat depression and anxiety in the post-ACS patient include the serotonin selective reuptake inhibitors, anxiolytics, and benzodiazepines.

Sexuality Concerns

Patients are often confused about returning to sexual relations after either an MI or a cardiac surgical intervention. Most patients can return to a healthy sexual life after a cardiac event. If a patient successfully finishes a cardiac rehabilitation program, the risk of experiencing an additional risk as a result of sexual activity is 20 in a million. The energy expended during a sexual encounter is equivalent to walking at a fast pace on level ground. It is currently believed that a patient should be ready to resume sexual activity within 6 to 8 weeks of an MI or after being cleared by a postmyocardial treadmill test. Many patients wait longer because of fear of another event. Patients should be warned to avoid sexual activity for several hours after eating a heavy meal, after excessive alcohol intake, in extreme temperatures, or while wearing restrictive clothes. Sexual dysfunction after an MI is often attributed to depression and/or medication side effects (Katz, 2007).

Complications

Many complications can occur as the result of an episode of ACS. The four main conditions are congestive heart failure, cardiogenic shock, dysrhythmias, and pericarditis.

Heart Failure

Heart failure is one of the more common complications of a coronary event. The more common events that lead to heart failure are left ventricular dysfunction due to decreased blood supply and decreased ventricular wall motion; the rupture of the intraventricular septum; the rupture of the papillary muscles, causing valvular dysfunction; and a right ventricular infarction. These etiologies cause a reduction in the amount of blood the heart can eject. Due to the increased preload and afterload, the heart muscle will transform into a more global organ called ventricular remodeling. The patient will often present with crackles in the lungs, wheezing, and tachypnea. If pulmonary complications occur due to the heart failing, the patient will produce frothy sputum, which is often pink tinged. Upon auscultation of the heart an S_3 sound will be appreciated depending on the heart muscle damage; the patient will often appear disoriented due to poor tissue perfusion. The patient is often watched and monitored closely in the critical care areas with specialized hemodynamic monitoring (O'Donnell, 1996). Special attention is made of the following hemodynamic values:

- Pulmonary artery pressures
- Pulmonary artery wedge pressures
- Right atrial pressures
- Pulmonary vascular resistance
- Systemic vascular resistance
- Cardiac output
- Cardiac index
- Central venous pressure

These measurements will guide the administration of fluids and pharmacological therapy. (See Chapter 6 ∞ for a complete discussion of therapy.)

Cardiogenic Shock

Cardiogenic shock needs to be assessed and treated quickly. This is the leading cause of mortality among the complications of ACS. It often occurs in patients when 40% or more of the left ventricle is damaged (O'Donnell, 1996). The patient usually presents with:

- Tachycardia
- Hypotension
- Decreased urine output (less than 0.5 mL/kg/hr)
- Cold, clammy skin
- Agitation

The patient is treated with morphine sulfate to ease pulmonary congestion and pain. Oxygen is applied to increase myocardial oxygen supply. The patient may require intubation and ventilatory assistance. The nurse will monitor the hemodynamic parameters and together with the physician will titrate the appropriate medications. If the client does not respond to drug therapy, the use of the intra-aortic balloon pump to increase perfusion to the myocardium is often recommended (see Chapter 6). ∞

Dysrhythmias

Dysrhythmias can occur in up to 95% of all patients with an MI and are frequently the cause for post-MI mortality. The location of the MI is important to determine the type of dysrhythmias the patient will demonstrate. Careful hemodynamic monitoring of the patient is essential for proper treatment of the patient. (See Chapter 4 ∞ for treatment of dysrhythmias.)

Anterior MIs are associated with the release of catecholamines, which increase HR, contractility, and BP. This type of MI often produces tachydysrhythmias, including sinus tachycardia and supraventricular tachycardias. The supraventricular tachycardias can include atrial fibrillation, atrial flutter, paroxysmal atrial tachycardia, and accelerated AV junctional rhythms. Ventricular irritability is also common for the patient with an anterior MI. A common cause for ventricular irritability is hypokalemia. The patient needs to be monitored frequently for the potassium level, and replacement should be given if the level falls below 3.5 mg/dL.

Inferior and posterior infarctions are associated with a parasympathetic response. In addition to the signs and symptoms of nausea, vomiting, and hypotension, this type of MI produces bradycardias and junctional escape rhythms.

AV blocks are also associated with acute MIs. These conduction defects are also associated by location of the myocardial damage. First-degree and second-degree type 1 occur often in inferior MIs. These rhythms are often transient and require no treatment.

Second-degree type II AV blocks are more likely to occur with anterior or anterioseptal MIs. Third degree of complete heart block is associated with inferior and anterior MIs. These blocks are less common, but more life-threatening for the patient, because they indicate that a large portion of the left ventricle has been damaged. Second-degree and third-degree heart blocks are often treated with a temporary pacemaker until the dysrhythmia resolves, or the patient is able to receive a permanent pacemaker (see Chapter 4). ∞

Pericarditis and Postcardiotomy Syndrome

Pericarditis is an inflammation of the pericardium and it is often characterized by chest pain and ECG changes. The pain is located in the anterior precordium, which can

TABLE 7–18

Differentiation Between Angina, Myocardial Infarction, and Pericarditis

ANGINA	MYOCARDIAL INFARCTION	PERICARDITIS
Substernal chest discomfort radiating to left arm	Substernal chest discomfort radiating to left arm, jaw, or back	Substernal chest discomfort increasing with inspiration
Pain relieved with rest or nitroglycerin	Pain relieved with morphine sulfate	Pain relieved with ASA and NSAIDs
No specific associated symptoms	Associated symptoms include: nausea, diaphoresis, dyspnea, fear and anxiety, fatigue, dysrhythmias	Associated symptoms include: friction rub, elevated white count, elevated temperature, dysrhythmias

radiate to the upper abdomen, upper arms, and back. The pain usually increases with inspiration and is relieved by having the patient lean forward (Table 7–18). When pericarditis occurs after a cardiac surgical procedure, it is often called postpericardiotomy syndrome. In addition to pericarditis the patient also presents with a low-grade fever, pericardial effusions, pleuritis, and an elevated white count. It is thought to be an autoimmune response.

ACUTE CORONARY SYNDROME SUMMARY

Although CHD remains the leading cause of death in the United States, dramatic improvements in patient outcomes and survival rates have occurred over the past 20 years. This is primarily due to the advent of cardiac reperfusion strategies and advances in medication ther-

Pericarditis and postpericardiotomy are often accompanied by pericardial friction rubs. This syndrome presents days to weeks after an MI or cardiac surgery and usually resolves without intervention, but many health care professionals treat it with the use of anti-inflammatory medications (aspirin (ASA), NSAIDs, and corticosteroids) to reduce the inflammation and pain (Prince & Cunha,1997).

apy. The nurse has essential responsibilities for the early identification and management of the patient experiencing an acute coronary event, care of the patient following intervention and/or surgery, and preparing the patient for cardiac rehabilitation and self-care.

VISUAL MAP   Assessment and Management of the Patient with Anginal Pain

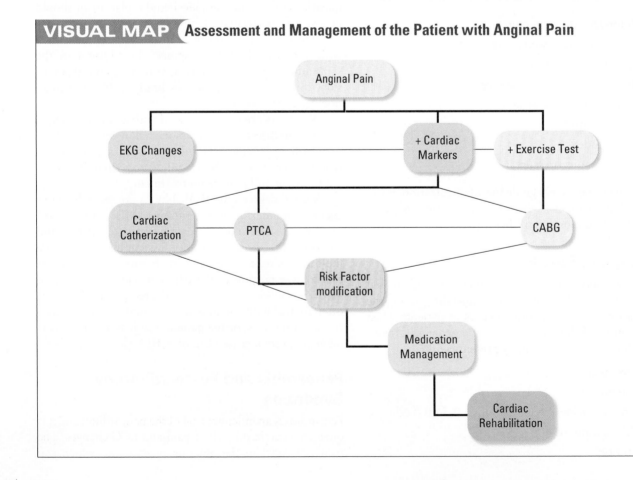

CASE STUDY

A 59-year-old male and successful business manager is transported to the hospital after experiencing chest pain at work. Upon arrival to the ED, you notice the patient clutching his chest and moaning. He states that the pain is in the middle of his chest and radiating to his jaw and left arm. You obtain a partial history from the patient.

Subjective data:
- States he has been working overtime for the past week, trying to obtain a multimillion dollar contract for his firm
- States he has been told to lose weight but has not had the time to go on a diet or exercise
- Recently divorced
- He has two children in college and one teenage son
- Is borderline diabetic

Objective data:
- Weight: 250 lb (114 kg)
- Height: 5 feet 11 inches
- Diaphoretic, pale, and short of breath
- BP 170/100
- Pulse 110 bpm and slightly irregular

- Respiratory rate 24
- Temperature 99

Diagnostic studies:
- ECG shows ST elevation in leads V_1–V_4
- Cardiac-specific enzyme troponin I is 12
- Total cholesterol level 275 mg/dL, LDL 120 mg/dL, HDL 35 mg/dL
- Creatinine phosphokinase 300
- Blood glucose 130

1. What are some of the causes of his chest pain?
2. What is the significance of the ECG results?
3. What is the possible pathophysiology of the patient's condition? How is it different from ACS?
4. What factors are contributing to the patient's medical condition?
5. What other lab values would the nurse need to evaluate? Why?
6. What should the immediate management strategies be for this patient? Why?

See answers to Case Studies in the Answer Section at the back of the book.

CRITICAL THINKING QUESTIONS

1. What is an STEMI? How is it differentiated from other causes of ACS?

2. Why is aspirin given to the patient immediately upon arrival to the ED?

3. What is troponin and why is it a useful test in patients with chest pain?

4. What are the electrolyte disturbances the nurse needs to be aware of with the ACS patient? Which is the most important? How is it treated?

5. How is pain managed in the ACS patient?

6. What are the complications of an MI? What are the causes of these complications?

7. What are the advantages of fibrinolytic therapy for the patient?

8. Why would a patient undergo a CABG surgery rather than a PCI?

See answers to Critical Thinking Questions in the Answer Section at the back of the book.

EXPLORE MEDIALINK
http://www.prenhall.com/perrin

Additional interactive resources for this chapter can be found on the Web site at http://www.prenhall.com/perrin. Click on "Chapter 7" to select activities for this chapter.

Case Study: Acute Coronary Syndrome

Nursing Care Plan

NCLEX Review Questions

MediaLinks:
- American Heart Association
- FDA: U.S. Food and Drug Administration
- FDA Heart Health Online: Coronary Artery Disease
- Medline Plus: Coronary Artery Disease

- National Heart Lung and Blood Institute
- Diseases and Conditions Index
- Coronary Artery Disease
- Texas Heart Institute
- Heart Information Center: Coronary Artery Disease
- WebMD
- Heart Disease: Coronary Artery Disease

MediaLink Applications

REFERENCES

Abando, A., & Hood, D. (2004). Peripheral arterial interventions. *Journal of Vascular Surgery, 40,* 287–290.

American College of Cardiology. (2002). *ACC/AHA 2002 guidelines update for the management of patients with unstable angina and non-ST segment elevation myocardial infarction.* Retrieved December 18, 2006, from http://www.acc.org/qualityandscience/clinical/guidelines/unstable/incorporated/index.htm

American Diabetes Association. Diabetes and Cardiovascular Disease. Retrieved June 29, 2008, from http://www.diabetes.org/diabetes-statistics/heart-disease.jsp

American Heart Association. (2006). *Acute coronary syndrome.* Retrieved December 18, 2006, from http://www.americanheart.org/presenter.jhtml?identifier=3010002

Antman, E., Anbe, D., Armstrong, P., Bates, E., Green L., Hand, M., et al. (2004). ACC/AHA guidelines for the management of patients with ST-elevation myocardial infarction-executive summary: A report of the American College of Cardiology/American Heart Association Task Force on Practice Guidelines. *Circulation, 110* (5), 588–636.

Aschenbrenner, D., & Price, C. (2007). Drug watch. *American Journal of Nursing, 107*(2), 35.

Attebring, M., Hartford, M., Hjalmarson, A., Caidahl, K., Karlsson, T., & Herlitz, J. (2004). Smoking habits and predictors of continued smoking in patients with acute coronary syndromes. *Journal of Advanced Nursing, 46*(6), 614–623.

Arthur, H. (2006). Depression, isolation, social support, and cardiovascular disease in older adults. *Journal of Cardiovascular Nursing, 21*(5s), 52–57.

Carson-De Witt, R., & Frey, R. (2006). Obesity. In *Gale encyclopedia of medicine* (3rd ed., vol. 4, pp. 2655–2661). Detroit, MI: Gale.

Chan, D., Chau, J., & Chang, A. (2005). Acute coronary syndromes: Cardiac rehabilitation programmes and quality of life. *Journal of Advanced Nursing, 49*(6), 591–599.

Corbett, J. (2004). *Laboratory tests and diagnostic procedures with nursing diagnoses.* Upper Saddle River, NJ: Prentice Hall.

Desmarais, P., & Cox, C. (2006). Q-wave versus non Q-wave myocardial infarction. Morbidity and mortality patterns after cardiac rehabilitation. *Journal of Cardiovascular Nursing, 21*(2), 118–122.

DeVon, H., & Ryan, C. (2005). Chest pain and associated symptoms of acute coronary syndrome. *Journal of Cardiovascular Nursing, 20*(4), 232–238.

Dulak, S. B. (2004). Men's health heart disease. *RN, 67*(11), 42–48.

Fesmire, F., Peterson, E., Roe, M., & Wojcik, J. (2003). Early use of glycoprotein IIb/IIIa inhibitors in the ED treatment of non-ST-segment elevation acute coronary syndromes: A local quality improvement initiative. *The American Journal of Emergency Medicine, 21*(4), 302–308.

Fletcher, G., Mills, W., & Taylor, W. (2006). Update on exercise testing. *American Family Physician, 74*(10), 1749–1754.

Gibbons, R., Balady, G., Bricker, J., Chaitman, B., Fletcher, B., et al. (2002). ACC/AHA 2002 guideline update for exercise testing. *Circulation, 116*(14), 1883–1892.

Goldich, G. (2006). Understanding the 12-lead ECG part II. *Nursing, 36*(12), 36–42.

Householder-Hughes, S. (2006, February). Non-ST-segment elevation acute coronary syndromes: Management strategies for optimal outcomes. *Critical Care Nurse Supplement,* 8–36.

Jensen, B. (2003). The illness experience of patients after a first time myocardial infarction. *Patient Education and Counseling 51*(2), 123–131.

Katz, A. (2007). Sexuality and myocardial infarction. *American Journal of Nursing, 107*(3), 49–52.

Klieman, L., Hyde, S., & Berra, K. (2006). Cardiovascular disease risk reduction in older adults. *Journal of Cardiovascular Nursing, 21*(5s), 27–39.

Lackey, S. A. (2006). Suppressing the scourge of AMI: Learn the seven key steps for improving survival and your role in implementing them. *Nursing, 36*(5), 37–42.

Lipid levels. (2006). In *Gale encyclopedia of medicine* (3rd ed.,vol. 2, pp. 867–870). Detroit, MI: Gale.

Marenzi, G., Assanelli, E., Manana, I., Lauri, G., Compodonico, J., Grazi, M., et al. (2006). N-Acetylcysteine and contrast induced nephropathy in primary angioplasty. *New England Journal of Medicine, 354*(26), 2773–2782.

Martin, C., & Turkelson, S. (2006). Nursing care of the patient undergoing coronary artery bypass grafting. *Journal of Cardiovascular Nursing, 12*(2), 2, 109–117.

Mc Cance, K., & Huether, S. (2005). *Pathophysiology, the biologic basis of diseases in adults and children* (5th ed.). St. Louis, MO: Elsevier.

Metules, T., & Bauer, J. (2005). Unstable angina: Is your care up to snuff. *RN, 68*(2), 22–28.

Moriarity, M. (2004). Women's health heart disease. *RN, 67*(1), 32–43.

O'Donnell, L. (1996). Complications of MI: Beyond the acute stage. *American Journal of Nursing, 96*(9), 24–31.

Prince, S., & Cunha, B. (1997). Postpericardiotomy syndrome. *Heart and Lung, 26*(2), 165–168.

Reigle, J. (2005). Evaluating the patient with chest pain: The value of a comprehensive history. *Journal of Cardiovascular Nursing, 20*(4), 226–231.

Robinson, S. (2004). Is it an MI? What the leads tell you. *RN, 67*(5), 18–51.

Roberts, R., Rogers, W., Mueller, H., Lambrew, C., Diver, D., et al. (1991). Immediate versus deferred beta blockade following thrombolytic therapy in patients with acute myocardial infarction. Results of the Thrombolysis in Myocardial Infarction (TIMI) II-B Study. *Circulation, 83*(2), 422–437.

Smith, S., Allen, J., Blair, S., Bonow, R., Brass, L., Fonarow, G., et al. (2006). AHA/ACC Secondary Prevention for patients with coronary artery disease and other atherosclerotic vascular diseases. *Circulation, 113*(19), 2363–2372.

Wilson, B., Shannon, M., Shields, K., & Stang, C. (2008). *Prentice Hall nurse's drug guide 2008.* Upper Saddle River, NJ: Prentice Hall.

Care of the Patient Following a Traumatic Injury

Kelley D. Taylor, RN, MSN

Learning Outcomes

Upon completion of this chapter, the learner will be able to:

1. Compare and contrast blunt and penetrating trauma.

2. Describe elements of the primary and secondary assessments.

3. Discuss airway problems that may develop in a trauma patient.

4. Compare and contrast manifestations and management of various types of thoracic trauma.

5. Recognize the manifestations of hemorrhagic shock and plan management strategies.

6. Explain cardiac tamponade.

7. Identify the patient with a spinal cord injury and describe management of the injury.

8. Describe elements of an abdominal assessment of the patient with a traumatic injury. Identify when surgery may be required.

9. Analyze the benefits of family presence during trauma resuscitation and care.

10. Discuss ways a nurse might provide comfort to the trauma patient.

Abbreviations

ABCs	Airway, Breathing, Circulation
ABGs	Arterial Blood Gases
ALI	Acute Lung Injury
AVPU	**A**lert, Responds to **V**erbal Stimuli, Responds to **P**ainful Stimuli, **U**nresponsive
BiPAP	Bi-level Positive Airway Pressure
CDC	Centers for Disease Control and Prevention
DPL	Diagnostic Peritoneal Lavage
EMS	Emergency Medical Services
FAST	Focused Assessment with Sonography
GCS	Glasgow Coma Scale
MAP	Mean Arterial Pressure
MODS	Multiorgan Dysfunction Syndrome
MVA	Motor Vehicle Accident
MVC	Motor Vehicle Crash
PEA	Pulseless Electrical Activity
RTS	Revised Trauma Score

Trauma is the number one cause of death in the United States for people ranging in age from 1 to 44. In addition, there are two cases of permanent disability for every death. As populations grow, the number of traumas also increases and care of the trauma patient becomes a frequent occurrence. In order to provide competent care, the nurse should understand the different types of traumatic injury and anticipate the associated body system injuries that can occur. Only by providing such evidence-based care can the nurse obtain the best outcomes for trauma patients.

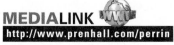

MEDIALINK
http://www.prenhall.com/perrin
See the Companion Website for chapter-specific resources at www.prenhall.com/perrin.

VISUAL MAP Traumatic Injury Overview

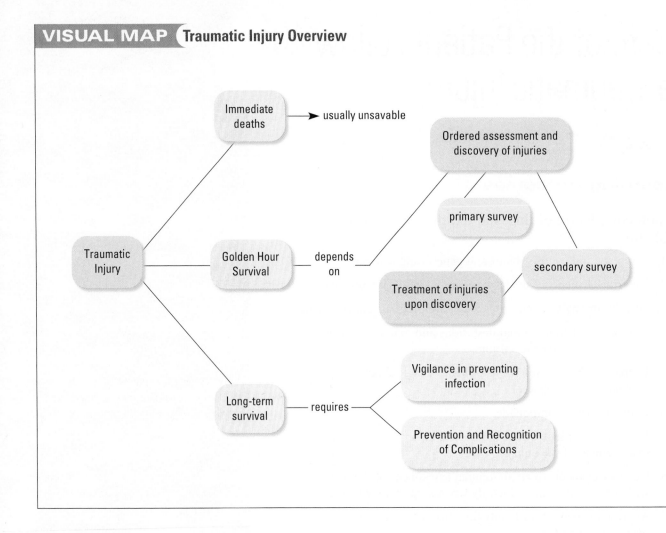

Principal Types of Trauma

Trauma is defined as a physical injury or wound caused by external forces. The National Trauma Data Bank reported that in 2005 the types of trauma were:

- Motor vehicle accident (MVA)—41.3%
- Falls—27.2%
- Burns—2%
- Gunshot wounds—5.6%
- Drowning—0.1%

Mechanisms of Injury

The preparation of care for the trauma patient includes a report on the mechanism of injury. The mechanism of injury is the energy transferred from the environment to the person. The different types of energy sources cause differing types of injuries to the body.

Types of energy sources include:

- Mechanical or kinetic energy
- Thermal energy
- Chemical energy
- Electrical energy
- Radiant energy
- Oxygen deprivation that is a cause, not an agent

Body tissue is injured when the energy source is beyond the body's resistance to tolerate that source. For example, a person striking his leg on a desk corner may develop a bruise. The body tissue is intact; however, the underlying vessels are ruptured. The skin tissue was able to resist or tolerate the strike to the leg but the underlying vessels did not tolerate the energy source. The types of tissues injured in a trauma are important. The four different types of tissues that may be damaged are epithelial, connective, muscle, and nerve.

The energy sources violating the body can be further categorized as internal and external forces (mechanical energy). An external force equation that is important to remember is:

amount of force = mass of object or body
+ velocity at which it is moving

The types of external force injuries are deceleration and acceleration. Deceleration occurs when a force stops or decreases the velocity of the moving victim, whereas acceleration is an increase in speed, for example, a pedestrian being struck by a car. Other types of forces include bullets, fists, stabbing, explosions, or blasts (may have blunt force or penetration injuries). Internal forces cause stress and strain on the body. Stress is the force applied to deform the body, and strain is tissue damage that results from stress. The different types of stress include tensile (tissue cells separated), compression (pressed together), and shearing (stress resulting from tangential force).

Types of Injuries

Injury to the different body systems is classified in two categories: blunt and penetrating trauma. In blunt trauma the skin remains intact with widespread injury underlying the area of impact. Penetrating trauma is an open injury or disruption of the skin. The most common penetrating injuries are lacerations, punctures, and amputations.

Trimodal Distribution of Trauma Deaths

Trauma deaths occur in three peaks related to the onset of the trauma. In the first peak, deaths occur within minutes of the injury due to major neurological or vascular injury. Medical treatment rarely improves the outcome. The second peak occurs during the golden hour due to intracranial hematoma and major thoracic or abdominal injuries. "Golden hour" is a term used in trauma care that refers to the first hour following the initial traumatic injury. Patient survival rates increase with the proper care in the golden hour. The third peak occurs days to weeks after the trauma due to sepsis and multiple organ failure (Eachempati, Reed, St. Louis, & Fischer, 1998; Whitehorne, 1989). Nurses are able to prevent death and disability by their

actions during the golden hour as well as by their vigilance in preventing sepsis and multiple-organ failure.

Trauma Center Classifications

The management of trauma has become a large part of hospital-based practice. Hospitals are assigned a number between 1 and 4 designating the type of care available to trauma patients. Trauma center classifications are:

- Level 1—Regional trauma center; capacity to provide tertiary care
- Level 2—Hospital provides definitive care but not as intricate as Level 1
- Level 3—Primary care is provided; the patient is stabilized and prepared for transfer for definitive care
- Level 4—Community hospital or health station in a remote area; patient is prepared for transfer

Emergency Medical Services are required by law to transport patients in life or death situations to the nearest hospital. The receiving facility may not be equipped to care for the patient. If the hospital is unable to provide adequate care, the patient is assessed and prepared for transfer to an appropriate facility that can deal with the patient's injuries (Emergency Nurses Association [ENA], 2000).

Trauma Teams

Research and outcome-related studies favor trauma teams to decrease the mortality and morbidity related to trauma by improving and expediting the trauma process. The trauma team is horizontally organized to care for the trauma patient. Trauma teams have been demonstrated to significantly reduce resuscitation times due to the

---

SAFETY INITIATIVES   **Improving Prehospital Intubation of Trauma Patients**

PURPOSE: To ensure that trauma patients receive the best possible airway management during the "golden hour"

RATIONALE: Endotracheal intubation (ET) has been used for airway management by paramedics for some time. Recently, questions have arisen as to the safety and effectiveness of both ET and rapid sequence intubation when performed outside of the hospital (Wang & Yealy, 2006). In one study, 25% of ET tubes were misplaced, 66% of these in the esophagus. More often, misplacement rates vary from 5.8% to 12%. In addition, ET has resulted in deleterious physiological responses from hyperventilation. Because few studies have confirmed the current practice of out-of-hospital intubation, this initiative reviews whether and which system level improvements might be endorsed, beginning with the question, "Should we intubate at all?" (Wang & Yealy, 2006).

HIGHLIGHTS OF RECOMMENDATIONS:
Consider increasing the number of successful intubations required for paramedics to graduate (the current standard for paramedics is 5 and for emergency physicians, 35) and limiting ETs to a well-prepared cadre of paramedics.
  Consider the use of waveform capnography in the field to ensure correct placement of the ET tube.
  Consider the addition of sedatives or neuromuscular blocking agents to the out-of-hospital protocol.
  Consider the use of alternative airways such as Combitube and laryngeal mask airway instead of ET.

Source: Wang, H., & Yealy, D. (2006). Out of hospital endotracheal intubation: Where are we? *Annals of Emergency Medicine, 47*(6), 532–541.

 Available: http://www.alaced.org/ haemrems/EMSINTUBATION.pdf

overlapping of care and allocating of tasks. This type of approach emphasizes a consistent effort in the care of trauma patients. Tasks are assigned prior to patient arrival. The members of the trauma team include the emergency department doctor, a registered nurse (RN) in charge of delegating tasks, an EMT-P or RN, a critical care aide, an emergency department technician, department secretary, x-ray technician, case manager/social worker, laboratory technician, and a respiratory therapist.

Preparation for the Patient's Arrival

Emergency Medical Services will call the receiving facility with a report about the patient en route to that facility. The primary nurse assigned to the patient begins preparing to receive the patient. The preparation includes:

- Raising the stretcher height for ease in transfer of the patient.
- Applying a trauma drape to the stretcher.
- Preparing intravenous equipment for a second or third intravenous line to be inserted. Intravenous fluids and tubing are primed; the rapid infuser is set up at the bedside.
- Collecting vials for laboratory blood specimen; arranging them on a bedside table.
- Alerting a respiratory therapist if the trauma patient is currently intubated or intubation is anticipated.
- Advising the nursing supervisor about the incoming trauma patient for the arrangement of hospital admission to the appropriate unit.
- Briefing the emergency department doctor on the trauma patient and the anticipated time of arrival.
- Notifying the on-call surgeon of the impending trauma patient's arrival. Depending on the injuries initially reported, other specialists may be called; for example, orthopedics, cardiologist, urologist.
- Alerting the x-ray department, which provides a portable x-ray machine for the initial x-rays.
- Mobilizing the trauma team in preparation for the patient's arrival if the receiving facility has a trauma team.
- Setting up a chest tube insertion kit if the initial report deems this necessary.
- Gathering other supplies that might be required such as a nasogastric tube and a Foley catheter.

The Primary Nurse Assigns Tasks. Before the patient arrives, the primary nurse works with the trauma team to assign tasks to each member. If no trauma team exists at the receiving facility, the primary nurse assigns tasks to other emergency department nurses, paramedics, and technicians. The assigning of tasks and assessments of the trauma patient should be organized similar to the assignment of tasks and assessments during a code. A common practice is to assign an RN or paramedic to the right side of the stretcher and one to the left side of the stretcher. The RN on the right side would have certain tasks and assessments to do as well as the RN on the left side. One example of how to assign these tasks and assessments is:

RN assigned to the right

- Inserts an intravenous catheter and infuses fluid and/or blood through this (if a rapid infusor is used, one RN or paramedic is assigned to watch the rapid infusion and add more fluids as necessary due to the short time frame fluids infuse with this piece of equipment)
- Draws blood samples for laboratory testing
- Assesses the patient's extremities and trunk for injuries
- Assists with insertion of a chest tube

RN assigned to the left

- Assesses the patient's airway, breathing, circulation (ABCs)
- Applies electrodes for 12 lead ECG
- Applies the blood pressure cuff, pulse oximeter, and takes a temperature
- Inserts the Foley catheter, if needed, and after the medical doctor (MD) has performed a digital rectal exam

Beginning Triage Process. Once the trauma patient has arrived, the assigned RN listens to report as she begins the triage process. The **primary survey** of airway, breathing, circulation, and disability is a continual assessment. If the trauma patient is in need of resuscitation, this would be occurring concurrently with the initial assessment. Evaluation is an ongoing process and the trauma patient is constantly assessed and reassessed. The trauma patient is stabilized then admitted to the receiving hospital or transferred to another facility better equipped to handle the patient's injury.

Initial Assessment and Management

The nurse working in the emergency setting performs an initial assessment of the trauma patient as soon as he arrives. The initial assessment, along with the report from the emergency medical response team, helps the nurse to focus on injuries that are life threatening and anticipate any acute conditions that may arise. The initial assessment identifies the extent and severity of the injuries. The nurse and members of the trauma team continue to reevaluate the elements in the primary survey (airway, breathing, circulation, and disability) throughout the patient's stay in the emergency department. It is important to remember that care of a trauma patient is based on assessment with treatment upon discovery. In other words,

Nursing Diagnoses

PATIENT FOLLOWING A TRAUMATIC INJURY

- Ineffective airway clearance related to tracheobronchial obstruction
- Impaired gas exchange related to altered oxygen supply
- Deficient fluid volume related to active fluid loss due to bleeding
- Acute pain related to trauma
- Risk for infection related to inadequate primary defenses
- Risk for ineffective tissue perfusion: peripheral, renal, gastrointestinal, cardiopulmonary, or cerebral related to hypovolemia, reduced arterial flow, and cerebral edema

the trauma patient is assessed in an orderly fashion and the treatment of each life-threatening injury is initiated upon discovery of that injury.

Priorities of Care— Primary Assessment

The priorities of care of any patient are the same: airway, breathing, circulation, and disability (neurovascular status). The trauma patient is no exception to the ABCs of care. The purpose of the primary survey is to perform a quick assessment that identifies any life-threatening problems (ENA, 2000; Sheehy, 1984):

- **A** stands for airway. The airway is maintained with C-spine precautions (the neck is stabilized with a hard cervical collar or manually held in line). (See Figure 8-1.) An ET is the preferred method of maintaining a patent airway.

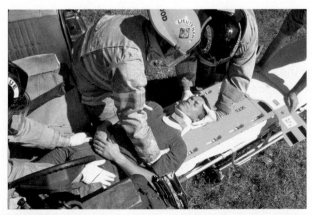

Figure 8-1 Immobilization of the cervical spine at the scene of the accident is essential to prevent further injury to the spinal cord. The combined use of a hard cervical collar, head blocks, and tape best restricts flexion, extension, rotation, and lateral bending of the neck.

- **B** stands for breathing. Is the trauma patient breathing on her own? What is the method of injury? The trauma patient may have the ability to maintain her own airway on arrival but this could change quickly. A manual ventilation bag may be attached to the end of the ET and the patient ventilated manually until she arrives at the accepting facility where a ventilator is set up and attached to breathe for the patient.

- **C** stands for circulation. Is the trauma patient maintaining her circulation? Circulation is assessed through blood pressure, palpating for pulses, checking the skin color, and monitoring oxygen saturation. Are there any obvious sources of bleeding?

- **D** is the next letter (the mnemonic follows the alphabet). Disability refers to the neurovascular status of the trauma patient. What is the level of consciousness of the patient? What are the size, shape, equality, and reactivity to light of the patient's pupils? Is the patient alert? Does the patient respond to verbal stimuli or painful stimuli? Is the patient unresponsive?

Secondary Assessment

As the primary survey and reevaluation process are underway, the secondary assessment begins. Continuing with the alphabet:

- **E** is for expose/environment, which consists of removing the clothing of the patient to check for other injuries while at the same time preventing heat loss with heated blankets, overhead warmers, or warmed intravenous fluids.

- **F** is for a full set of vital signs. F also pertains to having family members present during this phase of the patient's treatment.

- **G** refers to giving comfort measures. Comfort comes in the form of physical and emotional comfort. Physical comfort might consist of pain relief both in the form of pharmacological or alternative methods—if possible, repositioning the patient, distracting the patient, and touching the patient. Emotional comfort may be provided in the form of reassurance both physically and verbally, listening to the patient, and relaying information to the patient's family and friends.

- **H** represents head-to-toe assessment and medical history. The major part of the assessment has been completed but a head-to-toe assessment is very important to identify any additional injuries. The head-to-toe inspection consists of a systematic inspection beginning with the patient's head and face moving down the neck to the clavicles, shoulders, chest, abdomen, and flanks then moving on to the pelvis and perineum and on to the extremities. The head-to-toe assessment is comprised of a visual as well as manual assessment and auscultation of the appropriate areas.

H also stands for the patient's medical history. A responsive patient is very helpful in giving information to the medical team. An unresponsive patient is more difficult to assess. Family members are usually willing to divulge information; however, the patient does not always arrive with family in tow.

- I, the final letter of the mnemonic, stands for inspection of posterior surfaces. Often, the trauma patient arrives at the receiving facility on a back board. It is important to log roll the patient to inspect the posterior surfaces, making note of any injuries and informing the attending physician.

Trauma Scoring Systems

The **revised trauma score (RTS)** is a physiological scoring system, with high interrater reliability and demonstrated accuracy in predicting death. It is scored from the first set of data obtained on the patient, and consists of the **Glasgow Coma Scale (GCS)**, systolic blood pressure (SBP), and respiratory rate (RR) (Table 8–1).

The RTS may be used as a simple sum of the different values. However, it is often calculated with weighting for the various categories. When it is weighted, the RTS is calculated as

$$0.9368 \text{ GCS} + 0.7326 \text{ SBP} + 0.2908 \text{ RR}$$

Values for the weighted RTS range between 0 and 7.8408. The higher the RTS for the patient, the greater the probability of survival. Patients with scores higher than 5 are likely to survive with excellent care, whereas patients with scores less than 4 should be treated in a trauma center. Patients with scores of 0 or 1 are unlikely to survive (Trauma Care International).

Initial Treatment

Resuscitation is the most obvious initial treatment. The ABCs are referred to frequently during the initial assessment phase and thereafter. While the primary survey is in progress, a variety of interventions may be initiated and monitoring devices attached.

- One hundred percent oxygen (O_2) is administered via nonrebreather mask or ventilator while O_2 saturation and arterial blood gases are obtained.

- The patient is placed on a cardiac monitor with an automatic blood pressure cuff inflating at least every 5 minutes. An ECG is obtained. Intravenous fluids are infusing and blood products are administered as needed.

- X-rays of the suspicious areas are obtained initially. The patient may undergo a computerized tomography (CT) scan or magnetic resonance imaging (MRI) to determine further injuries.

- A nasogastric tube may be placed to decompress the stomach. A urinary catheter will probably be inserted to monitor output. However, every orifice should be visualized and palpated before any sort of tube is inserted. It is particularly important that the urethral meatus be visualized before a catheter is inserted to rule out the likelihood of urethral damage (Sparnon & Ford, 1986).

Detailed Description of the Primary Survey

The trauma patient is assessed and treated accordingly as quickly as possible. The description of each element of the A–I mnemonic may seem lengthy and time consuming when in reality this assessment is done very quickly. Typically, there is more than one nurse along

TABLE 8–1

The Revised Trauma Score

The revised trauma score (RTS) is a physiological scoring system, with high interrater reliability and demonstrated accuracy in predicting death. It is scored from the first set of data obtained on the patient, and consists of Glasgow Coma Scale, systolic blood pressure, and respiratory rate.

GLASGOW COMA SCALE (GCS)	SYSTOLIC BLOOD PRESSURE (SBP)	RESPIRATORY RATE (RR)	CODED VALUE
13–15	>89	10–29	4
9–12	76–89	>29	3
6–8	50–75	6–9	2
4–5	1–49	10–5	1
3	0	0	0

Source: Courtesy Trauma.org.

with at least one physician assessing and inspecting simultaneously. The mnemonic helps to systematically organize the assessment process of the trauma patient.

A: Airway

The number one priority with all patients is airway. To prevent hypoxemia, the patient requires an unobstructed, protected airway for adequate ventilation. Trauma patients should always be administered supplemental O_2 because the quickest killer of the injured is inadequate delivery of oxygenated blood to the brain and organs. To assess the airway, the nurse asks the patient's name. If the patient is able to articulate the answer clearly, his airway is patent. Then the mouth is inspected for blood or foreign materials and the neck for hematomas or tracheal deviation.

The nurse recognizes that patients with the following conditions will most likely lack an adequate airway and require an artificial airway to be placed and secured:

* Apnea
* Glasgow Coma Scale less than 9 or sustained seizure activity
* Unstable midface trauma with airway injuries
* Large flail segment or respiratory failure
* High aspiration risk
* Inability to otherwise maintain an airway or oxygenation

Treatment may be endotracheal intubation or placement of a surgical airway such as a cricothyroidotomy or emergent tracheostomy. Placement of an ET is shown in Figure 8-2.

Early Airway Problems

It is important for the nurse to recognize, anticipate, and prevent problems associated with the airway. Early airway management problems include:

* Failure to recognize the need for an airway
* Inability to establish an airway
* Failure to recognize an incorrectly placed airway

The nurse must assess and reassess the trauma patient to maintain and protect the airway. The nurse should always check correct placement of an airway! Correct airway placement may be confirmed by:

* Using a carbon dioxide (CO_2) detector. It is attached to the ET tube and changes color upon detection of CO_2, confirming ET tube placement.
* Listening for bilateral lung sounds and watching for bilateral expansion of the chest.
* Obtaining a chest x-ray.

Other problems in early airway management are displacement of a previously established airway, failure

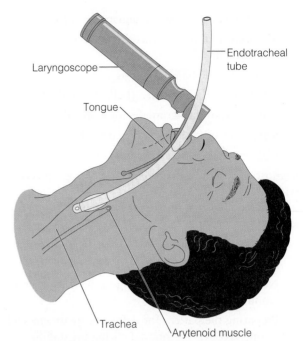

Figure 8-2 Placement of the oral endotracheal tube for intubation. When the ETT is in place, air or oxygen can be blown into the external opening of the tube and enter the trachea.

to recognize the need for ventilation, and aspiration of gastric contents. By continually reassessing the patient, a displaced airway can be identified and corrected quickly. An oral gastric tube can be inserted after an airway is established. The oral gastric tube is attached to low continuous suction to aid in prevention of aspiration of gastric contents. The need for continual reassessment cannot be stressed enough!

Assessment and Management of Midface Trauma

The patient with maxillofacial trauma is in need of aggressive management and is usually more comfortable sitting up. Typically, maxillary trauma is associated with multisystem injury and the possibility of a compromised airway. Maxillary trauma is categorized as follows:

Le Fort I is a transverse fracture that involves a detachment of the entire maxilla above the teeth at the level of the nasal floor.

Le Fort II is a pyramidal fracture involving the triangular segment of the midface and nasal bones.

Le Fort III is a complete disjunction of the cranial attachments from the facial bones. These facial fractures are not always well defined and may occur as partial or complete fractures and in conjunction with one another. The nursing assessment should take into consideration the mechanism of injury while examining the face and head. Manifestations of a facial fracture may include:

* Epistaxis
* Pain on the injury site

- Facial swelling, facial asymmetry or distortion
- Malocclusion, intraoral ecchymosis, midface maxillary mobility
- Periorbital edema/ecchymosis
- Cerebrospinal rhinorrhea (LeFort II and III)
- Symptoms of intracranial and/or spinal injury
- Symptoms of multisystem injuries (Frakes & Evans, 2004)

Diagnostic procedures would include radiographs of individual facial bones.

Nursing interventions for the patient with maxillofacial trauma include:

- Positioning the patient for optimal airway clearance and constant assessment of airway patency
- Noting the degree of swelling to the face and the amount of blood loss
- Preparing the patient for definitive treatment such as open reduction, internal wiring for stabilization, and administering prophylactic antibiotics
- Administering analgesics as prescribed (Frakes & Evans, 2004)

Collaborative Management

Neck trauma is recognized for the potential for **hemorrhage** and disruption of the larynx or trachea. Neck trauma may also involve **spinal cord injury,** which is discussed later in this chapter. A trauma patient with laryngeal trauma typically exhibits:

- Hoarseness in speech
- Laryngeal fracture palpable along with crepitus
- Pain with swallowing, cough, or hemoptysis

The nurse assesses the neck for:

- Ecchymosis
- Abrasions
- Loss of thyroid prominence

The nurse must ensure ABCs. The patient should have a CT scan for diagnostics because soft tissue neck films are not sensitive to laryngeal injury. The nurse should monitor arterial blood gas (ABG) values, assist with cricothyrotomy or tracheotomy when the patient cannot be intubated, and administer high-humidity oxygen. The following are indications for cricothyrotomy:

- Maxillofacial trauma
- Laryngeal fractures
- Facial or upper airway burns
- Severe oropharyngeal hemorrhage

B: Breathing

A variety of chest wall injuries may result in ineffective breathing for the patient with a traumatic injury. Thoracic trauma usually affects breathing due to the location of the lungs in the thoracic cavity. The thoracic cavity extends from the top of the sternum to the diaphragm. The structures contained within this cavity include the lungs, heart, esophagus, trachea, thoracic aorta, 12 thoracic vertebrae, inferior and superior vena cavae, vagus nerves, phrenic nerves, and other vascular structures. The diaphragm is included inferiorly in the thoracic cavity.

Chest wall injury is extremely common following blunt trauma. It varies in severity from minor bruising or an isolated rib fracture to severe crush injuries leading to respiratory compromise. Because trauma to the thoracic area is the second leading cause of traumatic death, it is essential that the nurse assess the trauma patient thoroughly for chest wall injuries.

Assessing for Breathing

When assessing the trauma patient for breathing, the nurse watches for:

- Spontaneous breathing
- The rise and fall of the chest (depth and symmetry)
- Skin color

By standing at the foot of the bed, the nurse can watch the chest rise and fall and ascertain if it is symmetrical. The RR and pattern should be noted: Is the patient breathing slowly, too fast, or about the normal rate? Is the patient using accessory muscles and/or abdominal muscles to aid in breathing? The nurse auscultates the lungs. The patient should have bilateral breath sounds. The nurse also checks for jugular vein distension and the position of the trachea. Percussion of the chest may yield additional information. ABGs should be monitored because thoracic trauma often results in hypoxia, hypercarbia, and acidosis.

Ineffective Breathing. It is extremely important to identify when chest injury is present because it has an incidence of 45% to 65% and a mortality of up to 60% in trauma patients. Assessment findings that indicate potentially life-threatening problems include:

- The absence of spontaneous ventilation
- Absent or asymmetric breath sounds (which may indicate either pneumothorax or ET malposition)
- Dyspnea with accessory muscle and/or abdominal muscle use
- Hyperresonance or dullness to chest percussion (suggesting tension pneumothorax or hemothorax)
- Gross chest wall instability or defects that compromise ventilation such as a flail chest or sucking chest wound

In addition, the patient may have:

- Altered mental status due to lack of oxygenated blood to the brain
- Cyanosis, especially circumoral cyanosis

These findings should all be treated upon discovery.

Nursing Management

The goal of care is to restore normal breathing patterns. Interventions are directed toward the specific injury or the underlying cause of the respiratory distress.

Basic nursing interventions for the patient with ineffective breathing are to:

- Provide supplemental O_2: Give 100% O_2 via non-rebreathing mask if the patient has a chest wall injury.
- Prepare the patient for intubation.
- Evaluate specific respiratory dysfunctions and provide appropriate interventions.

The treatment of patients with chest wall injuries can be extensive and prolonged. Patients with thoracic trauma are more likely to require longer periods of mechanical ventilation and hospitalization than other trauma patients. The initial injury may lead to the development of systemic inflammatory response syndrome, acute lung injury (ALI), nosocomial infections, and multiorgan dysfunction syndrome (MODS), which are discussed in Chapter 17. ∞ Therefore, the nurse is vigilant in implementing the ventilator bundle and using other measures to prevent sepsis (see Chapter 17). ∞

Assessment Findings and Management of Rib Fractures

Rib fractures might be identified when the nurse systematically examines the chest. Bruising or seat belt signs may be visible, and palpation of these areas may reveal the crepitus associated with broken ribs. Awake patients will usually complain of pain with palpation or on inspiration.

Although simple rib fractures may require no specific therapy, the nurse should carefully assess for indications of underlying trauma. Fractures of the lower ribs may be associated with spleen or liver injuries. Injuries to upper ribs are infrequently associated with injuries to adjacent great vessels. When multiple rib fractures are present, the nurse should assess for a flail chest and/or pulmonary contusions.

Assessment Findings and Management of Flail Chest

A flail chest occurs when there are at least two fractures of two or more adjoining ribs. This results in a segment of the thoracic cage that is not attached to any of the other ribs. The flail segment moves paradoxically to the rest of the chest wall: inward during inspiration and outward during expiration (Figure 8-3). Large flail segments involve a greater proportion of the chest wall and may extend bilaterally or involve the sternum. In these cases the disruption of pulmonary mechanics may be enough to require mechanical ventilation. Signs and symptoms include:

- Dyspnea
- Pain in the chest wall
- Paradoxical movement of a section of the chest wall

The presence of a flail chest indicates an underlying pulmonary contusion (Ciraulo, Elliott, Mitchell, & Rodriguez, 1994). It is often the size and severity of the contusion that determines whether the patient will need mechanical ventilation and for how long. Initially, the flail chest is splinted. However, this is only a short-term measure. Nonoperative management includes intubation and mechanical ventilation with aggressive pain management

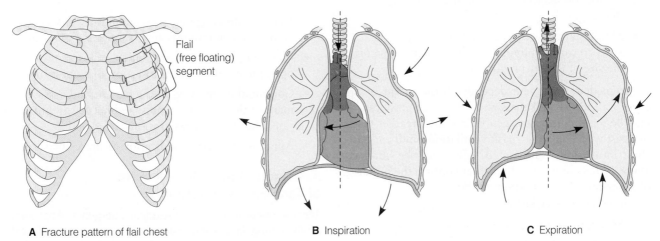

A Fracture pattern of flail chest   **B** Inspiration   **C** Expiration

Figure 8-3 Flail chest with paradoxical movement.

and frequent pulmonary care (Gundez, 2005). This strategy is aimed at preventing the development of pneumonia, which is the most common complication of chest wall injury (Yeo, 2001).

Pain relief is essential therapy for any rib fractures. Strapping the chest to splint rib fractures was utilized in the past but it prevents adequate chest wall movement and clearance of secretions. The nurse provides the patient with sufficient pain relief so that he is able to cough and deep breathe. After the emergent period, the best analgesia for a severe chest wall injury is a continuous epidural infusion of a local anesthetic because it provides adequate pain relief without the risks of respiratory depression (Harrahill, 1998).

Assessment and Management of Pneumothorax

A pneumothorax occurs when air enters the pleural space causing loss of negative intrapleural pressure and a total or partial collapse of the lung on the affected side. Open pneumothorax or a sucking chest wound refers to a traumatic injury in which the pleural cavity is exposed to the external environment through an open chest wall wound (Figure 8-4).

There are several important considerations for the nurse who is assessing the patient with a possible pneumothorax (Yamamoto, 2005):

- A closed pneumothorax occurs without external signs and may be difficult to identify (Figure 8-5).

- The classic finding of a pneumothorax is resonance on percussion.

- However, it is more commonly identified by the palpation of subcutaneous emphysema and rib fractures.

- In the trauma patient, tracheal shift from midline generally indicates a pneumothorax or pleural effusion.

- The need to auscultate breath sounds is basic. The nurse is listening for diminished or absent breath sounds that could indicate collapse of the lung.

- Manifestations vary from only changes in the x-ray to cardiopulmonary collapse depending on the size of the pneumothorax.

Immediate treatment depends on the extent of the chest wall injury and the size of the pneumothorax. It may be to administer oxygen via a nonrebreather mask or assist with bag-valve mask ventilations until endotracheal intubation is attempted. ABGs may be obtained along with a chest x-ray to further confirm the presence of a pneumothorax (Lettieri, 2006).

Interventions include:

- Maintaining ABCs

- Administering supplemental oxygen

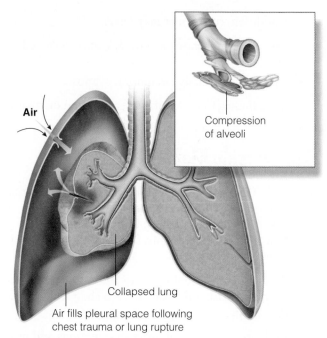

Air

Compression of alveoli

Collapsed lung

Air fills pleural space following chest trauma or lung rupture

Figure 8-4 Open pneumothorax.

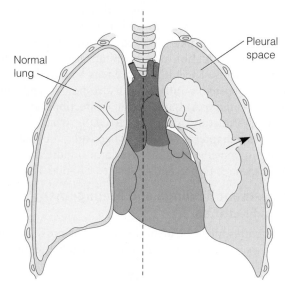

Normal lung

Pleural space

Figure 8-5 Closed pneumothorax.

- Placing a dressing that is taped on three sides over an open pneumothorax for temporary management

- Preparing the patient with either a closed or an open pneumothorax for insertion of a chest tube

- Continual monitoring of the patient and assessment of the vital signs, pulse oximetry, rhythm, rate, and depth of respirations

- Administering pain medication as prescribed

Assessment and Management of Tension Pneumothorax

Tension pneumothorax is a surgical emergency. An injury, often a lung laceration, allows air to enter the pleural space but not to exit, resulting in progressive accumulation of air in the pleural space. The pressure from the accumulating air may become so great that the patient may have a total lung collapse, and a mediastinal shift may occur (Figure 8-6). Because the pressure in the chest is elevated, tension pneumothorax leads to impairment of venous return to the heart and a fall in cardiac output. The classic signs of a tension pneumothorax are:

- Deviation of the trachea away from the side with the tension
- One hyperexpanded side of the chest that moves little with respiration
- Absent breath sounds on the affected side
- Hyperresonance to percussion on the affected side
- Acute respiratory distress
- Crepitus
- An elevated central venous pressure

The patient is almost always tachycardic and tachypneic and may be hypoxic. These signs are followed by hypotension and circulatory collapse with the possibility of traumatic arrest and pulseless electrical activity (PEA).

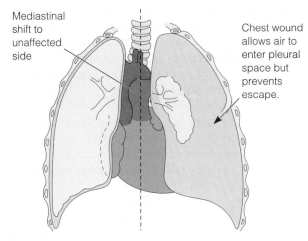

Mediastinal shift to unaffected side

Chest wound allows air to enter pleural space but prevents escape.

Figure 8-6 Tension pneumothorax.

The treatment for tension pneumothorax is the immediate insertion of a chest tube. Although some sources recommend blind needle thoracostomy (Figure 8-7), many physicians believe that unless the situation is truly emergent, the disadvantages outweigh the benefits. As long as the emergency department (ED) is prepared for emergent chest tube insertion, most patients can wait the few moments needed to complete the preparation for chest tube insertion. However, in some situations, needle thoracostomy can be life saving (Lettieri, 2006).

Tension hemothorax is similar to a tension pneumothorax except that blood is in the pleural space and is usually caused by a rupture of a blood vessel. Management of the tension hemothorax is also insertion of a chest tube.

Assessment and Management of Hemothorax

A hemothorax is a collection of blood in the pleural space and may be caused by blunt or penetrating trauma (Figure 8-8). Because most hemothoraces are the result of rib fractures and lung parenchymal or venous injuries, the bleeding is usually self-limiting. The classic signs of a hemothorax are:

- Decreased chest expansion
- Dullness to percussion
- Reduced breath sounds on the affected side

There is usually not a mediastinal or tracheal deviation unless there is a massive hemothorax. In fact, the signs may be subtle in the supine trauma patient in the ED, and many smaller hemothoraces will only be diagnosed after imaging studies.

The majority of hemothoraces stop bleeding so chest tube drainage is all that is required to treat the patient. For this reason, the nurse anticipates that the sanguinous drainage from the chest tube of a patient with a hemothorax will decrease in a stepwise fashion, such as 3-2-1. If the drainage does not subside, the nurse should notify the trauma surgeon (Richardson, Miller, Carrillo, & Spain, 1996).

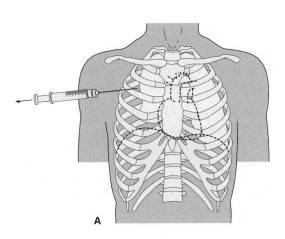

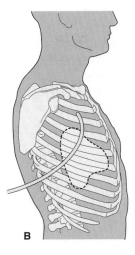

Figure 8-7 A needle thoracostomy may be used in the emergency treatment of a tension pneumothorax. *A,* A large gauge needle in introduced, and air and fluid are aspirated. *B,* Alternatively, a chest tube may be inserted and connected to a chest drainage system.

A   B

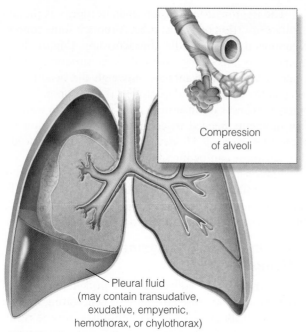

Figure 8-8 Hemothorax.

Pleural fluid
(may contain transudative,
exudative, empyemic,
hemothorax, or chylothorax)

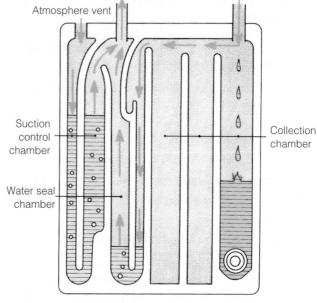

Figure 8-9 A closed-chest drainage system.

Connect to external
suction source

Connect to
chest tube

Atmosphere vent

Suction
control
chamber

Water seal
chamber

Collection
chamber

Building Technology Skills

Chest tubes are drainage systems that allow air, as in a pneumothorax, or fluid or blood, as in a hemothorax, to drain out of the pleural space. The goal is to remove the air, blood, or fluid from the pleural space, thereby reestablishing subatmospheric intrapleural pressure. The lung will then reexpand.

Technological Requirements

A chest tube is a tube inserted in the chest cavity attached to a closed drainage system that is usually attached to suction. The suction allows material (the air, blood, or fluid) to be removed from the lung without allowing air to be sucked into the pleural space. There are three chambers in a closed drainage system: a collection chamber, a water seal chamber, and a suction control chamber (Figure 8-9).

The insertion site of the chest tube depends on the type of drainage. Chest tubes from which air will be draining are placed high and anterior between the ribs, whereas fluid drainage chest tubes are placed low and posterior. The reason is that air tends to rise while fluid falls to the basal region of the pleural space. The most common complication of chest tubes is malposition. Therefore, chest tube placement should be confirmed with an x-ray.

Nursing Responsibilities

When caring for the patient with a chest tube, the nurse should:

Secure the chest tube site and dressing. Palpate the site of chest tube insertion for crepitus, document the extent of crepitus, and reassess for changes.

Maintain the level of the drainage system below the level of the chest and ensure that the tubes are free flowing (unkinked with no dependent loops). Maintain suction at the prescribed level.

Monitor the amount of drainage at least hourly immediately after insertion—the drainage normally decreases in a step-wise fashion, for example, 3, 2, 1. The nurse should notify the physician if the expected decrease in drainage does not occur.

Identify the presence of fluctuation in the drainage tubing and gentle bubbling in the water seal chamber with respiration (sometimes called tidaling). When tidaling ceases, it may indicate that the lung has fully expanded or there is a blockage in the chest tube so a chest x-ray may be indicated.

C: Circulation

As the assessment mnemonic continues, C, circulation, is the next priority for the trauma patient.

The circulation assessment includes:

- Palpating for carotid, brachial, radial, femoral, popliteal, and pedal pulses.

- The central pulses (carotid and femoral) are palpated first. If the patient exhibits these pulses, then his systolic blood pressure is usually at least 60 to 80 mm Hg systolic. If the patient has more peripheral pulses, such as radial and pedal, the blood pressure is usually higher than 80.

- The nurse notes the quality and rate of the pulse.
- The nurse documents the skin color of the patient, along with temperature and degrees of diaphoresis.
- The nurse inspects the patient for any signs of external bleeding, noting if it is controlled and auscultates the blood pressure.
- The nurse inspects the neck veins for distention or collapse and auscultates for heart sounds.

The objective of the assessment is to determine if the patient's circulation is effective.

Absent Circulation

Cardiopulmonary resuscitation is initiated if the trauma patient is displaying signs of no circulation (no pulse, no blood pressure). Advanced cardiac life support, which includes medication and intravenous fluids and/or blood, is also initiated, along with cardiopulmonary resuscitation (refer to Chapter 7). ∞ The trauma patient may need definitive surgical care at this point.

Signs and Symptoms of Ineffective Circulation

A trauma patient may exhibit tachycardia or loss of consciousness as symptoms of ineffective circulation. The patient may have uncontrolled external bleeding that needs to be controlled with direct pressure. Other signs and symptoms of ineffective circulation include distended or abnormally flattened jugular veins; pale, cool, diaphoretic skin; and distant heart sounds. The cause of ineffective circulation is often fluid volume deficit. Important causes of ineffective circulation in the trauma patient include hypovolemia (possibly from hemorrhage) and cardiac tamponade.

Collaborative Management

The first priority is to control any uncontrolled bleeding by placing pressure above the site, if possible. At least two large-bore intravenous catheters, preferably 14 to 16 gauge, are inserted, and infusion of lactated Ringer's solution is initiated. Lactated Ringer's solution is preferred for infusion in the trauma patient due to the close resemblance of the electrolyte composition of blood and plasma. Lactated Ringer's is an isotonic solution. The blood or intravenous (IV) fluids may be infused using a rapid infuser, which is an IV pump that simultaneously warms the fluid and can infuse a liter of fluid in approximately 2 minutes.

While the IVs are being inserted, another team member should be drawing blood for the laboratory. It is especially important to draw blood for type and crossmatch. The patient may need a blood transfusion; if there is no time to wait for the patient's blood type, type O blood, the universal donor, is provided. If a patient had a low blood pressure prior to hospital arrival, the Emergency Medical Service (EMS) team might have applied pneumatic antishock garment. This is rarely done in the hospital setting.

Shock

Shock is a clinical disorder evidenced by inadequate tissue and organ perfusion and oxygenation In the acute care setting it is imperative that the cause of the shock be identified and rectified. Shock in the trauma patient is most commonly caused by hemorrhage. Shock does not result from isolated brain injuries. The patient who is cool to the touch and tachycardic is considered to be in shock until proven otherwise. It is important that the nurse recognize the signs and symptoms of shock in order to correct the problem as quickly as possible (Figure 8-10). Tachycardia is one of the first signs of shock; however, an elderly patient is less likely to exhibit tachycardia when in shock. Because the body may compensate for shock with vasoconstriction, the blood pressure may remain normal until 30% of the blood is lost.

Hemorrhagic Shock

This is the most common form of shock in trauma patients. The trauma patient who is tachycardic and cool to the touch is assumed to be in hypovolemic shock. The normal adult blood volume is 7% of the ideal body weight. Thus, a 70-kg adult would have a blood volume of approximately 5 liters. The health care professional is expected to recognize shock and manage the bleeding by assessing the patient's circulation, controlling or stopping the bleeding, and treating the hypovolemia with fluid and/or blood replacement while watching for fluid shifts (Levett, Vercueil, & Grocott, 2006). The fluid shifts may be caused by bleeding into the injury or by third spacing. Third spacing occurs when fluid shifts from the vascular space into an area where it is not readily accessible as in extracellular fluid. The fluid remains in the body but is unavailable for use. This causes an isotonic fluid volume deficit. Because hemorrhage is the most common cause of shock, it is important to be aware of the different classifications of hemorrhage.

Pathophysiology of Blood Loss

The body will try to compensate for fluid volume deficit by progressively constricting the blood vessels in an attempt to preserve the vital organs. The heart rate speeds up in order to sustain cardiac output. The body releases

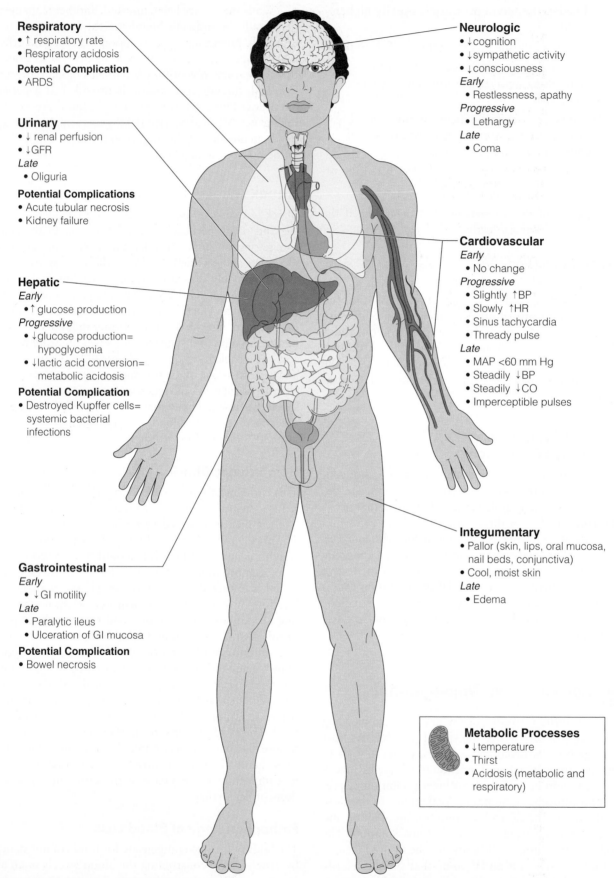

Respiratory
- ↑ respiratory rate
- Respiratory acidosis

Potential Complication
- ARDS

Urinary
- ↓ renal perfusion
- ↓GFR

Late
- Oliguria

Potential Complications
- Acute tubular necrosis
- Kidney failure

Hepatic
Early
- ↑ glucose production

Progressive
- ↓glucose production= hypoglycemia
- ↓lactic acid conversion= metabolic acidosis

Potential Complication
- Destroyed Kupffer cells= systemic bacterial infections

Gastrointestinal
Early
- ↓GI motility

Late
- Paralytic ileus
- Ulceration of GI mucosa

Potential Complication
- Bowel necrosis

Neurologic
- ↓cognition
- ↓sympathetic activity
- ↓consciousness

Early
- Restlessness, apathy

Progressive
- Lethargy

Late
- Coma

Cardiovascular
Early
- No change

Progressive
- Slightly ↑BP
- Slowly ↑HR
- Sinus tachycardia
- Thready pulse

Late
- MAP <60 mm Hg
- Steadily ↓BP
- Steadily ↓CO
- Imperceptible pulses

Integumentary
- Pallor (skin, lips, oral mucosa, nail beds, conjunctiva)
- Cool, moist skin

Late
- Edema

Metabolic Processes
- ↓temperature
- Thirst
- Acidosis (metabolic and respiratory)

Figure 8-10 Multisystem effects of shock.

catecholamines to increase the heart rate and the strength of cardiac contraction. The catecholamine epinephrine causes vasoconstriction, whereas the catecholamine norepinephrine promotes vasoconstriction by increasing peripheral resistance, which increases the blood pressure and perfusion. The body releases other hormones with vasoconstrictive properties (Baldwin & Morris, 2002).

Classifications of Hemorrhage

- Class I hemorrhage is characterized by a 15% loss of total blood volume (up to 750 mL in an average size adult) for which the patient is usually able to compensate.
  - Tachycardia may be the only symptom of a class I hemorrhage although the patient may have a heart rate less than 100.
  - Blood pressure, pulse pressure, capillary refill, urine output, and mental status are usually all normal but the patient may be slightly anxious.
  - This patient would benefit from a crystalloid infusion.
- Class II hemorrhage is marked by a 15% to 30% loss of blood volume (750 to 1,500 mL).
  - The signs and symptoms are tachycardia accompanied by a decrease in pulse pressure, anxiety on the part of the patient, and a mild increase in urine output.
  - Systolic blood pressure is usually normal; mean arterial pressure (MAP) has usually dropped 10 to 15 mm Hg.
  - A class II hemorrhage patient requires crystalloid fluid resuscitation.
- Class III hemorrhage is marked by 30% to 40% blood loss (1,500 to 2,000 mL). It is classified as a moderate hemorrhage and the patient is usually obviously ill.
  - The patient will exhibit: a heart rate greater than 120, tachypnea, mental status changes, a fall in the systolic blood pressure, and a drop of 20 mm Hg in the MAP, which means the body is not compensating for the fluid volume deficit
  - The class III hemorrhage patient will require a colloid fluid resuscitation and probably blood replacement.
- Class IV hemorrhage is considered an emergent state with greater than 40% blood loss (more than 2,000 mL).
  - The signs and symptoms are: heart rate greater than 140, tachypnea, pronounced mental status changes, low systolic blood pressure with a MAP less than 60, pale cold skin with delayed capillary refill.
  - Heart rate greater than 140

- Blood replacement is required along with a crystalloid fluid resuscitation.
- Intervention needs to occur promptly to preserve oxygenation and end-organ perfusion.

Nursing Management

The first line of treatment for the patient with hemorrhagic shock is fluids and blood replacement therapy. Because the nurse followed the ABCs, the patient should already be receiving supplemental oxygen. The trauma patient may be tachypneic in order to maintain the body's acid-base balance so oxygenation is essential. The nurse needs to carefully monitor the patient's acid-base balance and bicarbonate is provided cautiously. If the patient continues to actively bleed, the trauma team will attempt to stop the bleeding either with external pressure or surgically. Figure 8-11 displays points where pressure may be applied in an attempt to control bleeding.

Fluids

The preferred fluid for resuscitation is lactated Ringer's, which is classified as a crystalloid. Normal saline may be used; however, this fluid may increase the chloride levels of the patient and may lead to acidosis secondary to

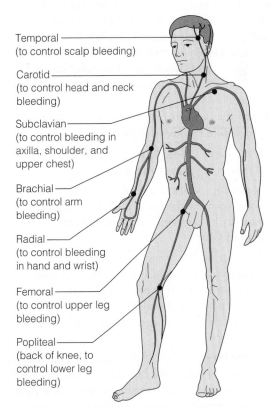

Temporal (to control scalp bleeding)

Carotid (to control head and neck bleeding)

Subclavian (to control bleeding in axilla, shoulder, and upper chest)

Brachial (to control arm bleeding)

Radial (to control bleeding in hand and wrist)

Femoral (to control upper leg bleeding)

Popliteal (back of knee, to control lower leg bleeding)

Figure 8-11 The major pressure points used to control bleeding.

bicarbonate loss. D_5W is contraindicated because this fluid will dilute sodium and should be avoided in all trauma patients (Levett et al., 2006). Fluids from the colloid classification may be administered later. The fluids should be infused through a large-bore IV in a peripheral line. In trauma cases in which large amounts of fluid need to be infused quickly, a rapid infuser may be used. Rapid infusers are pieces of equipment that are capable of warming fluid and infusing 1 liter of fluid in approximately 2 minutes. Large-bore catheters are required because small peripheral lines are not capable of delivering the large amounts of fluids needed for the trauma patient. Once volume has been adequately replaced, the physician may consider administering vasopressor drugs, along with fluids, for hypovolemic shock.

Blood

Patients with large blood losses due to trauma or who do not respond adequately to a crystalloid fluid bolus should be considered for a blood transfusion (Parillo, 2004). Traditionally transfusion of hypovolemic patients was directed toward maintaining a hemoglobin concentration of at least 10 g/dL. Using this value as the only indicator for administration of blood probably resulted in unnecessary and excessive administration of blood products. Current thought is that transfusion requirements should be based on the patient's hemoglobin in conjunction with physiological needs determined by the hemodynamic stability of the patient and the mixed venous partial pressure of oxygen (PvO_2). During trauma resuscitation hemodynamic stability and rate of blood loss are the key indicators. If the hemoglobin is greater than 8 g/dL, and blood loss has stopped, transfusion is less likely to be indicated. If the hemoglobin is less than 6 g/dL, transfusion is usually necessary. When the hemoglobin is between the two values, PvO_2 is useful in determining transfusion requirements.

When the nurse is preparing to administer blood to a patient with a traumatic injury:

- The patient should have a large-bore IV catheter in place (16 gauge to 18 gauge).
- IV tubing specifically used for blood is obtained along with the doctor's order, the signed transfusion consent form, and 500 mL of normal saline.
- If time is of the essence Type O negative packed cells are used because Type O is the universal donor. It is preferable to type, screen, and match the patient's blood. The patient is then given blood that is a match to his own blood type.
- Before blood or blood products are transfused, two nurses check the blood bank number on the armband of the patient and on the blood then both sign that this has been done.

- In nonemergent situations the blood is infused slowly over the first 15 to 30 minutes because this is when a transfusion reaction is most likely to occur.
- The nurse begins the transfusion with a baseline set of vital signs (temperature included) and takes vital signs every 5 minutes for the first 15 minutes along with a patient assessment.
- If any of the reactions that are discussed next occur, the blood infusion is stopped immediately and normal saline is infused. The nurse notes the reason for the cessation of the transfusion and the patient's vital signs, and the blood is placed in a biohazard bag along with the tubing and returned to the laboratory for further testing. Samples of the patient's blood and urine are obtained and sent to the laboratory. The doctor is alerted to the situation.

Common Types of Transfusion Reactions.

The most common types of transfusion reactions and the reasons for their development and their manifestations are:

- Hemolytic transfusion reaction—These reactions occur in 1 per 40,000 transfusions when mismatched blood has been transfused into the patient, resulting in destruction of the transfused red blood cells (RBCs). There is a grave risk of kidney damage or failure. Signs and symptoms include fever, chills, dyspnea, tachypnea, lumbar pain, hematuria, oliguria, tightness in the chest.
- Febrile reaction—This reaction is thought to result from the recipient having preformed antibodies to the donor white blood cells (WBCs) or platelets. However, it may also result from the presence of cytokines in stored blood. The signs and symptoms include chills, fever, nausea, and lumbar pain.
- Allergic—Antibody reaction to allergens is one of the most common types of transfusion reactions, occurring in 3% to 4% of all transfusions. The patient has an allergic reaction to the blood that is manifested as itching, hives, wheezing, vertigo, bronchospasm, anaphylaxis, dyspnea, and/or generalized edema.
- Circulatory overload—This results from infusion of large amounts of blood, especially to clients with cardiac disease or extreme age. The signs and symptoms include pulmonary edema, shortness of breath (SOB), cough, rales, cyanosis, and increased central venous pressure (CVP).

Massive Transfusion

Massive transfusion may be necessary in the trauma patient. It is arbitrarily defined as the replacement of a patient's total blood volume in less than 24 hours, or as the administration of more than half the patient's estimated blood volume in an hour. While administering sufficient blood to restore an adequate blood volume, the nurse must ensure that the patient's blood composition remains within safe limits for hemostasis, oxygen-carrying capacity, oncotic pressure, and biochemistry. The administration of so many units of blood may result in the following additional complications:

- Thrombocytopenia occurs because platelet function declines rapidly in stored blood. However, 1.5 times the patient's blood volume must be replaced before this becomes a clinical problem.

- Coagulation factor depletion often develops. It is unclear if this is a response to disseminated intravascular coagulopathy (DIC) or to deficiencies of coagulation factors in stored blood.

- O_2 delivery changes occur because the hemoglobin in stored blood has a high affinity for O_2, which limits O_2 delivery to the tissues.

- Hypocalcemia develops because each unit of blood contains citrate, which binds ionized calcium. With massive transfusions, patients may develop hypocalcemia and exhibit transient tetany and hypotension.

- Hyperkalemia may develop because the potassium concentration of blood increases during storage.

- Acid-base disturbances vary with the metabolism of the patient. Acidosis may develop from lactic acid in the stored blood, or alkalosis may result when citrate is metabolized to bicarbonate.

- Hypothermia may develop if cool blood is administered quickly. Hypothermia causes additional metabolic problems because it leads to a reduction in citrate and lactate metabolism (resulting in hypocalcemia and metabolic acidosis), an increase in affinity of hemoglobin for O_2, resulting in a further reduction in O_2 delivery to the tissues, and platelet dysfunction.

Patients with penetrating trauma who are hemodynamically unstable (do not respond to volume replacement) require immediate surgery. They should be taken to the operating room as soon as it is possible. When the wounds may be penetrating multiple cavities (e.g., both the thorax and the abdomen) so that the surgeon is unclear about the source of the bleeding, diagnostic peritoneal lavage (DPL) or focused assessment with sonography for trauma (FAST) scan may be used to determine the presence of free intraperitoneal fluid. For the DPL, an aspiration of frank blood, or lavage fluid with a red cell count greater than 100,000/mL, confirms the presence of intraperitoneal hemorrhage.

Ineffective Circulation Due to Cardiac Tamponade

Another condition that can result in inadequate circulation following trauma is cardiac tamponade. Cardiac tamponade results from injury to the heart or great vessels with fluid accumulating in the pericardial space.

The signs and symptoms of cardiac tamponade in the trauma patient are classically presented as **Beck's triad**. Beck's triad is:

- Hypotension
- Muffled heart tones (due to the accumulation of fluid around the heart)
- Increase in CVP (seen as jugular vein distension)

An additional sign is a paradoxical pulse. Paradoxical pulse is most clearly seen when the patient has an arterial line but may also be palpated at any pulse point or auscultated with the blood pressure. In paradoxical pulse, blood pressure (and therefore the force of each heartbeat felt as a pulse) is at least 10 mm Hg higher on expiration than on inspiration.

When cardiac tamponade develops, intrapericardial pressure is elevated and impairs the filling of the heart during diastole (Figure 8-12). This causes pronounced hypotension. The amount of fluid that results in tamponade depends on the rapidity of accumulation of the fluid. In the acutely ill patient, less than 100 mL of fluid in the pericardial space can produce an emergent life-threatening situation. The patient with chronic cardiac tamponade is usually ill but not emergently ill because

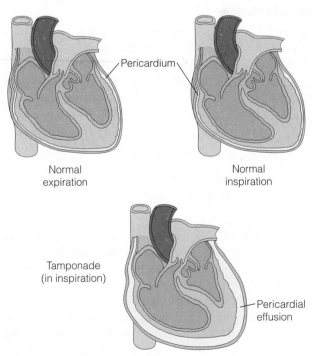

Normal expiration

Normal inspiration

Pericardium

Tamponade (in inspiration)

Pericardial effusion

Figure 8-12 Cardiac tamponade.

the pericardium can stretch slowly and accommodate up to a liter of fluid. Chronic cardiac tamponade is generally caused by malignancies.

Treatment of Cardiac Tamponade. Treatment of cardiac tamponade is directed at relieving the pressure and compression by removing the accumulated fluid. This is done by pericardiocentesis (inserting a needle in the pericardial cavity and aspirating the fluid) or by surgically creating a "window" or opening in the pericardium. Pericardiocentesis is an emergent procedure. The patient is placed with the head and torso elevated at a 45-degree angle. A 16- or 18-gauge, 6-inch or longer, over-the-needle catheter is attached to a 60-mL syringe. Under either ECG or fluoroscopic guidance, the physician inserts a needle attached to an ECG electrode at a 45-degree angle, lateral and to the left side of the xiphoid, 1 to 2 cm inferior to the xiphochondral junction. Blood is aspirated during introduction of the needle until as much nonclotted pericardial blood as possible is withdrawn. If the pericardial blood has clotted, the "open window" is necessary for treatment. Typically, pericardial blood does not clot and the aspiration of this blood will benefit the patient. The nurse observes the patient's ECG closely during insertion of the needle to identify any ST or T-wave changes that would indicate ischemia from the needle touching the myocardium. Following the procedure, the nurse assesses the patient for redevelopment of symptoms because pericardiocentesis does not treat the underlying problem; it merely removes the accumulated fluid.

D: Disability

A brief neurological assessment is necessary to determine level of consciousness. In this assessment, it is important to assess the pupils for size, shape, equality, and reactivity to light. The AVPU scale is used to rapidly determine level of consciousness. This scale is a mnemonic that consists of:

> A—alert
>
> V—responds to verbal stimuli
>
> P—responds to painful stimuli
>
> U—unresponsive

Once again, it is important to continue to monitor the patient's ABCs. If the patient is unresponsive or has a decreased level of consciousness, the nurse should conduct a further investigation during the secondary assessment to attempt to find the cause for the decreased level of consciousness. If the patient exhibits signs and symptoms of brain herniation or neurological deterioration, the nurse might consider hyperventilating the patient while awaiting further treatment. See Chapter 9 ∞ for a detailed description of care of the patient with cerebral trauma.

In addition, the nurse rapidly assesses the patient for spontaneous movement of the extremities. If the patient is awake and responsive, the presence of paraplegia or quadriplegia usually indicates spinal cord injury.

Spinal Cord Injuries

Motor vehicle crashes (MVC) or motor vehicle accidents (MVA) are the number one cause of spinal cord injury. The mechanism of injury is usually blunt force from deceleration and/or acceleration. These forces cause the spinal column to move beyond the usual range of motion. When the vertebral column is deformed there may be injury or secondary edema of the spinal cord, resulting in the loss of neurological function. Five percent of patients with spinal cord and/or vertebral column injury will worsen neurologically in the emergency department. Concurrent injuries associated with spinal cord trauma are closed head injuries, long bone fractures, and thoracic and abdominal injuries. The patient's inability to feel pain makes it more likely that potentially serious injuries in other areas of the body may not be identified.

▌ Collaborative Management

The patient with suspected spine injury is immobilized using a backboard and hard cervical collar or head blocks until the injury is ruled out. It is imperative to immobilize and stabilize the head and neck to prevent further damage to the neck and spine. A suspected spinal injury is ruled out by a combination of conventional x-rays, computerized tomography (CT) scan, and the patient's statement of no pain. If the spinal injury is ruled out the patient is "cleared" and the cervical collar and backboard are removed (Sherrin, 2005).

If the patient has a cervical spinal cord injury, he will require extra vigilance in the reassessment of his breathing. Some patients such as those with C4 and above spinal cord injuries may have required immediate intubation and ventilation. However, patients with lower level cervical injuries, especially those who are older than 40, smokers, and those who have associated chest trauma, may develop difficulty breathing as they tire and may need bi-level positive airway pressure (BiPAP) or intubation and ventilation for support of respiration. These patients will continue to need aggressive nursing care to prevent, identify, and treat atelectasis and pneumonia throughout their hospitalization.

Patients with spinal cord injury often develop neurogenic shock because the sympathetic innervation to the vasculature is disrupted, resulting in pronounced vasodilation. The characterizations of neurogenic shock include venous pooling (poor blood volume distribution), shunting in microcirculation or decrease in venous resistance, and faulty distribution of blood flow.

This vasodilation compounds the physiological effects of hypovolemia. The classic presentation of neurogenic shock is:

- Hypotension with bradycardia
- No cutaneous vasoconstriction
- Normal pulse pressure (the difference between the diastolic and systolic pressures; normal pulse pressure is about a 40-point difference).

Treatment of hypotension presumes hypovolemia and the patient is immediately provided with crystalloid fluids. If volume repletion does not restore an adequate blood pressure, vasopressors might be started, usually norepinephrine. Treatment for the patient with a confirmed spinal cord injury is evolving. If there is a cervical spinal cord injury, skeletal tongs may be applied to maintain alignment of the spine and to relieve muscle spasm pain (Figure 8-13). Inducing hypothermia is showing some early promising results at preserving spinal cord function. In experimental studies, moderate hypothermia (33°C/92°F) may be induced and maintained for a 48-hour period following the injury. If the patient has a nonpenetrating spinal cord injury, therapy might include high-dose steroids.

Steroid therapy is currently controversial because the risks of use may outweigh the potential benefits. The rationale for use is that steroids limit spinal cord edema and ischemia. If utilized, steroid therapy is initiated within 3 hours of the spinal cord trauma and continued for 24 hours. If the steroid therapy is initiated within 3 to 8 hours following the trauma, the therapy should continue for 48 hours.

Musculoskeletal Trauma

Fractures account for more than half of all trauma admissions. Musculoskeletal injuries can involve bone, muscles, nerves, soft tissue, and/or blood vessels. Blunt trauma or penetrating injuries may be involved in trauma to the musculoskeletal system. Large amounts

---

COMMONLY USED MEDICATIONS

METHYLPREDNISOLONE

Expected Action and Dose: Suppress inflammation and normal immune response. Steroid dosing is generally 30 mg/kg over 15 minutes initially, followed 45 minutes later with 5.4/kg/hr for 23 hours.

Nursing Responsibilities: The nurse assesses the patient for signs of adrenal insufficiency, monitors intake and output, assesses the patient for changes in level of consciousness and headache, and prevents infection.

Side and/or Toxic Effects: Depression/euphoria, hypertension, anorexia, peptic ulcer, thromboembolism, decreased wound healing, ecchymoses, and increased likelihood of infection (side effects are more common with high-dose/long-term therapy).

---

of blood may be lost in bone fractures depending on the bone involved. Femur fractures may lose up to 1,500 mL of blood, whereas a fracture of the humerus can cause as much as 750 mL of blood to be lost. If the fracture is a closed fracture this fluid and blood accumulates in the area of the fracture. The different types of fractures are:

- Open fracture is where skin integrity at or near the site is disrupted.
- Closed fracture is when the skin remains intact.
- Complete fracture is a total interruption of the bone continuity.
- Incomplete fractures are incomplete interruptions in the continuity of the bone.
- Comminuted fractures are a splintering of the bone into fragments.
- Greenstick involves a buckling or bending of the bone.
- Impacted fracture is where the distal and proximal bone sites are wedged into each other.
- Displaced fractures involve the distal and proximal ends of bone fracture sites becoming misaligned.

Nursing Management

The first intervention with an open musculoskeletal fracture is to stop the bleeding by applying pressure or traction. X-rays of the pelvis, chest, and lateral C-spine are usually obtained. The nurse checks the joints above and below any fracture for dislocations. The nurse should always assess the suspected fracture for bleeding, deformity, color, movement, tenderness, temperature, sensation, capillary refill, and crepitus. If necessary, the nurse prepares the patient for joint reduction and/or bone realignment. After a reduction or realignment, it is important for the nurse to reassess the patient for the presence of pulses in that extremity.

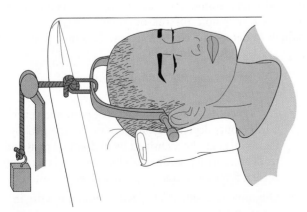

Figure 8-13 Cervical traction may be applied by several methods, including Gardner-Wells tongs.

Compartment Syndrome

Compartment syndrome occurs as blood or fluid enters the fascia, causing an increase in pressure in the fascial compartment. The increased pressure has a tourniquet-like effect, decreasing circulation and resulting in ischemia. Compartment syndrome usually develops within 2 hours following fractures to the lower extremities. The signs and symptoms are:

- Unusually severe pain for the injury associated with motion
- Decreased motion
- Swelling and tension, with decreased capillary refill in the tissue
- Paresthesia

Collaborative Management

The treatment is to release the pressure by removing the source of constriction on the extremity or performing a fasciotomy. A fasciotomy is a surgical procedure in which the surgeon makes an incision through the skin and subcutaneous tissues into the fascia of the affected compartment. This allows unrestricted swelling, and circulation is restored. The open wound is packed and dressed daily until secondary healing occurs, then the surgeon may debride the wound and apply a skin graft.

Pelvic Fracture

The nurse can become suspicious of a pelvic fracture from the description of the injury. Common causes of pelvic fractures include motorcycle accidents, pedestrian accidents vs. motor vehicle accidents, and falls greater than 12 feet. Pelvic fractures are classified into two categories: stable and unstable. A stable pelvic fracture reveals no deformities. An unstable pelvic fracture involves the pelvic ring being fractured and displaced in two places. Pelvic fractures usually involve large blood loss and can be life threatening. A patient with a 2-cm separation pelvic fracture can lose 1.3 liters of blood, whereas one with a 5-cm separation can lose up to 5 liters of blood (Smith, Scalea, & Ma, 2006). Therefore, the nurse carefully assesses the patient with a pelvic fracture for hypovolemia and shock.

Pelvic fractures may be open or closed, with open fractures having a significantly higher mortality rate. The nurse might stabilize a pelvic fracture with a sheet or pelvic sling to decrease bleeding. Eventually, the patient with a pelvic fracture may need surgery to stabilize it or may need pins inserted externally to stabilize with traction. However, some avulsive pelvic fractures heal with bed rest.

Detailed Description of the Secondary Assessment

The secondary assessment continues with the alphabet mnemonic E through I.

E—Stands for Expose

Expose the patient to assess for any unseen injuries. E also stands for **environment**; keep the patient covered to prevent heat loss. The trauma patient is prone to hypothermia due to the clothing being removed, blood and body fluids on the skin, and the uncovering of the patient for assessment. Hypothermia must be prevented and reversed. The nurse should consider using a Bair hugger, a device that forces warm air into an inflatable mattress placed over the patient to warm the body, and that warms the fluids administered to the patient. The patient should be kept dry and breezes in the room avoided.

Abdominal Trauma

The abdominal cavity may be assessed during the **secondary survey** either as part of E, exposure, or H, head-to-toe assessment. The abdominal cavity lies between the thorax and the pelvis. The liver, spleen, kidneys, and pancreas are the solid organs in the abdominal cavity. **Hollow organs** in this cavity include the stomach, small bowel, large bowel, and bladder. Assessment of the patient with abdominal injuries can be particularly difficult because the signs and symptoms of abdominal trauma can be difficult to distinguish, the abdominal cavity can hold large amounts of fluid before becoming distended, and abdominal assessment of the trauma patient is often hampered by alcohol intoxication, illicit drug use, brain injury, and/or fractured ribs. However, abdominal assessment is essential because unrecognized abdominal injury can cause preventable death. Therefore, the nurse carefully assesses for blood loss, absent bowel sounds, abdominal tenderness, and specific patterns of pain that are linked to the various abdominal injuries.

Conservative, nonoperative management is becoming the norm when the patient is initially stable following abdominal trauma. If such an approach is taken, the nurse is responsible for the ongoing assessment of the patient to detect any complications. This includes:

- Hourly assessment of vital signs including CVP with attention to any indication of ongoing bleeding.
- Assessment for the development of peritonitis every 1 to 4 hours depending on the status of the patient. Peritonitis may be identified by abdominal pain and tenderness with guarding, abdominal rigidity, tachycardia, fever, or decreased or absent bowel sounds.
- Ongoing assessment of specific abdominal organ functioning.

If the patient develops signs of hemodynamic instability or peritonitis during this period of observation, the surgeon should be notified and a laparotomy may be scheduled.

Traumatic Injury of the Liver. The liver is often injured in abdominal trauma due to its size and location in the abdomen. It is more frequently involved in penetrating trauma (80% of the time) than blunt trauma (20% of the time). Liver injury is often manifested by:

- Upper right quadrant pain
- Rebound tenderness
- Hypoactive or absent bowel sounds
- Abdominal wall muscle rigidity
- Hemorrhage
- Cullen's sign (bluish discoloration of the periumbilical skin caused by intraperitoneal hemorrhage)
- Grey Turner's sign (blue discoloration of the skin around the flanks or umbilicus in a patient with hemorrhagic pancreatitis)

Collaborative Management

To identify the extent of bleeding and the likelihood of liver involvement, a hemoglobin and hematocrit, liver enzyme studies, and coagulation studies are required. Radiologically, a flat plate of the liver and CT scan are ordered. Liver injuries are identifiable by CT scan and are graded from I to VI. A grade I injury is a nonexpanding subcapsular hematoma often resulting from a laceration of the liver. The surface area of the liver involved becomes greater as the grade gets higher, with a grade IV resulting in disruption involving 25% to 75% of the liver parenchyma or an entire hepatic lobe. Grade VI, the highest grade, represents hepatic avulsion.

The majority of patients who sustain liver trauma, patients with grades I to III liver injuries, are currently treated conservatively because almost 90% of hepatic injuries have stopped bleeding by the time the patient reaches surgery. In addition, blood transfusion requirements and intra-abdominal complications are significantly lower in patients who do not receive surgery. The nurse is responsible for the ongoing monitoring of the patient. It is essential that the nurse carefully assess the patient for any worsening of the initial symptoms and indications of ongoing bleeding and alert the physician because these may indicate the need for surgical intervention.

Due to the vascularity of the liver and its ability to store blood, some injuries to the liver can result in hemorrhage and hemorrhagic shock. Therefore, patients with grades IV through VI injuries may be managed surgically. The postsurgical patient is also closely monitored

for the manifestations of bleeding and hypotension that include rapid, thready pulse and increase in abdominal girth along with diaphoresis.

Splenic Injury. The spleen is capable of storing 100 to 300 mL of blood, roughly 4% of total blood volume. An enlarged spleen increases the blood storing capacity. Therefore, damage to the spleen can result in hemorrhage.

Signs and symptoms of splenic injury include:

- Signs of hemorrhage and/or hypovolemic shock
- Kehr's sign, which is pain referred to the left shoulder
- Upper left quadrant tenderness
- Muscle wall rigidity in the abdomen

Collaborative Management

The current management of splenic injury also favors nonoperative management. The nurse must observe the patient carefully during the first hours and days post trauma. If the patient has stable hemodynamic signs, stable hemoglobin levels, and requires 2 units or fewer of blood, she usually does not require surgery.

However, some patients continue to bleed and require surgical intervention. Efforts are usually made to preserve the spleen so it may be wrapped in a procedure called splenorrhaphy, or gel foam may be used for angioembolization. Following these procedures the nurse observes the patient carefully for any sign of rebleeding. Surgical removal of the spleen is a lifesaving last resort. The patient usually recovers over a period of about 5 days and a nasogastric tube is usually required for the first 2 days. One of the most important considerations for the patient whose spleen has been resected is that she is at risk for infections by encapsulated organisms such as pneumococcus. Therefore, she must receive at least a vaccination against pneumococcus but possibly vaccinations against haemophilus and meningococcus as well. Immunizations may be administered anywhere from 24 hours to 2 weeks after injury.

Trauma to the Kidneys

Renal trauma is present in approximately 10% of all abdominal injuries, and 90% of renal trauma is due to blunt injury. However, major renal trauma is more often associated with penetrating trauma than with blunt trauma. When a patient has major blunt abdominal trauma or penetrating flank and back wounds, the nurse should suspect renal injury.

Contusion to the kidneys is the most common blunt trauma kidney injury. The nurse assesses such patients for ecchymosis over the flank, abdominal or flank tenderness

flow such as when there is an increase in cerebral metabolism, a drop in cerebral oxygen levels, or an increase in cerebral carbon dioxide levels.

Munro Kelly Hypothesis

A rigid skull surrounds the brain, providing protection. However, it leaves no room for expansion to occur in any of the volumes in the skull without an increase in the intracranial pressure or a decrease in one of the other volumes. This is known as the **Munro Kelly hypothesis**.

> Intracranial Volume (VIC) = Volume brain + Volume blood + Volume CSF + Volume lesion

It states that changes in the volumes that are normally in the skull, the brain, the blood, and the cerebrospinal fluid (CSF) as well as the presence of any abnormal lesion such as a brain tumor, an aneurysm, or a hematoma have an effect on the intracranial pressure. Normally, the intracranial pressure is kept in a range between 5 and 15 mm Hg by a mechanism known as compliance. When the volume of one of the components increases, the body may respond by:

- Displacing CSF into the lumbar cistern
- Reabsorbing more CSF
- Compressing veins and shunting blood out of the venous sinuses (Josephson, 2004)

These compensatory mechanisms allow for small increases in the volumes of components in the skull to occur without a significant increase in intracranial pressure. However, the mechanisms can only accommodate a certain amount of extra volume; when that is exceeded, intracranial pressure can rise rapidly. Figure 9-1 displays an example of a volume-pressure curve showing how the intracranial pressure remains within the normal range as long as compliance is normal, then increases rapidly once the compensatory mechanisms have been exhausted. When intracranial pressure rises, cerebral perfusion can be affected.

Cerebral Perfusion Pressure

Cerebral perfusion is dependent on the blood pressure and the intracranial pressure (CPP). It is the difference between the pressure of the incoming blood (best measured as the mean arterial pressure [MAP]) and the force opposing perfusion of the brain, the intracranial pressure (ICP). The formula is:

$$CPP = MAP - ICP$$

Normally, values for CPP should be greater than 50 to 60. A CPP less than 40 to 50 usually results in the loss of autoregulation and leads to hypoxia of cerebral tissue. From the formula, it can be seen that factors that decrease the MAP or increase the ICP can result in a reduction in perfusion of the brain.

Increased Intracranial Pressure

Increased intracranial pressure (IICP) is a higher than normal level of pressure within the cranial cavity. Because it may result in a decrease in CPP, prolonged or severe increases can result in tissue ischemia and neural tissue damage. As noted previously, normal ICP ranges between 5 and 15 mm Hg.

Primary Causes of Increased Intracranial Pressure

Primary causes of IICP are underlying brain disorders. They may be associated with slow processes (such as a slow-growing brain tumor) where the brain initially compensates for the growth of the tumor and the ICP rises slowly. Or they may be sudden devastating increases in the volume within the cranial cavity, such as following trauma or a cerebral hemorrhage, where compensatory mechanisms are inadequate and ICP rises precipitously. The following is a list of common brain disorders that result in increases in ICP:

- Brain tumor or other space-occupying lesion
- Trauma
- Nontraumatic cerebral hemorrhage
- Ischemic stroke
- Hydrocephalus
- Postoperative cerebral edema
- Meningitis

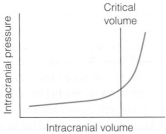

Figure 9-1 A volume-pressure curve.

Nursing Diagnoses

PATIENT EXPERIENCING AN INTRACRANIAL DYSFUNCTION

- Decreased intracranial adaptive capacity related to brain injury
- Ineffective tissue perfusion: cerebral related to increased intracranial pressure and decreased cerebral perfusion pressure
- Acute pain related to trauma
- Risk for aspiration related to reduced level of consciousness and depressed cough and gag reflexes
- Risk for injury related to seizure disorder

Secondary Causes of Increased Intracranial Pressure

The secondary causes are extracranial or systemic processes that contribute to increases in ICP. If these conditions are allowed to exist, they often contribute to secondary injury, producing ongoing increases in ICP and additional damage to the patient who has sustained a brain injury. However, they are often remediable. How to manage them is discussed in detail throughout this chapter. These secondary causes include:

- Airway obstruction
- Hypoxia or hypercarbia from hypoventilation
- Hypertension or hypotension
- Position
- Hyperthermia
- Seizures
- Metabolic disorders including hyponatremia

Focused Assessment of a Patient with a Potential for Increased Intracranial Pressure

One of the most important aspects of caring for a patient with a neurological disorder is ongoing and accurate neurological assessment. An accurate initial assessment establishes the patient's baseline neurological status, whereas ongoing assessments are essential to determining how the patient is progressing. Critical care nurses often perform ongoing assessments on an hourly basis. Components of an "hourly" neurological assessment usually include at least: the Glasgow Coma Scale or another assessment of level of consciousness, pupillary response to light, motor function, and vital signs. Assessment of cranial nerves, reflexes, and sensation may be added if indicated. On occasion, the nurse might be involved with assessing brainstem functioning.

Glasgow Coma Scale

The **Glasgow Coma Scale** (GCS) assesses both level of consciousness and motor response to a stimulus (Table 9–1). Although there have been concerns expressed about its reliability and sensitivity it is still widely used. When using the GCS, the nurse utilizes the patient's best response to obtain the score for each section.

The first section is eye opening. The nurse notes if the patient opens her eyes when the nurse approaches (scored as 4).

- If the patient does not, the nurse might say "Good morning, Mrs. Jones" and wait for her to open her eyes (scored as 3).
- If the patient does not open her eyes to her name then the nurse applies noxious stimuli (such as pressure on the trapezius or a sternal rub) and waits to see if the patient opens her eyes (scored as 2).

TABLE 9–1

Glasgow Coma Scale

RESPONSE	SCORE
Eye opening	
Spontaneous	4
To speech	3
To pain	2
Never	1
Motor response	
Obeys commands	6
Localizes pain	5
Normal flexion	4
Abnormal flexion	3
Extension	2
Nil	1
Verbal response	
Oriented	5
Confused conversation	4
Inappropriate words	3
Incomprehensible sounds	2
None	1

- If the patient does not attempt to open her eyes to any stimulus, it is scored as a 1.

The second section is motor response. The nurse asks the patient to obey a simple one-step command such as "Hold up your thumb" or "Hold up two fingers." If the patient does not respond, the nurse might ask the patient to follow the command again while demonstrating the action. If the patient follows the command, it is scored as a 6.

- If the patient does not follow a command then the nurse will need to determine how the patient responds to a noxious stimulus. The nurse might apply pressure on the trapezius; if the patient reaches toward the nurse's hand to push it away or pulls her shoulder away, the nurse scores it as a 5. Scoring the motor response a 5 means that the patient has clearly identified where the nurse is applying the stimulus and attempted to remove it.
- If instead the patient squirms when the nurse applies the noxious stimuli, moving her entire body although not seeming to be able to identify where the stimulus is applied, it is scored as a 4.
- If the patient assumes a position of abnormal flexion, also called decorticate posturing

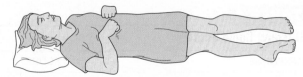

Figure 9-2 Decorticate posture is also known as abnormal flexion.

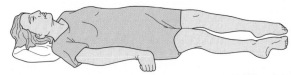

Figure 9-3 Decerebrate posture is also known as abnormal extension.

(shown in Figure 9-2), either on one or both sides, it is scored as a 3. This is an abnormal finding, and if it is a new finding the nurse should notify the physician after verifying it.

- With severe injuries, the patient might assume a position of abnormal extension known as decerebrate posturing either on one side or bilaterally (shown in Figure 9-3), which is scored as a 2. This is an ominous sign.

- If the patient does not respond at all to the stimulus, it is scored as a 1.

The last section is verbal response. Initially the patient is asked her name, the year, and her location. If she is able to respond accurately to these, she is scored a 5.

- If she responds to the question with inaccurate information (e.g., gives the incorrect year or says "I am in a department store"), she is scored a 4.

- If she replies with words unrelated to the question, she is scored a 3.

- If she only moans or groans in response, she is scored a 2.

- If she does not respond at all or has an endotracheal tube, she is scored a 1.

The score is then totaled with a range from 3 to 15. In general a score of 13 to 15 indicates mild or no brain injury, a score of 9 to 12 indicates moderate injury, and a score of 8 or less indicates severe injury.

Pupillary Function

The nurse begins by assessing the patient's pupils for size and shape. The size of the pupil may be affected by factors other than the patient's neurological status. A small pupil may be the result of a very bright room, medications for glaucoma, or administration of opiates. Neurologically, it may be the result of damage to the pons. A dilated pupil may result from fear, anxiety, or cocaine use. Neurologically, it may indicate brainstem

compression and is sometimes referred to as a "blown" pupil. There is early research that indicates that an ovoid pupil may be an indication of impending herniation.

Next, the nurse checks each pupil separately for response to light. Normally, pupils react briskly and completely to light. A nonreactive (fixed) pupil that is dilated usually indicates damage to the oculomotor nerve (III) and impending herniation. A fixed but small pupil may indicate damage to the pons. Figure 9-5, page 214, displays how neurological signs, including pupillary changes, may change as ICP increases.

Motor Assessment

If the nurse has utilized the GCS then he has already completed the initial portion of a motor assessment, which is motor response to stimuli. The next section is presence and strength of movement in each of the extremities. If the patient is able to follow simple commands, the nurse asks the patient to lift and hold her arms extended in front of her with the palms up and her eyes closed. A weakness is often revealed when one arm "drifts" down. The nurse grades the strength of movement in the extremities on the scale utilized by his agency. One commonly used easy scale is:

- Patient lifts and holds extremity against resistance
- Patient lifts and holds extremity against gravity
- Patient lifts and extremity falls back
- Patient moves extremity but cannot overcome gravity (moves on bed)
- Patient's muscle shows a trace of movement
- No movement noted

Although the nurse can assess the arms simultaneously, the legs are usually assessed separately. It is important that the nurse assess the movement in all four of the extremities and compare the strength of movement on both sides of the body.

If the patient is unable to move to command, the nurse notes if she is moving all her extremities spontaneously. If necessary, the nurse applies a noxious stimulus to one of the patient's nail beds on each of her extremities. This allows the nurse to determine whether the patient can sense the noxious stimulus, if the patient is able to move each extremity to withdraw from the stimulus, and the strength of the movement.

Although it is not voluntary movement, sometimes while the critical care nurse is assessing the ability of a patient to withdraw from a noxious stimulus, he will also check for the presence of a Babinski reflex. To elicit this reflex, the nurse strokes along the outer edge of the sole of the foot then across the ball of the foot with a dull object. The presence of the Babinski response, dorsiflexion of the big toe often accompanied by fanning of the other toes, is an abnormal finding.

A complete motor assessment would also include assessment of coordination. However, this is not ordinarily a part of an "hourly" neurological assessment. It would be included if the patient had had surgery on the cerebellum or experienced difficulty with coordination following posterior fossa surgery. Simple tests of coordination are the finger nose test and the rapid alternating movement test.

Selected Cranial Nerve Assessment

A complete cranial nerve assessment is time consuming so it is not always practical or necessary for nurses to perform one on every patient. However, nurses often test specific cranial nerves when caring for their patients. The following is a list of important cranial nerves to assess and ways to assess them.

- The II (optic) and III (oculomotor) nerves are assessed every time the nurse checks a patient's pupils. When the nurse checks for a direct response, he checks the third cranial nerve, and when he checks for a consensual response, he checks the second. It is also important to check the second cranial nerve by assessing the visual field of a patient who has a pituitary tumor, an aneurysm, or a stroke.

- Portions of the V (trigeminal) and VII (facial) cranial nerves can be assessed by checking for a corneal reflex. This is important to check in an unresponsive patient to determine if the patient is able to protect her corneas. It is also important to check following surgery on acoustic tumors.

- The nurse may need to check the VIII (acoustic) cranial nerve because it is one of the more common types of cranial nerve tumors. The nurse assesses the patient's hearing and asks the patient if she is experiencing tinnitus or dizziness.

- The nurse recognizes that the IX (glossopharyngeal) and X (vagus) nerves are intact when the patient exhibits cough and gag reflexes. When appropriate, the nurse may elicit these reflexes by touching the back of the tongue or throat with a tongue blade.

Evaluation of Brainstem Functioning

When a patient is comatose, the nurse may be asked to assist with evaluation of the oculocephalic and/or oculovestibular reflexes. The doll's eyes reflex, or oculocephalic reflex, occurs only in comatose patients. Before attempting to elicit the doll's eyes reflex, the nurse must be certain that the patient's spinal cord has been cleared. The doll's eyes reflex is produced by turning the patient's head left or right. When the reflex is present, the eyes of the patient remain stationary while the head is turned (Figure 9-4). If a comatose patient does not have a doll's eyes reflex, there is usually damage in the area of the pons and/or the medulla.

The oculovestibular reflex, or cold calorics, is performed only after determining that the tympanic membrane is intact. The head of the patient's bed is elevated 30 degrees, then 50 mL of cool saline is injected into an ear. The saline has the same effect as if the patient's head were turned to the opposite side of the injection. Thus, the patient's eyes will look toward the ear of injection for a sustained period. If the reflex is absent, there is most likely a lesion in the pons or the medulla. In a partially awake patient, the reflex will induce eye deviation and nystagmus in the direction of the noninjected ear.

Clinical Findings Associated with Increased Intracranial Pressure

When the volume of a lesion in the skull increases slowly, such as a slow-growing brain tumor, the body compensates for changes in the volume by shifting another volume (such as the CSF or blood). This controls and limits the rise in ICP. The patient usually demonstrates signs and symptoms of dysfunction of the area of the brain the tumor is encroaching on. For example, depending on the location of the tumor, the patient might develop weakness in her arm and hand. However, the increase in pressure is limited so the patient only experiences mild signs and symptoms of IICP such as headache, nausea, or papilledema.

Head in neutral position

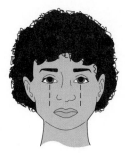

Eyes midline

Head rotated to client's left

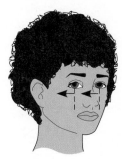

Doll's eyes present: Eyes move right in relation to head.

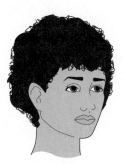

Doll's eyes absent: Eyes do not move in relation to head. Direction of vision follows head to left.

Figure 9-4 Oculocephalic reflex: Also known as doll's eye movements, characteristic of altered level of consciousness.

Nevertheless, once the expansion of the lesion has reached a certain point, or if the lesion is expanding rapidly, the body cannot compensate sufficiently and ICP increases precipitously as displayed in Figure 9-1. Rapidly increasing ICP is dangerous because of the likelihood of secondary injury to the brain and because if it continues unabated, it may result in herniation of the brain.

Downward herniation of the brain occurs when ICP is sufficiently elevated to push a portion of the brain downward through the tentoral notch, placing pressure on and distorting the midbrain. There are three types of downward herniation: uncal, central, and tonsillar. Clinical signs vary among the types of herniation. Figure 9-5 displays a constellation of vital and neurological signs

that may occur with uncal herniation and notes how it may differ from central. A triad of vital sign changes known as the Cushing response—bradycardia, hypertension (accompanied by a widened pulse pressure), and hyperventilation—may occur. It is extremely important to note that these changes in vital signs, dilation of the pupils, abnormal posturing, and absence of doll's eyes are very late signs indicating a significant amount of damage. Suspected herniation is an emergency and requires immediate response from the health care team. If intervention is not forthcoming, the patient will probably die. Discussion of the patient who is pronounced dead by neurologic criteria (brain death) is discussed in Chapter 15, ∞ under care of the transplant donor.

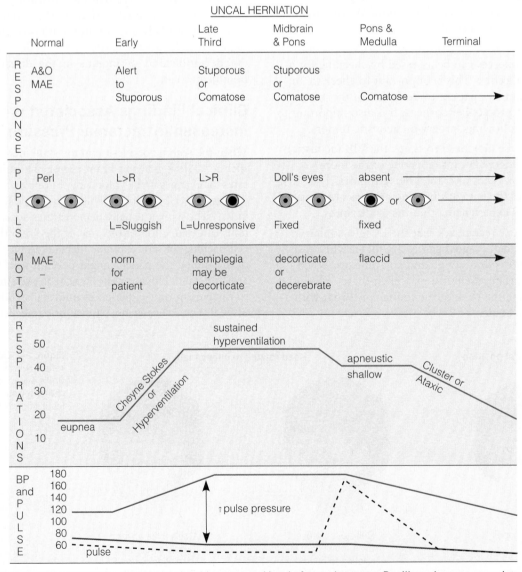

Figure 9-5 In central herniation, the changes begin with motor and level of consciousness. Pupillary changes occur later. The classic Cushing response is an increase in ↑PP, slow pulse ↓P, and respiratory variations. These are often very late signs.

Building Technology Skills

Intracranial Pressure Monitoring

Thus far the assessment of the patient with IICP has been described purely in terms of subjective signs and symptoms. Because some of these signs may occur only after ICP is gravely elevated and the signs can be difficult to interpret, it is important to have objective data to correlate with the neurological signs. ICP monitoring obtains objective measurement of ICP to correlate with the neurological findings and to guide therapy. ICP monitoring is useful because it can be continually displayed and is more likely to detect IICP than a CT scan.

Indications

ICP monitoring may be indicated in severely ill but salvageable patients with:

- Severe head injury with a GCS between 3 and 8
- Subarachnoid hemorrhage
- Hydrocephalus
- Brain tumors
- Stroke
- Meningitis

Principles of Treatment

ICP monitoring is used to identify a potentially dangerous ICP (ICP greater than 20 for 5 to 10 minutes), to determine when to institute therapy, and to evaluate the effectiveness of the therapy. According to the AANN (2005), "monitoring of ICP allows for observation of both the shape, height, and trends of individual and consecutive ICP waveforms that may reflect intracranial compliance, cerebrovascular status, and cerebral perfusion." The Brain Trauma Foundation (2007) has determined that data obtained from ICP monitoring are useful for determining prognosis and guiding therapy.

Methods

ICP monitoring devices may be inserted into a variety of spaces including the anterior horn of the lateral ventricle; the subdural, epidural, or subarachnoid spaces; and the brain parenchyma. There are three common types of sensing devices: fiberoptic, electronic sensor, and fluid-filled strain gauges. Figure 9-6 displays the location of various devices and the Brain Trauma Foundation ranking by preference.

According to the Brain Trauma Foundation (2007), the ventricular catheter connected to an external strain gauge is the most accurate, low-cost, reliable method of monitoring ICP. In addition, unlike some of the other sensors, it can be used to drain CSF and can be recalibrated in place. Due to the emergent nature of the situation, ventricular catheters may be inserted in the intensive care unit (ICU), emergency department (ED), or operating room

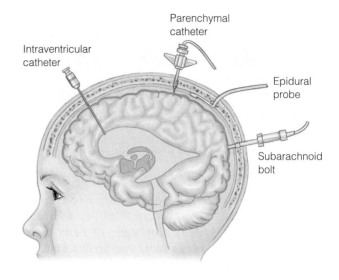

Figure 9-6 Location of types of intracranial pressure monitoring devices.
Numbers indicate location and BTF ranking by preference:
1. Intraventricular
2. Intraparenchymal
3. Subarachnoid
4. Epidural

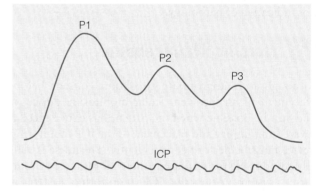

Figure 9-7 Contours of the normal ICP wave: P1, P2, P3.

(OR) by a neurosurgeon utilizing aseptic technique. After the scalp is prepped, the neurosurgeon uses a twist drill to create a burr hole through the skull over the patient's nondominant hemisphere. The ventricular catheter is then inserted through the burr hole and the brain tissue into the lateral ventricle. Once in place and connected, the catheter transmits ICP waveforms to the transducer, which converts the impulses into visible tracings or digital values on a monitor screen. Normal ICP ranges between 5 and 15 mm Hg. The normal ICP waveform has three peaks of decreasing height (P1, P2, and P3) that correlate with the arterial waveform (Figure 9-7).

There are three common variations in ICP waveforms termed A, B, and C waves (Figure 9-8). The first and most clinically significant are "A" waves, also known as plateau waves. "A" waves are elevations of ICP up to 50 to 100 mm Hg that last for 5 to 20 minutes.

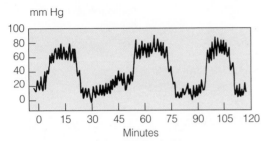

Figure 9-8 Common variations in ICP waveforms: A, B, and C waves.

They have a rapid onset and often occur from an already elevated baseline. "A" waves are significant because they are often accompanied by signs of neurological deterioration and may indicate impaired CSF flow, decreased compliance, or impending herniation.

Also clinically significant are "B" waves, which are rhythmic oscillations that occur once or twice a minute. They result in ICP increases of 20 to 50 mm Hg and may occur on a normal or elevated baseline. They are significant because they tend to occur when cerebral compliance is decreased and often precede "A" waves. "C" waves are smaller rhythmic oscillations that occur four to eight times per minute. Although ICP may increase up to 20 mm Hg, they tend to occur normally and are not indicative of pathology.

Nursing Management

Although it is appropriate to obtain consent before placement of an intraventricular monitoring device, it may not be possible when the patient has experienced a severe brain injury and placement of the ICP monitoring device must be performed emergently. The nurse is usually responsible for setting up and calibrating the monitoring system. After the ICP monitoring system is established, the nurse assesses, reports, and records the patient's initial pressures (MAP, ICP, and CPP), waveforms, and neurological status.

While an ICP monitor is in place, the nurse:

- Performs hourly neurological checks and compares them to the patient's baseline.
- Monitors MAP, ICP, and CPP (MAP-ICP) at least hourly.
- Validates that ICP waveforms and values are accurate. Especially if the values have changed, the nurse verifies the readings, correlates them to neurological findings, and notifies the physician. Some of the reasons ICP readings may be inaccurate are if the stopcocks are turned incorrectly, the transducer is incorrectly positioned, there is air in the monitoring line, or the catheter has become obstructed. Problematic malfunctions of the ventricular strain gauge monitoring system occur in 6% to 16% of patients and are one of the more common complications of

ICP monitoring. One of the disadvantages of a fiberoptic catheter tip device is that obstruction may occur as often as 40% of the time.

- Maintains strict aseptic technique when working with the system.
- Ensures that the dressing at the insertion site is clean, dry, and occlusive. The dressing should cover only the insertion site and should be changed if it is damp.
- If the nurse suspects there is a CSF leak (identified by the presence of a damp dressing with a halo or glucose in the leaking fluid), she checks the system for leaks and notifies the physician.

Complications

The most common complication, occurring in 1% to 27% of patients with ICP monitoring devices, is infection. Infections develop with increasing frequency during the first 10 days following insertion but then decrease in frequency. They are more likely to occur if the system is opened, irrigations are performed, or prophylactic bacitracin flushes are given. If infection develops, the patient may:

- Have a fever
- Report a headache
- Demonstrate signs of meningitis
- Have cloudy CSF drainage

The nurse anticipates that the CSF will be cultured, the patient will be treated with antibiotics, and the patient may undergo removal of the ICP monitoring system. The Brain Trauma Foundation (2007) does not recommend preventing infection by either routine changing of the catheter or administration of antibiotics throughout the time the monitoring system is in place.

Another complication, occurring in 1% to 2% of patients with a ventriculostomy catheter, is hemorrhage during insertion of the catheter followed by hematoma formation. It is more likely to occur in patients with coagulation abnormalities. Usually the patient must be taken to the OR for repair.

Primary Cause of Increased Intracranial Pressure: Traumatic Brain Injury

In the United States an average of 1.4 million traumatic brain injuries (TBIs) occur each year, resulting in 1.1 million visits to the ED, 235,000 hospitalizations, and 50,000 deaths. Head injuries represent 2% to 3% of all cause deaths and 26% to 68% of trauma deaths. Overall men are about twice as likely as women to experience TBI. Children aged less than 4, adolescents, and adults over the age of 75 are more likely to be hospitalized and/or die from TBI. The leading causes of TBI are falls, motor vehicle crashes, struck by or against events, and assaults—all forms of blunt

Gerontologic Considerations

Because older adults have age-related brain atrophy, they are less likely to present with the generalized symptoms of IICP such as headache and papilledema and more likely to present with mental status changes.

In spite of having a significant intracranial injury, older adults may present with a normal level of consciousness, absence of neurological deficit, and no evidence of open or depressed skull fracture—especially if they are receiving anticoagulant therapy.

Adults over the age of 75 are more likely to be hospitalized and die from TBI.

Patients with acute subdural hematomas older than 65 who are comatose on admission have significantly higher mortality rates than other patients (Roger, Butler, & Benzel, 2006).

Chronic subdural hematomas are more common in older adults. This may be attributed to age-related brain atrophy resulting in more subdural space so that the older adult is less likely to be affected initially by a small subdural bleed.

If an older patient with a traumatic brain injury develops hypernatremia (serum sodium greater than 160 mmol/L), he is at increased risk for renal failure, heart failure, and pulmonary edema than a younger adult.

The prevalence of epilepsy increases with age, and there are about 570,000 persons over the age of 65 with epilepsy.

trauma. Sports and recreation events are a major source of concussions and are thought to be severely underestimated in the national data sets because only between 8% and 20% of people sustaining such injuries lose consciousness and seek medical assistance (Langlois, Rutland-Brown, & Wald, 2006). These large numbers of injuries are especially problematic because TBI is one of the most disabling of injuries. Langlois et al. (2006) estimated that about 5.3 Americans are living with long-term or lifelong disability following hospitalization for a TBI. In addition, in the first 3 years post injury, patients recovering from a TBI are more likely to report binge drinking, develop epilepsy, and die.

Predisposing or Risk Factors

Blunt trauma is the most common cause of TBI. Motor vehicle crashes account for 50% of TBIs, whereas falls (21%), assaults (12%), and sports-related injuries (10%) account for the majority of the rest. The remaining injuries are explained by penetrating injuries such as gunshot wounds and blast injuries. Although blast injuries are uncommon in the United States, they are the leading cause of TBI among active duty military in war zones.

There are clearly established ways to prevent TBI-related deaths. Wearing a lap belt reduces mortality in motor vehicle crashes by 50%. Wearing a motorcycle helmet reduces fatalities also by 50%. More impressively, wearing a bicycle helmet can reduce mortality from TBI in bicycle crashes by 85% (Nolan, 2005).

Pathophysiology and Manifestations of Primary Brain Injuries

In TBI, the primary injury is a result of the initial impact to the head causing direct damage to the cerebral parenchyma and resulting in axonal injury. The severity of the injuries is often classified according to the GCS. A **mild injury** (GCS 13–15) is usually associated with a loss of consciousness or amnesia for less than an hour. A **moderate head injury** (GCS 9–12) may be associated with a loss of consciousness for up to a day, whereas a **severe head injury** (GCS less than or equal to 8) is usually associated with loss of consciousness for more than 24 hours. The specific injuries are described next.

Concussion and Mild Brain Injury

Mild TBIs account for 75% of all diagnosed head injuries. The Centers for Disease Control and Prevention (CDC) estimates that mild brain injuries (MBIs) cost nearly $17 billion each year and refers to them as a "silent epidemic." MBIs often result from falls or blunt trauma but may be especially common from sports-related injuries. Concussion, a type of MBI, is caused by the sudden deceleration of the brain against the fixed skull and is not associated with underlying parenchymal damage. In MBI, the exact neural mechanisms are unclear but most likely include release of neurotransmitters, mitochondrial dysfunction, diminished glucose metabolism, and transient hyperkalemia.

Despite the realization that the GCS lacks sensitivity, it is still commonly used for patients with TBI. A patient with a GCS score of 15 is considered to have mild injury. Amnesia is a hallmark of MBI, so patients should be asked to describe the circumstances surrounding the injury. Patients may be stratified for further evaluation and treatment based on the Canadian CT Head Rule (CCTHR depicted in Table 9–2). According to Clement et al. (2006),

TABLE 9-2

Canadian CT Head Rule

High-Risk for Neurological Intervention
  GCS score less than 15 at 2 hours after injury
  Suspected open or depressed skull fracture
  Any sign of basalar skull fracture
  Age older than 65 years
Medium Risk for Brain Injury on CT
  Amnesia before impact of greater than or equal to 30 minutes
  Dangerous mechanism
Dangerous mechanism is defined as pedestrian struck, an occupant ejected, or a fall from greater than 3 feet.
The rule is not applicable for a nontrauma patient, a patient with a GCS less than 13, a patient less than 16 years of age, a patient with a bleeding disorder or taking an anticoagulant, and a patient with an open skull fracture.

Source: Divisions of Emergency Medicine, University of British Columbia, Vancouver, Canada.

less than 1% of patients with a GCS of 15 require surgical intervention, and these can all be identified as being at high risk for neurological intervention on the CCTHR.

Problems experienced by patients with MBIs include headache and memory loss, which are not visible, are difficult to detect, and may result in functional loss (Bay & McLean, 2007). Postconcussion syndrome, the persistence of memory or attention deficits accompanied by disordered sleep, headaches, irritability, dizziness, or personality changes beyond 6 months, occurs in 20% to 80% of people with MBI. Headache and dizziness can be difficult to manage and are associated with delayed return to work. There is evidence that repeated MBIs have a cumulative effect, especially if the repeat injury occurs before the patient has fully recovered from the first injury. This has implications for when patients should be allowed to return to their normal activities—especially participation in sports.

Cerebral Contusions and Diffuse Axonal Injuries

Contusions and axonal injuries often result from acceleration/deceleration injuries such as a fall or a motor vehicle collision. Contusions develop as the brain accelerates against the fixed skull, causing disruption of the underlying cerebral parenchyma and blood vessels. This is known as a coup injury. After impacting the skull, the brain may recoil and impact the skull on the opposite side, causing additional damage to the cerebral parenchyma known as a countercoup injury. The severity of the contusion is related to the amount of energy that is transferred on impact. Cerebral edema develops 24 to 72 hours in response to the brain tissue injury and may result in IICP. The most common locations for cerebral contusions are the frontal and temporal lobes.

Diffuse axonal injury results from deceleration and shearing between the different densities of white and gray matter in the brain. Axonal injuries are graded from I to III with Grade I being found in patients with milder injuries, Grade II consisting of tear hemorrhages and axonal injuries in the cerebral hemispheres, and Grade III including abnormalities of the brainstem in addition to the Grade II injuries. Axonal edema and degeneration may continue for the first 2 weeks following injury. Initial neuroimaging may be normal with edema, atrophy, and petechial hemorrhages becoming evident with time. The patient manifestations are dependent on the location and extent of the injury.

Skull Fractures

Skull fractures may occur in response to a blunt, penetrating, or blast injury. Common types of skull fractures include:

- Linear fractures are nondisplaced and occur from a low-velocity impact.
- Depressed skull fractures are fractures in which depression of the bone has developed at the point of impact. They may be closed (without direct

penetration of the brain) or open (penetrating the dura). These patients usually require surgery for repair of the skull, debridement of bone fragments, and repair of the dura. Postoperatively, the nurse must assess the patient carefully for CSF leaks and the development of meningitis.

- Basilar fractures occur at the base of the skull. Patients may develop a dural tear and have CSF draining from their nose and/or ears. See the earlier discussion for management of a CSF leak. Eventually, the patient may develop "raccoon eyes" and Battle's sign, which are ecchymoses about the eyes and behind the ears.

Vascular Injuries

Vascular injuries may result from bleeding of the arteries and veins between the brain and the skull or in the brain tissue. Bleeding that occurs between the brain and the skull is a surgical emergency because the enlarging hematoma may compress the adjacent blood vessels, causing cerebral ischemia, or distort surrounding brain tissue.

Epidural Hematomas. **Epidural hematomas** occur in 1% to 2% of TBIs. They usually occur in conjunction with a skull fracture and result from a laceration of the middle meningeal artery, causing bleeding between the dura mater and the skull (Figure 9-9). Approximately half of the patients who suffer this injury demonstrate the classic presentation of an initial loss of consciousness followed by a lucid interval then a sudden reloss of consciousness with rapid deterioration in neurological status. Because the origin of the bleeding is arterial, the hematoma accumulates rapidly and must be evacuated immediately. Patient outcomes are often good if the condition is identified promptly and the patient is taken to the OR for immediate surgical evacuation of the hematoma.

Subdural Hematomas. **Subdural hematomas** occur in 10% to 20% of TBIs. In blunt trauma, they

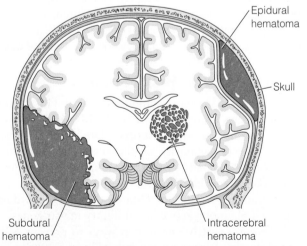

Figure 9-9 Hematomas: epidural, subdural, and intracerebral hematomas.

usually are the result of countercoup injuries, occurring on the opposite side of the skull from the injury just below the dura (see Figure 9-9). In contrast to an epidural hematoma, this hematoma is usually the result of venous bleeding, often originating with the stretching of bridging veins. Subdural hematomas are classified as acute, subacute, and chronic.

Acute subdural hematomas are collections of thick, jellylike blood that accumulate within the first 24 to 48 hours after blunt trauma. Patients usually present with a loss of consciousness and deteriorating scores on the GCS. In addition, they may have focal signs such as hemiparesis or dysphagia. If allowed to continue to expand, the hematoma can have a mass effect, causing an increase in ICP, midline shift of the brain, and even herniation. Acute subdural hematomas can be rapidly identified on computerized tomography (CT) scan and require emergent craniotomy for evacuation of the thick, coagulated blood. Patients older than 65 with acute subdural hematomas who are comatose on admission have significantly higher mortality rates than other patients (Roger et al., 2006).

Subacute subdural hematomas usually develop over days to weeks following the injury. The clot usually has liquefied and surgical evacuation may be performed on an elective basis.

Chronic subdural hematomas are more common in older adults. This may be attributed to age-related brain atrophy resulting in more subdural space so that the older adult is less likely to be affected initially by a small subdural bleed. However, during the 2 to 3 weeks following the injury, the hematoma liquefies, enlarges, and develops fibrous membranes. As the hematoma enlarges, the patient usually develops nonspecific symptoms such as headache, confusion, and speech deficits. The hematoma can be identified on CT scan. Treatment may involve drainage via burr holes (Figure 9-10) or craniotomy depending on how medically stable the patient is and the characteristics of the hematoma.

Postcraniotomy for subdural hematoma, the most common complication, occurring in 25% of patients, is a reaccumulation of the hematoma. This occurs more commonly in older adults who tend to have slow expansion of their brains after evacuation of the hematoma. Often, soft drains, such as Jackson Pratt drains, are placed for drainage. The nurse handles these aseptically and monitors the output. The nurse also assesses the patient's neurological signs and immediately identifies and reports any change from baseline.

Subarachnoid Hemorrhage. **Subarachnoid hemorrhage**, bleeding between the arachnoid and pia mater, may result from rupture of a preexisting or a traumatic cerebral aneurysm. Assessment and management of the patient with a subarachnoid hemorrhage from an aneurysm is described in Chapter 10. ∞

Intracranial Hemorrhage. Intracranial hemorrhages result in bleeding into the parenchyma or ventricles

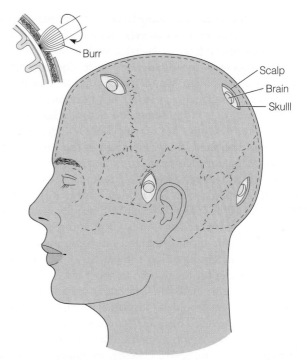

Figure 9-10 Possible location of burr holes.

of the brain. Cerebral contusions and edema usually accompany them. Management is described in the section Collaborative Management on the following page.

Assessment of the Patient with a Severe Traumatic Brain Injury

Guidelines for assessing a newly admitted trauma patient are described in Chapter 8. ∞ In addition, for the patient with a TBI, the nurse completes the GCS and assesses the pupillary response to light, motor function, and vital signs. Assessment of cranial nerves, reflexes, and sensation may be added if indicated. On occasion, the nurse might also be involved in assessing brainstem functioning of the patient with a severe TBI. How to assess these elements was discussed earlier in this chapter in the section Focused Assessment of a Patient with a Potential for Increased Intracranial Pressure.

There are several findings from the initial neurological assessment that predict death and disability for a patient with a severe TBI. The factors most predictive of outcome are:

- Patient age
- Admission motor score on the GCS
- Admission pupillary response
- Findings on the CT scan
- The presence of hypotension (Cremer, Moons, van Dijk, van Balen, & Kalkman, 2006)

Patients who were older, had lower motor scores, had one or both nonreactive pupils, or had a blood pressure (BP) less than 90 systolic were more likely to have unfavorable outcomes. Hypotension was even more likely to result in a poor outcome if it was associated with hypoxia.

Findings from the initial assessment should be acted upon with the patient's underlying condition in mind. Older adults may appear relatively normal, having a normal level of consciousness, no neurological deficit, and no skull fracture. Yet they may actually have a significant intracranial injury, especially if they are receiving anticoagulant therapy. Approximately 35% to 50% of patients who experience a TBI are under the influence of alcohol. Sperry et al. (2006) demonstrated that alcohol intoxication does not result in clinically significant changes in patient scores on the GCS, and recommends that appropriate monitoring and interventions be instituted immediately based on the patient's GCS and not delayed waiting for the patient to sober up.

According to the Brain Trauma Foundation (2007), ICP monitoring should be instituted in all salvageable patients with severe TBIs (GCS scores 3–8) who have abnormal CT scan findings such as hematoma, swelling, herniation, or compressed cisterns. In addition, it is indicated in patients with severe brain trauma with normal CT scan findings if they are over the age of 40, exhibiting posturing, or have a systolic BP less than 90 mm Hg. The details of ICP monitoring are described earlier in the chapter. The rationale for recommending ICP monitoring is that "only part of the damage occurs at the moment of impact and significant reductions in morbidity and mortality can be achieved in patients with severe TBI by using intensive management protocols" (S-37).

Collaborative Management

In TBI, although the primary neurological injury can be life threatening, it is often management of the secondary injuries that determines the patient's outcome. Secondary injuries are the physiological responses to the initial neurological insult. If the patient develops an uncontrolled increase in ICP, autoregulation may be impaired and viable cerebral tissue may not be adequately perfused. If the patient becomes hypotensive, the CPP will fall and brain tissue may be in peril. The neurons' response to this reduction in blood supply and ischemia are responsible for the secondary brain injury. When the cerebral cells are deprived of oxygen and they are forced to utilize anaerobic pathways of metabolism, normal processes fail. The sodium-potassium pump fails, allowing sodium and water to enter cells. At the same time the cell membrane breaks down. Both these factors result in edema formation (Josephson, 2004). With insufficient energy available for cellular functioning, excitatory

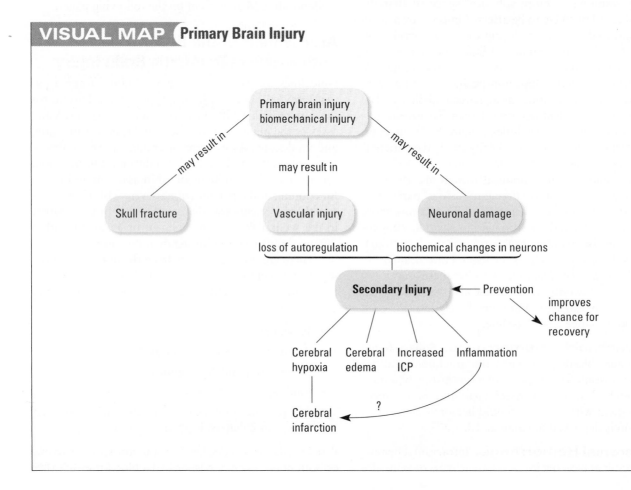

VISUAL MAP   **Primary Brain Injury**

neurotransmitters are released, there is an influx of calcium into the neurons, oxygen-free radicals are generated, and inflammatory mediators are released. These processes contribute to a downward spiral, with cerebral edema increasing, ICP rising, perfusion of the brain decreasing, and cerebral ischemia worsening. Thus, the development of secondary injuries contributes significantly to disability and death post TBI.

The goal of collaborative management for the patient with a severe head injury is maintaining sufficient blood flow and oxygenation to meet the brain's metabolic needs, thus avoiding secondary injury while the brain recovers from the traumatic event. Initial management of the trauma patient is described in Chapter 8. ∞ According to the Brain Trauma Foundation (2007), protocols for immediate management of the severely head-injured patient call for:

- Early intubation
- Transport
- Prompt fluid resuscitation
- CT scanning
- Immediate evacuation of any intracranial mass lesion
- Management in an ICU with ICP monitoring

When these measures are instituted, patient mortality has been reduced from about 50% to between 30% and 40% (AANN, 2005). Therefore, when the patient arrives in the critical care unit, he may have been intubated, has usually undergone initial CT scanning, and may have had emergent surgery and/or an intraventricular catheter placed for monitoring and drainage of CSF.

Provision of Adequate Oxygenation

The critical care nurse recognizes that patients with severe TBIs will be at risk for respiratory compromise. Rangel-Castillo and Robertson (2006) state that 60% of patients with severe head injuries have breathing abnormalities such as periodic respirations. Almost 40% of comatose head-injured patients are hypoxic from respiratory dysfunction and require intubation and mechanical ventilation. It is imperative that the critical care nurse monitor the patient's pO_2 and oxygen saturation because hypoxia, defined by the Brain Trauma Foundation (2007) as a pO_2 less than 60 or an O_2 saturation less than 90%, are associated with increased morbidity and mortality. If the patient has not already been intubated, the nurse attempts to improve the patient's oxygenation through positioning and oxygen administration. Should that not be feasible, she anticipates the likelihood of emergent intubation to maintain effective airway management and ventilation to ensure adequate oxygenation.

Intubation and mechanical ventilation of the head-injured patient are not benign procedures and may be associated with problems for the severely head-injured person. Intubation can be a noxious procedure and may increase ICP. Therefore, many institutions utilize rapid sequence intubation (Josephson, 2004). According to Josephson, rapid sequence intubation might include:

- Supporting the patient's respirations with 100% O_2 via bag-valve mask
- Administration of lidocaine to inhibit central responses that can increase ICP
- Administration of a sedative hypnotic agent
- Administration of a rapid-acting neuroblocking agent
- Checking for jaw relaxation after 30 seconds; if it is present, intubation
- Confirmation of tube placement
- Sedation of patient with chosen agent

Mechanical ventilation alone may have adverse effects on ICP. The critical care nurse will need to monitor the patient to determine that he is optimally ventilated. Davis et al. (2006) determined that mechanically ventilated head-injured patients who were either hypercarbic or hypocarbic had worse outcomes. It is postulated that a low pCO_2 results in vasoconstriction contributing to cerebral ischemia, whereas a high pCO_2 induces vasodilation and increases ICP. This finding highlights how essential it is that the nurse review the patient's blood gases and determine that the patient is adequately ventilated. Improved survival for ventilated patients occurred when their pCO_2 ranged between 30 and 49.

The critical care nurse recognizes that suctioning the patient's endotracheal tube may result in transient reductions in oxygenation. In addition, suctioning is a noxious procedure and for both these reasons may impact ICP. Therefore, the nurse:

- Preoxygenates the patient prior to suctioning
- May medicate the patient prior to suctioning with lidocaine or opiates
- Limits the duration of each suctioning pass to less than 10 seconds and the number of passes
- Observes the effect of positive end expiratory pressure (PEEP) on the patient's blood pressure (BP) and ICP to be certain that they are not deleteriously affected. PEEP may have an adverse effect on the patient's ICP by either decreasing the venous return from the head or by decreasing the BP. The higher the ICP, the higher the PEEP must be to have an effect on venous return.

Provision of Adequate Perfusion

Because cerebral blood flow is dependent on the BP, the Brain Trauma Foundation (2007) states that the BP should be monitored and hypotension should be avoided. Although the Brain Trauma Foundation believes that it would be preferable to identify a target BP, preferably a target MAP, it states that there is not an adequate research base to support such a goal. Therefore, the Brain Trauma Foundation guidelines specify that a systolic BP less than 90 mm Hg should be avoided. However, the Brain Trauma Foundation has not been able to establish an optimal (target) BP nor has it been able to identify when the BP might be too high. Many patients with TBI and/or IICP will present with hypertension associated with sympathetic hyperactivity. In patients with intracranial lesions, this BP is usually not treated because the higher pressure is probably maintaining cerebral perfusion. In other hypertensive brain-injured patients, the BP may decrease in response to adequate sedation.

Although a target BP may not be identifiable, a systolic BP less than 90 mm Hg in a patient with a TBI is clearly a predictor of a poor outcome. Initial management usually involves ensuring that the patient is euvolemic. There is controversy about how fluids should be utilized to achieve an adequate BP. In general, physicians avoid providing hypotonic crystalloids, such as D_5W or 0.45% normal saline, to patients with TBIs because they worry about the potential for worsening cerebral edema. In addition, patients with TBI who receive large volumes of fluid are at much higher risks for the development of adult respiratory distress syndrome (ARDS). Isotonic crystalloids such as 0.9% saline or Ringer's solution are most commonly used. Normal saline is preferred because it is inexpensive, iso-osmolar, and has no free water. The administration of free water is avoided because sodium disturbances are common in TBI patients and hyponatremia is associated with poor outcomes. Although a sufficient research base is not yet available for the Brain Trauma Foundation to include it as a recommendation, there have been successes reported utilizing 250 mL of hypertonic saline to expand intravascular volume and correct hypotension while limiting cerebral edema. One drawback of using hypertonic saline as a resuscitation fluid is that health care providers must know the serum sodium prior to beginning the infusion.

Maintenance of Adequate Cerebral Perfusion

Maintenance of a systolic pressure greater than 90 mm Hg is only one of several factors necessary to maintain adequate perfusion of the brain. As noted previously, CPP is defined as the MAP minus the ICP.

$$CPP = MAP - ICP$$

Therefore, any factor that increases the ICP will have an impact on cerebral perfusion. At this point, it is clear that a low CPP (less than 50) should be avoided because it is associated with a loss of autoregulation, the brain's ability to call for an adequate BP to enhance cerebral perfusion, and with poor patient outcomes. The Brain Trauma Foundation states there is even clearer evidence that increasing the CPP to values greater than 70 by providing fluids and vasopressors (which was once recommended) should be avoided due to the high risk of ARDS and the likelihood that a CPP greater than 70 has detrimental

effects on the brain. Thus, it believes that an optimum value for a CPP lies between 50 and 70, possibly about 60. Based on the equation, CPP can be increased by either increasing MAP (see previous text) or decreasing ICP.

Managing Intracranial Pressure

According to the Brain Trauma Foundation (2007), there is clear evidence that treatments to reduce ICP should be initiated when the ICP threshold rises above 20 mm Hg. Sustained increases in ICP to greater than 20 mm Hg for 10 minutes or longer are associated with poor patient outcomes. A variety of therapies may be attempted to reduce ICP.

Nursing Care

A patient who is agitated and in pain may have a significant increase in his BP and ICP. The Brain Trauma Foundation (2007) notes that the use of sedation is a common management strategy even though it has not been shown to affect patient outcomes. Often benzodiazepines are utilized to control agitation associated with mechanical ventilation because they are generally well tolerated and can reduce cerebral metabolism (see Chapter 1). ∞ The exception to this is midazolam, which in 33% of patients results in a reduction in MAP and an increase in ICP, both dangerous in the patient with a TBI. Therefore, the Brain Trauma Foundation recommends using a test dose to determine the effect on a patient before midazolam therapy is initiated. An alternative for a ventilated patient is propofol, a sedative-hypnotic anesthetic, which decreases ICP but does not improve mortality. One advantage of propofol is that in most patients, the dose may be lowered or discontinued, and within about 10 minutes an accurate neurological assessment can be obtained. Long-term and high-dose use are associated with significant morbidity, specifically the propofol infusion syndrome. See Chapter 1 for details. ∞

The patient with a head injury may experience significant pain either from the head injury or from other injuries incurred in the traumatic event. Morphine is most widely used because it has a high level of efficacy and safety yet is minimally sedating. It can be given as a continuous infusion and titrated as needed for additional pain. If necessary for a neurological assessment, it can be reversed with Narcan. Fentanyl is used cautiously because it results in a mild but definite increase in ICP, according to the Brain Trauma Foundation (2007).

Osmotherapy

The osmotically active agents currently being used to decrease ICP are mannitol and hypertonic saline. Adamides et al. (2006) state that class II and III evidence suggest that both may be effective. The current controversies include: Which of the two therapies is superior, what dose is best, and whether osmotherapy improves outcome in patients with TBI.

COMMONLY USED MEDICATIONS

MANNITOL (OSMITROL), AN OSMOTIC DIURETIC

Desired Effect: Mannitol decreases ICP while reducing cerebrovascular resistance and increasing cerebral blood flow. The reduction in ICP from mannitol begins almost immediately after administration probably due to its plasma expanding effect and a decrease in the rigidity and volume of the red blood cells. The result is an increased blood flow to cerebral tissue. After 15 to 30 minutes, a delayed osmotic effect develops with the direct removal of water from brain parenchyma. Onset of diuresis is in 1 to 3 hours with a duration of effect of up to 6 hours. The Brain Trauma Foundation (2007) states, "Mannitol is effective for control of raised ICP at doses of 0.25 to 1 g/Kg body weight" (p. S14). Nonetheless, some centers utilize low-dose mannitol at scheduled 2-hour increments in an attempt to obtain a lower and smoother ICP. The use of continuous infusions or prolonged administration of mannitol is often avoided because it is theoretically possible that mannitol could accumulate in the cerebral tissues and result in a rebound edema.

Nursing Responsibilities:
- The nurse identifies when the patient's ICP warrants treatment with mannitol (usually for a sustained ICP greater than 20).
- The nurse monitors the patient's neurological signs and ICP following administration of mannitol.
- If the 15%, 20%, or 25% solutions are utilized, then the nurse administers mannitol through an in-line filter.
- Mannitol may cause hypotension after rapid administration, especially in volume-depleted patients. Therefore, it is important that the patient be euvolemic and the nurse administer a bolus dose no more rapidly than over 15 to 30 minutes.
- Mannitol increases the osmolality of the blood with optimal osmolality between 300 and 320 mOsm. If repeated doses of mannitol are given, the nurse monitors the serum osmolality every 4 to 6 hours and ensures that it remains less than 320 mOsm.
- The nurse also monitors the urine output to ensure that it is at least 30 to 50 mL/hr and reviews the lab results, looking specifically for hyponatremia and hypokalemia.

Potential Side and/or Toxic Effects: Even though side effects of mannitol are rare when administered as directed, the patient needs to be closely monitored for the adverse effects that can occur from its use. The most common adverse effects are hypotension, congestive heart failure, pulmonary edema, and electrolyte imbalances (hyponatremia and hypokalemia).

HYPERTONIC SALINE

Desired Effect: Theoretically, hypertonic saline decreases ICP while increasing CPP. The principal effect is probably mobilization of water and reduction in the cerebral water content. It also increases BP because of its plasma expansion effect and may have beneficial effects on the brain's microcirculation. The Brain Trauma Foundation (2007) states that current evidence is not strong enough to make a recommendation on its use, concentration, or administration in IICP. In practice and in several studies, it has been associated with reductions in ICP and improved patient outcomes. The initial effects of the infusion on the ICP should be visible within 15 minutes of beginning the infusion.

Nursing Responsibilities:
- Hypertonic saline is available in 2%, 3%, 5%, 7.5%, and 23% solutions. In solutions up to 7.5%, it may be administered via continuous infusion at rates from 30 mL to 150 mL/hr, adjusted according to serum sodium levels. In acute elevations of ICP, a bolus dose of 30 mL of 23% might be given over 15 minutes.
- Any concentration greater than 2% should be administered by central line. The nurse monitors the patient's neurological signs and ICP to determine if the dose has been effective.
- Serum sodium levels are monitored at least every 6 hours and levels are maintained within the 145 to 155 mmol/L range.
- The nurse should assess the patient's volume status, including weight, central venous pressure, and intake and output (I&O) because patients are less likely to develop adverse side effects from hypertonic saline when they are euvolemic.
- Serum osmolarity should be measured at least every 12 hours and maintained at less than 320 mOsm/L (Mortimer & Janick, 2006).

Potential Side and/or Toxic Effects: The most potentially dangerous effect occurs in patients with chronic hyponatremia. Administration of hypertonic saline may result in central pontine myelinolysis when serum sodium levels rise too quickly. There is rapid demyelination of the pons, resulting in a decreased level of consciousness and quadraparesis that may be difficult to identify in the TBI patient. Therefore, the serum sodium is monitored at least every 6 hours and not allowed to rise any more rapidly than 10 to 20 mEq/L per day. The patient with hyponatremia may be treated with 0.9% saline until the serum sodium is normal, then therapy with hypertonic saline might be instituted (Mortimer & Janick, 2006).

If the patient develops hypernatremia (serum sodium greater than 160 mmol/L), he is at increased risk for renal failure, heart failure, and pulmonary edema. Older adults may develop these treatment-related adverse effects more readily than younger adults (Mortimer & Janick, 2006).

Cerebrospinal Fluid Drainage

CSF drainage can be accomplished through an external drainage system that is connected to an intraventricular catheter and a pressure transducer as shown in Figure 9-11. Information about the catheter and intracranial pressure monitoring is available earlier in the chapter. Unlike mannitol and hypertonic saline, CSF drainage has a negligible effect on cerebral blood flow. However, CSF drainage does lower intracranial pressure immediately by draining fluid from the ventricle. It also may decrease ICP on a more long-term basis by allowing edema fluid to drain into the system. Drainage of even a small amount of fluid can result in a significant reduction in ICP. This leads to controversy about how and when drainage should occur. Some argue that CSF should be drained for a prescribed amount of time (such as 10 minutes) when the ICP exceeds 20 mm Hg. Others argue that CSF should be drained continuously. However, when CSF is drained continuously, and the brain is diffusely swollen, the drainage of CSF may cause the ventricles to collapse.

The nurse has specific responsibilities when caring for a patient whose CSF is being drained through an external ventricular drain (EVD).

- First the transducer and stopcock must be leveled at the tragus of the ear or higher as determined by the neurosurgeon.
- If continuous drainage is being utilized, it is essential that the level be maintained as the patient moves or is repositioned.

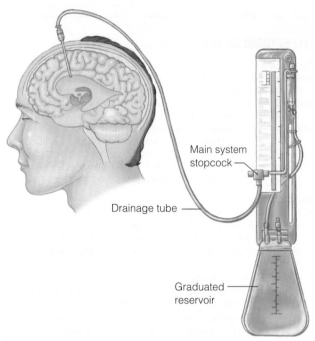

Figure 9-11 Cerebral spinal fluid drainage system.

- The amount of drainage as well as the color, clarity, and presence of sediment are noted at least hourly.
- Also hourly, the nurse accurately determines the ICP by temporarily turning off continuous drainage.
- To institute drainage in an intermittent system, the nurse turns the stopcock to allow drainage and is diligent about ensuring that CSF is drained only as prescribed. Too rapid draining of CSF can be life threatening.
- Routine changing of CSF collection bags has been associated with an increase in infections so collection bags are changed only when necessary.

Hyperventilation

Hyperventilation, causing a purposeful reduction in the pCO_2 for the patient with increased ICP, has been associated in the long term with vasoconstriction, a decrease in cerebral perfusion, and poor patient outcomes. Thus, hyperventilation is not recommended for routine management of ICP. However, acute hyperventilation is useful in neurological emergencies (Adamides et al., 2006). Hyperventilation decreases the pCO_2, inducing vasoconstriction and resulting in a rapid reduction in ICP. Thus, when a patient has a sudden deterioration in neurological signs or acute severe elevations in ICP with herniation appearing to be imminent, short-term hyperventilation may be lifesaving. It may provide time for a CT to be performed, a pathology to be identified, and definitive therapy to be planned.

High-Dose Barbiturate Therapy

High-dose barbiturate therapy might be considered when the elevated ICP is refractory to other treatments or when the patient has uncontrolled seizures. Although barbiturate therapy does decrease ICP, it is not as effective as mannitol. It most likely decreases ICP by decreasing cerebral metabolic rate, reducing cerebral blood flow, and inhibiting damage from oxygen free radicals. However, it is associated with significant side effects and complications. Patients receiving high-dose barbiturate therapy are dependent on their nurses because their vital functions are depressed (Josephson, 2004).

- Most patients who are placed in a barbiturate coma respond with a drop in BP sufficient to impact CPP. Therefore, hemodynamic stability is essential before high-dose barbiturate therapy is instituted. If necessary, vasopressors may be initiated to maintain an adequate BP.
- Once high-dose therapy is instituted, it is no longer possible to perform conventional neurological assessments such as the GCS; therefore, the patient must have an ICP monitoring device in place to guide therapy.
- There is suppression of the ventilatory drive with high-dose barbiturate therapy. Therefore, the patient must be ventilated and carefully observed for the development of hypoventilation and hypoxia.
- Infection, specifically ventilator-associated pneumonia, is a common complication, so the nurse should institute the ventilator bundle.
- Patients often develop hypothermia; therefore, the nurse identifies the optimal temperature for the patient, monitors the patient's temperature, and initiates appropriate measures to maintain the temperature.
- Many patients develop a significant ileus that is not responsive to prokinetic agents (Bochicchio et al., 2006). Therefore, the nurse assesses the patient carefully for the presence of bowel sounds and anticipates that it may be necessary to initiate parenteral nutrition.
- Patients often lack a corneal reflex. Therefore, the nurse must take measures to protect the patient's corneas.

Prophylactic Hypothermia

Therapeutic hypothermia can reduce ICP most likely by decreasing levels of excitatory neurotransmitters, free radical production, and cerebral edema. It also reduces the cerebral metabolic rate (Adamides et al., 2006). Initial studies on patients who had moderate hypothermia (33°C) induced for 48 hours after TBI did not show any difference in patient outcomes at 6 months between patients treated with hypothermia and patients treated with standard protocols. Therefore, the Brain Trauma Foundation (2007) does not recommend it for routine use at present. However, it may be attempted when there are no other ways to reduce ICP. In addition, questions remain about whether hypothermia would result in better outcomes if it were continued beyond 48 hours or if slightly lower temperatures were utilized. If the critical care nurse is caring for a patient with induced hypothermia, he must be vigilant about preventing, identifying, and treating shivering because shivering can increase ICP. The nurse also assesses the patient for the following adverse effects: cardiac arrhythmias, coagulopathies, pulmonary infections, hypothermia-induced diuresis, and electrolyte imbalances.

Collaborative Management

Surgery to evacuate a mass lesion such as a brain tumor, an expanding hematoma, a depressed skull fracture, or an aneurysm is accepted and necessary practice for the patient with IICP. Postoperative care for such surgery is described in Chapter 10. ∞ However, other surgeries are more controversial.

Decompression Craniectomy

When primary measures fail to control high ICP, second-line therapies are started. These second-line therapies include high-dose barbiturates, hyperventilation, and induction of moderate hypothermia. When these therapies have all failed, removal of a variable amount of skull bone (known as decompressive craniectomy) may be attempted (Sahuquillo & Arikan, 2006). Because opening the dura in addition to opening the skull results in further reductions in ICP, some physicians favor opening the dura and covering the dural defect with synthetic dura or pericranium (duroplasty) as well. The duroplasty leaves a space into which the intracranial volume can expand (Tazbir, Marthaler, Moredich, & Kereszles, 2005). Although such procedures decrease the ICP immediately in 85% of patients with intractably elevated ICP, there is no clear evidence that they improve the long-term neurological outcomes for adult patients. However, there are ongoing randomized studies to determine the long-term effectiveness of decompression craniectomy for patients with TBI and cerebral infarction.

Indications for craniectomy are changing. The current indication is a continuing deterioration in neurological status despite treatment with signs of early herniation such as a unilateral fixed pupil or a dilated pupil. Once signs of late herniation such as bilateral pupil changes and extensor posturing are present, the patient is less likely to be a good candidate for craniectomy (Tazbir et al., 2005).

Postoperatively, the patient is critically ill and usually has an ICP monitoring device in place. Even with the presence of a duroplasty, CSF may still be drained if necessary. The nurse continues the methods to maintain adequate cerebral oxygenation and perfusion described previously. Placing the patient's head on the side of the craniectomy is contraindicated because it has the potential to push the cranial contents inward, increasing ICP. If there is a duroplasty, positioning the patient on that side may stress the suture line and allow a CSF leak (Tazbir et al., 2005). The nurse needs to assess the patient for development of complications such as infection, hydrocephalus, subdural fluid collection, seizures, and CSF leak.

Prevention of Seizures

Seizure types and management are described in more detail at the end of this chapter. However, because between 10% and 25% of patients experiencing a severe TBI develop early-onset seizures, specific concerns for these patients are highlighted now. Seizure activity in the first week following a traumatic injury may cause secondary brain damage as a result of increased metabolic demands, raised ICP, and excess neurotransmitter release. Therefore, about 60% of neurosurgeons initiate therapy with phenytoin post TBI because it is effective in preventing early seizures. Antiseizure prophylaxis is associated with significant risks to the patient, including rashes, Stevens-Johnson syndrome, hematologic abnormalities, ataxia, and behavioral abnormalities. Some surgeons only initiate therapy if the patient is likely to experience an early seizure. Risk factors include:

GCS less than 10

Cortical contusion

Depressed skull fracture

Subdural, epidural, or intracerebral hematomas

Penetrating head wounds

A seizure within the first 24 hours postinjury

There is no indication that prophylactic anticonvulsants are effective in preventing late-onset seizures or in preventing disability (Schierhout & Roberts, 2006). If prophylactic phenytoin therapy has been instituted, it is usually discontinued a week after the trauma if the patient has not had a seizure.

Nursing Care

The way the critical care nurse provides care to the patient with IICP can have a pronounced effect on the ICP. The nurse intervenes to decrease ICP whenever possible and avoids activities that have been demonstrated to increase it.

Avoiding Situations That Increase Intracranial Pressure

The patient's position has been shown to have an effect on ICP. Maintaining the head of the patient's bed at a 30-degree elevation allows adequate cerebral perfusion while promoting venous return from the head. Thus, it is the preferred position for the patient. In addition, it is important to keep the body and neck in alignment without knee elevation and to make certain that the cervical collar or endotracheal tube ties are not too tight to maintain good venous outflow.

When nursing activities are delivered in a traditional "cluster" fashion, with one activity following another, the patient's ICP may rise with the first activity and continue to rise with each additional activity. Whenever possible, it is preferable to intervene (for example, suction the patient) then allow the patient's ICP to return to baseline before continuing with other activities (such as turning) that may increase the ICP.

When a patient engages in a Valsalva maneuver, such as when he strains when having a bowel movement or pushes himself up in bed, his ICP usually rises. Many neurosurgeons will provide orders for a variety of stool softeners or laxatives. The nurse then uses whichever is necessary to ensure that the patient has a daily soft bowel movement without straining.

Keeping external stimulation to a minimum has been demonstrated to limit the rise in ICP. This may include noxious stimuli like suctioning and turning that should be performed when necessary but only as necessary. It also includes discussion around the patient by both the family and the health care team. Some studies have demonstrated a rise in a patient's ICP when discussions about the patient were conducted around him that did not include him.

Promotion of Comfort

The management of sedation and pain in the TBI patient is discussed in the Collaborative Management section of this chapter because pain management is an integral component of management of ICP.

Provision of Adequate Nutrition

Patients with TBI have a metabolic rate that is increased to 120% to 240% of expected. Even if the patients are sedated or paralyzed, their metabolic needs are 100% to 120% of expected (Brain Trauma Foundation, 2007). There is evidence to suggest that patients have better outcomes when they receive full caloric replacement by the ninth day post injury. Therefore, the Brain Trauma Foundation recommends that these patients should begin enteral feedings (either jejeunal or gastric) by 72 hours post injury so that they can receive their full caloric needs by day 7. Enteral feedings are recommended because they are usually well tolerated and are less likely to be associated with infection than parenteral nutrition. Most patients with a TBI will tolerate gastric feedings if they are started at 25 mL/hr and increased by 25 mL every 12 hours until the dose that meets full caloric needs is reached. However, if a patient is unable to tolerate enteral feedings (as are most patients in barbiturate coma) then parenteral nutrition should be instituted. Provision of enteral and parenteral nutrition is discussed in detail in Chapter 1. ∞

Hyperglycemia can worsen ischemic brain injury. Therefore, the patient with a severe TBI injury should be closely monitored to maintain a blood glucose between 80 and 120 mg/dL, and intensive insulin management might be initiated.

Maintenance of Normothermia

Hyperthermia is common in patients with IICP or severe TBI. It is defined as a dysfunction of thermoregulatory mechanisms leading to an unregulated rise in temperature and is different from fever that is a response to an infection. The patient lacks the compensatory cooling mechanisms, and the elevated temperature may persist until physical cooling is instituted. Patients with increased ICP may develop hyperthermia but they may also develop fever. Unfortunately, an elevated temperature can further increase ICP by increasing cerebral metabolism, cerebral blood flow, and axonal swelling. It is associated with an increase in neurological deficits. Therefore, the critical care nurse must be vigilant in identifying and treating hyperthermia and fever in the TBI patient. It is advantageous to maintain a brain temperature between 36°C and 37°C (96.8°F and 98.6°F). Some centers measure brain temperature directly but many rely on core temperatures through pulmonary artery (PA) catheters and bladder or rectal probes. A common conversion is that the PA temperature is usually 0.4°C less than the brain temperature, whereas rectal and bladder temperatures may underestimate the brain temperature by 0.1°C to 2°C.

There is no standard determination of when to initiate management of an elevated temperature. Thompson, Kirkness, and Mitchell (2006) noted that some authorities recommend initiating therapy at 37.5°C (99.5°F) yet the policies in most institutions do not call for treatment until the temperature exceeds 38.5°C (101.3°F). However, what Thompson et al. found to be most discouraging was that despite institutional policies and the known hazard of an elevated temperature in patients with IICP, only 5% of patients in their study were normothermic. There were documented nursing interventions to decrease an elevated temperature identified in only 31% of the patients.

It is the responsibility of the critical care nurse to initiate management of an elevated temperature at the appropriate time. Treatment modalities include both antipyretics and physical means of cooling. Interventions to reduce fever should be assessed in terms of potential risks. Acetaminophen is one of the most commonly used antipyretics. It is inconsistently absorbed in critically ill patients with administration via nasogastric tube, often resulting in higher levels of the drug. Repeated therapy at recommended doses can result in drug accumulation, and hepatotoxicity has developed in some patients. Antipyretics are ineffective in those patients who have a disorder of the thermoregulatory system and physical cooling may be needed.

Holtzclaw (2002) stated that physical cooling is justified when the patient's thermoregulatory mechanisms are impaired or when the patient has neurological damage. Treating hyperthermia preserves brain function because the metabolic needs of the brain are reduced by about 10% for each degree Celsius the patient's temperature is lowered. Patients may be cooled by convective airflow blankets, infusions of cool fluids, or indwelling cooling catheters such as Setpoint. However, external cooling (hypothermia) blankets are still commonly utilized to cool patients.

Of particular concern when instituting physical cooling is the potential for the patient to shiver. Shivering causes an increase in the metabolic rate of 100% to 200% and increases body temperature. Thus, it should be prevented. According to Holtzclaw (2002), in order to prevent shivering, the nurse might:

- Use higher temperatures on the cooling blanket (as high as 23.9°C [75°F]) so that the patient's temperature does not drop as rapidly.
- Wrap the patient's arms and legs in cloth towels and position them so they are off the blanket.
- Place a bath blanket between the patient and the hypothermia blanket to prevent burning the patient's skin.
- Sedate or even paralyze the patient.

Most patients are also treated with an antipyretic. According to Axelrod and Diringer (2006), if seriously ill febrile patients are externally cooled and sedated or paralyzed to suppress shivering, they may have a more rapid reduction of fever than if treated with antipyretic medications alone. The utilization of such an external cooling blanket requires continuous, accurate assessment of the patient's core or brain temperature. Usually the blanket is turned off when the patient's temperature is about 1°C above the desired temperature to allow the temperature to drift toward the goal.

Providing Support for the Patient and Family

Most families and patients define the moment of a severe TBI as the time when the life of the patient and family were turned upside down (Lefebvre & Lever, 2006). Some family members describe the experience as "waiting to wake up from a nightmare." In any case, a TBI marks a dramatic change in the life of the patient and family.

In a study by Lefebvre and Lever (2006), most family members believed that the way they were provided the "bad news" of the injury had a significant impact on their adjustment. They reported that information was often insufficient, imprecise, or simply not provided. They believed they "endured long waits, were left to their own devices, and received only a trickle of information" (p. 714).

Health care providers in the same study, although acknowledging the feelings of the family, stated they believed that part of the problem was related to the families' state of shock and inability to recall information. However, the problem was worsened by the uncertainty of the prognosis and the health care providers not knowing what to say. They told Lefebvre and Lever (2006) about their "fear of being wrong; they were afraid of upsetting the family further or giving them false hope" (p. 715).

Marks and Daggett (2006) developed a critical pathway for meeting the needs of families of patients with severe TBI. It begins with health information and management. On the first day, the family meets with the physician and nurse to discuss the patient's injury and plan of care. At that time a primary nurse contact and family contact person are identified. As the ICU stay progresses, the primary nursing contact is responsible for discussing new topics as the family expresses a need to know.

The next aspect of family care identified in the pathway is provision of emotional support. Throughout the patient's stay, all members of the staff are encouraged to answer questions, explain equipment, and assess for and reinforce positive coping behaviors. Contacts are made with the chaplain and social services as appropriate.

Another aspect of family care identified is involvement in patient care. As the patient stabilizes, the nurse demonstrates appropriate ways the family can touch and speak to the patient. After the patient has fully stabilized, the family, if willing, may be taught how to deliver oral hygiene, assist with turning, assist with physical therapy, or provide coma stimulation.

Institution of Coma Stimulation

Coma stimulation is a treatment (such as an auditory, a tactile, an olfactory, or a gustatory stimulus) that is varied in intensity and frequency in an attempt to increase the patient's arousal and awareness (Gerber, 2005). In the past, it was not attempted until rehabilitation, but now it may be started in the critical care unit after 72 hours if the patient is stable. According to Gerber, it is important that the stimulation be provided when the patient has just completed a sleep/rest period, the room is uncluttered and quiet, and the patient is stable. The stimulation might be as simple as providing mouth care, changing position, or providing the patient with his favorite type of music. During the stimulation, only one person should be speaking at a time and only one mode of stimulation provided at a time. The patient's family can become involved in coma stimulation by stroking the patient's hand, brushing his hair, and bringing in familiar objects from home. A Cochrane Review by Lombardi, Taricco, De Tanti, Telaro, and Liberati in 2006 determined that there is no reliable evidence to support, or rule out, the effectiveness of multisensory programs in patients in a coma or vegetative state.

Complications

Patients develop a wide range of complications post TBI.

Pulmonary Complications: Pneumonia and Adult Respiratory Distress Syndrome

Aspiration resulting in pneumonia occurs in as many as 40% of patients following TBI, usually between the second and fourth day post injury. Aspiration may occur immediately after the injury if the patient has been vomiting, or it may happen during intubation. This is an additional reason for the use of rapid sequence intubation in the head-injured patient. When the patient is ventilated, in order to prevent ventilator-associated pneumonia, the nurse institutes the ventilator bundle.

ARDS may develop following pneumonia or excessive fluid volume replacement. At one time, it was recommended that a patient with a TBI have a CPP greater than at least 70. To achieve this goal, patients received large amounts of volume to increase their MAP. Although this did not improve their cerebral function, it did increase their likelihood of developing ARDS and is therefore no longer an accepted mode of management. The early manifestations and management of ARDS is discussed in Chapter 3. ∞

Deep Vein Thrombosis

Patients with severe TBIs are at an elevated risk for deep vein thrombosis (DVT) because many of them have abnormalities in coagulation. Additional risks for DVT are common and include immobility in the acute care setting, paralysis, and concurrent orthopedic injuries. The result is that DVT occurs often in patients with TBI, occurring in 7% to 20% of patients during their rehabilitation (Carlile et al., 2006). One of the major concerns is that the patient who develops a DVT while immobile during acute care hospitalization will have a pulmonary embolus when mobilized in rehabilitation.

The Brain Injury Foundation (2007) recommends the use of intermittent pneumatic compression stockings until the patient is ambulatory unless prevented by lower extremity injury. Low molecular weight and fractionated heparin have been used in conjunction with stockings but they increased the risk of bleeding. Therefore, there are no guidelines for their use in patients with TBI at this time. The critical care nurse should remember that the prevention of DVT is essential in the care of the TBI patient and institute the use of compression stockings or boots as soon as possible.

Sodium Imbalances

Disturbances of the pituitary with either profound deficiencies of antidiuretic hormone (ADH), diabetes insipidus (DI), or excessive release of ADH—syndrome of inappropriate ADH (SIADH)—may develop. With the absence of ADH that occurs in DI, the patient excretes large volumes of dilute urine, and the serum sodium increases. It is more likely to develop following

---

SAFETY INITIATIVES   **Reducing Surgical Complications: Venous Thromboembolism (VTE) Prophylaxis**

PURPOSE: To reduce the incidence of deep vein thrombosis (DVT) and subsequent pulmonary embolism in hospitalized patients

RATIONALE: If prophylaxis is not provided to surgical patients, between 10% and 40% of them will develop a DVT. Surgical patients are at increased risk for DVT because of immobility, pain, and the effects of pain-relieving medications. Nursing assessments for the common manifestations of DVT have been shown to be unreliable in the early stages. If a pulmonary embolism results from the DVT, there is the potential for significant patient morbidity and instantaneous death. In one study, 32% of patients who died suddenly during the first 30 days postoperative died from a pulmonary embolism. Therefore, prophylaxis for all surgical patients is a prudent course of action.

HIGHLIGHTS OF RECOMMENDATIONS:
- Develop standard order sets for DVT prophylaxis, which might include the following elements:
  - A plan for active and passive lower extremity activity, including flexion and extension of the ankle, knees, and hips unless contraindicated.
  - Early and aggressive ambulation unless contraindicated.

- Graduated compression stockings or intermittent pneumatic compression devices, which should be worn at all times when the patient is inactive except during skin care and bathing. They should be measured to ensure correct fit. Foot pumps might be used instead but these also should be worn whenever the patient is inactive (which includes when the patient is resting in a chair or away from the unit for a test).
- Anticoagulant therapy per specific protocol or physician order.
- Develop protocols for providing prophylaxis automatically, based on the surgical procedure.
- Provide education and training for staff on the importance of VTE prophylaxis.
- Educate patients preoperatively about the prophylaxis they will receive and steps they can take to reduce risk.

Sources: Institute for Healthcare Improvement: Reduce Surgical Complications Campaign; and National Guideline Clearinghouse: Prevention of Deep Vein Thrombosis

 Available: http://www.ihi.org/IHI/Programs/Campaign/SurgicalComplications.htm and http://www.guideline.gov/summary/summary.aspx?ss=15&doc_id=9266&nbr=4960

pituitary surgery or in patients with such severely elevated ICP that they are likely to suffer from brain death and be considered as transplant donors. Management of DI is discussed in more detail in Chapter 15 ∞ and may involve administration of fluids and exogenous vasopressin.

SIADH is excessive release of ADH from the pituitary that occurs following severe head trauma, a brain tumor, or meningitis. The patient excretes excessive amounts of ADH, too much water is reabsorbed, and the intravascular volume expands. The excessive intravascular water results in a relative deficiency of serum sodium. The nurse carefully monitors the patient's hydration status and serum sodium. Treatment might be fluid restriction or careful sodium replacement.

Recovery

There are a variety of factors that may predict a patient's recovery during the first few weeks and months after a TBI. These include the duration and severity of the coma (as measured by the GCS), the duration of post-traumatic amnesia, the location and size of contusions and hemorrhages in the brain, and the severity of other injuries.

Recovery after brain injury results from several different mechanisms. Initially, the patient may show improvement as cerebral edema decreases. Next, over a period of several weeks to months, damaged brain cells may begin to function again. Finally, the patient may develop new pathways, and undamaged areas of the brain may take over some of the functions of permanently damaged areas. It is very difficult to predict any specific patient's precise recovery. In general, the more severe the patient's injury, the longer the recovery period, and the more likely the survivor will have a neurological impairment. Also, the longer a patient remains unresponsive, the longer the recovery time.

Primary Cause of Increased Intracranial Pressure: Meningitis

Meningitis is inflammation of the meninges and the underlying subarachnoid space that contains the CSF. Depending on the development and duration of symptoms, meningitis may be classified as acute, subacute, or chronic. Acute meningitis is particularly dangerous because in less than a day a patient may become severely ill with signs and symptoms of meningeal inflammation and systemic infection. The patient can decompensate very quickly and require emergency care, including antimicrobial therapy within minutes of ED arrival to survive. Fortunately, 75% of patients present subacutely. Although they still require urgent ED diagnosis and care, there is time for treatment. Chronic meningitis, the least common type, characteristically develops over several weeks. Although meningitis may be infectious or noninfectious, this section focuses on acute bacterial meningitis, the most common type.

Risk Factors

Common risk factors include:

- Circumstances that promote exposure to infectious organisms such as crowded living conditions and dormitories
- Presence of infections such as otitis media, sinusitis, or dental abscess
- Neurological injury, surgery, or invasive procedure but especially penetrating head trauma or a basal skull fracture with a dural tear
- IV drug use, especially if it results in endocarditis

Pathophysiology

Bacteria gain access to the central nervous system (CNS) and cause disease in several ways. First, bacteria may colonize or establish a localized infection in the host, usually in the nasopharynx. From this site, the organisms gain access to the CNS via the bloodstream or by spreading from adjacent structures such as the sinuses. Bacteria may also enter through a hole in the dura following trauma, surgery, or an invasive procedure. Once in the CSF, infectious agents survive and flourish because host defenses such as antibodies and white blood cells are not abundant there. Replicating bacteria and increasing numbers of white cells account for the characteristic changes in CSF cell count, protein, and glucose. Exudates extend throughout the CSF, damaging cranial nerves such as VIII, resulting in hearing loss; obstructing CSF pathways, causing hydrocephalus; and inducing vasculitis, causing localized brain ischemia (Lazoff, 2005).

As ICP continues to rise and brain edema progresses, autoregulation of cerebral blood flow is impaired and blood flow begins to fall. Without medical intervention, a cycle of decreasing cerebral perfusion, cerebral edema, and increasing ICP proceeds unchecked. Septic shock may develop, which also impairs cerebral blood flow, and the patient can die from systemic complications or from diffuse CNS ischemic injury. With treatment, "morbidity and mortality depend on the pathogen, patient's age and condition, and severity of acute illness" (Lazoff, 2005).

Before the widespread use of HiB vaccine, *H. influenzae* meningitis was the most common cause of bacterial meningitis. Now it represents less than 7% of all cases. The rate for *N. meningitidis* has remained constant at 14% to 25%, accounting for most of the cases among 2- to 18-year-old patients. It is carried in the nasopharynx of otherwise healthy individuals and initiates invasion by penetrating the airway epithelial surface. *S. pneumoniae,* accounting for 47% of all cases, is now the most common cause of meningitis in all age groups. It colonizes the human nasopharynx in 5% to 10% of healthy adults and causes meningitis by escaping the local host defenses and seeding the CSF through bacteremia or through direct extension from sinusitis or otitis media. It is the most common cause of meningitis in patients with basilar skull fractures and CSF leaks. Pneumococcal meningitis has the highest rates of mortality (21%) and morbidity (15%).

Manifestations

The classic presentation of meningitis includes fever; headache; neck stiffness; photophobia; nausea; vomiting; and changes in mental status such as irritability, lethargy, confusion, and coma.

- The triad of fever, neck stiffness, and change in mental status is found in two thirds of patients.
- Signs of meningeal irritation are observed in approximately 50% of patients with bacterial meningitis. They include:
  - Kernig's sign: In a supine patient, the nurse begins with the patient's hip flexed to 90 degrees while the knee is flexed at 90 degrees. Extending the knee produces pain in the hamstrings and resistance to further extension.
  - Brudzinski's sign: With the patient supine and extremities extended, the nurse passively flexes the patient's neck. The patient responds with flexion of the hips when there is meningeal irritation.
  - Nuchal rigidity: the patient experiences resistance and pain with passive flexion of the neck.
- Cranial nerve palsies may be observed as exudates encase the nerve roots. The most common findings are deafness associated with cranial nerve VIII and defects of cranial nerves IV, VI, and VII.
- Focal neurological signs may develop as a result of ischemia from vascular inflammation and thrombosis.
- Seizures occur in approximately 30% of patients.
- Papilledema and other signs of increased ICP may be present.

Assessment

The development of acute bacterial meningitis is a medical emergency. Therefore, many EDs have triage protocols to identify patients at risk. When a patient complains of the symptoms and displays the classic signs of meningitis on focused neurological assessment, the patient should bypass the usual history taking and proceed immediately to definitive diagnosis and emergent management.

Diagnostic Criteria

If acute bacterial meningitis is suspected the physician performs a lumbar puncture urgently. Examination of the CSF in patients with acute bacterial meningitis reveals the following:

- Cloudy or even purulent appearance
- White blood cell count of 1,000 to 10,000 with more than 80% polymorphonuclear cells

- Glucose less than 40 mg/dL in 60% of patients (normally 40 to 70 mg/dL) and
- Elevated protein level (normally 20 to 50 mg/dL)

CSF is sent immediately for Gram stain, culture, and sensitivity. The Gram stain permits rapid identification of the bacterial cause in 60% to 90% of patients, allowing treatment to begin with an antibiotic that is likely to be effective. CSF bacterial cultures and sensitivities are also sent. They identify the bacterial cause in 70% to 85% of cases and ensure that the most appropriate antibiotic therapy is provided (Razonable & Keating, 2005).

Additionally, cultures of the blood, urine, nose, and throat may be sent to assist in identifying the appropriate pathogen. A complete blood count (CBC) is sent, which usually reveals leukocytosis. If a focal neurological deficit is present, a CT scan is often obtained.

Collaborative Management

The goal of care is provision of an appropriate antibiotic, possibly in conjunction with steroids, within 30 minutes of identification of acute bacterial meningitis. When patients are treated aggressively, and CSF is sterilized rapidly, the signs and symptoms may resolve completely. Ideal antibiotic therapy is based on a clearly identified organism on CSF Gram stain. However, if there is likely to be a delay, for example, in obtaining a lumbar puncture, empiric antibiotic therapy based on the known predisposing factors is started as soon as possible. This is necessary because delays in instituting antibiotic treatment in individuals with bacterial meningitis can lead to significant morbidity and mortality. Once the pathogen has been identified and susceptibilities determined, the antibiotic(s) may be modified for optimal treatment (Razonable & Keating, 2005).

Steroids are currently recommended as adjunctive treatment of bacterial meningitis. Dexamethasone is believed to interrupt the neurotoxic effects resulting from the lysis of bacteria during the first days of antibiotic use. Therefore, when steroids are given, they should be administered prior to or during the administration of antibiotics on the first 2 days of therapy.

Nursing Care

Patients with *N. meningitides* will require isolation for infection control. Prophylaxis is recommended for close contacts of a patient with *N. meningitidis* or *H. influenzae* type B meningitis. Contacts should be instructed to contact a health care provider or ED immediately at the first sign of fever, sore throat, rash, or symptoms of meningitis. In addition, some forms of meningitis must be reported to state and federal health agencies.

Avoiding Situations That Increase Intracranial Pressure

The nurse performs a baseline neurological assessment, including at least GCS, pupillary response to light, motor activity, hearing, and the presence of seizure activity. The assessment is repeated hourly at first and compared to the baseline to detect any changes. If the patient is relatively stable,

> elevating the head of the bed to 30 degrees,
>
> controlling straining at stool,
>
> preventing coughing, and
>
> avoiding systemic hypotension by providing adequate volume will assist in preventing increases in ICP. For patients who are less stable, refer to the section on managing ICP in the trauma patient earlier in this chapter for additional management strategies.

Promotion of Comfort

Relief of pain is also important in preventing increases in ICP. Patients often describe the headache as initially severe and getting progressively worse before treatment. Elevating the head of the bed may help to decrease the headache. Short-acting, reversible analgesic agents are preferred for pain relief.

Photophobia may be pronounced and can be a major source of discomfort for these patients. Therefore, they should be placed in a darkened room or a cloth is placed over their eyes.

Maintenance of Normothermia

A fever can increase ICP. It is therefore important to identify and treat fever in a patient with meningitis. The patient should have her temperature taken every 2 hours. Antipyretics such as acetaminophen can be utilized initially for fever. If an appropriate antibiotic is provided and an antipyretic administered, the fever may respond quickly. However, if it persists, external cooling, as discussed earlier in the chapter, may be necessary.

Common and Life-Threatening Complications

Complications from meningitis can be severe. During the acute phase, approximately 30% of patients with bacterial meningitis develop seizures. If a seizure occurs, it is treated aggressively because seizure activity increases ICP. One recommended management strategy is lorazepam 0.1 mg/kg IV.

Two potentially life-threatening complications that are associated primarily with meningococcal meningitis are Waterhouse-Frederichsen syndrome and disseminated intravascular coagulation (DIC). Waterhouse-Frederichsen syndrome is an adrenal hemorrhage that results in adrenal insufficiency, hypotension, and circulatory collapse. It is treated with immediate replacement of adrenal corticosteroids and supportive therapy. DIC is discussed in Chapter 17. ∞

Seizures

Seizures are defined as "stereotyped behavior associated with electrographic abnormalities in the EEG" (Kohrman, 2007).

Overview

When a seizure occurs, the electrical system of the brain malfunctions. Instead of discharging electrical energy in an orderly manner, the brain cells fire repeatedly and haphazardly. If the entire brain is involved at once, the surge of energy may cause a loss of consciousness and massive contractions of the muscles. If instead only part of the brain is affected, the seizure may present as any activity that the brain can control. It may cloud awareness; block normal communication; or produce a variety of undirected, uncontrolled, unorganized movements (Cavazos & Lum, 2005). Most seizures last for only a minute or two. However, the person may remain confused and drowsy for a period of time afterward (postictal phase). Epilepsy is the occurrence of at least two seizures without an identifiable cause.

Predisposing Conditions or Risk Factors

In the United States approximately 300,000 people have a first convulsion each year. Many of these people will have a single, one-time seizure (such as a febrile seizure or a treatable seizure) and require no ongoing treatment. Treatable causes of seizures include:

> Hypernatremia/hyponatremia
>
> Hyperglycemia/hypoglycemia
>
> Hypercalcemia/hypocalcemia
>
> Hypomagnesemia
>
> Hypophosphatemia
>
> Meningitis
>
> Toxins: pertussis, salmonella, Shigella
>
> Drug or alcohol intoxication or withdrawal (Kohrman, 2007)

There are a variety of other identifiable causes of seizures as well. Other known causes of seizures include:

> Hypoxia
>
> Brain tumors
>
> Fever
>
> Head injury

Between 70,000 and 128,000 new cases of epilepsy (seizures without an identifiable cause) are diagnosed each year. Currently there are 2.7 million people in the United States with active epilepsy (a history of the disorder plus a seizure or use of anticonvulsant medicine within the past 5 years). The prevalence increases with age, and there are about 570,000 persons over the age of 65 with epilepsy.

Pathophysiology and Manifestations

Seizures result from a spontaneous electrical discharge initiated by highly excitable cortical neurons. This increased electrical activity may occur in response to a stimulus such as dehydration, fatigue, flashing lights, hypocarbia, emotional stress, or monthly hormonal fluctuations. The neuronal excitement may remain in one site (focal or partial), spread slowly (secondarily generalize), or generalize immediately at the onset. The clinical signs and symptoms of a specific seizure depend on the location and extent of the spread of the discharging neurons. Seizure classifications are displayed in Table 9–3.

Critical care nurses commonly see focal seizures after a patient has had a head injury or brain surgery. The nurse might notice that the patient's hand was twitching rhythmically. If the seizure then progressed up the arm, along the side of the body, and finally encompassed the entire body, it would be a secondarily generalized seizure. The most recognizable primary generalized seizure is the tonic-clonic seizure. Tonic-clonic seizures, also referred to as grand mal seizures, consist of several motor behaviors. The first is generalized tonic extension

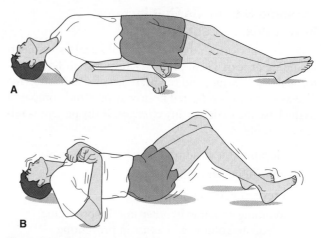

Figure 9-12 Tonic-clonic seizures in grand mal seizures. *A,* Tonic phase. *B,* Clonic phase.

of the extremities lasting for 10 to 20 seconds, followed by clonic rhythmic movements lasting 20 to 30 seconds then prolonged postictal confusion (Figure 9-12). The critical care nurse is less likely to notice the other common type of generalized seizure, an absence seizure, which is a period of impaired consciousness that lasts for approximately 20 seconds.

Assessment with Intervention upon Discovery

If the nurse observes a seizure then her first priority is to intervene to protect the patient and prevent aspiration. This usually involves:

- Lowering the patient to the floor or bed if he is not in a bed
- Cushioning the patient's head
- Loosening any tight clothing
- Padding or removing objects that the patient might strike
- It does not involve inserting a tongue blade, restraining the patient, or interfering with the course of the seizure.

During the minute or two that the seizure lasts, the nurse observes the seizure. While the nurse is observing the seizure, or if the nurse is obtaining a history from a witness after the seizure, the nurse considers the following:

- Was there any warning that a seizure might occur? If so, what kind of warning occurred (e.g., Did the patient have a sensory aura)?
- Was there any trigger (e.g., Was the patient looking at flashing lights)?
- What did the patient do during the seizure? Was there a tonic phase? Were there rhythmic contractions of muscles? Where did they start? How did they progress?

TABLE 9–3

Classification of Seizures

I. Partial seizures
  A. Simple partial seizures: No change in the level of consciousness
    1. With motor signs
      a. Focal (may occur with march [Jacksonian] or without march)
      b. May be versive, postural, or phonatory
    2. With somatosensory or special-sensory symptoms such as visual, auditory, olfactory, gustatory, or vertiginous
    3. With autonomic symptoms or signs
    4. With psychic symptoms such as illusions, or structured hallucinations
  B. Complex partial seizures: Impairment of consciousness may develop after the seizure begins or at the onset of the seizure
  C. Partial seizures evolving to secondarily generalized seizures
    1. Simple partial seizures evolving to generalized seizures
    2. Complex partial seizures evolving to generalized seizures
    3. Simple partial seizures evolving to complex evolving to generalized seizures
II. Generalized seizures
  A. Absence seizures
    1. Typical absence seizures
    2. Atypical absence seizures
  B. Myoclonic seizures
  C. Clonic seizures
  D. Tonic seizures
  E. Tonic-clonic seizures
  F. Atonic seizures

- Was the patient able to relate to the environment during the seizure and/or does the patient remember the seizure?
- How long did each phase of the seizure last?

Once the seizure ends, the nurse may turn the patient on his side and make sure that the patient starts breathing. She checks for a return to consciousness and determines the patient's orientation. The patient's vital signs including temperature and oxygen saturation are obtained. The nurse should also determine:

- How the patient felt after the seizure
- If the patient was incontinent or drooling
- How long it took for the patient to get back to his baseline condition

If the seizure does not end after a minute or two, or if it occurs in a patient post head surgery or brain injury, it will require aggressive management. Management is described later in the chapter.

When the nurse is obtaining a history from the patient or family member, the nurse should ask:

- Has this ever happened before?
- If so, how frequently do these seizures occur?
- What has the patient been doing for the seizures and has he shown any response to therapy?

Diagnostic Criteria

A single generalized seizure that follows a pattern familiar to the patient and terminates without treatment may not require any diagnostic follow-up. When a patient with a known seizure disorder has seizures with increasing frequency, follow-up may involve determining the blood level of the patient's antiseizure medication. However, when a patient has a first seizure or develops status epilepticus, there is usually a diagnostic work-up to determine the cause of the seizure.

- Laboratory studies may be performed to check for:
  - Any of the electrolyte imbalances described previously that can cause treatable seizures (particularly sodium imbalances)
  - Hypoglycemia (a blood glucose is obtained as soon as possible)
  - Anticonvulsant levels in a patient with a history of seizures
  - Levels of alcohol and drugs of abuse
- For patients with new-onset seizures, noncontrast CT is indicated because it quickly detects any brain lesion or the presence of acute hemorrhagic stroke.
- An electroencephalogram (EEG) is obtained to evaluate the brain's electrical activity.
- A lumbar puncture (LP) is indicated if CNS infection is suspected.

Collaborative Management

Recurrent unprovoked seizures are usually managed with an anticonvulsant. However, if the patient has had only a single unprovoked seizure, the likelihood of him having another is small. Therefore, anticonvulsants are not recommended for a single seizure and the patient is told to avoid triggers such as sleep deprivation, flashing lights, and dehydration.

Seizure control is the key to quality of life for a patient with recurrent seizures (Kohrman, 2007). Approximately 70% of patients with epilepsy will become seizure-free with an appropriate anticonvulsant and will remain seizure-free even after they are weaned from the medication. Weaning usually begins if the patient has been taking medication for 2 to 5 years and is seizure-free. An additional 10% to 15% of patients with epilepsy will remain seizure-free while continuing to take medication. However, between 15% and 20% of people will continue to have seizures despite appropriate, even aggressive, anticonvulsant therapy.

The goal of anticonvulsant therapy is to attain seizure control with a minimum of side effects. General principles of seizure control include:

- Use of a single anticonvulsant to minimize side effects
- Once a day dosing (if possible) to enhance patient compliance
- Slow increases in the dose of the medication until control of seizures is achieved or the patient experiences intolerable side effects (Kohrman, 2007)

Anticonvulsants

The type of seizure and the specific epileptic syndrome play a role in the selection of the initial anticonvulsant. First-line antiseizure medication recommendations for long-term therapy of specific types of seizures include:

- Valproic acid, topiramate, or lamotrigine for primary generalized tonic-clonic seizures
- Carbamazepine for partial-onset seizures
- Ethosuccimide for absence seizures

However, the anticonvulsant phenytoin is often utilized in critical care because it is effective against both generalized and partial-onset seizures and is one of the most effective drugs for treating acute seizures and status epilepticus.

Ketogenic Diet

A ketogenic diet may be utilized to prevent seizures. It is a high-fat diet consisting of four parts fat to one part protein and carbohydrate. The diet may work because ketogenesis results in the production of an endogenous anticonvulsant and is about as effective as standard anticonvulsant therapy. It is primarily used in children and

COMMONLY USED MEDICATIONS

PHENYTOIN (DILANTIN) Phenytoin is an anticonvulsant that works by blocking the repetitive action of the sodium channel.

Desired Effect: Phenytoin has a long half-life. Therefore, a loading dose is utilized when beginning therapy. The oral loading dose is 15 to 18 mg/kg usually followed by a 300 mg/day maintenance dose. When phenytoin is administered in emergent situations, the loading dose is 10 to 20 mg/kg IV (maximum dose 1.5 gm). In an emergency situation, it may take 15 to 20 minutes for a seizure to be controlled by IV phenytoin, so an IV benzodiazepine is usually administered concomitantly.

Nursing Responsibilities:

- IV phenytoin must be administered carefully. It is very alkaline so it is essential to verify the patency of the IV before administering the drug. It must be given into an IV of normal saline because it will precipitate in dextrose and it is appropriate to flush the line before and after with NS. Phenytoin is administered no faster than 25 to 50 mg/min, because faster administration may result in bradycardia, hypotension, heart block, and ventricular fibrillation.
- The nurse monitors the ECG and BP during administration and for at least half an hour afterward.

Potential Side and/or Toxic Effects: Adverse effects are common with long-term use and may result in patients, especially adolescent females, discontinuing the medication. The effects include hirsutism, acne, and gingival hyperplasia. Patients may also develop hematologic abnormalities such as agranulocytosis and aplastic anemia. A potentially severe but rare adverse effect is the development of Stevens-Johnson syndrome. Phenytoin may therefore be discontinued if the patient develops a rash.

There is a narrow therapeutic window, and toxic effects may begin just above the therapeutic level (10 to 20 mcg/mL). Initially the patient may present with nystagmus then develop ataxia, tremors, and drowsiness.

Because IV administration of phenytoin is associated with so many problems, fosphenytoin (Cerebyx) might be given instead. The dose of fosphenytoin is always expressed as phenytoin equivalents (PE). If fosphenytoin is being administered for status epilepticus, the loading dose is 15 to 20 mg PE/kg. It may be given into an IV of D_5W or NS and administered at a rate of 100 to 150 mg PE/min. The patient may become hypotensive if this rate is exceeded. The patient is transferred to oral phenytoin as soon as possible.

young adults. After at least 6 years on the diet, the children in one study experienced more than a 90% decrease in seizures. However, some of the children found the diet intolerable and many experienced side effects, such as slowed growth, kidney stones, and fractures.

Invasive and Surgical Management

A patient has medically refractory epilepsy when three different anticonvulsants have failed to control the patient's seizures despite attaining adequate serum concentrations. If another anticonvulsant is attempted in the patient with medically refractory epilepsy, the likelihood of success is less than 5%. Therefore, such a patient may be referred for possible invasive or surgical management.

Invasive management might be implantation of a programmable vagus nerve stimulator. It intermittently stimulates the vagus nerve, resulting in altered brain excitability and decreasing the frequency and severity of seizures. It is similar to anticonvulsants in its ability to prevent seizures, and the stimulator may be activated by a magnet if the patient senses a seizure is about to occur. Problems are infections at the implantation site, voice changes when the device is activated, and, in rare circumstances, bradycardia or asystole.

Current surgical procedures are safe and effective (Kohrman, 2007). Preoperatively, the epileptogenic zone is usually mapped using video-EEG monitoring with intracranial electrodes. Mapping of motor, sensory, and speech areas is also performed. Several curative surgeries are possible, including lobectomy, lesionectomy, hemispherectomy, and callosectomy. Outcomes of temporal-lobe surgeries are better than those for surgeries in other areas. If a patient has unilateral temporal-lobe seizures, the likelihood of no seizures at 2 years is 85% (Cavazos & Lum, 2005). After surgery, the nurse performs regular neurological assessments, paying particular attention to visual field defects and mild memory deficits in the patient who has had a temporal lobectomy and paresis or urinary incontinence in the patient who has had a callosectomy.

Nursing Care

Nursing care is related to the patient's underlying illness and likelihood of having a recurrent seizure. The nurse may need to help some patients prepare for additional testing to determine the cause of their seizures. These patients may be quite anxious and may need the opportunity to verbalize their anxiety. The nurse will be able to reassure other patients that recurrence of a seizure is unlikely as long as they follow their medical regimes carefully. This is especially true for the diabetic with hypoglycemia or the patient in congestive heart failure (CHF) with hyponatremia. Those patients with recurrent unprovoked seizures will need referral to a neurologist and thoughtful education.

Education of the Patient and Family

The information provided to patients and their families needs to be specific to the patients' epileptic syndrome and medication. However, there are some general categories of information that patients and families need. These include:

- Information about epilepsy
- How to care for the patient before, during, and after a seizure
- When to contact a health care provider for a seizure and when to go to the ED
- Information about the patient's anticonvulsant medication, such as how often drug levels should be monitored, the potential for status epilepticus if the medication is stopped abruptly, and the adverse and toxic effects of the specific anticonvulsant
- Safety considerations such as wearing a Medic Alert bracelet and restrictions on driving, swimming, and climbing in high places

Life-Threatening Complication: Status Epilepticus

Status epilepticus has been defined as 20 to 30 minutes of continuous seizure activity or seizures occurring in succession for 20 to 30 minutes without a return to consciousness. Any type of seizure may occur continuously but is much easier to recognize when a major motor seizure does not terminate. Approximately 150,000 identified cases of status epilepticus occur each year resulting in over 40,000 deaths. The mortality rate is highest in elderly patients who develop status epilepticus following a stroke. People who survive following an episode frequently have cognitive declines.

There are three general categories of causes of status epilepticus. In roughly one third of cases, the patient has a known seizure disorder. According to Huff (2005), in this circumstance, noncompliance with medications is the rule rather than the exception. In another third of cases, the episode of status epilepticus is the first seizure the patient has experienced. The final set of causes includes a variety of toxic and metabolic conditions as well as events such as stroke that cause damage to the cerebral cortex (Huff, 2005).

A variety of physiological events occur during status epilepticus. There is a surge of catecholamines so the patient often develops hypertension, tachycardia, cardiac arrhythmias, and hyperglycemia. The patient's body temperature may increase when there is vigorous muscle activity. Lactic acidosis, which occurs even after a single generalized motor seizure, is common in status epilepticus. In the early phases of status epilepticus, neuronal loss has been linked to rapid and chaotic firing. Later the cerebral metabolic needs are increased and often exceed available oxygen and glucose delivery, resulting in potentially irreversible neuronal destruction. These events progress until the seizure is terminated. Thus, termination is necessary to preserve brain functioning as well as to resolve the hypertension, tachycardia, hyperthermia, and lactic acidosis. Most seizures terminate spontaneously. Why the seizure(s) continue in status epilepticus is unknown.

Collaborative Management

Aggressive supportive care and prompt termination of seizure activity are the goals of treatment. Specific protocols vary according to the institution. However, some general guidelines for management are:

- It is essential to stay with the patient, observe the seizure, and recognize if it does not terminate after the usual minute or two. When a seizure does not terminate after 4 to 5 minutes, the nurse must take action.
- The first priority in status epilepticus, as always, is airway and oxygenation; for some patients, a nasopharyngeal airway is sufficient with provision of oxygen by nasal cannula. For other patients, endotracheal intubation is necessary.
- ECG, BP, and O_2 saturation monitoring are necessary and are initiated (if not already in place). An IV of normal saline is started. Labs are drawn to check the likely causes of seizure activity, including glucose, electrolytes, levels of the patient's prescribed anticonvulsant, and toxicologies. A blood glucose is obtained. If it is not possible to obtain a blood glucose or hypoglycemia is suspected, 50 mL of D50 are given. Thiamine may be given to the patient suspected of alcohol misuse.
- "Seizures beget seizures" is an accepted clinical axiom (Huff, 2005). Therefore, early treatment of status epilepticus is the rule. Anticonvulsant medications are administered if seizure activity does not terminate after 4 to 5 minutes. IV administration is the preferred route because it allows therapeutic levels to be attained more rapidly.
  - The initial drug of choice is a benzodiazepine, usually lorazepam (2 to 4 mg IV over 1 minute) because it terminates seizures 75% to 80% of the time. The dose may be repeated after 5 to 10 minutes if the seizure has not stopped. The nurse monitors the patient's BP, respirations, and O_2 saturation closely because the major adverse effects are respiratory depression, hypotension, and sedation.
  - A phenytoin, phenytoin sodium or fosphenytoin (Cerebyx), is usually administered concomitantly to maintain seizure control. (See earlier discussion.)
- If the seizure continues beyond 20 to 30 minutes, the patient is intubated, a Foley catheter is inserted, an EEG is obtained, and the patient's temperature is monitored.
  - Failure to respond to optimal doses of a benzodiazepine and phenytoin is defined as refractory status epilepticus. There is no consensus on the best third-line drug, and protocols vary greatly. The alternatives include phenobarbital, midazolam, propofol, pentobarbital, valproate, and lidocaine.

Once control of the seizure is attained, the nurse will need to continue to monitor the patient's respiratory rate, O_2 saturation, and monitor pattern. The elevated heart rate, BP, and temperature should return to baseline, usually without treatment. In fact, the patient may become hypotensive following administration of the anticonvulsant medications. As the patient awakens, the nurse will need to orient him to his surroundings and explain what has occurred. An EEG may be obtained to verify there is no ongoing seizure activity.

VISUAL MAP Life-Threatening Brain Injury

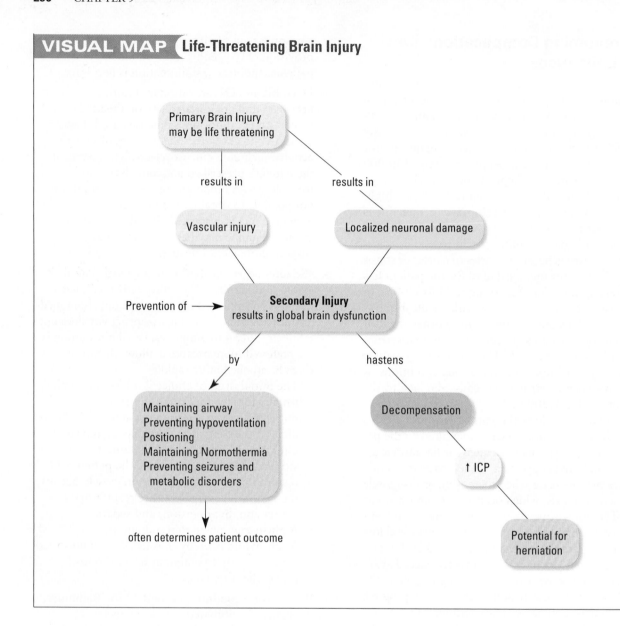

INTRACRANIAL DYSFUNCTION SUMMARY

The nurse has important roles in the care of the patient with IICP. It is usually the nurse, while performing hourly nursing assessments, who is responsible for evaluating the patient's ongoing neurological status. It is also the nurse who is responsible for providing care in a fashion that prevents secondary brain injury. Once the patient has survived the initial injury, the patient's outcome is often determined by the way that care is delivered and secondary brain injury is avoided.

CASE STUDY

Adam Simmons, 25 years old, was in a snowmobile accident. He was found lying against a tree unresponsive. In the field his blood pressure was 132/72, pulse 74, and respirations 14. When he arrived at the hospital, his pupils were unequal and reacted slowly. He moved his left side only to noxious stimuli and did not move his right side at all. His BP was 170/70, pulse 60, and respirations 22.

1. What do these findings most likely indicate and why did the vital sign changes occur?

2. Mannitol 50 gms was ordered immediately. What was its purpose? What are the nursing implications of administering mannitol emergently?

3. Adam was taken to CT scan then immediately to the OR for evacuation of an epidural hematoma. Why does discovery of an epidural hematoma require emergent surgery?

4. On transfer to the ICU following surgery, Adam was receiving Diprivan (propofol) for sedation. Why might sedation have been required? What are the advantages and problems of using propofol for sedation in the patient with IICP?

5. In the ICU, Adam had an ICP monitor and an external ventricular drain that was to be maintained 5 cm above the tragus and drained continuously. What are the nursing responsibilities associated with maintaining such a system?

6. Adam's ICP suddenly increased to 40. His pupils became fixed and he exhibited decerebrate posturing. How should the nurse have responded?

See answers to Case Studies in the Answer Section at the back of the book.

CRITICAL THINKING QUESTIONS

1. How does the brain maintain a relatively normal intracranial pressure when a patient has a slowing expanding subdural hematoma?

2. Why do secondary insults (secondary causes of increased intracranial pressure) have such an impact on patient outcome?

3. Which of the components of the Glasgow Coma Scale is most predictive of patient outcome in traumatic brain injury?

4. What is the clinical significance of a patient developing an intracranial pressure of 34 and a cerebral perfusion pressure of 50? How should the nurse respond to such findings?

5. Why is traumatic brain injury a significant public health concern?

6. What is the difference in patient presentation and collaborative management between subdural and epidural hematomas?

7. What are the initial priorities in the collaborative management of a patient with a traumatic brain injury?

8. What measures can a nurse utilize to prevent shivering when using external cooling to decrease a patient's temperature?

9. What are the early manifestations of meningitis? What should a nurse do if she suspects a patient has meningitis?

10. How should a nurse respond when a patient with a traumatic brain injury has a seizure?

See answers to Critical Thinking Questions in the Answer Section at the back of the book.

EXPLORE MEDIALINK

http://www.prenhall.com/perrin

Additional interactive resources for this chapter can be found on the Web site at http://www.prenhall.com/perrin. Click on "Chapter 9" to select activities for this chapter.

Case Study: Traumatic Brain Injury

Nursing Care Plan

NCLEX Review Questions

MediaLinks:
• Brain Trauma Foundation Guidelines

• Brain Trauma Research Center
• Epilepsy Foundation
• The Brain Injury Recovery Network
• The Brain Trauma Foundation
• The Precise Neurological Exam

MediaLink Applications

REFERENCES

Adamides, A. A., Winter, C., Lewis, P. M., Cooper, D. J., Kossmann, T., & Rosenfeld, J. V. (2006). Current controversies in the management of patients with severe traumatic brain injuries. *Australasian Journal of Surgery, 76*, 163–174.

American Association of Neuroscience Nurses (AANN). (2005). Guide to the care of the patient with intracranial pressure monitoring. Accessed March 1, 2008, from: http://www.aann.org/pubs/guidelines.html

Axelrod, Y., & Diringer, M. (2006). Temperature management in acute neurologic disorders. *Critical Care Clinics, 22*(4), 267–285.

Bay, E., & McLean, S. A. (2007). Mild traumatic brain injury: An update for nurse practitioners. *Journal of Neuroscience Nursing, 29*(1), 43–51.

Bochicchio, G. V., Kochicchio, K., Nehman, S., Casey, C., Andrews, P., & Scales, T. (2006). Tolerance and efficacy of enteral nutrition in traumatic brain-injured patients induced into barbiturate coma. *Journal of Parenteral and Enteral Nutrition, 30*(6), 503–506.

Brain Trauma Foundation. (2007). Guidelines for the management of severe traumatic brain injury. *Journal of Neurotrauma, 1*(Suppl. 1), S1–106. Retrieved June 2007, from http://www2.braintrauma.org/guidelines/downloads/JON_24_Suppl.pdf

Carlile, M., Yablon, S., Mysiw, W., Frol, A., Lo, D., & Diaz-Arrista, R. (2006). Deep venous thrombosis management following traumatic brain injury: a practice survey of the traumatic brain injury models. *Journal of Head Trauma Rehabilitation, 21*(6), 483–490.

Cavazos, J. E., & Lum, F. (2005). Seizures and epilepsy. *EMedicine.* Retrieved February 29, 2008, from http://www.emedicine.com/neuro/topic415.htm

Clement, C., Steill, I. G., Schuli, M., Rowe, B., Brison, R., Lee, J., et al. (2006). Clinical features of head injury patients presenting with a Glasgow Coma Scale score of 15 and who require neurosurgical intervention. *Annals of Emergency Medicine, 48*(3), 245–251.

Cremer, O. L., Moons, K. G. M., van Dijk, G. W., van Balen, P., & Kalkman, C. J. (2006). Prognosis following severe head injury: Development and validation of a model for prediction of death, disability, and functional recovery. *The Journal of Trauma Injury, Infection, and Critical Care, 61*, 1484–1491.

Davis, D., Idris, A., Sise, M., Kennedy, F., Eastman, A., Velkey, T., et al. (2006). Early ventilation and outcome in patients with severe to moderate traumatic brain injury. *Critical Care Medicine, 34*(4), 1202–1208.

Gerber, C. S. (2005). Understanding and managing coma stimulation: Are we doing everything that we can. *Critical Care Nursing Quarterly, 28*(2), 94–108.

Holtzclaw, B. J. (2002). Use of thermoregulatory principles in patient care: Fever management. *The Online Journal of Clinical Innovations, 31*(5), 1–64.

Huff, J. S. (2005). Status epilepticus. *EMedicine.* Retrieved February 29, 2008, from http://www.emedicine.com/emerg/topic554.htm

Josephson, L. (2004). Management of increased intracranial pressure: A primer for the non-neuro critical care nurse. *Dimensions of Critical Care Nursing, 23*(5), 194–206.

Kohrman, M. H. (2007). What is epilepsy? Clinical perspectives in diagnosis and treatment. *Journal of Clinical Neurophysiology, 24*(2), 87–95.

Langlois, J., Rutland-Brown, W., & Wald, M. M. (2006). The epidemiology and impact of traumatic brain injury. *Journal of Head Trauma Rehabilitation, 21*(5), 375–378.

Lazoff, M. (2005). Meningitis. *eMedicine.* Retrieved February 29, 2008, from http://www.emedicine.com/emerg/topic309.htm

Lefebvre, H., & Lever, M. J. (2006). Breaking the news of traumatic brain injury and incapacities. *Brain Injury, 20*(7), 711–718.

Lombardi, F., Taricco, M., De Tanti, A., Telaro, E., & Liberati, A. (2006). Sensory stimulation for brain injured individuals in coma or vegetative state. *Cochrane Database of Systematic Reviews, 2006*(4).

Marks, J. P., & Daggett, L. M. (2006). A critical pathway for meeting the needs of families of patients with severe traumatic brain injury. *Journal of Neuroscience Nursing, 38*(2), 84–89.

Mortimer, D. S., & Janick, J. (2006). Administering hypertonic saline to patients with severe traumatic brain

injury. *Journal of Neuroscience Nursing, 38*(3), 142–146.

Nolan, S. (2005). Traumatic brain injury: A review. *Critical Care Nursing Quarterly, 28*(2), 188–194.

Rangel-Castillo, L., & Robertson, C. (2006). Management of intracranial hypertension. *Critical Care Clinics, 22*, 713–732.

Razonable, R., & Keating, M. R. (2005). Meningitis. *eMedicine.* Retrieved from http://www.emedicine.com/med/topic2613.htm

Roger, E. P., Butler, J., & Benzel, E. C. (2006). Neurosurgery in the elderly; Brain tumors and subdural hematomas. *Clinics in Geiatric Medicine, 22*, 623–644.

Sahuquillo, J., & Arikan, F. (2006). Decompression craniectomy for acute traumatic brain injury. *Cochrane Database of Systematic Reviews, 2006* (4).

Schierhout, G., & Roberts, I. (2006). Anti-epileptic drugs for preventing seizures following acute traumatic brain injury. *Cochrane Database of Systematic Reviews, 2006* (4).

Sperry, J. L., Gentilello, L., Minei, J. P., Diaz-Arrastia, R. R., Friese, R. S., & Shafi, S. (2006). Waiting for the patient to "sober up": Effect of alcohol intoxication on Glasgow Coma Scale score of brain injured patients. *The Journal of Trauma, Injury, and Critical Care, 61*, 1305–1311.

Tazbir, J., Marthaler, M. Y., Moredich, C., & Kereszles, P. (2005). Decompressive hemicraniectomy with duraplasty: A treatment for large-volume ischemic stroke. *Journal of Neuroscience Nursing, 37*(4), 194–199.

Thompson, J. J., Kirkness, C. J., & Mitchell, P. H. (2006). Intensive care unit management of fever following traumatic brain injury. *Intensive and Critical Care Nursing, 23*, 91–96.

Care of the Patient with a Cerebral or Cerebrovascular Disorder

Kathleen Schuler, MSN, RN
Kathleen Perrin, PhD, RN, CCRN

Learning Outcomes

Upon completion of this chapter, the learner will be able to:

1. List the common manifestations of brain tumors and explain their causation.

2. Explain why glucocorticoids are administered to patients with brain tumors.

3. Compare and contrast the care of patients with supratentoral, posterior fossa, and pituitary tumors.

4. Summarize strategies used to prevent common complications post craniotomy.

5. Compare and contrast the mechanisms of hemorrhagic and ischemic strokes.

6. Describe emergent management of the patient with an ischemic stroke.

7. Compare and contrast intracerebral hemorrhage and subarachnoid hemorrhage.

8. Describe the three most common complications following rupture of an aneurysm and subarachnoid hemorrhage.

9. Discuss screening for dysphagia in the stroke survivor.

chapter 10

Abbreviations

ADLS	Activities of Daily Living
ASA	American Stroke Association
BAC	Brain Attack Coalition
HPA	Hypothalamic-Pituitary-Adrenocortical
NIH	National Institutes of Health
NINDS	National Institute for Neurological Disorders and Stroke
PSC	Primary Stroke Center
TPP	Thrombotic Thrombocytopenic Purpura

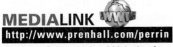

MEDIALINK
http://www.prenhall.com/perrin

See the Companion Website for chapter-specific resources at www.prenhall.com/perrin.

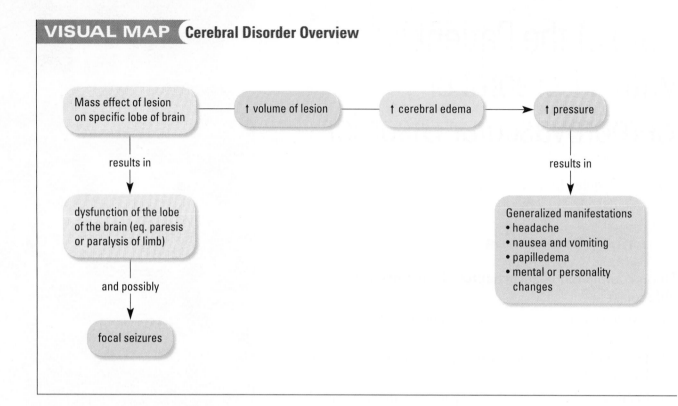

VISUAL MAP Cerebral Disorder Overview

Mass effect of lesion on specific lobe of brain → ↑ volume of lesion → ↑ cerebral edema → ↑ pressure

results in

dysfunction of the lobe of the brain (eq. paresis or paralysis of limb)

and possibly

focal seizures

results in

Generalized manifestations
• headache
• nausea and vomiting
• papilledema
• mental or personality changes

Cerebrovascular disorders are the leading cause of disability and the third leading cause of death in the United States. Identification and prompt treatment of stroke can lead to improved outcomes, yet only 29% of patients present for treatment within the necessary amount of time. Patients often do not recognize the focal signs of brain injury (whether they are associated with brain tumors or strokes) and wait to present for treatment until more dramatic symptoms have developed. Nurses ought to be able to identify focal signs of cerebral disorders and encourage patients to present for treatment.

Anatomy and Physiology Review

In order to understand cerebral and cerebrovascular disorders it is important to have an understanding of the anatomy and physiology of the brain. This chapter includes a brief review of the functions of various parts of the brain, its vascular supply, and the blood-brain barrier. Chapter 9 ∞ reviews the metabolic requirements of the brain, the Munro Kelly hypothesis, and cerebral perfusion pressure as well as the primary and secondary causes of increased intracranial pressure.

Functions of the Lobes of the Brain

The locations and functions of various lobes of the brain are displayed in Figure 10-1.

In order to understand the neurological deficits that a patient may develop from a brain tumor or a cerebrovas-

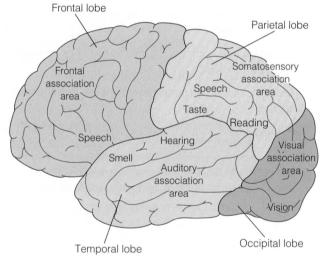

Figure 10-1 Functions of the lobes of the brain.

cular accident, the nurse must understand the functions of various portions of the brain.

Activity of the Brain

As explained in the previous chapter, the brain is one of the most metabolically active organs in the body and is dependent on a consistent blood flow to meet its oxygen and energy requirements. When there is a disruption in cerebral blood flow, neuronal cellular injury or death may occur. Figure 10-2 displays cerebral blood flow, indicating which vessels perfuse which portions of the brain. Understanding which blood vessel perfuses each portion of the brain helps the nurse understand why

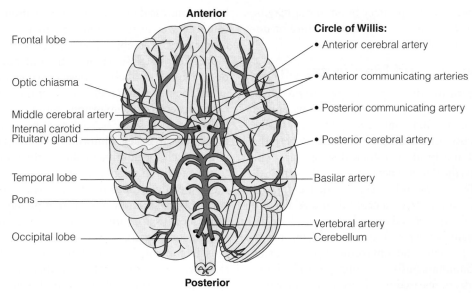

Figure 10-2 Cerebral blood flow.

deficits result from certain types of brain attacks or from an aneurysm in a specific blood vessel.

Not only does the brain require a constant blood supply, it also requires a very stable chemical environment in order for the nerve cells to communicate with one another. Glial cells form a layer around blood vessels called the blood-brain barrier to provide just such protection for the brain. The blood-brain barrier protects the brain from foreign substances in the blood that may injure the brain, as well as from hormones and neurotransmitters in the rest of the body. Large molecules and molecules with high electrical charge do not pass through the blood-brain barrier easily. However, lipid-soluble molecules cross rapidly into the brain. Thus, the blood-brain barrier helps to maintain the stable chemical environment required for the brain to function.

Cerebral Disorder: Brain Tumors

It is difficult to document the incidence of primary brain tumors in the United States. The most accurate estimate for 2004 was that approximately 41,000 people were diagnosed with tumors that originated in the brain and about 100,000 people developed metastatic brain tumors. Of the 360,000 people surviving with brain tumors, 75% had initially been diagnosed with a benign tumor and 23% with a malignancy.

Risk Factors

Genetic mutations and deletions of tumor suppressor genes increase the risk for some types of brain cancer. In rare cases, inherited diseases such as neurofibromatosis and retinoblastoma are also associated with brain tumors. Exposure to vinyl chloride is an environmental risk factor for brain cancer. Vinyl chloride is a carcinogen used in

manufacturing plastic products such as pipes, wire coatings, furniture, car parts, and housewares. It is also present in tobacco smoke. People who work or live in close proximity to manufacturing and chemical plants that produce vinyl chloride have an increased risk for brain cancer. Low-dose radiation and radiotherapy for childhood cancers and leukemia have also been associated with the development of brain tumors.

Types and Characteristics of Brain Tumors

Brain tumors are classified as primary or metastatic. Approximately 100,000 metastatic brain tumors are diagnosed each year, most arising from the lungs, breast, and skin. Primary brain tumors may be either benign or malignant.

Astrocytomas, the most common types of primary brain tumor, account for 50% to 75% of malignant brain tumors. Astrocytomas are graded from 1 to 4 according to tissue histology. Grade I tumor cells are well defined and almost normally shaped. They have a low incidence of brain infiltration. Grade I and grade II tumors are considered to be low-grade tumors and have the most favorable survival rates. However, there is the possibility that a grade II tumor will transform to a higher grade (Gonzalez & Gilbert, 2005). Higher-grade (III and IV) tumor cells are abnormally shaped and have a pronounced ability to infiltrate normal brain tissue.

The most common benign brain tumors arise from the meninges; called **meningiomas**, they account for about 25% of primary brain tumors. They are usually well circumscribed, may be attached to the dura, and are associated with an excellent prognosis when gross-total resection is possible. Other common benign brain tumors arise from nerve sheaths (acoustic neuromas) or the pituitary (pituitary adenomas). A noncancerous primary brain tumor may be life threatening if it compromises a vital structure or undergoes malignant transformation.

Pathophysiology and Manifestations

Brain tumors appear to cause symptoms by several different mechanisms. The first two mechanisms, invasion of the brain parenchyma and compression of brain tissue, result in dysfunction of the area of the brain where the tumor is located and focal neurological symptoms. The next mechanism is the development of cerebral edema. Although not fully understood, cerebral edema appears to develop once tumors have increased in size beyond 1 mm. The new blood vessels that feed the tumor lack the normal blood-brain barrier and are more permeable to macromolecules, proteins, and ions, resulting in vasogenic cerebral edema. Simultaneously, macrophages and inflammatory mediators are released that increase vascular permeability and edema. The final two mechanisms by which brain tumors cause symptoms are obstruction of the flow of cerebrospinal fluid, resulting in hydrocephalus, and herniation. These mechanisms cause symptoms related to the increased mass within the cranial cavity and the increased intracranial pressure (IICP). Manifestations that result from this increase in intracranial pressure (ICP) are called generalized symptoms. Patients with brain tumors commonly have the following signs and symptoms.

Approximately 40% of people with a primary brain tumor describe a headache as their initial symptom, whereas 80% of people will complain of headache by the time of diagnosis. These headaches are typically worse in the morning with improvement after the patient arises. The headache may worsen with coughing, exercise, or with a change in position such as bending or kneeling and often do not respond to the usual headache remedies.

Nausea and vomiting occur in about 30% of patients and may accompany headache. Drowsiness and visual problems such as blurred or double vision or loss of peripheral vision occur in about 25% of patients. A swollen optic nerve (papilledema) is a clear sign of IICP. This sign is common in young children, in persons with slow-growing tumors, and in patients with tumors in the posterior fossa. Some authorities argue that because older adults have age-related brain atrophy, they are less likely to present with generalized symptoms of IICP such as headache and papilledema and more likely to present with mental changes.

Mental and/or personality changes can be caused by the tumor itself, by IICP, or by involvement of the parts of the brain that control personality. These can range from problems with memory (especially short-term memory), speech, communication, and/or concentration changes to severe intellectual problems and confusion. Changes in behavior, temperament, and personality may also occur, depending on where the tumor is located.

Seizures are a common presenting symptom of brain tumors resulting from tumor irritation of brain tissue. The likelihood of a patient developing a seizure from a brain tumor is dependent on the location and type of the tumor as well as the age of the patient. Slow-growing tumors near the cerebral cortex (such as meningiomas) are more likely to cause seizures, and older adults with brain tumors are less likely to develop seizures than younger adults. Seizures in patients with brain tumors may present as generalized convulsions with loss of consciousness. However, focal seizures, such as muscle twitching or jerking of an arm or leg, abnormal smells or tastes, problems with speech, or numbness and tingling, may also occur.

In addition to the general symptoms listed, other more specific symptoms, known as focal symptoms, occur in approximately one third of patients with brain tumors. Focal symptoms include hearing problems such as ringing or buzzing sounds or hearing loss, decreased muscle control, lack of coordination, decreased sensation, weakness or paralysis, difficulty with walking or speech, balance problems, or double vision. Because the symptoms are usually caused by invasion or compression from the tumor, these focal symptoms can help identify the location of the tumor. Figure 10-3 displays the focal symptoms that often develop from brain tumors originating in specific structures of the brain. The tracts of the central nervous system cross near the base of the skull, so a tumor on one side of the brain causes symptoms on the opposite side of the body.

Focused Assessment

History taking is the first, important step in nursing assessment of a patient with a brain tumor. The nurse questions the patient about any symptoms she might be experiencing. Even if the patient does not mention them, the nurse questions the patient concerning the presence of any of the symptoms described previously, paying special attention to the time of day when they occurred and what exacerbated them. For example: Was the headache severe on awakening? Did it improve as the day progressed? What happened when the patient bent down? The nurse will need to question the patient concerning any indications of focal symptoms or seizures. Depending on the symptoms the patient describes, the nurse will also need to pay special attention in the nursing assessment to the patient's ability to perform activities of daily living (ADL). Finally, the nurse completes a baseline neurological assessment as described in Chapter 9 ∞ with particularly careful emphasis on the areas affected by the tumor.

Magnetic resonance imaging (MRI) and computerized tomography (CT) scanning are standard imaging tools for diagnosis and guided treatment of brain tumors. In fact, the introduction of MRI was one of the most important advances in the diagnosis and care of patients with brain tumors. According to Agulnik and Mason (2006), it allows for "assistance with pre-operative diagnosis, localization for operative planning, and tumor surveillance for progression and response to therapy" (p. 1253). MRI scans are utilized more often than CT scans because they are more sensitive and are capable of detecting tumors too

Common Manifestations of Brain Tumors Located in Specific Areas of the Brain

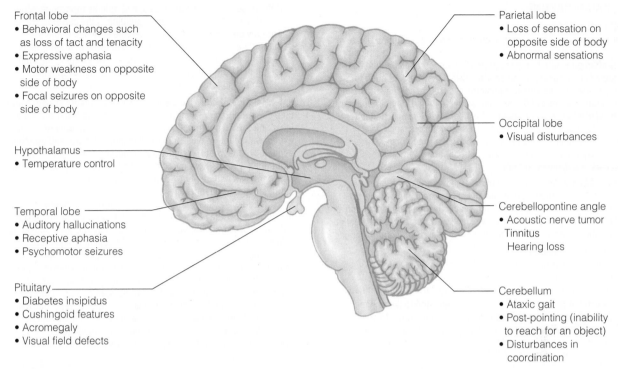

Frontal lobe
• Behavioral changes such as loss of tact and tenacity
• Expressive aphasia
• Motor weakness on opposite side of body
• Focal seizures on opposite side of body

Hypothalamus
• Temperature control

Temporal lobe
• Auditory hallucinations
• Receptive aphasia
• Psychomotor seizures

Pituitary
• Diabetes insipidus
• Cushingoid features
• Acromegaly
• Visual field defects

Parietal lobe
• Loss of sensation on opposite side of body
• Abnormal sensations

Occipital lobe
• Visual disturbances

Cerebellopontine angle
• Acoustic nerve tumor
   Tinnitus
   Hearing loss

Cerebellum
• Ataxic gait
• Post-pointing (inability to reach for an object)
• Disturbances in coordination

Figure 10-3 Focal symptoms that develop with damage to specific areas of the brain.

small to be noted on CT scans. Positron emission tomography (PET) scans also have a role in grading a tumor for prognosis, localizing a tumor for biopsy, and mapping brain areas prior to surgery.

Collaborative Management

The collaborative management of the patient with a brain tumor is aimed at reducing the edema surrounding the tumor, decreasing the tumor mass, and dealing with any possible spread of the cancer. Management may involve steroids, biopsy or resection of the tumor, radiation therapy, and chemotherapy.

Medical Management

Glucocorticoids are the mainstay of treatment for vasogenic cerebral edema. These agents decrease the tissue swelling associated with brain tumors and manage some of the troublesome signs and symptoms patients experience, including headaches, seizures, motor deficits, and altered mental status. The decrease in cerebral edema may occur because glucocorticoids directly affect vascular endothelial cell function and restore normal capillary permeability. In addition, dexamethasone may cause cerebral vasoconstriction. Since 1961, glucocorticoid therapy with dexamethasone has been the standard treatment for tumor-associated edema. Dexamethasone has been the corticosteroid of choice because of its high-potency, low-mineralocorticoid effect that makes it less likely to result in sodium retention and 48-hour half-life.

Surgical Management of the Patient with a Craniotomy

Surgical management has three separate goals: decompression of the surrounding brain, removal or reduction of the tumor mass, and diagnostic tissue sampling (Roger, Butler, & Benzel, 2006). The extent of tumor resection is predictive of patient outcome for most types of brain tumors and resection is usually first-line treatment. The amount of tissue resected ranges from gross total to partial (also known as debulking) to biopsy only with the best outcomes resulting when gross total resection is possible. The amount of tissue that can be resected is dependent on the invasiveness of the tumor, its location in the brain, and the patient's health status.

Prior to surgery, the nurse ensures that the consent form has been signed and that all preoperative procedures have been completed. It is wise to explain to the patient how much hair will be clipped because this can be upsetting to the patient. It is also helpful to explain to the family that the patient may be in surgery for an extended period. The nurse also clearly documents the patient's neurological findings so that they can be used as a baseline for postoperative assessment. Elements of a neurological assessment are described at the beginning of Chapter 9 and in Table 9–1. ∞

Once in the operating room (OR), the hair on the scalp is clipped and an incision is made. Then a circular piece of the skull bone is removed and the dura is opened to expose the brain. After the brain is exposed, the surgeon may do some mapping to identify precisely

COMMONLY USED MEDICATIONS

DEXAMETHASONE

INTRODUCTION

Dexamethasone (Decadron), a glucocorticoid, is indicated for use in patients who have symptomatic cerebral edema from brain tumors. It is often provided during the perioperative period and while the patient is undergoing radiation. However, it may be continued for as long as it alleviates patient symptoms of cerebral edema. The usual initial dose is 10 mg of IV dexamethasone followed by maintenance dosing of 4 mg IV every 6 hours. Postoperative dosing is dependent on the type and location of the tumor. Some tumors, such as metastatic tumors, have more glucocorticoid receptors and are more responsive to dexamethasone treatment, whereas others, such as menigiomas, are not.

Desired Effect: Administration of dexamethasone can produce a reduction in cerebral edema and an improvement in neurological symptoms within 8 to 48 hours of the initial dosing, most commonly in 12 to 24 hours (Nahaczewski, Fowler, & Hariharan, 2004). The decline in cerebral edema and ICP can persist for as long as 72 hours.

Nursing Responsibilities:
- Side effects from glucocorticoid therapy are common, so it is important to determine that the patient is among the 70% to 80% of patients who benefit from the therapy if it is to be continued.
- To avoid adverse effects, the dose is adjusted to the minimum that will control the patient's symptoms. Even at the lowest appropriate dose, typical doses given to patients with brain tumors have the potential to suppress the hypothalamic-pituitary-adrenocortical (HPA) axis.

- If the dose is to be discontinued, it should be tapered to allow the HPA axis time to recover. In addition, if the steroids are abruptly discontinued, rebound edema may occur and the patient may have an abrupt return of neurological symptoms. Tapering schedules for dexamethasone vary depending on the length of time the patient has been on the steroid and the patient's symptoms.

Potential Side and/or Toxic Effects: Adverse effects are dose and time dependent with as many as 50% of patients experiencing at least one toxic symptom. Common effects include euphoria, with excessive feeling of well-being and insomnia; increased appetite, especially for sweets; weight gain; hyperglycemia, particularly in diabetics; hypertension; muscle weakness in the legs (the patient may complain of inability to climb stairs or arise from chairs); stomach ulcer; and increased risk of infection.

The nurse may need to educate the patient and family concerning muscle weakness because they may fear that it is an indication of worsening neurological function. Dietary counseling is important to prevent excessive weight gain and high blood sugars. Nurses should encourage the patients to take steroids with food and avoid aspirin and nonsteroidal anti-inflammatory agents to prevent gastric ulceration and bleeding. When patients with brain tumors receive steroids for a prolonged period, their CD4 count may drop sufficiently to predispose them to opportunistic infections. Nurses should inspect the mouths of these patients to detect the presence of oral and esophageal candidiasis. To prevent the development of *Pneumocystis* pneumonia, Bactrim might be administered.

---

what function is performed by parts of the brain near the surgical site. There are several ways to "map" the brain. Some are used during surgery; others may have been performed preoperatively. Mapping may involve:

- Stimulating brain tissue with tiny electrical currents

- Measuring brain waves as they are stimulated

- Using ultrasound probes inside or near brain structures

- Probing the brain with special computerized "wands"

- Using PET or single photon emission computed tomography (SPECT)

Cortical mapping allows the surgeon to identify and avoid "eloquent" areas of the brain.

Most tumors have been located precisely by MRI and CT preoperatively. When surgery is performed, it is usually computer assisted with specialized equipment to aid in the positioning of the patient and the delivery of the treatment. Called surgical navigation, this approach allows for precise, limited craniotomy with minimal disruption of normal tissue. In addition to traditional surgery, alternative methods of tumor destruction may be utilized. These treatment methods can be directed at the tumors so exactly that little or no nearby normal tissue is damaged. Thermal destruction instruments, such as lasers, can be placed in the exact spot to destroy tumor tissue. Ultrasonic aspiration may be used to break up tumor tissue and evacuate it from the brain.

If tumor removal is possible, then portions of the resected tumor are sent to pathology for a definitive diagnosis. When the tumor may not be resected, the biopsy is usually performed stereotactically using either a CT- or MRI-based frame. These systems allow precise placement of the biopsy probe within the tumor mass.

Alternatives to surgery are also available. The following procedures are considered ablative procedures because they cause cell death and necrosis of the tumor over time. They are most appropriate for people with smaller tumors in nonaccessible areas. Multiple small doses of external radiation can be aimed at the tumor (stereotactic radiosurgery or "gamma knife"). The blood supply to the tumors can be identified by angiography then a variety of plugs can be introduced to block the artery, causing the tumor to die from lack of blood flow.

Nursing Care

Postoperatively, the nursing care of the craniotomy patient is centered on assessment of the patient's neurological status. The nurse compares the findings to the preoperative baseline to detect any changes that might indicate postoperative problems. Historically most patients were transferred to an intensive care unit (ICU) for 24 hours following cranial surgery so that they could be carefully observed with a neurological exam every hour after they stabilized. One recent study calls such management into question. It found that complications are

TABLE 10-1

Common Types of Cranial Surgeries

TYPE OF SURGERY	SUPRATENTORAL	POSTERIOR FOSSA	TRANSPHENOIDAL
Type of Tumor	May be either a metastatic or a primary brain tumor.	Primary brain tumors often of the cerebellum, perhaps of the acoustic nerve.	Pituitary tumors.
Age of patient	Majority of adult tumors.	55–70% of pediatric tumors. 15–20% of adult tumors.	10% of adult tumors.
Surgical Considerations	Mapping may be used to avoid "eloquent" areas of the brain.	Small enclosed space near critical brain structures, including the brainstem, the cerebellum, and cranial nerves.	Approach is through the nose and sinuses. Pituitary sits on the optic chiasma.
Nursing Considerations	Patients are usually positioned with their head of the bed elevated 30 degrees postoperatively. Patients are not turned to the side of the tumor if a large tumor has been removed. At a minimum the Glasgow Coma Scale, pupillary response and strength, movement and sensation in extremities should be assessed	Level of the head of patient's bed varies by institution from flat to 60-degree elevation. Prevent patient from pronounced flexion or extension of the neck post-op. Assess function of cranial nerves (V, VII, VIII, IX, and X). Evaluate coordination.	Maintain head of the bed elevated 30–45 degrees. Provide a moustache dressing. Assess for CSF leakage on dressing. Discourage patient from sneezing and blowing the nose. Assess for visual field defect. Assess pituitary function and identify presence of diabetes insipidus.

most common during the first 4 hours following surgery then again after 24 hours.

Initially the patient is monitored to be certain that she recovers from anesthesia and returns to her baseline neurological status. Once the patient has recovered from anesthesia, changes in neurological status are identified and reported to the appropriate person. A change in neurological status could be indicative of increasing edema around the tumor site; this usually responds to an increase in the dose of dexamethasone. Deterioration in neurological status might also be an indication of a generalized increase in ICP; management of ICP is described in Chapter 9. ∞ Rarely, deterioration in neurological status postoperatively is associated with postoperative hemorrhage and the patient must be returned to the OR. Nursing assessments and interventions specific to patients with common types of cranial surgeries are displayed in Table 10–1.

Positioning

Postoperatively patients are usually positioned with the head of their bed elevated 30 degrees. This facilitates venous drainage from the head and neck, preventing increases in ICP and increasing patient comfort. If a large tumor was resected, the patient is usually not permitted to turn her head to the operative side because it may cause a shift in cerebral contents. If the patient has had posterior fossa surgery, a stiff dressing or cervical collar may be applied to prevent the patient from hyperflexing or extending her neck, causing stress on the surgical site.

Promotion of Comfort

There is disagreement concerning the amount of discomfort experienced by patients post craniotomy. When medical records were scrutinized in one study, 58% of

postcraniotomy patients had neither complained of any discomfort nor received any analgesia. Although the brain itself does not have any nocioreceptors, stretching of the dura and increasing pressure in the skull can cause pain.

According to Roberts (2004), codeine phosphate is the most commonly used analgesic post craniotomy. However, she believes that it is an unpredictable prodrug that does not equate to a safe and effective method of providing analgesia post craniotomy. She argues that the justification for withholding morphine in postcraniotomy pain (it may alter the patient's respiratory rate and neurological signs) is largely based on anecdotal evidence. With these factors in mind, Roberts suggests critical care nurses actively assess their postcraniotomy patients for pain and consider the pharmacological properties of the analgesics being used. In addition, she believes it is time for the neurosurgical community to reevaluate pain-management strategies and develop an evidence base for pain management in the postcraniotomy patient.

Postoperative Complications

Four of the potentially serious complications following cranial surgery are systemic venous thromboembolism, cerebrospinal fluid leaks, meningitis, and seizures.

Symptomatic Venous Thromboembolism

Symptomatic **venous thromboembolism (VTE)** occurs in 3% to 60% of patients during the first 6 weeks after surgery for a malignant glioma. After this 6-week interval, 24% of patients will develop VTE during the remainder of the course of their treatment (Bachelor & Byrne, 2006).

Risk factors for development of VTE include age older than 60, leg weakness, large tumor size, surgery lasting longer than 4 hours, and tumor histology. Bachelor notes that a biologic factor secreted by some types of malignant brain tumors may be one of the causes of the coagulation abnormality.

Therefore, prophylaxis for VTE is recommended for most patients following surgery for malignant primary brain tumors. Pneumatic compression boots and graduated compression stockings have been shown to decrease the occurrence of VTEs without increasing ICP. An alternative is the use of compression boots prior, during, and for 24 hours after the surgery followed by low-dose heparin 5,000 units twice a day or enoxaparin 40 mg/day. Prophylaxis is especially important because management of VTE in patients post brain tumor surgery has been controversial.

Controversy surrounds whether anticoagulation is contraindicated in patients who have had brain tumors. Case studies in the past documented central nervous system (CNS) hemorrhages in patients who had been anticoagulated. Therefore, some physicians recommend placement of inferior vena cava filters as alternatives to anticoagulation. Unfortunately, according to Bachelor and Byrne (2006), brain tumor patients treated with filters have a 12% recurrence of pulmonary embolism and a 62% complication rate. Therefore, Bachelor and Byrne recommend the use of properly regulated anticoagulation with heparin followed by warfarin for patients who develop VTE following surgery for most types of brain tumors.

The critical care nurse needs to maintain the compression boots or stockings during the immediate postoperative period. Studies have shown that compression devices are often removed for longer than necessary for bathing, moving, or transport. Although the nurse assesses the patient for such evidence of deep vein thrombosis as leg discomfort, swelling, warmth, and a positive Homan's sign, he recognizes that patients with VTE are asymptomatic 80% of the time.

Cerebrospinal Fluid Leaks

Cerebrospinal fluid (CSF) leakages occur when there is a tear in the dura, allowing an opening to develop between the subarachnoid space and the outside. The critical care nurse can identify a CSF leak by clear fluid containing glucose leaking from the patient's ear or nose and forming a halo as it settles on a pillowcase. These leaks may be problematic because they may result in CSF depletion. If so, the patient will complain of a headache, which is usually more severe when the patient is in the upright position and is alleviated when the patient is supine. Most CSF leaks heal spontaneously within a week. However, on occasion, surgery is required to seal the dura. While the leak continues:

- If the CSF leak is from the nose, the patient is positioned with the head of the bed elevated slightly with a moustache dressing applied to catch the leaking CSF.

- The patient should not be suctioned nasally and packing should not be inserted into the nose.
- If the CSF is leaking from the ear or surgical wound, the patient may be positioned on that side, depending on the surgeon's preference, and a sterile dressing is applied.

The major concern with a CSF leak is that there is an open pathway to the subarachnoid space and the patient has the potential to develop meningitis.

Meningitis

Approximately 9% of patients developed **meningitis** post craniotomy in one study (Reichert & Medeiros, 2002). Gram-negative bacilli were the most common etiologic agents. Several risk factors were identified, including postoperative external ventricular shunt, remote site infection, and repeat operation. Meningitis that developed post craniotomy resulted in a high mortality rate (nearly 30%) and a longer hospital stay for the patients who survived. Therefore, the critical care nurse:

- Uses aseptic technique when caring for external ventricular shunts, wound drains, and surgical sites.
- If the patient has had a repeat operation, the nurse is especially diligent in observing for the manifestations of meningitis. These include fever, chills, increasing headache, neck stiffness, and photophobia.

Seizures

Seizure types and management are described in detail at the end of Chapter 9. ∞ However, because between 30% and 70% of patients with brain tumors develop seizures, specific concerns for those patients are highlighted now. The risk of seizure development is partially dependent on the type of brain tumor. Patients with low-grade, slow-growing gliomas are most likely to develop seizures. Of patients who develop seizures, approximately 50% have tonic-clonic seizures, including status epilepticus. Even if they receive optimal treatment, the majority of patients with brain tumors continue with some type of seizure, most commonly a focal seizure. Unfortunately, side effects of treatment with antiepilepsy drugs occur more frequently in patients with brain tumors than in other patients with seizures (Vecht & van Breemen, 2006). Consensus statements about the use of medications for patients with brain tumors have been developed by the American Academy of Neurology that state:

- Antiepilepsy prophylaxis should not be routinely used in patients who have not had a history of seizures.
- Antiepilepsy prophylaxis can be provided for the first week following brain surgery. However, after a week, antiepilepsy drugs should be discontinued for patients who do not have a history of seizures.

If anticonvulsant medication is required, Vecht recommends either levetiracetam (Keppra), unless the patient has renal dysfunction, or lamotrigine (Lamictal), unless the patient has liver dysfunction. These medications have been shown to have few side effects in patients with brain tumors who are also receiving radiation and chemotherapy agents. Anticonvulsant medications are discussed in detail at the end of Chapter 9. ∞

Recovery

Recovery depends on a variety of factors, including patient age, the location of the tumor, the histology of the tumor, the amount of tumor resected, the patient's neurological status, and the radiation dose. Radiation is one of the most effective treatments for gliomas and is the foundation for nearly all treatment regimens for malignant brain tumors. The current standard of care according to Gonzalez and Gilbert (2005) is localized field radiation with a total dose of 60 Gy in 30 fractions. Usually, patients begin radiation treatments within 2 to 4 weeks after tumor resection. Treatments are given daily for 4 to 6 weeks.

Adjunctive chemotherapy may be also provided, usually after the completion of radiation therapy. Grade III anaplastic astrocytomas are often treated with procarbazine, lomustine, and vincristine, whereas grade IV glioblastoma multiforme tumors are usually treated with carmustine, paclitaxel, and temozolomide. For older patients with glioblastoma multiforme, important questions have arisen about the timing of chemotherapy. Specifically, should chemotherapy for older individuals be delayed until there is evidence that the tumor is growing again after radiation therapy, thus allowing the patient time to recover strength? Or, should chemotherapy begin immediately after radiation therapy with different therapy provided when the tumor starts to grow again? De Angelis (2005) noted that even with the most aggressive surgery, radiation,

and chemotherapy regimens, glioblastoma multiforme (the most common type of malignant brain tumor in adults) kills patients within a median of 1 year post diagnosis.

Currently, a variety of approaches are being evaluated for their ability to overcome the blood-brain barrier and make chemotherapy more effective. First, drugs such as mannitol may open the barrier and allow chemotherapy agents to pass through. Additionally, disc-shaped wafers soaked with carmustine may be placed directly into the surgical cavity after a tumor is removed. High-dose chemotherapy may be delivered directly into arteries in the brain. Finally, enclosing highly potent anticancer drugs in protective microspheres may allow the drugs to enter tumors without unduly increasing the risk for severe toxicity.

Cerebrovascular Disorders

Cerebral vascular accident (CVA), also referred to as a **brain attack** or **stroke**, is a decrease in blood flow and oxygen to brain cells with the subsequent loss of neurological functioning. Causes of CVA are classified as ischemic (disruption of blood flow to part of the brain due to a thrombus or embolus), which accounts for 80% of CVAs, and hemorrhagic (loss of blood flow due to rupture of cerebral vessels), which accounts for 20%. The extent of damage to the brain cells varies according to the length of time blood flow is disrupted, the area of the brain affected, and the size of the area involved. An extensive disruption of blood flow to the brain can result in severe disability or death. CVA is the leading cause of disability and the third leading cause of death in the United States. Forty-seven percent of patients who survive an initial CVA die within a year, usually from complications or a recurrent stroke.

The American Stroke Association (ASA), *Healthy People 2010*, and the Brain Attack Coalition (BAC) all recommend the establishment of acute stroke units in order to improve patient outcomes (Adams et al., 2007; Alberts et al., 2005). The Joint Commission (JCAHO) on Accreditation of Healthcare Organizations (Joint Commission) has developed a Primary Stroke Center (PSC) certification program promoting timeliness and specific guidelines for provision of acute stroke services. The Joint Commission designates hospitals to be a Stroke Center of Excellence when they have shown they offer the best possible outcomes for stroke patients (Wojner-Alexandrov & Malkoff, 2006).

Risk Factors

The single most important risk factor for stroke is age. For each successive 10 years after age 55, the rate of stroke doubles in both women and men. Patients older than 80 years of age are likely to die in the hospital after stroke. An increased blood pressure is a substantial risk for stroke. Hypertension is acknowledged as a sign of physiological and structural abnormalities of vascular function. Atrial fibrillation (AF) is the most common dysrhythmia associated with ischemic stroke. Blood clots can develop in the quivering of the atria. Because these clots are a common cause of embolic strokes, most patients in AF now receive an anticoagulant.

Increased total cholesterol and decreased high-density lipoprotein can increase the risk of an ischemic stroke due to plaque build-up in the artery walls. Hyperinsulinemia or increased insulin resistance may result in arterial stiffening, which can increase the risk of ischemic stroke.

Modifiable risk factors include high-fat diet, obesity, smoking, and lack of exercise.

Pathophysiology and Manifestations of Cerebral Vascular Accident

Because the brain is so metabolically active, pathophysiologic changes begin minutes after a reduction in blood flow and oxygen supply to the cerebral neurons. Cellular metabolism stops as glucose, glycogen, and adenosine triphosphate (ATP) are depleted, resulting in failure of the sodium-potassium pump. Cerebral blood vessels swell, resulting in further decreased blood flow. Vasospasm and increased blood viscosity can result in obstruction to blood flow, even after circulation is restored. When brain cells are damaged, function of the body parts they control are impaired or lost, causing paralysis, speech and sensory problems, memory and reasoning deficits, coma, and, possibly, death. The degree of damage to the brain cells depends on the size of a perfusion deficit, the amount of brain tissue that is infarcted, and the type of stroke.

The two major categories of CVA, hemorrhage and ischemia, are totally opposite conditions. Whereas hemorrhage is defined as rupture of a blood vessel and too much blood within the closed cranial cavity, ischemia is defined as too little blood supply with inadequate oxygen and nutrients to part of the brain. These categories can be broken down into the following classifications: intracerebral hemorrhage, subarachnoid hemorrhage, and brain ischemia. Each of the following classifications has different causes, symptoms, outcomes, and treatments.

Hemorrhagic Stroke

Intracerebral hemorrhage (ICH) is usually derived from bleeding of small arteries or arterioles directly into the brain, forming a localized hematoma that spreads along white matter tracts. Blood accumulates over minutes to hours as the hematoma enlarges, resulting in the progressive development of neurological symptoms. In contrast to brain embolism and subarachnoid hemorrhage, the neurological symptoms do not begin immediately and are not maximal at onset. The most common causes of ICH are hypertension, trauma, illicit drug use (particularly amphetamines and cocaine), vascular malformations, and bleeding diathesis. ICH results from hypertension when the arteries in the brain become brittle, susceptible to cracking, and rupture.

Subarachnoid hemorrhage (SAH) is rupture of an aneurysm that releases blood directly into the CSF under arterial pressure. The blood spreads rapidly within the CSF, immediately increasing ICP. If bleeding continues, deep coma or death may result. Typically the bleeding lasts only a few seconds but there is risk of rebleeding. The classic symptom is a sudden, severe headache that begins abruptly and is described as "the worst headache of my life."

Ischemic Stroke or Brain Attack

Ischemic stroke or brain attack includes the following subtypes: thrombotic, embolic, and hypoperfusion.

Thrombotic Brain Attacks

Thrombotic brain attacks or strokes occur when the pathologic process promotes thrombus formation in an artery, causing a stroke due to decreased blood flow. Disease of the arterial wall, dissection, or fibromuscular dysplasia may cause the obstruction. Atherosclerosis is the most common cause of occlusion within the large extracranial and intracranial arteries that supply the brain.

Embolic Brain Attacks

Embolic brain attacks or strokes are caused by particles that arise from another part of the body, resulting in blockage of arterial blood flow to a particular area of the brain. Embolic strokes commonly originate from a source in the heart, aorta, or large vessels. The onset of symptoms is abrupt and maximal, because the embolus suddenly blocks the involved area of the brain. Embolic strokes are divided into four categories related to the cause:

- Known source is cardiac
- An arterial source

- Possible cardiac or aortic source based on transthoracic and/or transesophageal echocardiographic findings
- Unknown source in which these tests are negative or inconclusive

Systemic Hypoperfusion

Systemic hypoperfusion is a general circulatory problem that can occur in the brain and possibly other organs. Decreased perfusion can be due to cardiac arrest, arrhythmia, pulmonary embolism, pericardial effusion, or bleeding. Hypoxemia may further decrease the amount of oxygen carried to the brain. Symptoms of brain dysfunction are diffuse and less specific as compared to strokes that are thrombotic or embolic in nature.

Manifestations

Strokes, also known as brain attacks, typically manifest with the sudden onset of focal neurological deficits resulting from damage to the injured portion of the brain. Classic signs and symptoms include:

- Sudden confusion
- Difficulty understanding or speaking
- Sudden loss of vision out of one eye
- Sudden severe headache
- Sudden weakness of the face, arm, or leg, especially affecting one side of the body

The public should be encouraged to respond to these symptoms just as they would to the development of chest pain and immediately activate the Emergency Medical Services (EMS) system. The Cincinnati Prehospital Stroke Scale (Table 10–2) is a valid tool that can be performed by emergency medical personnel in less than 1 minute. Facial droop, arm drift, and speech are assessed, with any abnormal findings indicating an acute stroke.

TABLE 10–2

The Cincinnati Prehospital Stroke Scale

The Cincinnati Prehospital Stroke Scale is a system used to diagnose the presence of a stroke in a patient. If any one of the three tests shows abnormal findings, the patient may be having a stroke and should be transported to a hospital as soon as possible.
1. *Facial droop:* Ask the person to smile or show his teeth.
   - Normal: Both sides of face move equally
   - Abnormal: One side of face does not move as well as the other (or at all)
2. *Arm drift:* Ask the person to close his eyes and hold his arms straight out in front for about 10 seconds.
   - Normal: Both arms move equally or not at all
   - Abnormal: One arm does not move, or one arm drifts down compared with the other side
3. *Speech:* Ask the person to say, "You can't teach an old dog new tricks," or some other simple, familiar saying.
   - Normal: Patient uses correct words with no slurring
   - Abnormal: Slurred or inappropriate words or mute

Manifestations of a brain attack are usually specific to the area of the brain that has been affected (refer to Figure 10-3). Each of the four major neuroanatomic stroke syndromes results from disruption of the vascular distribution to specific areas of the brain.

Middle cerebral artery (MCA) occlusions commonly produce

- hemiparesis,
- hypesthesia on the opposite side of the body,
- hemianopsia (blindness in one half of the visual field), and
- gaze preference toward the side of the lesion.

Anterior cerebral artery occlusions primarily affect frontal lobe function and can result in

- disinhibition,
- speech perseveration,
- altered mental status,
- impaired judgment,
- contralateral weakness, and
- urinary incontinence.

Posterior cerebral artery occlusions affect vision and thought, producing:

- homonymous hemianopsia,
- cortical blindness,
- visual agnosia,
- altered mental status, and
- impaired memory.

The last type of stroke syndrome, vertebrobasilar artery occlusion, is difficult to detect because it results in a wide variety of cranial nerve, cerebellar, and brainstem deficits.

Assessment

Time is of the essence in the assessment of brain attack patients. A focused history and neurological exam along with diagnostic tests should detect the stroke mechanism and guide therapy. The single most important point in the patient's history is the onset of symptoms and should be established as soon as possible. Additional important information to obtain is any recent medical, surgical, trauma, or transient ischemic attack (TIA) events. The nurse reviews the patient's history to identify any risk factors for strokes and obtains a complete list of medications the patient is taking, especially anticoagulant and antiplatelet agents.

The neurological examination attempts to confirm the findings from the history and provides a quantifiable, objective way to evaluate neurological changes. The National Institutes of Health (NIH) Stroke Scale (Table 10–3) is performed as soon as a stroke is suspected. It is a valid, reliable tool that measures the severity of neurological dysfunction in stroke patients and permits the assessment

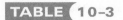

National Institutes of Health Stroke Scale

CATEGORY	DESCRIPTION	SCORE	
1a	Level of consciousness (LOC)	Alert	0
		Drowsy	1
		Stuporous	2
		Coma	3
1b	LOC questions (month, age)	Answers both correctly	0
		Answers 1 correctly	1
		Incorrect on both	2
1c	LOC commands (open-close eyes, grip and release hand)	Obeys both correctly	0
		Obeys 1 correctly	1
		Incorrect on both	2
2	Best gaze (follow finger)	Normal	0
		Partial gaze palsy	1
		Forced deviation	2
3	Best visual (visual fields)	No visual loss	0
		Partial hemianopia	1
		Complete hemianopia	2
		Bilateral hemianopia	3
4	Facial palsy (show teeth, raise brows, squeeze eyes shut)	Normal	0
		Minor	1
		Partial	2
		Complete	3
5	Motor arm left* (raise 90°, hold 10 seconds)	No drift	0
		Drift	1
		Cannot resist gravity	2
		No effort against gravity	3
		No movement	4
6	Motor arm right** (raise 90°, hold 10 seconds)	No drift	0
		Drift	1
		Cannot resist gravity	2
		No effort against gravity	3
		No movement	4
7	Motor leg left* (raise 30°, hold 5 seconds)	No drift	0
		Drift	1
		Cannot resist gravity	2
		No effort against gravity	3
		No movement	4
8	Motor leg right* (raise 30°, hold 5 seconds)	No drift	0
		Drift	1
		Cannot resist gravity	2
		No effort against gravity	3
		No movement	4
9	Limb ataxia (finger-nose, heel-shin)	Absent	0
		Present in 1 limb	1
		Present in 2 limbs	2
10	Sensory (pinprick to face, arm, leg)	Normal	0
		Partial loss	1
		Severe loss	2
11	Extinction/neglect (double simultaneous testing)	No neglect	0
		Partial neglect	1
		Complete neglect	2
12	Dysarthria (speech clarity to "mama, baseball, huckleberry, tip-top, fifty-fifty")	Normal articulation	0
		Mild to moderate dysarthria	1
		Near to unintelligible or worse	2
13	Best language** (name items, describe pictures)	No aphasia	0
		Mild to moderate aphasia	1
		Severe aphasia	2
		Mute	3
	Total	—	0–42

*For limbs with amputation, joint fusion, etc., score 9 and explain.
**For intubation or other physical barriers to speech, score 9 and explain. Do not add 9 to the total score.

of changes in neurological deficits over time. An experienced nurse can score all of the items in 7 minutes. The NIH Stroke Scale examines visual, motor, sensory, cerebellar, inattention, language, and level of consciousness (LOC) functioning. A maximum score of 42 signifies a severe stroke, whereas a score of 0 indicates a normal exam.

Diagnostic Criteria

All patients with a suspected brain attack or CVA should have the following tests as soon as possible following admission to the emergency department:

- Noncontrast brain CT or brain MRI (see neuroimaging)
- Electrocardiogram (ECG) used to diagnose any cardiac dysrhythmias or myocardial infarction (MI)
- Complete blood count (CBC) including platelets (Platelet count used to rule out thrombotic thrombocytopenic purpura [TPP].)
- Cardiac enzymes and troponin
- Electrolytes, urea nitrogen, creatinine (Hyponatremia [Na less than 135 mEq/L] is found in 10% to 40% of patients with subarachnoid hemorrhage.)
- Serum glucose (Hypoglycemia can present with neurological deficits mimicking stroke and severe hypoglycemia can cause neuronal damage. Hyperglycemia is common in patients with acute ischemic stroke and is associated with a poorer prognosis.)
- Prothrombin time (PT) and international normalized ratio (INR)—anticoagulant use is a common cause of intracerebral hemorrhage
- Partial thromboplastin time (PTT)
- Oxygen saturation

Neuroimaging

In the evaluation of the acute CVA patient, imaging studies are necessary to rule out hemorrhage as a cause of the presenting symptoms. They are also beneficial to determine the degree of brain injury and to identify the vascular lesion accountable for the ischemic deficit. Brain imaging studies are imperative to differentiate ischemic stroke from hemorrhage and to determine vascular distribution of the ischemic lesion.

Computerized Tomography. CT is the current minimal standard imaging study to rule out hemorrhagic events and to identify patients who are eligible for rtPA therapy. It should be performed within 45 minutes and interpreted within 20 minutes of the patient's arrival to the hospital emergency department. If the CT scan is positive for a hemorrhagic stroke, an immediate neurosurgical consult should be ordered. In the case of ischemic stroke, intravenous thrombolysis (rtPA) should be administered if the time since the onset of symptoms is less than 3 hours and the patient is eligible based on criteria.

Magnetic Resonance Imagery. MRI can immediately provide information in regard to blood flow in vascular territories and specific brain regions. More specifically, it can determine the size of a perfusion deficit and identify brain tissue that may be ischemic but not infarcted.

Magnetic Resonance Angiography. Magnetic resonance angiography (MRA) is a noninvasive and effective test to visualize abnormalities of the intracranial and the extracranial cerebral circulation.

Catheter Angiography. Catheter angiography (CA) is considered the "gold standard" for detecting cerebral aneurysms, arteriovenous malformations (AVMs), and arteriovenous fistulae (AVFs). It can also measure the exact degree of stenosis in extracranial and intracranial arteries.

Carotid Ultrasound. Carotid ultrasound is a noninvasive and inexpensive test used to detect occlusions of the extracranial carotid and vertebral arteries. It can be used in patients in whom an MRA is contraindicated (pacemaker, metal implants, etc.) or who are unable to receive contrast material.

Transcranial Doppler. Transcranial Doppler (TCD) is a noninvasive and low-cost technique for imaging the large intracranial vessels at the base of the skull. It is used in patients with acute cerebral ischemia to detect intracranial stenosis and occlusions. It may also be used to detect vasospasms in patients with neurological deterioration from a subarachnoid hemorrhage.

Transthoracic and Transesophageal Echocardiography. Transthoracic echocardiography (TTE) and transesophageal echocardiography (TEE) use may be indicated based on the high percentage of strokes that are of cardioembolic origin. TTE is a routine test used to view the heart for the presence of clots, valvular abnormalities, and left ventricular function. TEE is a highly sensitive test for detecting cardiac and aortic lesions that may cause ischemic strokes.

Collaborative Management

In recent years, brain attack has changed from being called a cerebrovascular accident to an infarct of specific causality. By understanding the underlying mechanism, appropriate measures can be instituted to improve acute care and foster positive long-term outcomes. The immediate goals of collaborative management for the patient with a CVA include minimizing brain injury and preventing medical complications.

Emergent Care

Treatment is ideally administered in an ICU where the multidisciplinary team is able to foresee and respond rapidly to complications related to airway patency and breathing pattern, cardiovascular status (cardiac rhythm and rate, blood pressure), and serious neurological deficits.

Airway and Breathing Management

The goal of airway management is to prevent hypoxia, hypoventilation, and worsening cerebral injury. Impaired consciousness may result in partial airway obstruction or aspiration of saliva and other secretions. Positioning the patient on his side may help to open the airway. However, intubation may be required in some patients to reestablish adequate ventilation. Patients who require intubation are usually sicker, and 50% die in the first 30 days following the stroke. The nurse should monitor all CVA patients' oxygen saturations. High-flow oxygen (O_2) therapy is indicated when arterial blood gas (ABG) or O_2 saturation less than 92% suggests hypoxia. Hypoventilation may cause an elevation in carbon dioxide, which could lead to cerebral vasodilation and further increase ICP.

Cardiac Monitoring

Ongoing cardiac monitoring is imperative for detecting signs of related acute cardiac ischemia. The ECG can detect chronic arrhythmias such as AF that may have precipitated an embolic event. The stroke itself can cause arrhythmias when the sympathetic response results in demand-induced myocardial ischemia. Lastly, there may be centrally mediated changes in the ECG when large strokes occur, particularly with a subarachnoid hemorrhage.

Blood Pressure Management

Acute management of blood pressure (BP) will vary depending on the type of brain attack. A neuroimaging study with CT or MRI is vital to help determine how to manage the BP of stroke patients.

Ischemic Brain Attack. Hypertension occurs frequently with acute ischemic stroke and needs to be closely monitored. In patients experiencing an ischemic stroke, the perfusion pressure distal to the occluded vessel is reduced and the cerebral vessels are dilated. The mean arterial pressure (MAP) is commonly elevated in patients with an acute stroke due to an immediate sympathetic response or chronic hypertension. The elevated BP may be necessary to maintain brain perfusion, and rapid lowering it could cause neurological deterioration.

The ASA (Adams et al., 2007) states that management of arterial hypertension is controversial. Many patients have a spontaneous decline in BP within the first 24 hours so antihypertensive agents may be restricted to use only when the systolic blood pressure (SBP) is greater than 220 mm Hg or the diastolic blood pressure (DBP) is greater than 120 mm Hg. When the BP remains elevated, the nurse should first investigate if there are other factors such as pain or discomfort from bladder distention that are contributing to the patient's hypertension. When treatment is determined to be necessary,

cautious lowering of the BP by about 15% during the first 24 hours after the onset of brain attack is recommended with continual reassessment of neurological function.

Special recommendations apply to BP control in patients with ischemic stroke who are eligible for thrombolytic therapy (Adams et al., 2007). Before lytic therapy is started, it is suggested that SBP be less than or equal to 185 mm Hg and DBP be less than or equal to 110 mm Hg. To accomplish this, the nurse might administer labetolol (Normodyne) 10 to 20 mg IV over 1 to 2 minutes. The dose may be repeated once. The goal is to maintain the BP below 180/105 for a minimum of 24 hours after intravenous tPA treatment. If the blood pressure does not drop to an appropriate level, the patient is no longer a candidate for thrombolytic therapy.

Hemorrhagic Brain Attack. An elevation in BP may increase the bleeding in patients with a hemorrhagic stroke. The benefits and risks of BP management are examined to determine the appropriate treatment. Decreasing the BP in patients with ICH or SAH may produce benefits by preventing further bleeding and additional vascular damage. When ICP monitoring is in place, the BP may be reduced to lower levels because the cerebral perfusion pressure may be calculated (see Chapter 9). ∞ In patients with ICH and normal cerebral perfusion, the BP can be lowered by at least 15% without causing ischemia to the tissue surrounding the affected area.

There is not sufficient evidence to support a specific therapy for hypertension in the patient with a SAH. An elevated BP can aggravate a SAH because the direct force across the plugged bleeding area is related to the pressure difference between the CSF and the systemic blood pressure. In contrast, the risk of rebleeding from an aneurysm may be reduced by lowering the BP; however, ischemia may result due to inadequate cerebral perfusion. The recommendation of BP control for ICH is to maintain the SBP between 140 and 160 mm Hg and to carefully monitor the patient for signs of cerebral hypoperfusion, which is caused by a fall in BP. A SBP of greater than 170 mm Hg should be treated with intravenous medications such as labetalol (Normodyne), nicardipine (Cardene), or nitroprusside (Nitropress).

Determining Diagnosis

Time is crucial in the evaluation of the stroke mechanism because it will determine therapy choices. In most cases, a patient history, physical examination with NIH stroke scale, and noncontrast CT scan are adequate. Differential diagnosis is necessary to rule out conditions that mimic CVA, such as drug overdose, migraine, head trauma, brain tumor, systemic infection, hypoglycemia, hyponatremia and TTP. A thorough history will determine if the patient is on anticoagulant therapy, a common cause of intracerebral hemorrhage.

Acute Care After Diagnosis Is Determined

The goal of acute stroke management is rapid and efficient care. After assessment of the patient's airway, breathing, and circulation (ABCs) and a stroke evaluation, it should be determined if the patient is suffering an ischemic stroke and is a candidate for thrombolytic therapy. If the patient is eligible, therapy should be administered within 1 hour from the patient's presentation to the emergency department (ED). The National Institute for Neurological Disorders and Stroke (NINDS) has recommended the following time benchmarks for the potential thrombolysis candidate:

Door to doctor	10 minutes
Access to neurological expertise	15 minutes
Door to CT scan completion	25 minutes
Door to CT scan interpretation	45 minutes
Door to treatment	60 minutes
Admission to monitored bed	3 hours

Ischemic Brain Attack

In the United States, the vast majority of strokes, more than 80%, are ischemic. Revascularization (reestablishment of blood flow through the artery) is the most critical aspect of treatment for a patient with an ischemic stroke.

Collaborative Management

When patients arrive for medical assistance within the first hours following the onset of symptoms, it may be possible to utilize a thrombolytic to reestablish blood flow through the involved cerebral artery. *Thrombolysis*, the administration of recombinant tissue-type plasminogen activator (rt-PA or alteplase), ideally dissolves the clot in the cerebral artery, restores blood flow, and improves neurological functioning. Alteplase should be given as soon as possible after the onset of symptoms but usually within 3 hours. Administration after 3 hours is more likely to result in cerebral hemorrhage. However, a patient might be considered for either intravenous or intra-arterial thrombolysis up to 6 hours after the development of symptoms if imaging tests show a substantial "at-risk" brain that is underperfused but not yet infarcted and there is an occlusive thromboembolus. Patients who are candidates for thrombolysis have:

- Had an ischemic stroke with a measurable defect
- A blood pressure in the acceptable range (less than 185/110)
- A defect that is not minor, isolated, or clearing spontaneously
- Had onset of the defect within the previous 3 hours

COMMONLY USED MEDICATIONS

THROMBOLYTIC THERAPY rt-PA (TISSUE PLASMINOGEN ACTIVATOR, RECOMBINANT) ALTEPLASE, ACTIVASE

Desired Effect: rt-PA is an enzyme that is used to restore blood flow, minimize the ischemic penumbra, and limit infarction volume. It binds to the fibrin in a thrombus and converts the trapped plasminogen to plasmin, which triggers local fibrolysis and clears the blocked artery, restoring circulation. The usual dose of rt-PA is 0.9 mg/kg (maximum dose 90 mg) administered over 60 minutes with the first 10% given over 1 minute. Onset of action is prompt with patency of the vessel usually occurring within 1 to 2 hours.

Nursing Responsibilities:

- The nurse reviews the criteria and determines that the patient is a candidate for thrombolysis.

- Patients may not be able to consent to thrombolytic therapy due to their neurological impairment. This should not prevent them from receiving the therapy, and both patients and their families need to be advised of the possible risks and benefits.

- It is best to establish a separate IV for administration.

- The patient receiving rt-PA should be admitted to ICU. Focused neurological assessments and measurements of BP are required:
  - Every 15 minutes during administration of the medication
  - Every 30 minutes for the first 6 hours following administration
  - Every hour for the first 24 hours

- The infusion should be discontinued if the patient develops severe headache, hypertension, or nausea and vomiting because these may indicate intracranial bleeding.

- The nurse should delay placing an nasogastric (NG) tube, Foley, or arterial line during administration of the thrombolytic.

- A follow-up CT scan is indicated 24 hours after administration.

Potential Side and/or Toxic Effects: Bleeding is the most common side effect. It may be internal such as GI or GU or may be external such as at intravenous (IV) sites or from the gums and nose. Approximately 6% of patients receiving thrombolytic therapy develop intracranial hemorrhage usually during the first 36 hours.

- Not had head trauma, an MI, or a CVA within the previous 3 months
- Not had a urinary or GI bleed within the previous 3 weeks
- Not had major surgery in the past 2 weeks
- No bleeding abnormalities

Invasive and Surgical Management

Blood flow to ischemic cerebral tissue may also be reestablished by interventional radiology, a specialty that uses an endovascular approach and views the blood vessels that supply the nervous system from inside the vessel. Two endovascular approaches to help restore normal blood flow are thrombolysis and embolectomy. In an arterial thrombolysis, alteplase may be administered directly to the site of the clot for up to 6 hours after onset of symptoms. *Embolectomy* restores blood flow in stroke patients by removing the clot. A catheter is guided up through the femoral artery to the site of the clot and then a special wire with loops in it is deployed. The wire threads through the embolus and grasps onto it so that it can be removed. The procedure can be performed within 8 hours of symptom onset but is considered experimental.

Other surgical options for preventing and treating an ischemic stroke include carotid endarterectomy, angioplasty, and carotid stenting. Carotid endarterectomy is a procedure that cleans out and opens up the narrowed artery. The surgeon scrapes away the plaque from the wall of the artery, allowing for increased blood flow to the brain. Angioplasty is a procedure performed in a cardiac catheterization lab or radiology suite. Using fluoroscopy and a contrast agent, the physician obtains angiograms of the lesion to determine the baseline cerebral circulation. A puncture in the femoral artery is made and a catheter with a tiny balloon at the end is advanced through the artery to the blockage, then inflated to open the artery. Once the vessel is dilated, a stent may be placed inside the artery to hold it open and to maintain increased blood flow. Currently, stents can be used for asymptomatic patients with more than 80% carotid stenosis and symptomatic patients with more than 50% carotid stenosis (Strimike, 2007).

After the approximately 1 hour procedure, the nurse needs to carefully monitor the patient's BP, because unstable BP is a common occurrence. The patient is usually monitored because bradycardia develops frequently. At regular intervals beginning with every 15 minutes, the nurse assesses the patient's neurological status (see earlier), hemodynamic status, arterial puncture site for hematoma or bleeding, and peripheral pulses below the puncture site.

Hemorrhagic Brain Attack

In the United States, about 20% of all strokes are hemorrhagic. There are two primary types of hemorrhagic strokes: ICH and SAH.

Intracerebral Hemorrhages

Of the hemorrhagic strokes, up to 15% may be ICH. The mortality for ICH can exceed 50% with many of the patients dying in the first 2 days. The ASA (2007) recommends that patients with ICH be cared for in ICUs because patients experience frequent increases in ICP and usually have additional medical issues. Hydrocephalus is also a common complication of ICH. A ventriculostomy may need to be performed and an external ventricular drain inserted to drain CSF. Management of the ventilated patient with increased ICP and an external ventricular drain is discussed in Chapter 9. ∞

Therapy targeted to management of the intracerebral hematoma is limited. If the patient has been receiving an anticoagulant, the appropriate drug to reverse its effects might be administered. Protamine sulfate is used to reverse heparin-associated ICH with the dose dependent on the time since the cessation of heparin, whereas intravenous vitamin K is used to reverse the effects of warfarin. A craniotomy for hematoma removal might be performed, especially if the bleeding occurred near the surface of the brain. On the horizon are a variety of novel therapies, including injecting a thrombolytic inside the hematoma to facilitate endoscopic removal of the blood, new surgical approaches to removal of the hematoma, and using recombinant factor VIIa to reduce hematoma size.

Subarachnoid Hemorrhages

The most common cause of bleeding in the subarachnoid space is rupture of an aneurysm or an AVM. Aneurysms commonly arise at the bifurcations of major arteries. Most saccular aneurysms arise on the circle of Willis or the MCA bifurcation. Nearly 90% of intracranial aneurysms arise on the anterior (carotid) circulation. Common locations include the anterior communicating artery, the internal carotid artery at the posterior communicating artery origin, and the MCA bifurcation (Brisman et al., 2007).

Cerebral aneurysms occur in about 4% of the population. However, in most instances, the presence of an aneurysm is not known until the aneurysm ruptures and the patient presents with a SAH. The focused assessment of the patient with a ruptured cerebral aneurysm includes a careful neurological assessment with grading of severity by the Hunt and Hess scale. The scale uses clinical findings to measure the severity of the hemorrhage on admission and has been shown to correlate with patient outcome. The grades of the Hunt and Hess scale are:

- Grade 0—Unruptured aneurysm
- Grade 1—Asymptomatic or minimal headache and slight nuchal rigidity
- Grade 1A—No acute meningeal or brain reaction but with fixed neurological deficit
- Grade 2—Moderate-to-severe headache, nuchal rigidity, no neurological deficit other than cranial nerve palsy
- Grade 3—Drowsiness, confusion, or mild focal deficit
- Grade 4—Stupor, moderate-to-severe hemiparesis, possible early decerebrate rigidity, and vegetative disturbances
- Grade 5—Deep coma, decerebrate rigidity, and moribund appearance

Signs and symptoms of aneurysms other than those associated with SAH are relatively uncommon. However, a posterior communicating aneurysm may result in a third nerve palsy, and giant aneurysms may result in focal symptoms because of their mass effect.

Diagnostic Studies

Possible diagnostic studies include a noncontrast CT scan, an MRA, angiography, and TCD. These tests are described earlier in the chapter.

Mortality and morbidity are high following rupture of a cerebral aneurysm. Ten percent of patients with SAH die before reaching medical attention, whereas another

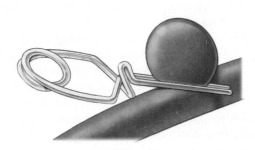

Figure 10-4 Aneurysm with clip.

50% die within the first month. Fifty percent of survivors have neurological deficits. Ruptured aneurysms are most likely to rebleed within the first day and the risk remains very high for 2 weeks if the aneurysm is not repaired. Therefore, ruptured aneurysms (less than grade 5) are usually repaired within 72 hours of hemorrhage to prevent rebleeding.

In the past, most patients were treated with craniotomy and surgical clipping of the aneurysm. In this procedure, after the patient is anesthetized, the skull is opened and the aneurysm is located. The neurosurgeon isolates the affected blood vessel and places a small, metal clip on the neck of the aneurysm, restricting its blood supply. The clip remains in place, preventing future bleeding (Figure 10-4).

Endovascular embolization is an alternative to surgery. Once the patient has been anesthetized, the doctor inserts a catheter into an artery (usually the femoral) and threads it to the site of the aneurysm. Using a guide wire, detachable coils of platinum wire are passed through the catheter and released into the aneurysm. The process is continued until angiography demonstrates that the coils have obliterated the aneurysm (Figure 10-5). The most common coils used in endovascular procedures are platinum Guglielmi detachable coils. The purpose of the coils is to induce thrombosis in the aneurysm via electrothrombosis. Electrothrombosis occurs because white and red blood cells, platelets, and fibrinogen are nega-

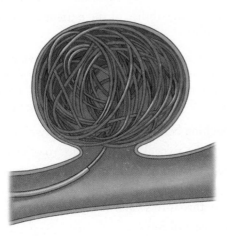

Figure 10-5 Aneurysm with Guglielmi coils.

tively charged. When the positively charged platinum coils are inserted in the aneurysm, they attract the negatively charged blood components and a clot is formed. Studies comparing the two techniques have found coiling to be safer but slightly less durable than clipping. However, if necessary, coiling may be performed more than once during a patient's lifetime.

Nursing Management

Nursing care after obliteration of a ruptured aneurysm is focused on accurate neurological assessments and prevention of complications. Following treatment, the patient remains at high risk for two of the major complications of aneurysm rupture: **vasospasm** and **hydrocephalus**.

Vasospasm

Now that early intervention limits the amount of rebleeding, vasospasm is the leading cause of disability and death following rupture of a cerebral aneurysm (Brisman et al., 2007). Vasospasm is defined as an angiographic narrowing of cerebral blood vessel(s) that can lead to delayed ischemia. It develops in between 17% and 40% of patients with a ruptured aneurysm. The Fisher grade, which describes the amount of blood seen on a noncontrast head CT, is useful for identifying the likelihood the patient will develop vasospasm. Fisher grades are:

1) No blood detected
2) Diffuse or vertical layers less than 1 mm thick
3) Localized clot or vertical layer greater than or equal to 1 mm
4) Intracerebral or intraventricular clot with diffuse or no SAH

Vasospasm is most likely to occur in patients with a Fisher grade 3 and a high grade on the Hunt and Hess scale. Most patients who have survived rupture of a cerebral aneurysm receive a calcium channel blocker (usually nimodipine [Nimotop] for 21 days). Initially nimodipine was administered because it was thought to prevent vasospasm. Although this mode of action has not been confirmed, nimodipine has been shown to have a neuroprotective effect after subarachnoid hemorrhage and is still administered routinely to patients.

The nurse assesses for the presence of vasospasm when doing routine neurological signs. A deterioration in mental status, such as restlessness or lethargy, and the development of focal neurological deficits, most likely hemiparesis or dysphasia, suggest the patient might be developing vasospasm. Symptoms may wax and wane, changing from minute to minute. They tend to become more apparent when the patient's BP drops and less obvious when the BP increases. TCD and CA studies might be utilized to confirm the diagnosis.

Aggressively Managed Vasospasm.
Vasospasm must be aggressively managed once it is detected to prevent permanent disability and death. Current management is hypertension, hypervolemia, and hemodilution (HHH) therapy (Kosty, 2005). The theory behind the treatment is that the only way to increase blood flow to cerebral tissue during vasospasm is to increase the BP. The simplest way to achieve all three aims of therapy simultaneously is through volume expansion. Precise parameters for volume expansion have not been defined so treatment varies between institutions. Most authorities recommend placement of a pulmonary artery (PA) line to guide fluid administration but target values for PA pressures and the fluid used to achieve volume expansion vary (Kosty, 2005). Hemodilution usually results from the hypervolemia. If the patient does not achieve a BP of 10 to 60 mm Hg above baseline or 150 to 200 mm Hg systolic (depending on institutional policy) by volume expansion alone, then hypertension might be attained by the use of a vasoactive drug such as dopamine (Intropin) or phenylephrine (Neo-Synephrine). When HHH therapy fails, transluminal balloon angioplasty is the method of choice, but intra-arterial papaverine may be used for vasospasm in the distal vasculature, where balloons may not be able to access.

Hydrocephalus. The third common major neurological complication following rupture of a cerebral aneurysm is hydrocephalus. It develops when blood in the subarachnoid space obliterates the arachnoidal villi, preventing absorption of CSF, or blood within the ventricles blocks the foramen of Monroe, preventing drainage of CSF. If hydrocephalus leads to an increase in ICP and deterioration of the patient's neurological status, an external ventricular drain might be emergently placed for CSF diversion (see Chapter 9). ∞ The nurse anticipates that the patient's neurological examination will improve dramatically after the drain has been placed and hydrocephalus has been treated. In about 20% of patients, the hydrocephalus is persistent and the patient requires a ventriculoperitoneal shunt.

Nursing Care

Ongoing neurological assessments and seizure precautions are necessary components of nursing care of the stroke patient (Frizzell, 2005). During the first few days, the nurse carefully assesses the patient's neurological status because cerebral edema usually peaks within 3 to 5 days post stroke. Cerebral edema sufficient to cause significant increases in ICP occurs in approximately 15% of stroke patients. IICP in the stroke patient is managed by the interventions described in Chapter 9. ∞ Initially, simple measures such as elevating the head of the patient's bed and providing sedation or analgesia are attempted. If more aggressive therapies such as osmotic diuretics or CSF drainage are required, the patient usually requires ICP monitoring.

Small-vessel hemorrhage or hemorrhagic transformation is a grave concern for patients with an embolic stroke. Patients who develop hemorrhagic transformation, like patients with progressive cerebral edema, will demonstrate acute clinical decline. Therefore, patients need to be thoroughly monitored for a decline in neurological status during the first week post stroke to identify and treat hemorrhagic conversion and diminish its neurological effects. The nurse also needs to be vigilant in identifying seizures. Partial seizures occur in 5% to 7% of ischemic stroke patients and 28% of patients following ICH and require treatment as described in Chapter 9. ∞

Once the patient is stable, admission to a stroke unit is effective in reducing complications, stroke reoccurrence, and disability. Management of patient care may be established through standing orders and a critical path care plan (Kavanagh, Connolly, & Cohen, 2006). Standardized admission orders prompt the physician to consider all facets of care and acts as a guide to determine the appropriate treatment plan. Patient care plans and critical paths should include neurological assessments, monitoring vital signs and lab values, medications, nutrients and fluids, and positioning. Additional important components of nursing care include screening for dysphagia, providing adequate nutrition, promoting patient comfort, preventing hyperthermia, and providing support to the patient and family.

Screening for Dysphagia

Dysphagia, difficulty swallowing, is very common post stroke and is a major risk factor for developing aspiration pneumonia. Dysphagia can occur when there is damage to the brain and results in muscle weakness of the mouth and throat. When dysphagia is present, there is an increased risk of aspirating saliva or food, which may result in pneumonia. To determine if a patient has a swallowing deficit, the nurse might use the following swallow screening criteria. Prior to swallow screening, the nurse should:

- Evaluate lung sounds and obtain the patient's most recent vital signs including temperature.
- Evaluate the ability of the patient to follow directions.

If the patient demonstrates any of the following problems at any time during the assessment, the nurse should cease the evaluation, keep the patient NPO, and ask the MD for a speech therapy order for a swallowing evaluation:

- Coughing before, during, or after swallowing
- Gurgly/wet vocal quality or any voice changes
- Need to swallow two or more times to clear
- Excessive length of time to move food to the back of the throat to swallow
- Pocketing of food
- Excessive secretions

VISUAL MAP Stroke

Stroke

Alert EMS

Does patient have 1) a facial droop 2) a drift 3) slurred speech

If Yes to ED as soon as possible

In first 45 minutes ED
nurse acts to:
• Protect airway
• Monitor cardiac rhythm
• Control BP
• Assess NIHSS
• Obtain lab tests
• Obtain CT scan

Scan indicates hemorrhagic stroke (20%)

Scan indicates ischemic stroke (80%)

ICH

SAH

< 3 hours since
symptom onset

> 3 hours since
symptom onset

Possibly reverse
anticoagulation

Clipping or
coiling in 72 hours

rt-PA if patient
meets criteria

Assessment for
vasospasm and
hydrocephalos

Supportive nursing care

The nurse should consider each of the following when doing a swallow screening:

1) Does the patient have facial weakness or a droop?

2) Does the patient have difficulty with arousal?

3) Does the patient have an absent gag reflex?

4) Given one bite of applesauce, does the patient cough or clear her throat?

5) Given one sip of water, does the patient cough or clear her throat?

6) Given consecutive sips of water, does the patient cough or clear her throat?

7) Given a graham cracker or saltine, does the patient have difficulty chewing, oral residue after swallowing, or cough and clear her throat?

8) Does the patient need to swallow more than one time per bite/sip?

9) Does the patient need more time to chew and/or initiate swallow?

If the answer is yes to any of the questions, the nurse should keep the patient NPO, alert the physician, and obtain an order for a swallowing evaluation by speech therapy.

Swallowing evaluations may include videofluoroscopy or barium swallow. *Videofluoroscopy* allows for accurate visualization of the sequence of events that comprise a swallow. Test analysis identifies abnormal movement of fluid/food such as pooling or aspiration. It may also detect any abnormal movement of anatomic structures and inability of muscle activities. It is essential to test the effects of various consistencies of food and positions to determine the patient's swallowing potential and ensure safety when feeding. A barium swallow may identify the presence of an aspiration and more subtle anatomic abnormalities. This test is especially useful if more than one abnormality is discovered.

Provision of Adequate Nutrition

Undernourished CVA survivors have a higher mortality rate 6 months post stroke than survivors who are well nourished. Undernourished survivors are also more likely to develop complications such as pneumonia, other infections, and GI bleeding during their hospital stay. During recovery, when anabolism exceeds catabolism, the goal is to replenish nutritional deficits by maintaining a positive nitrogen balance and replacing protein stores. A thorough nutritional assessment should include the patient's past and present weight, eating habits, blood testing, and a physical exam of the eyes, hair, skin, mouth, and muscles. An accurate intake and output (I & O) and calorie count should be monitored to determine if the patient's needs are being met. The American Heart Association (AHA)/ASA currently recommend that patients with acute stroke who cannot take fluids and food orally should receive hydration and nutrition via an NG tube or percutaneous endoscopic gastrostomy (PEG) tube while waiting for swallowing to resume (Adams et al., 2007). They believe that patients should be provided sufficient calories to meet their nutritional needs but should not require additional supplementation.

Monitoring Lab Values for Alterations in Blood Glucose

Alterations in blood glucose are common during the acute phase of stroke and are associated with adverse outcomes. All patients should be monitored for hyperglycemia and hypoglycemia with the goal of less than 145/dL.

Hyperglycemia, defined as a serum glucose level greater than 126 mg/dL, is common in patients with acute ischemic stroke. Hyperglycemia may intensify brain injury by increasing tissue acidosis and increasing blood-brain barrier permeability. The AHA/ASA guidelines recommend treatment with insulin for patients who have blood glucose levels greater than 140 to 185 mg/dL (Adams et al., 2007).

Hypoglycemia, defined as a serum glucose level less than 70 mg/dL, can cause focal neurological deficits that mimic stroke. It is essential to manage low blood glucose levels as they alone can cause neuronal damage. It may be necessary to administer glucose with stroke patients who take oral hypoglycemic agents or insulin.

Monitoring for Hyperthermia

Fever may promote further brain injury in patients with an acute stroke. One study showed that body temperature was independently related to the severity and size of the infarct of the initial stroke, and that for each 1°C increase in body temperature the relative risk of a poor outcome increased by 2.2. Treatment includes finding the source of fever and immediately treating with antipyretic agents. Patients who have sustained a stroke are often provided acetaminophen as soon as their temperature reaches 38°C (100.4°F).

Promotion of Patient Comfort

Areas that may need to be addressed are pain, incontinence, and constipation. When assessing pain, an appropriate scale should be used to determine the patient's level of pain. The Face Legs Activity Cry and Consolability (FLACC) Pain Scale is a behavioral scale that may be appropriate for patients who are cognitively impaired or have aphasia. Interventions to relieve pain may include positioning, complementary therapies, and medication.

Bladder distention may cause sufficient discomfort in a stroke patient to result in hypertension. Urinary catheterization might be initiated if monitoring output is necessary or if the patient is retaining urine and is uncomfortable. If possible, bladder programs should be used to control incontinence. During a bladder training program or when a catheter is discontinued, a bladder scan may be used to monitor post-void residual (PVR). If the PVR is greater than 400 cc, a straight catheterization is usually recommended. When the PVR is less than 100 cc for three consecutive times, then the bladder scan protocol may be discontinued. Frequent toileting will also help prevent incontinence and assist with increasing bladder tone.

Constipation and fecal impaction can be significant sources of discomfort for the patient post stroke. A GI assessment including history of bowel habits prior to the stroke should be obtained. Aside from monitoring bowel movements, interventions may include stool softeners, fiber, increased fluids, and frequent toileting.

Promoting Effective Communication

Communication with critically ill patients is described in Chapter 2. ∞ Communication can be a particularly frustrating experience for the stroke patient. The patient may be experiencing expressive aphasia and realize that she is unable to retrieve the words that she needs. Some ways that the nurse can enhance communication with a patient who has aphasia include:

Facing the patient when speaking so the patient can see the nurse's face

Speaking slowly and clearly rather than loudly

Using simple language and only making one statement at a time

Engaging the patient in conversation

Listening carefully and patiently

Complimenting the patient on any noticeable progress

Some nurse specialists recommend that patients sing their thoughts because they may be able to express themselves more fluently in song. Gradually, they move from singing to speaking in a sing-song voice to more fluent normal speech. If a patient does not wish to sing, the nurse needs to be patient, listening to the patient and allowing her to express herself but not allowing her to become overly frustrated when her speech is not fluent. Although the patient may not want to speak, she needs to be encouraged to attempt speech because it is only through practice that fluency will begin to return.

Providing Support for the Patient and Family

Ways that critical care nurses can provide support to the families of critically ill patients is discussed in Chapter 2. ∞ In particular, the nurse may need to advocate for the brain attack patient and her family by providing resources and by arranging for appropriate referrals. Resources may include educational materials (written, on-line sites, videos) and support groups for the survivor and caregivers. It is especially important when dealing with CVA patients that the nurse begins discharge planning on the day of admission. Determining patients' probable home care needs early will enhance the likelihood of their successful return to home.

Prevention and Management of Complications

Approximately half of the deaths after stroke are due to complications. The prevention of medical complications of stroke is an essential goal of the nursing management of the stroke patient. Common acute and subacute complications that may occur are MI, stroke reoccurrence, blood clots, aspiration pneumonia, gastrointestinal (GI) bleeding, urinary tract infection (UTI), alterations in serum glucose, hyperthermia, dehydration, malnutrition, falls, contractures, pressure sores, and constipation. In a study by Langhorne et al. (2000), the percentage of patients who developed the following complications during the first 30 months following a stroke were:

Falls	25%
Urinary tract infections	24%
Chest infection	22%
Pressure sores	21%
Depression	16%
Shoulder pain	9%
Deep vein thrombosis	2%
Pulmonary embolism	1%

In order to prevent complications in the stroke patient, the nurse should do the following.

Promote Safety

Falls have been documented as the most common complication of acute stroke. Hospitalized patients on bed rest may develop diminished bone density, which increases their risk of fractures. Stroke survivors may be at risk for falls due to paralysis, muscle weakness, and lack of coordination. They may also have poor judgment and be impulsive due to cognitive impairments. A fall risk assessment should be performed (see Safety Initiative) to determine the patient's level of risk. Physical therapy and occupational therapy consults will determine the individual's needs and physical abilities related to activities of daily living.

Monitor for Urinary Tract Infection

UTI is a common complication and occurs in about 11% of patients during the first 3 months post stroke. Following a stroke, patients have difficulty emptying their bladder and a catheter may need to be inserted. Indwelling catheters increase the risk of infection; therefore, they should only be used when necessary and if used discontinued as soon as possible. Nurses should monitor and report any signs or symptoms of infection.

Monitor Cardiac Status

Research has shown that angina, MI, and cardiac ischemia complicate 6% of acute strokes, and 1% of patients develop life-threatening medical events. Furthermore, the majority of the MIs in stroke survivors are asymptomatic,

SAFETY INITIATIVES | Prevention of Falls

PURPOSE: To update the issues, strategies, and tools to prevent falls among patients in acute care settings

RATIONALE: Fall-related injuries account for 6% of medical expenditures for people in the United States over the age of 65. Falls occur in all types of health care institutions, in all patient populations, and are the most common reason for completion of an incident report on a hospitalized patient. Consequences for the patient may include, at a minimum, fractures, soft tissue or head injury, anxiety, and depression. The morbidity, mortality, and financial burdens from patient falls make it one of the most serious risk management issues for health care institutions. Because most of the currently available data on fall prevention are from long-term care settings, recognition, evaluation, and prevention of falls in the hospital setting can present significant challenges for the acute care nurse.

HIGHLIGHTS OF RECOMMENDATIONS:
- Measure and track falls using a "fall rate" (The fall rate is the number of patient falls multiplied by 1,000 and divided by the number of patient days.) or other rate used to track falls such as the number of patients at risk, the number of patients who fell, and the number of falls/bed.
- Trends and rates in falls should take into account the fall risk of the patient population.

- Identify and classify the causes of falls (accidental, such as when a patient falls because of environmental factors; unanticipated physiological falls, such as when a patient has an unanticipated seizure and falls; or anticipated physiological falls, such as when a patient with a prior fall, weak gait, or has been identified as at risk for falling falls).
- Institute general safety interventions such as:
  - Instructing the patient to request assistance
  - Providing appropriate footwear, environmental surfaces, and lighting
  - Considering peak effects of medication that might affect the patient's level of consciousness, gait, or elimination when planning nursing care
- Conduct a risk assessment on admission and when the patient's status changes, using a validated tool such as the Morse Fall Scale.
- Provide risk fall assessments of the patient to all the patient's health care providers.
- Develop an individualized plan for falls prevention for each patient who requires one.
- Provide sitters as necessary for one-one observation of the patient under the direction of a registered nurse (RN).

Source: Premier Inc: Falls Prevention

 Available: http://www.premierinc.com/safety/topics/falls/

---

emphasizing the need for monitoring labs and ECGs with stroke patients. As noted earlier, a definitive diagnosis of MI contraindicates the use of thrombolysis in acute stroke. Ongoing cardiac monitoring by the nurse and evaluation of lab work is necessary to evaluate cardiac status.

Monitor for Altered Tissue Perfusion

Approximately 5% of hospitalized stroke survivors will develop a deep vein thrombosis (DVT) and about 2% will be diagnosed with a pulmonary embolus (PE). A DVT is a blood clot that develops in the deep veins of the legs. When the clot breaks off and travels to the lung, it is called a PE. Blood clots occur most often between the second and seventh day post stroke. A poststroke patient has an increased risk of developing a blood clot due to decreased mobility or paralysis. The major causes of DVT are venous stasis, hypercoagulability, and vessel injury. Anticoagulative therapy is the most common treatment for DVT; however, due to the risk of bleeding, hemorrhagic stroke survivors should be treated initially with compression boots or stockings. Aspirin is recom-

mended early in poststroke course to prevent a recurrent ischemic stroke. Dosages ranging from 160 mg to 325 mg daily may be started 24 to 48 hours post stroke but only in patients with no allergic or bleeding complications. Early range of motion and ambulation should be established as soon as the patient is stable to decrease the risk of DVT.

Monitor for Gastrointestinal Bleeding

Poststroke patients, particularly those who require a ventilator, have an increased risk of developing an upper GI bleed. To decrease the risk of bleeding, medication can be administered to lower the production of gastric acid (e.g., ranitidine hydrochloride).

Recovery

Recovery time and plans of care are specific to each individual. One study of stroke survivors found that "while most subjects experienced a dramatic increase in function in the first three months following stroke, many also suffered a subsequent decline. The slopes of these declines were highly variable, and correlated to new onset depression. Age was not found to be associated with functional decline, as opposed to common belief. Subjects who were younger, had social support, or had higher functional status or neurological status scores at three months were more likely to achieve full functional recovery" (Shaughnessy, n.d.).

CEREBRAL OR CEREBROVASCULAR DISORDER SUMMARY

Patients with cerebral dysfunction are very dependent on the ability of the nurse. Nurses caring for patients with cerebral or cerebrovascular disorders must be able to identify subtle changes in neurological function (such as those indicative of cerebral vasospasm) with sufficient certainty to notify the appropriate colleague and begin intervention.

Nurses must also be skilled in identifying those functions (such as swallowing) that patients are no longer able to perform and arranging for further assessment and appropriate management. In addition, the nurse must intervene to assist in the restoration of neurological functioning and prevent the development of complications.

CASE STUDY

Mr. Williams is a 75-year-old man admitted to the emergency department (ED), after his wife noted that his left leg and arm were weak and his speech was slurred. His wife also noticed that the left side of his face was "flat." She called 911 and he was transported via ambulance. The paramedics reported that his initial vital signs were: BP 180/100, pulse 60, and respirations 16. On admission, his temperature was 100°F (37.8°C) and Glasgow Coma Scale score was 9. He was able to speak and denied headache, chest pain, or shortness of breath. The admission assessment revealed a history of hypertension, carotid stenosis, and TIAs.

1. Prioritize a list of immediate nursing strategies.

2. What other information needs to be obtained as part of the admission assessment?

3. What are the likely risk factors contributing to his admission?

4. What diagnostic tests should be ordered?

   Mr. Williams's tests results show a thrombotic stroke affecting the right side of his brain.

5. What are some possible treatment options?

6. Identify some poststroke complications and teaching needs.

See answers to Case Studies in the Answer Section at the back of the book.

CRITICAL THINKING QUESTIONS

1. What are the most common generalized symptoms of a brain tumor? What is a focal symptom?

2. How does dexamethasone decrease cerebral edema for the patient with a brain tumor? What are the nursing implications associated with dexamethasone administration?

3. What are the nursing responsibilities in the post-op care of the patient with a pituitary tumor?

4. How should the nurse prevent a DVT in the patient who has a cerebrovascular disease?

5. What is the difference between a hemorrhagic and an ischemic stroke?

6. What are the four common stroke syndromes?

7. How would a nurse identify if a patient was developing vasospasm following a subarachnoid hemorrhage?

8. Why is screening for dysphagia essential in a stroke survivor? What are the steps in dysphagia screening?

See answers to Critical Thinking Questions in the Answer Section at the back of the book.

EXPLORE MEDIALINK
http://www.prenhall.com/perrin

Additional interactive resources for this chapter can be found on the Web site at
http://www.prenhall.com/perrin. Click on "Chapter 10" to select activities for this chapter.

Case Study: Stroke

Nursing Care Plan

NCLEX Review Questions

MediaLinks:
- American Brain Tumor Association
- American Stroke Association
- Brain Tumor Clinical Trials
- Brain Trauma Foundation Guidelines
- Information on Clinical Trials: Cerebrovascular Disorders
- MGH Brain Tumor Center

- National Brain Tumor Foundation
- National Institute of Neurological Disorders and Stroke
- National Institute of Neurological Disorders Stroke Scale Booklet
- National Stroke Association
- The Brain Tumor Society
- The Precise Neurological Exam
- Stroke Assessment Scales—Cincinnati Scale Pictorial
- Stroke Assessment Scales—Overview of Scales

MediaLink Applications

REFERENCES

Adams, H. P., del Zoppo, G., Alberts, M. S., Bhall, D., Brass, L., Furlan, A., et al. (2007). ASA/AHA Guidelines for early management of adults with ischemic stroke. *Stroke, 38,* 1655–1711. Retrieved: March 5, 2008, from http:// strokeahajournals.org/egi/content/full/38/ 5/1655

Agulnik, M., & Mason, W. P. (2006). The changing management of low-grade astrocytomas and oligodendrogliomas. *Hematology/Oncology Clinics of North America, 20,* 1249–1266.

Alberts, M., Latchaw, R., Selman, W., Shepard, T., Hadley, M., Brass, L., et al. (2005). Recommendations for comprehensive stroke centers, a consensus statement from the brain attack coalition. *Stroke, 36,* 1597–1610.

Bachelor, T. T., & Byrne, T. N. (2006). Supportive care of brain tumor patients. *Hematology/Oncology Clinics of North America, 20,* 1337–1361.

Brisman, J., Soliman, E., Kader, A., & Perez, N. (2007). Cerebral aneurysm. *eMedicine.* Retrieved March 5, 2008, from http:/ /www.emedicine.com/Med/topic3468.htm

De Angelis, L. M. (2005). Chemotherapy for brain tumors—A new beginning. *New England Journal of Medicine, 352*(10), 1036–1038.

Frizzell, J. P. (2005). Acute stroke: Pathophysiology, diagnosis, and treatment. *AACN Clinical Issues, 16*(4), 421–440.

Gonzalez, J., & Gilbert, M. (2005). Treatment of astrocytomas. *Current Opinion in Neurology, 18*(6), 632–638.

Kavanagh, D., Connolly, P., & Cohen, J. (2006). Promoting evidence-based practice: Implementing the American Stroke Association's acute stroke program. *Journal of Nursing Care Quality, 21*(2), 135–142.

Kosty, T. (2005). Cerebral vasospasm after subarachnoid hemorrhage: An update. *Critical Care Nursing Quarterly, 28*(2), 122–134.

Langhorne, P., Stott, D. J., Robertson, L., McDonald, J., Jones, L., McAlpine, C., et al. (2000). Medical complications after stroke: A multicenter study. *Stroke, 31,* 1223.

Nahaczewski, A. E., Fowler, S. B., & Hariharan, S. (2004). Dexamethasone therapy in patients with brain tumors—A focus on tapering. *Journal of Neuroscience Nursing, 24*(6), 340–343.

Reichert, M. C. F., & Medeiros, E. A. S. (2002). Hospital-acquired meningitis in patients undergoing craniotomy:

Incidence, evolution, and risk factors. *American Journal of Infection Control, 30*(3), 158–163.

Roberts, G. (2004). A review of the efficacy and safety of opioid analgesics post-craniotomy. *Nursing in Critical Care, 9*(6), 277–283.

Roger, E. P., Butler, J., & Benzel, E. C. (2006). Neurosurgery in the elderly; brain tumors and subdural hematomas. *Clinics in Geriatric Medicine, 22,* 623–644.

Shaughnessy, M. (no date). *The trajectory of functional recovery over 12 months following stroke.* Virginia Henderson International Library, Registry of Nursing Research. Retrieved June 8, 2007, from http://www.nursinglibrary.org/Portal/main .aspx?pageid=4024&sid=22060

Strimike C. Carotid artery stents. *American Nurse Today,* 2007 (1), 12–14.

Vecht, C. J., & van Breemen, M. (2006). Optimizing therapy of seizures in patients with brain tumors. *Neurology, 67*(Suppl. 4), S10–13.

Wojner-Alexandrov, A., & Malkoff, M. (2006). The United States stroke system: Credentialing and legislative efforts to improve acute stroke care. *International Journal of Stroke, 1*(2), 109.

Care of the Critically Ill Patient Experiencing Alcohol Withdrawal and/or Liver Failure

June Kasper, MSN, RN, CGRN

Learning Outcomes

Upon completion of this chapter, the learner will be able to:

1. Explain the relationship between the pharmacological effects of alcohol and the cause of withdrawal symptoms.

2. Discuss the essential components of a focused assessment to detect alcohol dependency.

3. Describe the clinical manifestations of alcohol withdrawal syndrome.

4. Discuss the advantages of utilizing the Clinical Institute Withdrawal Assessment for Alcohol Scale.

5. Discuss collaborative and nursing management of a patient experiencing alcohol withdrawal syndrome.

6. Differentiate between acute liver failure and chronic liver failure.

7. Explain the clinical significance of acetaminophen toxicity.

8. Describe collaborative management of a patient with acetaminophen toxicity.

9. Explain the relationship between portal hypertension and the development of decompensated liver disease.

10. Describe the clinical manifestations of decompensated liver disease.

11. Describe the collaborative management and nursing responsibilities for the patient with decompensated liver disease.

Abbreviations

ALF	Acute Liver Failure
AWS	Alcohol Withdrawal Syndrome
CIWA-Ar	Clinical Institute Withdrawal Assessment for Alcohol Scale Revised
DSM-IV-TR	Diagnostic and Statistical Manual of Mental Disorders Text Revision
FHF	Fulminant Hepatic Failure
HRS	Hepatorenal Syndrome
NAC	N-Acetylcysteine
NIAAA	National Institute for Alcohol Abuse and Addiction
TIPS	Transjugular Intrahepatic Portosystemic Shunt

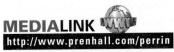

MEDIALINK

http://www.prenhall.com/perrin

See the Companion Website for chapter-specific resources at www.prenhall.com/perrin.

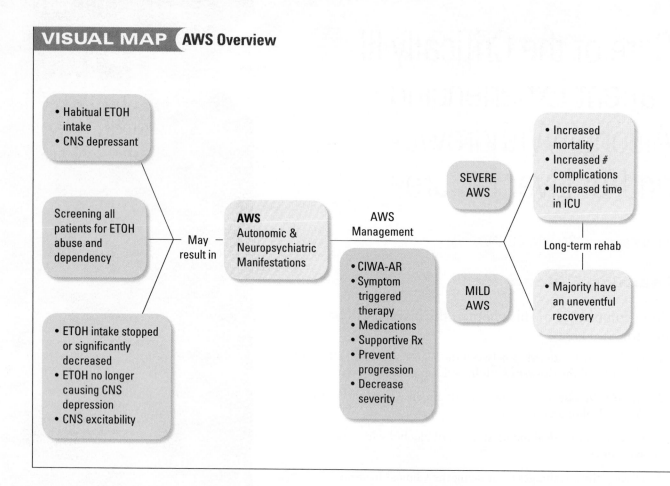

VISUAL MAP **AWS Overview**

- Habitual ETOH intake
- CNS depressant

Screening all patients for ETOH abuse and dependency

- ETOH intake stopped or significantly decreased
- ETOH no longer causing CNS depression
- CNS excitability

May result in

AWS
Autonomic & Neuropsychiatric Manifestations

AWS Management

- CIWA-AR
- Symptom triggered therapy
- Medications
- Supportive Rx
- Prevent progression
- Decrease severity

SEVERE AWS

MILD AWS

- Increased mortality
- Increased # complications
- Increased time in ICU

Long-term rehab

- Majority have an uneventful recovery

Alcohol, the most commonly abused substance in the United States, contributes to 100,000 deaths annually. Approximately eight million Americans are alcohol dependent and approximately 500,000 people per year will require pharmacological management for alcohol withdrawal (Weinhouse & Manaker, 2006). **Alcohol withdrawal syndrome** (AWS) may develop in individuals with habitual alcohol intake who stop or significantly decrease their alcohol consumption. As many as 20% of critical care patients experience AWS as either a primary or a secondary diagnosis. AWS can exacerbate other illnesses and complicate care. It is associated with increased mortality rates, complications, and length of time in an intensive care unit (ICU).

Acute liver failure (ALF), also referred to as fulminant hepatic failure (FHF), is a rare condition characterized by a rapid decline in liver function that occurs in a person without preexisting liver disease. Acetaminophen (Tylenol) overdosing is the leading cause of ALF in the United States. Acetaminophen overdoses are potentiated by alcohol use.

Cirrhosis is the end stage of chronic liver disease. It results from disorders such as hepatitis and alcohol misuse that damage liver cells over time. In the early stages, cirrhosis can be silent, causing few, if any, signs or symptoms. In the later stages, it is characterized by progressive deterioration in liver function and development of portal hypertension. Management involves treating the underlying disease in hopes of halting the process while preventing or treating complications and evaluating the patient for transplantation.

Anatomy and Physiology Review

The following key terms related to anatomy and physiology are foundational to understanding the chapter.

Neurotransmitters—Chemical substances that allow neurons to communicate with each other. In the brain, neurotransmitters either excite (accelerate) or inhibit (brake) impulses along the neurons. Normally there is a balance between excitatory and inhibitory neurotransmission.

Neuroreceptor—A site on or inside a neuron to which a hormone or neurotransmitter can initiate a chemical or electrical reaction.

Gamma-aminobutyric acid (GABA)—A CNS inhibitory neurotransmitter.

Gamma-aminobutric acid A (GABA A)—A neuroreceptor for GABA.

Glutamate—A CNS excitatory neurotransmitter that can interact with several receptors.

N-methyl-D-aspartate (NMDA)—One of the neuroreceptors for glutamate.

Depressant—A substance that slows down the nervous system and its transmission of messages.

Alcohol (ethanol)—A CNS depressant.

Alcohol Withdrawal Syndrome

When exposed to repeated doses of alcohol, the central nervous system (CNS) becomes accustomed to the depressant effects of the alcohol and produces adaptive changes in an attempt to function normally. In the absence of or with a significant decrease in the amount of alcohol, chaos erupts within the CNS. When alcohol is no longer acting as a depressant, the compensatory actions cause excessive CNS excitability. It is analogous to having an accelerator without a brake. The time course of withdrawal is determined by the time it takes to restore balance.

Alcohol abuse and dependency are defined by the Diagnostic and Statistical Manual of Mental Disorders Text Revision (DSM-IV-TR) as follows:

Alcohol abuse is a pattern of maladaptive behavior coupled with one or more of the following:

- Failure to fulfill school, social, or work obligations
- Recurrent alcohol use in physically hazardous situations
- Recurrent legal problems related to substance abuse
- Despite alcohol-related social and interpersonal problems, continues to use alcohol

Alcohol dependency (also known as alcoholism) is a pattern of maladaptive behavior associated with one or more of the following:

- Withdrawal symptoms
- Proof of tolerance
- Relentless desire to cut down or control use
- Occupational, social, and recreational tasks that are given up
- Alcohol taken in a larger amount than planned
- Time is spent obtaining, using, and recovering from the alcohol
- Alcohol use continues regardless of physical and psychological troubles

Patients who meet the criteria for abuse or dependency are at risk for AWS. AWS is defined by the DSM-IV as having two components:

- History of cessation or significant reduction in prolonged and heavy alcohol use

- The presence of two or more of the characteristic alcohol withdrawal symptoms:
  - Psychomotor agitation
  - Anxiety
  - Autonomic hyperactivity (tachycardia or sweating)
  - Increased hand tremor
  - Insomnia
  - Nausea or vomiting
  - Transient tactile, visual, or auditory hallucinations
  - Tonic-clonic seizure

The nurse should consider the clinical manifestations of AWS on a progressive continuum, where time frames and durations are not exact and often overlap. The pattern, severity, and exact manifestations may be inconsistent from patient to patient. Stages of withdrawal are described chronologically as early and late or according to severity in terms of minor and major or mild, moderate, or severe.

Severity is evaluated by the degree of autonomic hyperactivity and neuropsychiatric behavior and the occurrence of complications. It is not clear why some individuals experience a more severe clinical course. It is thought that severity is dose dependent associated with higher blood alcohol concentrations, longer durations of heavy alcohol consumption, and intensified by the stress of concurrent illnesses. Having a history of previous withdrawals also suggests that subsequent withdrawals can be progressively more severe. This is known as a "kindling effect." Other risk factors include liver dysfunction and use of other addictive drugs.

As the patient progresses through the continuum, the withdrawal manifestations become more intense. The majority of the patients experience minor withdrawal and have an uneventful recovery within a few days. Others may progress to major withdrawal and experience the most severe manifestations, including withdrawal seizures, alcoholic hallucinosis, withdrawal delirium, or delirium tremens (DTs).

Assessment and Management of the Patient with Alcohol Withdrawal Syndrome

Most important is the assessment and recognition of all patients who are at risk for AWS, regardless of the point of entry (McKinley, 2005). Critical to treatment is an accurate history, which can be a challenge in patients with an impaired cognitive status and an unknown past. The goals of management are to:

- Identify patients at risk for AWS
- Establish severity
- Decrease agitation and prevent withdrawal progression

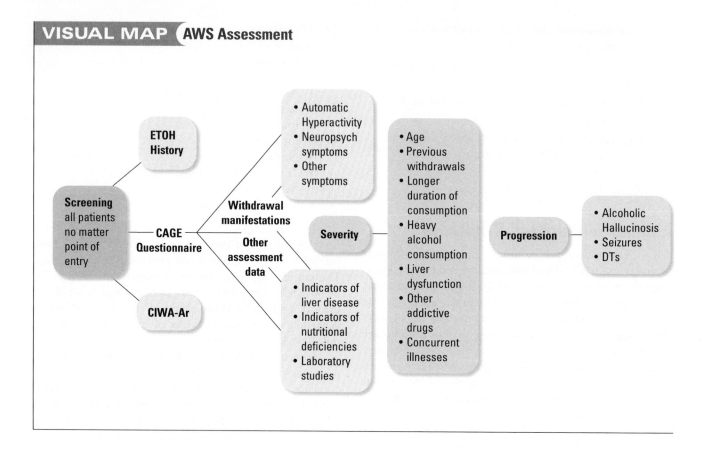

VISUAL MAP (AWS Assessment

- Screening all patients no matter point of entry
  - ETOH History
  - CAGE Questionnaire
  - CIWA-Ar
- Withdrawal manifestations
  - Automatic Hyperactivity
  - Neuropsych symptoms
  - Other symptoms
- Other assessment data
  - Indicators of liver disease
  - Indicators of nutritional deficiencies
  - Laboratory studies
- Severity
  - Age
  - Previous withdrawals
  - Longer duration of consumption
  - Heavy alcohol consumption
  - Liver dysfunction
  - Other addictive drugs
  - Concurrent illnesses
- Progression
  - Alcoholic Hallucinosis
  - Seizures
  - DTs

- Provide supportive care
- Maintain fluid and electrolyte balance
- Provide a safe and dignified environment
- Minimize effects on acute and chronic comorbid illnesses
- Prevent complications
- Initiate case management services for future rehabilitation treatment

Risk Assessment for Alcohol Withdrawal Syndrome

The nurse should obtain a complete history in a non-threatening manner from the patient and/or family. It is important to consider a patient's nonverbal responses, anxiety, and presence or absence of eye contact for clues. The nurse questions the patient and/or family related to:

- Current and past alcohol use and family history of alcohol problems.
  - Abuse and dependence are more prevalent in families where first-degree relatives have been afflicted (Gold & Aronson, 2006).
- Quantity and frequency or pattern of alcohol use.
  - Severity can depend on duration and quantity of consumption.

- Patients and families may underreport consumption and abuse or deny it. This common problem needs to be considered. It is helpful to educate the patient and family as to why this information is so important and how the accuracy of the information can better help them.
- The National Institute for Alcohol Abuse and Addiction (NIAAA, 2005) defines "low-risk"/moderate drinking and high-risk/heavy drinking (Table 11–1).
- It is important to obtain specific information related to the type and amount of alcohol consumed. The NIAAA defines a standard drink as containing 14 grams of alcohol (Table 11–2).
- Time of last alcohol ingestion.
- Characteristics of abuse and dependency as previously described.
- History of liver disease or other alcohol-related illnesses, previous withdrawals, psychiatric or behavioral issues, and alcohol-related injuries (trauma, falls, and collisions).
  - There is a high incidence of anxiety, depression, and other substance abuse with alcohol abuse and dependent individuals. Eighty percent of patients with alcohol abuse and dependency smoke (Gold & Aronson, 2006).

VISUAL MAP AWS Management

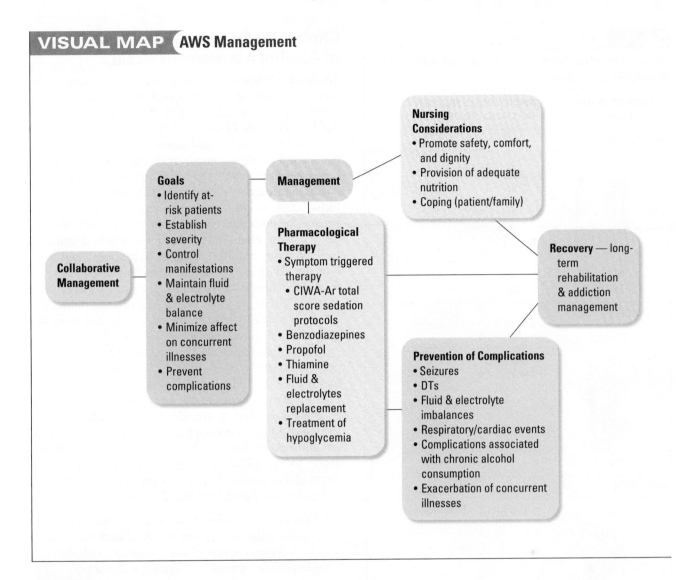

TABLE 11–1

National Institute for Alcohol Abuse and Addiction Risks

RISK FOR ALCOHOL PROBLEMS	NUMBER OF DRINKS FOR MEN	NUMBER OF DRINKS FOR WOMEN
Low-risk/moderate drinking	Less than three drinks daily	Less than two drinks daily
High-risk/heavy drinking	Greater than 14 drinks per week or more than 4 per occasion	Greater than 7 drinks per week or more than 3 per occasion

Source: National Institute for Alcohol Abuse and Addiction Risks.

The CAGE Questionnaire

Additionally, a standardized questionnaire should be utilized to detect dependency. There are several reliable and valid questionnaires available. One such questionnaire is the CAGE. It is a simple, fast, short, reliable, and valid questionnaire. The acronym helps the clinician to recall the following questions:

- Have you ever felt the need to CUT down on drinking?
- Have you ever felt ANNOYED by criticism of your drinking?

- Have you ever had GUILTY feelings about your drinking?
- Have you ever had an EYE opener first thing in the morning to steady your nerves or get rid of a hangover? (Ewing, 1984)

Scoring consists of 1 point for each positive answer. A score of 1 to 3 is highly suspicious for alcohol dependency and warrants further evaluation with an AWS withdrawal scale. The questionnaire will be of limited utility if the patient is unable to respond to the questions.

TABLE 11–2

National Institute for Alcohol Abuse and Addiction Standard Drink Equivalents

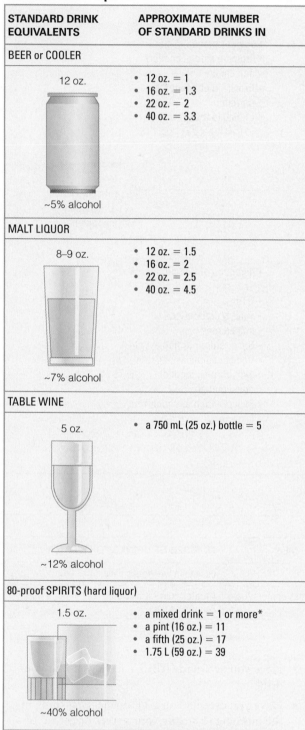

STANDARD DRINK EQUIVALENTS	APPROXIMATE NUMBER OF STANDARD DRINKS IN
BEER or COOLER	
12 oz. ~5% alcohol	• 12 oz. = 1 • 16 oz. = 1.3 • 22 oz. = 2 • 40 oz. = 3.3
MALT LIQUOR	
8–9 oz. ~7% alcohol	• 12 oz. = 1.5 • 16 oz. = 2 • 22 oz. = 2.5 • 40 oz. = 4.5
TABLE WINE	
5 oz. ~12% alcohol	• a 750 mL (25 oz.) bottle = 5
80-proof SPIRITS (hard liquor)	
1.5 oz. ~40% alcohol	• a mixed drink = 1 or more* • a pint (16 oz.) = 11 • a fifth (25 oz.) = 17 • 1.75 L (59 oz.) = 39

Source: From National Institute on Alcohol Abuse and Alcoholism (NIAAA) Publication. (2005). *A pocket guide for alcohol screening and brief intervention.* http://pubs.niaaa.nih.gov/publications/Practitioner/pocketguide/pocket_guide2.htm

*Note: Depending on factors such as the type of spirits and the recipe, one mixed drink can contain from one to three or more standard drinks.

Clinical Institute for Withdrawal of Alcohol Assessment Scale

To objectively assess and manage according to severity, the most frequently used withdrawal scale is the Clinical Institute Withdrawal Assessment for Alcohol Scale revised (CIWA-Ar) (Table 11–3).

The nurse assesses and scores 10 specific symptoms: nausea and vomiting, tremor, sweating, anxiety, agitation, headache, disorientation, tactile disturbances, visual disturbances, and auditory disturbances. Concurrently vital signs including temperature and pulse oximetry are evaluated. Patients are medicated when they cross a designated threshold of severity. Frequency of assessments will be determined by the severity, treatment, response to treatment, and overall acuity. The higher the score, the greater the patient's risk for severe withdrawal symptoms. The highest score attainable is 67 (refer to Table 11–3). Best practice utilizes the CIWA-Ar to guide pharmacological therapy and direct the level of care required as shown in Table 11–4.

Because alcohol is short acting, the nurse anticipates that signs and symptoms of minor withdrawal commonly appear within 6 to 12 hours of the last ingestion, peak in 24 to 36 hours, and resolve after 48 hours. In the patient whose liver is already compromised, AWS can last much longer secondary to poor metabolic function not allowing the liver to excrete toxins effectively. In addition to the CIWA-Ar scale, the nurse's history and physical assessment should also consider the following indicators associated with withdrawal:

- Autonomic manifestations: hyperventilation, tachycardia, palpitations, hypertension, increased body temperature, hyperreflexia, insomnia, restlessness, diaphoresis, tremors, mydriasis, and seizures
- Neuropsychiatric manifestations: anxiety, fear, anger, argumentive, belligerent, paranoid, impaired attention span, disorientation, tactile, auditory-visual hallucinations, global confusion
- Other manifestations: nausea, vomiting, diarrhea, anorexia, abdominal cramps, and recurrent infections

Nursing Management

The nurse also accesses for indications of liver disease and for nutritional deficiencies. Repeated excessive consumption of alcohol frequently results in deterioration of liver function. If the nurse suspects chronic alcoholism, she should assess the patient for the following indications of liver disease; these are described later in the chapter:

- Skin vascularization: spider angioma, palmar erythema
- Jaundice
- Ascites/peripheral edema

TABLE 11–3

Clinical Institute Withdrawal Assessment for Alcohol (CIWA-Ar)

Patient: _____   **Date:** (yy/mm/dd) _____/_____/_____   **Time:** (24 hr) _____

Pulse or heart rate: _____   **Blood Pressure:** _____

Nausea and Vomiting—Ask "*Do you feel sick to your stomach?*" "*Have you vomited?*" Observation.
- 0—no nausea and no vomiting
- 1—mild nausea with no vomiting
- 2
- 3
- 4—intermittent nausea with dry heaves
- 5
- 6
- 7—constant nausea, frequent dry heaves and vomiting

Tremor—Arms extended and fingers spread apart. Observation.
- 0—no tremor
- 1—not visible, but can be felt fingertip to fingertip
- 2
- 3
- 4—moderate, with patient's arms extended
- 5
- 6
- 7—severe, even with arms not extended

Paroxysmal Sweats—Observation.
- 0—no sweat visible
- 1—barely perceptible sweating, palms moist
- 2
- 3
- 4—beads of sweat obvious on forehead
- 5
- 6
- 7—drenching sweats

Anxiety—Ask "Do you feel nervous?" Observation.
- 0—no anxiety, at ease
- 1—mildly anxious
- 2
- 3
- 4—moderately anxious, or guarded, so anxiety is inferred
- 5
- 6
- 7—equivalent to acute panic states as seen in severe delirium or acute schizophrenic reactions

Agitation—Observation.
- 0—normal activity
- 1—somewhat more than normal activity
- 2
- 3
- 4—moderately fidgety and restless
- 5
- 6
- 7—paces back and forth during most of the interview, or constantly thrashes about

Tactile Disturbances—Ask "Have you any itching, pins and needles sensations, any burning, any numbness, or do you feel bugs crawling on or under your skin?" Observation.
- 0—none
- 1—very mild itching, pins and needles, burning, or numbness
- 2—mild itching, pins and needles, burning, or numbness
- 3—moderate itching, pins and needles, burning, or numbness
- 4—moderately severe hallucinations
- 5—severe hallucinations
- 6—extremely severe hallucinations
- 7—continuous hallucinations

Auditory Disturbances—Ask "Are you more aware of sounds around you? Are they harsh? Do they frighten you? Are you hearing anything that is disturbing to you? Are you hearing things that you know aren't there?" Observation.
- 0—not present
- 1—very mild harshness or ability to frighten
- 2—mild harshness or ability to frighten
- 3—moderate harshness or ability to frighten
- 4—moderately severe hallucinations
- 5—severe hallucinations
- 6—extremely severe hallucinations
- 7—continuous hallucinations

Visual Disturbances—Ask "Does the light appear to be too bright? Is its color different? Does it hurt your eyes? Are you seeing anything that is disturbing you? Are you seeing things that you know aren't there?" Observation.
- 0—not present
- 1—very mild sensitivity
- 2—mild sensitivity
- 3—moderate sensitivity
- 4—moderately severe hallucinations
- 5—severe hallucinations
- 6—extremely severe hallucinations
- 7—continuous hallucinations

Headache, Fullness in Head—Ask "Does your head feel different? Does it feel like there is a band around your head?" Do not rate dizziness or lightheadedness. Otherwise, rate severity.
- 0—not present
- 1—very mild
- 2—mild
- 3—moderate
- 4—moderately severe
- 5—severe
- 6—very severe
- 7—extremely severe

Orientation and Clouding of Sensorium—Ask "What day is this? Where are you? Who am I?"
- 0—oriented and can do serial additions
- 1—cannot do serial additions or is uncertain about date
- 2—disoriented for date by no more than two calendar days
- 3—disoriented for date by more than two calendar days
- 4—disoriented for place and/or person

Note: Table 11–4 on page 270 correlates the CIWA-Ar score with the severity of withdrawal.

Total CIWA-Ar Score _____

Rater's Initials _____

Maximum Possible Score = 67

Source: Sullivan, J.T., Sykora, K., Schneiderman, J., Naranjo, C.A., and Sellers, E.M. (1989). Assessment of alcohol withdrawal: The revised Clinical Institute Withdrawal Assessment for Alcohol scale (**CIWA-Ar**). *British Journal of Addiction, 84*:1353–1357.

TABLE 11-4

Clinical Institute Withdrawal Assessment of Alcohol Scale, Revised (CIWA-Ar)

SCORES	SEVERITY OF WITHDRAWAL
Less than 8–10	Minimal to mild withdrawal
8–15	Moderate symptoms
>15	Severe symptoms

Source: Sullivan, J.T., Sykora, K., Schneiderman, J., Naranjo, C.A., and Sellers, E.M. (1989). Assessment of alcohol withdrawal: The revised Clinical Institute Withdrawal Assessment for Alcohol scale (**CIWA-Ar**). *British Journal of Addiction, 84*:1353–1357.

Nursing Diagnoses

CRITICALLY ILL PATIENT EXPERIENCING ALCOHOL WITHDRAWAL

- Anxiety related to situational crisis: alcohol withdrawal
- Acute confusion related to the effects of alcohol
- Dysfunctional family processes: alcoholism related to abuse of alcohol
- Excess fluid volume related to portal hypertension
- Imbalanced nutrition less than body requirements related to suppression of appetite and inability to absorb nutrients
- Risk for injury related to alcohol intoxication or withdrawal and abnormal blood profile (increased serum ammonia)
- Risk for infection related to chronic liver disease
- Risk for deficient fluid volume related to loss of fluid from hemorrhage, vomiting, severe fluid shift, or diuresis

- Encephalopathy/impaired mental status
- Hepatomegaly

Repeated excessive consumption of alcohol often provides empty calories, suppressing the appetite, and causes early satiety (fullness), resulting in nutritional deficiencies and malnutrition. The nurse assesses for the following manifestations of nutritional deficiencies:

- Underweight
- Fatigue (folic acid/folate deficiency)
- Anemia (folic acid/folate deficiency
- Ataxia (thiamine deficiency/Wernicke's encephalopathy)
- Nystagmus (thiamine deficiency/Wernicke's encephalopathy)
- Peripheral neuropathy (thiamine deficiency)
- Ophthalmoplegia (thiamine deficiency/Wernicke's encephalopathy)
- Muscle weakness and wasting

Laboratory Studies

Additionally, the nurse would review the following laboratory studies:

- Toxicology screen (blood and urine) to include a blood alcohol concentration—will confirm recent alcohol ingestion and the presence of other abuse substances but not abuse or dependence.
- Complete blood count (CBC)—often reveals anemia but macrocytosis (elevated MCV between 100 and 110 fl) develops prior to the anemia in the majority of alcoholics. Also seen with chronic abuse is leukocytosis and thrombocytopenia.
- Serum glucose (normal 70 to 10 mg/dL)—hypoglycemia may accompany AWS and symptoms of AWS can mimic that of hypoglycemia. Less than 50 mg/dL is a critical value.
- Blood urea nitrogen (BUN) and creatinine—are evaluated for hydration status and renal function.
- Prothrombin time/international normalized ratio (INR)—can be increased with excessive alcohol consumption and liver dysfunction.
- Liver function tests—a variety of studies to assess liver function and the presence of liver disease are performed. Alcohol abuse is a common cause of abnormal liver function tests.

Because alcohol can affect all systems, the nurse anticipates tests may be ordered relative to nutritional deficiencies (e.g., serum iron, folate, protein, albumin) and other alcohol-related disorders. Diagnostic tests and physical characteristics help to support the diagnosis of alcohol abuse and dependence; however, normal tests and a physical exam do not rule out the diagnosis.

Assessment of the Patient with Severe Alcohol Withdrawal

As withdrawal severity increases, the critical care nurse expects that manifestations will be progressive, exaggerated, and potentially life threatening. Focused attention is on cardiac and respiratory status and neuropsychiatric indicators of the **delirium tremens (DTs)**. In severe withdrawal, the patient may need to be intubated and mechanically ventilated in order to adequately control symptoms.

Alcohol Withdrawal Seizures

Alcohol withdrawal seizures ("rum fits") commonly occur and can manifest anytime during withdrawal. They often appear early, within 6 to 48 hours of the last alcohol ingestion. Though they can occur in the absence of other signs and symptoms, they are usually part of the progression. Patients with a chronic heavy drinking history who have experienced previous episodes of withdrawal have an increased incidence of seizures. The nurse will identify high-risk individuals, assess characteristics of seizure activity, and implement seizure precautions and one-to-one observations as necessary.

Withdrawal seizures are likely to be brief, single, generalized, and tonic-clonic. Occasionally they present in small clusters. The majority of the seizures terminate spontaneously. Status epilepticus is rare and it should prompt further investigation for a differential diagnosis. The nurse monitors for fluid and electrolyte abnormalities and hypoglycemia, which may be associated with seizures. Patients who experience seizures predicatively have a more complicated withdrawal and an increased incidence of developing DTs.

Alcoholic Hallucinosis

Alcoholic hallucinosis can manifest from 12 to 24 hours after the last alcohol ingestion. With alcohol hallucinosis the patient experiences perceptual disturbances, usually visual, auditory, or tactile phenomena, without sensorial alterations. The patient is fully conscious, aware of the environment, acknowledging that the hallucinations are related to the substance dependence and withdrawal. Though the duration can be variable, lasting for days, they usually resolve in 24 to 48 hours. The nurse assesses the characteristics of the hallucinations along with orientation status to distinguish hallucinosis from the hallucinations characteristic of the DTs. DTs usually do not appear for 48 hours after the last alcohol ingestion.

Delirium Tremens

DTs, also called alcohol withdrawal delirium, is the most severe complication of withdrawal. It is seen in approximately 5% of the cases. Mortality varies depending on the comorbidities, but the average is about 1% (Mayo-Smith et al., 2004). Risk factors include older age of the patient, a concurrent illness, a previous history of DTs, and/or a history of sustained drinking.

The autonomic and neuropsychological manifestations are profoundly exaggerated. The nurse must recognize that the most characteristic distinction of the DTs is the disorientation and global confusion. The nurse must assess for marked agitation, hallucinations, and distractibility with accentuated response to external stimuli, and increases in heart rate, blood pressure, respiratory rate, and temperature. The hallucinations can be horrific, thus increasing agitation, confusion, and aggressiveness. Often patients become violent in an attempt to escape. Autonomic hyperactivity and instability evidenced by pronounced tachycardia greater than 120 beats per minute, temperature elevation of greater than 100°F (37.5°C), hypertension (often labile), and tachypnea can cause increased cardiac workload, oxygen delivery, and consumption. The nurse needs to assess for cardiac dysrhythmias, respiratory insufficiency, severe dehydration, and hyperthermia. If autonomic instability is not recognized and treated properly death may occur from respiratory and/or cardiovascular collapse. Patients with a core body temperature greater than 104°F (40°C) have

an increased risk of mortality (Weinhouse & Manaker, 2006). DTs are a medical emergency.

The timing and duration of the DTs on the continuum is variable. DTs typically occur within 48 to 72 hours after the patient's last alcoholic beverage and they can last for 48 to 72 hours (Mayo-Smith et al., 2004). Reports have indicated that DTs have lasted up to 14 days. Lingering cognitive dysfunction may last from 4 to 12 weeks. Knowing the approximate time frames enables the nurse to be more vigilant.

Collaborative Management

The nurse works collaboratively with the health care team (physician and appropriate health care disciplines) to establish alcohol abuse and dependence and risk for AWS, control autonomic hyperactivity, and identify neuropsychiatric behaviors. The goal is to prevent, recognize, and treat symptoms; halt progression; provide a safe and dignified withdrawal; and prevent and treat complications. Supportive care and pharmacological therapy are instrumental in accomplishing management goals.

Symptom-Triggered Therapy

Symptom-triggered therapy is the preferred method of medication administration for AWS (McKay, Koranda, & Axen, 2004). The nurse monitors the signs and symptoms, utilizing the CIWA-Ar assessment tool. Medication administration and dosing protocols are based on the total score. The goal is to achieve the therapeutic effect of the medication evident by light somnolence, no breakthrough or progression of manifestations, and hemodynamic stability (Puz & Stokes, 2005). The nurses' responsibilities include:

- Assessment of vital signs, including temperature and pulse oximetry. Actual frequency will depend on acuity, CIWA-Ar score, and medication administration and therapeutic response.

- Assessment of AWS symptoms (while the patient is awake) using the CIWA-Ar scale, the frequency as described above.

- Administer prescribed medications for clinically significant symptoms as established by the total CIWA-Ar score:
  - Best practice for the management of AWS supports development of specific order sets and treatment plans that include assessment parameters and appropriate interventions and outcome evaluation criteria based on the total score. Separate order sets for prophylaxis, actual AWS, and different levels of care may be developed.
  - Order sets establish the severity threshold or total score at which sedation is initiated. The nurse will see some variation as to what total

COMMONLY USED MEDICATIONS

SEDATIVE-HYPNOTICS: BENZODIAZEPINES

INTRODUCTION

Benzodiazepines are the foundation of pharmacological therapy for AWS. These agents serve as a substitute for alcohol by acting on inhibitory GABA mediators, replacing the depressant effects on the CNS. As a substitute for alcohol, they counteract hyperactivity; thus they are known to have "cross tolerance." In addition to their sedative-hypnotic effect, they also have anticonvulsant properties and less adverse effects than other drugs in this classification. Benzodiazepines have been proven to be safe and effective in preventing and reducing withdrawal severity, including seizures and delirium (Kennedy, 2004).

Desired Effect: A variety of benzodiazepines are available with similar efficacies and no one drug has proven superiority; therefore, the nurse may see some variation in clinical practice (Mayo-Smith et al., 2004). The choice of drug is based on the individual's clinical picture, comorbidities, and pharmacokinetic factors, including:

- Prophylaxis versus progressive AWS
- Age
- Route of administration
- Onset of action
- Duration (elimination, half-life)
- The presence of active metabolites
- History of previous withdrawals with seizures or DTs
- Impaired liver function

Benzodiazepines can be long acting, intermediate acting, or short acting. Diazepam (Valium) and clordiazepoxide (Librium) are long-acting agents. Lorazepam (Ativan) and oxazepam (Serax) are intermediate-acting agents, and midazolam (Versed) is a short-acting agent.

Generally, long-acting agents allow for a smoother course with less chance of breakthrough symptoms and a decreased risk of seizures or delirium. They are preferred in moderate to severe withdrawals.

Intermediate-acting agents, preferred for older adults and individuals with liver and severe lung disease, have a higher incidence of breakthrough symptoms and seizures.

Nursing Responsibilities:

- The nurse anticipates that the route of administration and dosing will be guided by the clinical picture and the kinetic properties of the benzodiazepine chosen. The therapeutic goal is to achieve light somnolence. Evidence of light somnolence is that the patient sleeps when not stimulated, yet is easily arousable when sleeping. Intravenous administration has the quickest onset. Continuous intravenous administration is acceptable but is usually reserved for severe, complicated withdrawals requiring intubation and ventilation.

- Dosing requirements are affected by age, severity of signs and symptoms, comorbidities, and tolerance. It must be noted that these drugs are replacing alcohol. General principles are to start early based on symptoms and history rather than wait for withdrawal to advance, and anticipate higher doses in order to counteract the tolerance. Once withdrawal is prevented or under control and the patient's overall condition stabilizes, the doses and dosing intervals will be adjusted to wean patients off the original substance.

- For severe withdrawal, the nurse can expect to be administering larger doses of intravenous benzodiazepines. In fact, massive doses may be required in some severe cases. Apprehension in administering the necessary massive doses often results in undertreatment of AWS. The patient receiving massive doses is monitored in an ICU setting for hemodynamic stability and airway protection. The patient with a critical concurrent illness who is intubated may receive a continuous intravenous infusion of a short-acting benzodiazepine like midazolam (Versed). However, there is no support that this method is more beneficial for AWS and it is more expensive (Mayo-Smith et al., 2004).

---

score receives sedation. Generally, sedation is initiated for a score between 8 and 10. Table 11-5 shows an example of a protocol based on CIWA-Ar scores.

Overall, symptom-triggered therapy has been as successful as fixed dosing schedules and studies have shown that it requires considerably less medication and shorter duration of treatment. It also limits both undersedation and oversedation. Low-dose benzodiazepines may be considered prophylactically for a patient who has a history of severe withdrawals. A low-dose, fixed schedule regimen may be ordered with routine CIWA-Ar assessments (at least every 4 hours). The fixed schedule can be transitioned to symptom-triggered therapy according to the total CIWA-Ar score. At any transition of care (change of shift, transfer), it is recommended that two nurses assess and complete the CIWA-Ar score together to ensure agreement and consistency of care.

Neuroleptic Agents

Neuroleptic agents (e.g., haloperidol [Haldol]) are not recommended as monotherapy for AWS. In comparison to benzodiazepines, they have been implicated in higher mortality, longer delirium, and more complications. They lower the seizure threshold, may interfere with heat dissipation, and are not cross-tolerant with alcohol. Earlier literature recommended consideration as an adjunct to benzodiazepine therapy when agitation, sensorial impairment, psychosis, and perceptual disorders are not well controlled (Mayo-Smith et al., 2004). Later sources recommend that they not be used in AWS (Weinhouse & Manaker, 2006).

It is important for the nurse to be aware of this, especially if a facility does not have an attentive AWS screening protocol. Too often, especially if a patient has a psychiatric history, agitation is not properly evaluated and is quickly treated with neuroleptic agents. The nurse must remember that patients with alcohol abuse and dependency have a high incidence of psychiatric and behavioral disorders.

Nursing Management

Thiamine (vitamin B_1) deficiency is frequently seen in alcohol-dependent individuals because of insufficient dietary intake, impaired gastrointestinal absorption, and impaired utilization. Thiamine is an essential for normal

TABLE 11–5

Lorazepam Therapy

Lorazepam (Ativan) every 30 minutes PRN-based on CIWA-Ar score:

TOTAL CIWA-AR SCORE	LORAZEPAM (ATIVAN) DOSE
10 or less	No therapy
11–14	1–2 mg IV or IM
15–19	3–4 mg IV
20 or greater	Call physician for dose
Reassess CIWA-Ar 30 minutes after initial dose of lorazepam (Ativan)	
Repeat dose based on above chart if score is greater than 10 and respiratory rate is greater than 12 breaths/minute	
Reassess CIWA-Ar 30 minutes after each repeated dose of lorazepam (Ativan)	
If no repeat dose of lorazepam (Ativan) is required, reassess CIWA-Ar every 2 hours × 2, then every 4 hours	
Call House Officer for: • CIWA-Ar score greater than "15" 30 minutes after dose of lorazepam (Ativan) • Heart rate less than 55 beats per minute or greater than 110 beats per minute • Diastolic blood pressure greater than 95 mm Hg • Systolic blood pressure greater than 180 mm Hg • Respiratory rate less than 12 breaths per minute or greater than 28 breaths per minute • Oxygen saturation less than 90% • Seizures • Expressed or suspected suicidal tendencies • Other: _____	

Source: Developed at Lahey Clinic Medical Center, Burlington, MA as a guideline for therapy. Revised: 04/28/06.

metabolism and utilization of glucose. As a cofactor for several enzyme systems, it plays a role in cerebral energy utilization and maintenance of nerve impulses. Alcohol also depletes liver glycogen stores and impairs glucogenesis (the formation of glucose from glycogen); thus, hypoglycemia may accompany AWS. Administration of intravenous (IV) dextrose without thiamine administration increases the patient's risk for developing an acute neurological complication called **Wernicke's encephalopathy** (confusion, abnormal gait, and paralysis of certain eye muscles). This is a complication of a nutritional deficiency, not AWS. **Korsakoff's syndrome** (selective memory disturbances, amnesia) occurs in the majority of the patients recovering from both Wernicke's encephalopathy and AWS. When the two occur together, it is referred to as Wernicke-Korsakoff syndrome.

AWS treatment protocols initiate the administration of thiamine immediately and prior to any IV dextrose infusion to prevent Wernicke-Korsakoff syndrome. Patient history and risk factors for severe withdrawal will influence the route of administration. The parenteral route is preferred because the oral route can have erratic absorp-

tion. The nurse can anticipate administrating thiamine 100 mg IM/IV as soon as possible. Generally, thiamine 100 mg is ordered daily in a liter of IV fluids for at least 3 days. Once a normal diet is tolerated, IV thiamine may be transitioned to dosages of 50 to 100 mg as tolerated orally. IV administration is safe with rare adverse effects. Larger doses of thiamine are administered to patients with Wernicke-Korsakoff syndrome. The nurse monitors the patient for any adverse effects of the medication and for signs and symptoms of Wernicke-Korsakoff syndrome.

Evidence-Based Interventions for the Treatment of Alcohol Withdrawal Seizures

The nurse should implement seizure precautions for all high-risk patients. Alcohol withdrawal seizures do not require treatment with an anticonvulsant. Benzodiazepines have anticonvulsant properties and are usually sufficient for both primary and secondary prevention and status epilepticus. Patients with a history of withdrawal seizures or a predicted severe withdrawal may have higher initial doses ordered and a slower tapering schedule. As described, alcohol withdrawal seizures are often self-limited and can terminate spontaneously.

Collaborative Management

The nurse works collaboratively with the health care team to promote fluid and electrolyte balance. Signs and symptoms of dehydration and overhydration have to be accurately monitored. Severe withdrawal, including the DTs, typically causes dehydration. The goal of management is to maintain fluid and electrolyte balance.

Assessment of Fluid Balance

Early stages of withdrawal are often marked by fluid retention secondary to the effect of alcohol on antidiuretic hormone (ADH). Alcohol inhibits the secretion of ADH, causing an increase in urine output. In withdrawal, ADH is no longer inhibited, causing fluid retention. In severe AWS, especially complicated by the DTs, dehydration is a concern secondary to the additional fluid losses from vomiting, diarrhea, hyperventilation, diaphoresis, and fever. The nurse realizes that vital signs may not be an accurate reflection of fluid status secondary to increased adrenergic stimulation from the withdrawal syndrome causing tachycardia, and hypertension and massive doses of sedatives causing hypotension. Therefore, the nurse evaluates the following for evidence of dehydration or overhydration:

Weight

Vital signs/other hemodynamic values (see Chapter 5) ∞

Intake and output

BUN, creatinine, and electrolytes

Skin and mucous membrane characteristics (warm, dry, moist, cool)

Presence/absence of edema

Lung sounds

Fluid Administration

Depending on the history and severity of the AWS, hydration is provided orally or intravenously. Typically a glucose-based solution (e.g., D5$\frac{1}{2}$ NS) is initiated to administer thiamine as previously discussed. Protocols may also provide for multivitamin and folic acid administration either orally or intravenously. The rate of the IV will depend on:

- Ability to take oral supplements
- Other comorbidities, acute illnesses
- Duration of severe withdrawal symptoms
- Presence of autonomic/hemodynamic stability
- Diagnostic evidence from serum electrolytes, BUN, creatinine, and urinalysis

Occasionally, severe cases may need aggressive fluid resuscitation. Patients admitted with the DTs already in progress may already have significant fluid losses. Boluses of an isotonic solution, typically normal saline, may be required in addition to the glucose/vitamin solution. Critically ill patients may have fluid administration guided by hemodynamic monitoring (central venous pressure or pulmonary artery pressures).

Assessment of Potassium Balance

A low serum potassium (hypokalemia less than 3.5 mEq/L) is a frequent finding in AWS related to inadequate intake, excessive diuresis, vomiting, and diarrhea. Manifestations of AWS can potentially mask the manifestations of hypokalemia. The nurse reviews the patient's serum potassium level and assesses for the cardiac signs of severe hypokalemia (less than 2.5 mEq/L), ventricular dysrhythmias, and electrocardiogram changes: flattened or inverted T wave, prominent U waves, prolonged QT and ST depression.

Potassium Administration

Typically, the nurse administers potassium chloride (KCl) as ordered for replacement. Route of administration depends on the patient's serum level, the need for prompt replacement, and the patient's ability to take and tolerate supplements orally. Potassium administration is guided by serum potassium levels, renal function, hydration status, and protocols for specific concentrations and rate of administration. (Commonly, potassium sulfate is added to a liter of maintenance fluid one or more times a day.)

Because alcohol-dependent patients may also have associated low serum phosphorus (hypophosphatemia less than 1.7 mEq/L), potassium phosphate may be ordered based on the degree of phosphate deficiency. If low serum magnesium exists with hypokalemia, administration of potassium will not completely resolve the deficit without magnesium replacement. If the patient's potassium level is between 3.0 and 3.5 mEq/L, the nurse can expect that it will take between 100 and 200 mEq of KCl to elevate the potassium level 1 mEq/L (Kee, 2005). IV potassium can cause pain at the IV site irritating the vein, causing phlebitis, and infiltration can irritate the tissue, causing sloughing. Serum levels and resolution of signs and symptoms will serve as evaluative criteria.

Assessment of Magnesium Imbalance

A low serum magnesium (hypomagnesemia less than 1.5 mEq/L) is associated with chronic alcohol ingestion related to poor nutritional status, malabsorption, and increased magnesium excretion. During withdrawal, magnesium shifts into the cells secondary to metabolic changes, including alcohol ketoacidosis, lactic acidosis, and hypoglycemia, decreasing serum levels (Al-Sanouri, Dikin, & Soubani, 2005). Magnesium's membrane-stabilizing properties promote potassium and calcium homeostasis and may offer protection against seizures and arrhythmias. The nurse evaluates the serum potassium and serum calcium levels concurrently because hypokalemia and a low calcium level (hypocalcemia total calcium less than 4.5 mEq/L) can cause hypomagnesemia. Similar to hypokalemia, hypomagnesemia manifestations can mimic AWS manifestations. The nurse reviews the serum magnesium level and assesses for the following manifestations of severe hypomagnesemia (less than 1 mEq/L):

- Neuromuscular irritability/tetany symptoms (tremors, spasticity, spasms, twitching)
- Anorexia, nausea, or vomiting
- Behavioral changes (mood changes, confusion, insomnia)
- Tachycardia, hypertension, and cardiac dysrhythmias
- Electrocardiogram changes: inverted or flat T wave
- Positive Chvostek's sign (observes spasm of the cheek and twitching of the corner of the lip in response to taping the facial nerve just in front of the ear)

Magnesium Administration

The nurse administers magnesium sulfate as ordered for a documented magnesium deficiency. A 10% magnesium sulfate (1 g/10 mL) solution is available for IV use. Currently there is no concrete evidence that magnesium specifically benefits alcoholic delirium. However, if there is no renal dysfunction and levels are routinely evaluated it is acceptable to include magnesium in IV replacement fluids (Mayo-Smith et al., 2004). Magnesium administration is guided by serum magnesium levels, renal function, hydration status, and protocols for specific concentrations and rate of administration.

The nurse anticipates that the patient may experience a hot flushed feeling with IV administration. Calcium gluconate should be available in case of magnesium toxicity. Serum levels and resolution of signs and symptoms will serve as evaluative criteria.

Assessment of Hypoglycemia (Decreased Blood Sugar Level)

Hypoglycemia is encountered in AWS because alcohol exhausts liver glycogen stores and impairs gluconeogenesis (the synthesis of glucose from protein or lipids). Long-term metabolism of alcohol alters the metabolism of glucose, amino acids, and fats, increasing the susceptibility to hypoglycemia. Alcoholic hypoglycemia has both adrenergic and CNS manifestations (see Chapter 13 for manifestations). ∞

Nursing Management

Management involves the administration of thiamine prior to IV glucose administration to prevent Wernicke-Korsakoff syndrome as discussed. The nurse can anticipate administering a dextrose-based IV solution (e.g., D5 $\frac{1}{2}$ NS) to prevent hypoglycemia. Acute hypoglycemic episodes are treated with 50% dextrose as any episode of hypoglycemia (see Chapter 13). ∞

Nursing Care

The nursing care of the patient with alcohol withdrawal is centered on providing a safe environment and assisting the patient and family to cope with the immediate situation.

The goals of nursing care are to promote safety, comfort, and dignity. The nurse recognizes that alcoholism is a medical disorder and cares for the patient in a respectful, nonjudgmental manner. The signs and symptoms of AWS can be uncomfortable, embarrassing, and often put the patient at significant risk for harm. Both the patient and the family will need support and understanding. The following interventions are implemented to decrease environmental stimulation and promote orientation and comfort:

- Quiet room; decreased lighting, sound, and activity
- Evaluation of visitation on an individual basis (see Chapter 2) ∞
- Avoidance of caffeine

- Environmental adjuncts (clock, calendar), frequent reorientation
- Education related to what to expect from the withdrawal to both patient and family
- Reassurance and positive encouragement
- Consistent caregivers whenever possible

The nurse will also implement interventions to promote safety and dignity:

- Accurate assessment and appropriate medication administration per protocols (vital signs and level of consciousness (LOC))
- One-to-one continuous observation and monitoring
- Institute fall protocols relative to disorientation and sedation
- Seizure precautions
- Aspiration precautions
- Physical restraints to prevent injury to self and staff (see Chapter 2) ∞
- Be safe; provide care as a team and dress appropriately with no dangling articles that can be pulled by a violent patient

Provision of Adequate Nutrition

One of the health dangers of alcohol abuse and dependence is malnutrition. Appetite is often suppressed by the euphoria and the empty calories of alcohol. Because alcohol affects all body systems, it can cause damage to the lining of the stomach and impair digestion. Because alcohol impairs absorption and metabolism, disrupts liver function, and increases the excretion of many nutrients, malnutrition can be present even when intake is adequate. In addition to protein energy malnutrition, there are significant deficiencies in vitamins, minerals, and electrolytes causing bone loss, bleeding tendencies, anemia, and neurological changes.

All patients diagnosed with alcohol abuse and dependence should have a nutritional consult. Damage to other organs must be a consideration in terms of requiring a special diet (cardiac, liver, renal dysfunction). As discussed, electrolyte replacement is guided by blood studies. Thiamine, multivitamins (MVI), and folate are routinely administered. Depending on the severity of the withdrawal, patients may be NPO because they are at high risk for aspiration pneumonia related to agitation, seizures, sedation, and impaired immune system secondary to alcohol abuse.

In the critical care units, nutritional status is monitored closely and short-term nutritional requirements are usually easy to meet by enteral or parenteral means. Long-term maintenance of nutritional status may be a challenge and will depend on the success of the patient's efforts to abstain from alcohol. A collaborative team

SAFETY INITIATIVES   Restraint Reduction

PURPOSE: To reduce restraint use in all settings in all hospitals with all patient populations

RATIONALE: The Final Rule is a regulation that "focuses on patient safety and the protection of patients from abuse." It supports "patients' rights in the hospital setting specifically the right to be free from the inappropriate use of restraints" with regulations that protect the patient when restraint is necessary. The use of restraint is not prohibited but "using restraints as a substitute for adequate staffing, monitoring, assessment, or investigation of the reason behind a patient's behavior . . . which may be indicative of unmet needs" is.

Harmful consequences occur either directly or indirectly from the use of restraints. Psychosocial consequences can develop, including anger, agitation, and depression. Some of the short-term physical consequences from the use of restraints are hyperthermia, new onset of bowel and bladder incontinence, new pressure ulcers, and an increased rate of nosocomial infections. Permanent injuries of the brachial plexus can occur from wrist restraints. At least a hundred deaths occurred in the nation's hospitals between 1999 and 2004 from the use of restraints, more than 40% of which were not reported to the appropriate governmental agency as required.

HIGHLIGHTS OF RECOMMENDATIONS:
A restraint is defined by the Final Rule as "any manual method, physical or mechanical device, material, or equipment that immobilizes or reduces the ability of a patient to move his or her arms, legs, body, or head freely. However, restraints are not devices such as orthopedically prescribed devices, surgical dressings or bandages, or devices to protect the patient from falling out of bed, or to permit the patient to participate in activities without the risk of physical harm." Thus, the Final Rule does not apply to measures (such as side rails) that might keep a patient who is recovering from anesthesia, sedated, or on a therapeutic bed from falling out of the bed. However, it does apply to patients who might be trying to leave their bed, because this might cause entrapment. The Final Rule states that clinical judgment determines whether side rails are considered restraints and governed by the Final Rule or not.

According to the Final Rule restraint may only be used when:

Less restrictive interventions have been determined to be ineffective to protect the patient or others from harm.

The type or techniques used are the least restrictive intervention that will be effective.

It is in accordance with a written modification to the patient's plan of care and implemented in accordance with safe and appropriate techniques as determined by hospital policy and state law.

In addition:

Restraint must be in accordance with the order of a physician or other licensed independent practitioner who is responsible for the care of the patient and is authorized to order restraint by hospital policy in accordance with state law.

The order may **never** be written as a standing order or on an as-needed basis.

The use of restraint must be discontinued at the earliest possible time, regardless of the length of time identified in the order.

Required documentation includes:
The patient's condition or symptoms that warranted the use of the restraint

The patient's response to the intervention, including monitoring the physical and psychological well-being of the patient who is restrained for respiratory and circulatory status, skin integrity, vital signs, and any special requirements specified by hospital policy associated with the 1-hour face-to-face clinical identification of specific behavioral changes that indicate that restraint is no longer necessary.

Source: Federal Regulation Volume 71 No 236 December 8, 2006, Final Rule Available: http://a257.g.akamaitech.net/7/257/2422/01jan20061800/edocket.access.gpo.gov/2006/pdf/06-9559.pdfKey Messages

Source: National Government Clearinghouse Available: http://www.guideline.gov/summary/summary.aspx?ss=15&doc_id=3515&nbr=2741#s26

---

effort is initiated with the patient and responsible support systems to develop a nutritional/diet teaching plan.

Assistance with Coping

Coping may be very difficult for the patient and the family. They are often dealing with withdrawal symptoms that involve violent and embarrassing behavior. Depending on its severity, AWS may be life threatening. Chances are the patient and family have been dealing with the social, legal, occupational, and interpersonal implications

of alcohol abuse and dependence for some time. Additionally, AWS is often coupled with an acute illness. The nurse needs to be sensitive to the needs of the patient and family. When the patient is adequately sedated, the family may be the priority. Often families experience guilt in response to the situation. The nurse should:

- Evaluate the patient and family's coping strategies.
- Provide reassurance regarding current and anticipated signs and symptoms, especially behavior.

- Encourage questions and discussion of negative feelings.
- Promote forgiveness.
- Provide education (consider level of learning and willingness and readiness to learn):
  - Related to duration and resolution of AWS
  - Related to other comorbidities influencing the patient's condition
- Collaborate with other members of the health team to evaluate for and initiate necessary referrals.

Prevention of Complications

Prevention of complications is crucial to patient recovery and positive patient outcomes. Mortality from AWS in the general population is related to development of the DTs. If the DTs are unrecognized or untreated, mortality is as high as 35%. With early recognition and treatment, mortality is less than 5% (Gossman, 2005). Other factors influencing mortality are older age, core temperature greater than 104°F (40°C), and preexisting pulmonary and liver disease. Additionally, the critical care patient may have the added burden of a critical illness coupled with AWS. The nurse needs to consider the effect of chronic alcohol abuse and dependence on all body systems and anticipate cardiac, respiratory, hepatic, neurological, renal, and gastrointestinal complications.

The nurses' role in prevention of complications for patients experiencing AWS is to limit the progression of AWS and ultimately to prevent the DTs. Concerns with severe AWS and the treatment of the DTs are the potential for massive doses of sedation, self-harm, and the physiological effects of autonomic hyperactivity. The nurse:

- Monitors airway and breathing status
- Monitors cardiac status for dysrhythmias, decreased myocardial perfusion, cardiovascular collapse
- Supports fluid and electrolyte status
- Takes prompt action for signs and symptoms refractory to pharmacological therapy

Chronic alcohol abuse and dependence affects all body systems. The nurse anticipates and assesses for the development of the following complications:

- Respiratory infections
- Acute respiratory distress syndrome (ARDS)
- Metabolic dysfunction (lactic acidosis, ketoacidosis, hypoglycemia, electrolyte abnormalities)
- Cardiovascular complications (cardiomyopathy, atrial and ventricular dysrhythmias, variant angina)

The nurse recognizes that long-term alcohol misuse is one of the leading causes of chronic liver disease and liver failure in the United States. Therefore, the nurse assesses the patient undergoing AWS for the development of any of the following manifestations of liver failure. These manifestations are described further elsewhere in the chapter:

- Hepatic encephalopathy
- Wernicke-Korsakoff syndrome
- Gastrointestinal bleeding
- Renal insufficiency/failure

Liver Failure

In the United States, the most common reasons for the development of liver failure are acetaminophen overdose, hepatitis, and alcohol misuse. These factors may precipitate liver failure singly or in conjunction with one another. In order for the nurse to understand the multitude of problems the patient with liver failure develops, the nurse must understand the complexity of liver structure and function.

Gerontological Considerations

ALCOHOL WITHDRAWAL AND MISUSE
Age-related changes can cause older adults to have a greater sensitivity to the effects of alcohol. A decrease in total body fluid results in higher blood alcohol concentrations.

Decreased hepatic blood flow, slower metabolism, and increased permeability of the blood-brain barrier cause an increase in the duration of exposure and significant effects from smaller amounts of alcohol in older adults.

It is estimated that interactions between alcohol and prescription medications result in problems for 17% of older adults.

Most at-risk older drinkers are Caucasian men aged 65 to 74, 25% of whom had a history of heavy drinking when they were younger.

The acute care alcohol-related admission rate for older adults is equal to the admission rate for myocardial infarction (MI) in older adults.

Although older men are more likely to be admitted with problems from alcohol misuse, older women are more likely to have been drinking alone so that significant others are not aware of their pattern of alcohol consumption.

LIVER DISEASE
The likelihood of serious complications developing from liver disease is greater in older adults because as a person ages, the liver is less able to recover from severe physiological stressors or to tolerate toxic accumulations.

It is likely that the liver cells of older adults are less able to regenerate following an insult.

It can be easy to miss hepatic encephalopathy when it develops in an older person because it may be mistaken for dementia or delirium.

VISUAL MAP   Liver Failure Overview

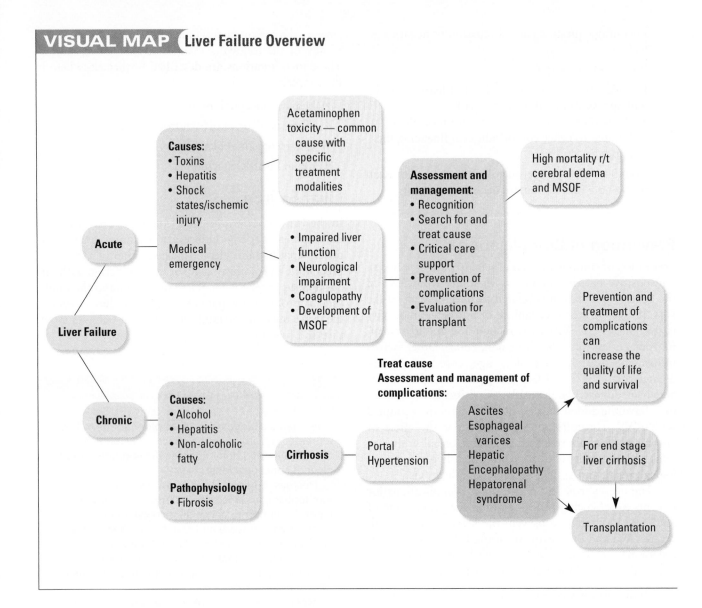

Anatomy and Physiology Review: Liver Anatomy

The largest internal organ, weighing about 3 to 4 pounds, the liver is located in the right upper quadrant of the abdomen, below the diaphragm. It is divided into a right and left lobe with the right lobe approximately six times larger than the left. Each lobe is divided into lobules. Approximately 1,500 mL of blood enters the liver each minute, making it the most vascular organ in the body.

The hepatic lobule is the functional unit of the liver, and an estimated one million lobules form the mass of the liver. They are 2 mm high and 1 mm in circumference (Figure 11-1). Each lobule consists of:

- Hepatocytes: the functional cells of the liver that secrete bile and perform a number of metabolic functions.

- Sinusoids: specialized vascular beds located between each row of hepatocytes that are lined with Kupffer cells and highly permeable endothelium.

- Kupffer cells: phagocytic cells that remove amino acids, nutrients, old red blood cells, bacteria, and debris from the blood. They detoxify toxins and other substances. They also play a role in maintaining vascular homeostasis through production of vasoactive mediators.

The liver receives blood from both venous and arterial sources and has a vast vascular network capable of storing a large volume of blood. The amount of blood stored at any one time depends on the pressure relationships between the arteries and the veins. Unlike other organs, the majority of the blood supply is venous.

- Hepatic portal vein: Supplies 75% of the blood flow and 50% of the oxygen. This blood originates

Normal liver

The liver contains multiple lobules made up of plates of hepatocytes, the functional cells of the liver, surrounded by small capillaries called sinusoids. These sinusoids receive a mixture of venous and arterial blood from branches of the portal vein and hepatic artery. Blood from the sinusoids drains into the central vein of the lobule. Hepatocytes produce bile, which drains outward to bile ducts.

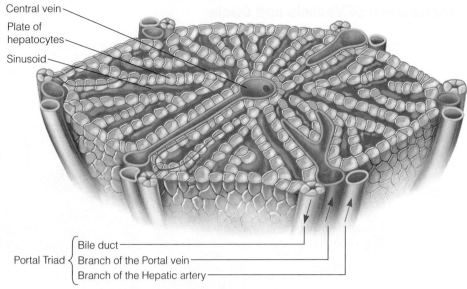

Figure 11-1 Normal liver.

from the capillaries of the entire gastrointestinal (GI) tract and though it carries some oxygen, it is full of nutrients that have been absorbed from the digestive tract. Oxygen and nutrients diffuse through the capillaries into the liver cells.

- Hepatic artery: Supplies 25% of the blood flow and 50% of the oxygen. It branches from the abdominal aorta, providing oxygenated blood.
- Hepatic vein: Blood from the sinusoids drain into a central vein then into the hepatic vein, which drains blood from the liver.
- Inferior vena cava: Blood from the hepatic vein flows to the vena cava to return to the right side of the heart.

As noted previously, each lobule contains a hepatic artery, a portal vein, and a bile duct, known as the portal triad. The hepatic duct is responsible for the transport of bile produced by the liver cells to the gallbladder and duodenum. The bile ducts in each lobule connect to small ducts that connect to larger ducts that eventually connect to form the main hepatic ducts (Figure 11-2).

Liver Physiology

The liver has more than 500 specific functions, including metabolic and hematologic regulation and the production of bile as summarized in the following list:

- Bile formation and secretion—helps to carry waste away and break down fats in the small intestine
- Metabolism of bilirubin, a by-product of aged red blood cells destruction
- Production of proteins for blood plasma (produces albumin, a protein responsible for maintenance of normal fluid balance in the body)

- Metabolism of carbohydrates, proteins, and fats
- Conversion of ammonia to urea, which is then excreted in the urine
- Coagulation and anticoagulation—producing blood proteins necessary for normal clotting
- Metabolic detoxification
- Metabolizing medications
- Storage of minerals and vitamins

Liver cells have the ability to regenerate themselves within 3 weeks.

Liver Failure

Liver failure can be acute, chronic, or acute superimposed on chronic. It can be caused by an acute injury wherein the patient will rapidly develop massive liver cell death, or it can be the result of a chronic disease. Patients with chronic liver disease may have a precipitating event that causes them to experience an acute deterioration in liver function; this is known as acute or chronic disease.

Etiology of Acute Liver Failure

The most common causes of acute liver failure (ALF) include:

- Toxins/drugs such as acetaminophen
- Viral hepatitis (inflammation of the liver)—though hepatitis A is the most common form of acute hepatitis, hepatitis B is the most common hepatitis that causes ALF
- Hypoperfusion/shock states/ischemic injury

The actual time line for development of ALF after the initial insult varies in the literature. The time frame,

Distribution of Vessels and Ducts

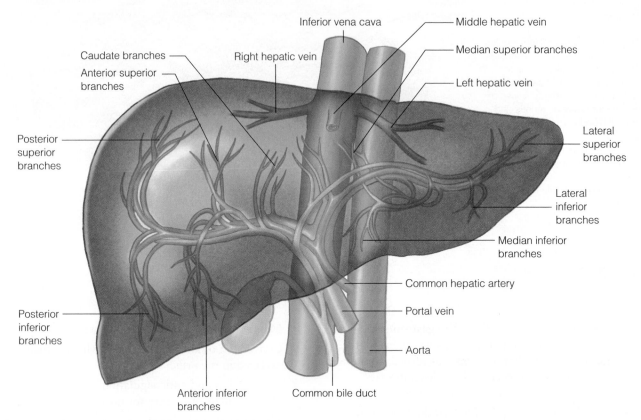

Figure 11-2 Distribution of vessels and ducts in the liver.

as defined by the American Association for the Study of Liver Diseases, is altered coagulopathy and mentation up to 26 weeks (Polson & Lee, 2005). Other sources define ALF as encephalopathy and coagulopathy within 8 weeks of the onset of illness (Fontana, 2006).

In ALF, the specific etiology guides management decisions and treatments and is one of the best prognostic markers. Other variables influencing the prognosis are the patient's age and degree of encephalopathy. In view of the significance of acetaminophen overdose as a cause of ALF, assessment and management of ALF are described.

Collaborative Management

ALF is a medical emergency with the potential for a high mortality rate resulting from the consequences of cerebral edema and the development of multisystem organ failure. The assessment and management of ALF involves recognition, prompt care in a critical care unit to support all systems and prevent complications, aggressive search for the precise etiology to guide treatments, and early evaluation of transplant criteria.

Patient History

Historical elements of the patient's history should focus on exposure to viral infections, drugs or other toxins, or other recent injuries or illnesses. The patient and family should be questioned specifically about acetaminophen intake.

Clinical Manifestations

Clinical manifestations may result from impaired liver function and the effects of liver dysfunction on other organs. The nurse assesses for nonspecific complaints commonly seen with early liver dysfunction such as nausea, vomiting, and malaise. Assessment for signs and symptoms of liver failure must also be considered.

The nurse assesses for characteristic indicators and for potential complications of ALF. The nurse assesses the following indicators of ALF:

- Neurological status—requires vigilant assessment because **hepatic encephalopathy (HE)**, cerebral edema, and increased intracranial pressure can rapidly progress to brainstem herniation and death.
  - Altered mental status, level of consciousness
  - Presence and stage of HE (HE is a condition characterized by a wide range of potentially

reversible neuropsychiatric manifestations. See page 300.)
- Evidence of cerebral edema, increased intracranial pressure (see Chapter 9) ∞
- Coagulopathy
  - Bruising or acute bleeding
  - Increased prothrombin time/INR
  - Thrombocytopenia
  - Signs and symptoms of disseminated intravascular coagulation (DIC) (see Chapter 17) ∞

The nurse also assesses for potential complications of ALF:

- Respiratory insufficiency/failure—related to degree of encephalopathy and increased risk for ARDS
- Hemodynamic instability—related to increased risk of bleeding (coagulopathy, stress ulceration), hypovolemia, circulatory impairment
- Infection/sepsis—related to decreased immune function and invasive procedures
- Hypoglycemia—related to decreased glucose synthesis
- Acid-base and electrolyte disturbances—metabolic acidosis, respiratory alkalosis, hypokalemia, hyponatremia, hypophosphatemia
- Renal failure—related to hypovolemia, increased risk for acute tubular necrosis
- Malnutrition—preexisting, prevention of catabolism

The nurse anticipates an extensive diagnostic work-up in an effort to evaluate cause and severity.

Collaborative Management

The nurse works collaboratively with the health care team (physician and appropriate health care disciplines) to treat the specific cause and to provide intensive supportive care to prevent, recognize, and treat complications.

Critical Care Monitoring

General management includes critical care monitoring because the patient's condition can deteriorate rapidly and because of the potential for multisystem organ failure:

- Respiratory support—possible mechanical ventilation for management of cerebral edema and ARDS (see Chapter 3). ∞
- Circulatory support—hemodynamic monitoring, fluid management, vasopressors (see Chapter 5). ∞
- Neurological support—HE is a major complication of ALF and prognostic marker. It is progressive unless the liver failure is resolved. Treatment

focuses on resolution of liver failure, decreasing ammonia levels as discussed, and monitoring intracranial pressure with subsequent interventions to decrease cerebral edema (see Chapter 9). ∞
- Coagulopathy—another major complication and prognostic marker. Replacement therapy for thrombocytopenia or increased prothrombin time is recommended in active bleeding and prior to invasive procedures.
- Gastrointestinal support—prevention of stress ulcers, provision of nutrition to prevent malnutrition.
- Renal support—volume replacement, avoidance of nephrotoxic drugs, continuous renal replacement therapy (CRRT), vasopressor support.
- Infection—aseptic care, monitor for infection/sepsis, appropriate cultures, antibiotic prophylaxis may be considered.
- Metabolic support—treat electrolyte and acid-base disorders, monitor blood glucose level, and treat hypoglycemia.

Liver transplantation has greatly improved survival rates and remains the most definitive treatment. Early consideration must be given to the likelihood of recovery without a transplant and the contraindications to transplantation. Prompt evaluation, referral, and transport to a transplant facility is imperative when prognostic markers show a high probability of death.

Acetaminophen Toxicity

Specific treatments for ALF have only been established for acetaminophen (Tylenol) overdose. Acetaminophen is easily available and the most widely used analgesic/antipyretic medication in the United States. As a component of many over-the-counter medications and prescription combinations, patients unknowingly may be taking several drugs that contain acetaminophen. In addition, because of easy access, it is a popular drug for intentional overdoses. In therapeutic doses, 1 to 4 grams/day for an adult, it has an excellent safety profile. However, it is a dose-dependent drug that can result in both fatal and nonfatal hepatotoxicity when overdosed, misused, or combined with large amounts of alcohol.

Age, malnutrition/fasting, dose, blood level, chronic alcohol intake, certain medications (antitubercular and antiepileptic drugs), time of presentation, and other comorbidities influence the metabolism of acetaminophen and increase the risk of toxicity. There is controversy related to the optimal dose of acetaminophen in individuals who regularly consume alcohol. Generally, the recommended dose of acetaminophen is 2 grams per 24 hours for individuals consuming two to three drinks a day.

VISUAL MAP Acetaminophen Toxicity Assessment and Management

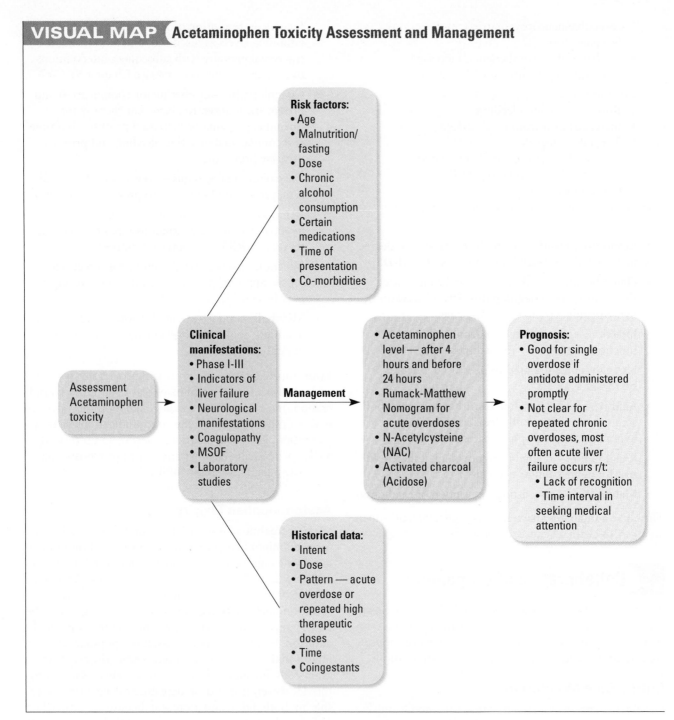

Risk factors:
- Age
- Malnutrition/ fasting
- Dose
- Chronic alcohol consumption
- Certain medications
- Time of presentation
- Co-morbidities

Assessment Acetaminophen toxicity

Clinical manifestations:
- Phase I–III
- Indicators of liver failure
- Neurological manifestations
- Coagulopathy
- MSOF
- Laboratory studies

Management

- Acetaminophen level — after 4 hours and before 24 hours
- Rumack-Matthew Nomogram for acute overdoses
- N-Acetylcysteine (NAC)
- Activated charcoal (Acidose)

Prognosis:
- Good for single overdose if antidote administered promptly
- Not clear for repeated chronic overdoses, most often acute liver failure occurs r/t:
  - Lack of recognition
  - Time interval in seeking medical attention

Historical data:
- Intent
- Dose
- Pattern — acute overdose or repeated high therapeutic doses
- Time
- Coingestants

Time of presentation is an important factor with patients who unintentionally poison themselves with repeated high doses. Additionally, individuals who consistently ingest excess alcohol have a lower toxic dose threshold. Both populations are at a higher risk for severe hepatotoxicity, hepatic coma, and death because they tend to seek medical attention later than the intentional suicidal group.

Acetaminophen is readily absorbed from the GI tract, primarily metabolized by the liver, and has a half-life of 2 to 4 hours. Thus, peak levels may not occur until 4 hours after an overdose. When acetaminophen (Tylenol) is taken in therapeutic doses, 90% is metabolized to a con-

jugate, which is excreted in the urine. A portion of acetaminophen that remains is excreted unchanged in the urine, and the remaining portion is metabolized into a toxic metabolite. Normally this toxic metabolite is conjugated by hepatic glutathione to form a nontoxic substance that is excreted in the urine.

When there is an acute overdose or the maximum daily dose is repeatedly exceeded, the normal pathways of metabolism become saturated and more of the toxic metabolite is produced. When the hepatic glutathione stores are depleted, the toxic substances accumulate, causing hepatic injury. The toxic single dose of acetaminophen is 7 to 10 grams (Farrell, 2006).

N-acetylcysteine (NAC) (Mucomyst) is an antidote that counteracts the effects of acetaminophen toxicity. When administered within 12 hours of ingestion of a single dose it can eliminate significant hepatic injury. NAC (Mucomyst) has several mechanisms of action:

- Limits the formation and accumulation of the toxic metabolite

- Increases glutathione stores

- Directly detoxifies the toxic metabolite to a nontoxic substance

- Has both anti-inflammatory and antioxidant effects that may limit tissue injury

- Has vasodilating and positive inotropic effects to improve microcirculatory blood flow and oxygen delivery (Burns, Friedman, & Larson, 2007)

The predicted risk of toxicity from a single acute overdose relies on the time of ingestion and serum acetaminophen level. Whether a level is toxic or nontoxic can only be interpreted when the time of ingestion is accurately accounted for. The Rumack-Matthew nomogram (refer to Figure 11-3) can be used to predict hepatic toxicity between 4 and 24 hours after an acute ingestion.

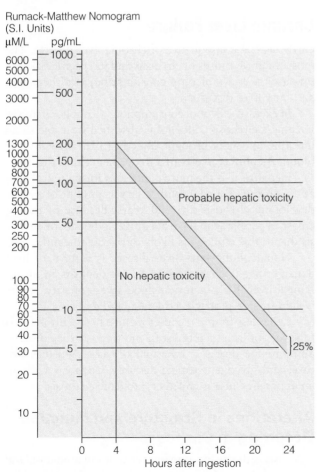

Rumack-Matthew Nomogram
(S.I. Units)

Figure 11-3 The Rumack-Matthew Nomogram.
(Used by permission of Clinical Toxicology, published by Informa Healthcare.)

The diagnosis and risk assessment for repeated high therapeutic doses is less concrete. The clinical manifestations are often subtle and nonspecific and do not predict the delayed hepatotoxicity. It depends on an insightful history, clinical manifestations, and laboratory studies. The acetaminophen nomogram cannot be used, and the acetaminophen level and the aminotransferase (AST/ALT) level will guide treatment. The prognosis is favorable for a single overdose if the antidote is administered promptly. Prognosis for repeated chronic overdose is not clear; most often ALF occurs because of the interval in seeking medical attention and lack of recognition.

Assessment and management of acetaminophen toxicity require prompt recognition or suspicion, supportive care, prevention of absorption, and antidotal treatment to promote drug elimination. It is also important to recognize the differences between a single acute overdose and repeated chronic overdoses. The goal is to administer the antidote within 12 hours of acute ingestion.

Assessment: Acetaminophen Toxicity/Acute Liver Failure

As mentioned, the nurse must review and investigate historical data related to acetaminophen intake. It is important to establish:

- Intent—Is it an intentional ingestion of a large amount of acetaminophen in an effort to commit suicide or an unintentional ingestion of high quantities therapeutically for pain over a period of time? If the patient's intent was to commit suicide, the patient needs to be placed on suicide precautions and have a psychiatric consult.

- Dose.

- Pattern—Single/repeated.

- Time of ingestion.

- Coingestants—It is important to establish the particular form of the drug or drugs (extended release, other drugs, or combination drugs).

The nurse realizes that the clinical manifestations of an acute acetaminophen overdose is generally delayed and seen in four phases (Goldberg & Chopra, 2005). Relative to the time frame the nurse would assess for:

- Phase I (0 to 24 hours)—Anorexia, nausea, vomiting, malaise, pallor, lethargy, diaphoresis. The patient may be dehydrated related to emesis. Many patients are asymptomatic. Laboratory studies are usually normal.

- Phase II (24 to 72 hours)—Right upper quadrant abdominal pain/tenderness on palpation, tachycardia, hypotension, hepatomegaly. Nausea and vomiting usually resolve temporarily. Patients may appear to improve clinically. AST and ALT begin to elevate by 24 hours with progressive elevation by 36 hours. Prothrombin time (PT), total bilirubin, and renal function tests may elevate.

- Phase III (72 to 96 hours)—Abdominal pain, nausea, vomiting.

    Manifestations of liver failure are jaundice, coagulopathy, hypoglycemia, hepatic encephalopathy, signs and symptoms of cerebral edema, increased intracranial pressure, and possible GI bleeding; may progress to multisystem organ failure and possibly death. Liver function tests peak. AST and ALT greater than 1,000 IU/L defines toxicity. Total bilirubin is often greater than 4.0 mg/dL. Death is common in this stage, typically from multisystem organ failure.

- Phase IV (4 to 14 days or longer)—Recovery phase typically begins by day 4 and is often complete by day 7. Severely ill patients may take several weeks to recover. Chronic liver impairment does not ensue.

The following laboratory studies are of particular interest in acetaminophen toxicity:

- Arterial blood gases—Evaluates blood pH. A pH less than 7.3 that does not respond to fluid administration indicates a poor prognosis and a high mortality rate without a transplant.

- Serum creatinine—Assesses renal function because renal failure often occurs with hepatic failure.

- Prothrombin time/INR—Elevates 24 to 72 hours after an acute ingestion due to liver cell damage. Early prognostic indicator.

- Serum total bilirubin—Elevates with hepatocellular injury. It starts in stage II and continues to elevate.

- Aminotransferases—Will elevate 24 to 72 hours after acute ingestion. Levels greater than 1,000 U/L define toxicity.

- Serum acetaminophen level—Acute single overdose patients need to wait to have this drawn until at least 4 hours after ingestion. A level drawn before 4 hours may not represent the peak value.

Collaborative Management

The nurse works collaboratively with the health care team and the regional poison control center to diagnose and treat acetaminophen toxicity. The goal of management is to promptly administer the antidote to prevent extensive hepatotoxicity and acute liver failure.

Evidence-Based Interventions for Acetaminophen (Tylenol) Toxicity

A serum acetaminophen level drawn 4 hours after but before 24 hours post acute single ingestion can be plotted on the Rumack-Matthew nomogram to estimate whether the patient is at "no risk," "possible risk," or "probable risk" of hepatotoxicity (Figure 11-3). This information determines whether antidotal treatment is indicated. The upper line is the "probable risk" line and the lower line is the "possible risk" line. The standard of care is to start antidotal treatment on all patients who fall above the "possible risk" line.

A level drawn before 4 hours does not represent the peak value and should not be used. If the ingestion was more than 4 hours earlier, a level is drawn immediately. Establishing the exact time of ingestion is crucial to using the nomogram because it plots the hours after ingestion against the acetaminophen level.

The nomogram is not useful in predicting acute liver failure or mortality. The following situations cannot be risk stratified with the nomogram:

- Delayed presentation, greater than 24 hours after ingestion
- An unknown time or duration of ingestion
- Ingestion of extended release products
- Repeated high therapeutic ingestions

If the time of ingestion was less than 4 hours, gastric lavage may be considered.

Chronic Liver Failure

Cirrhosis is a consequence of chronic liver disease. The most common causes of cirrhosis and its specific risk factors are excessive alcohol consumption, viral hepatitis, and fatty liver disease.

In excessive alcohol consumption (alcoholic cirrhosis/Laennec's cirrhosis), alcohol is absorbed from the small intestine and it is brought directly to the liver by the blood. Alcohol converts to a toxic chemical in the liver.

Hepatitis C is the more dangerous form of viral hepatitis (chronic B or C), with a larger amount of people developing cirrhosis after 20 years. Because of the increase in people who have hepatitis C, the rate of cirrhosis due to this etiology is likely to rise significantly.

Nonalcoholic fatty liver disease is a form of liver damage that is characterized by fat deposits in an inflamed liver. Risk factors include severe obesity, severe weight loss, hypertriglyceridemia, and diabetes.

Other less frequent causes include hemochromatosis (disorder of iron metabolism), end stage cardiac disease, autoimmune diseases, inherited diseases, Wilson's disease, and glycogen storage diseases. Cirrhosis without an apparent cause is called cryptogenic cirrhosis.

Alterations in Structure and Function Occurring in Cirrhosis

Cirrhosis is the result of many years of inflammation and various degrees of injury to the liver resulting in severe

COMMONLY USED MEDICATIONS

N-ACETYLCYSTEINE (NAC) (MUCOMYST)

Desired Effect: N-acetylcysteine (NAC) (Mucomyst) is the antidote for acetaminophen toxicity and is administered if the serum acetaminophen level drawn between 4 and 24 hours or more after a single ingestion falls above the "possible risk" line on the Rumack-Matthew nomogram. NAC (Mucomyst) is also recommended based on less concrete criteria and historical data. Overall, it is administered if the patient has risk factors for toxicity, suspected ingestion either single or repeated, and indications of hepatotoxicity or liver failure.

Nursing Responsibilities:
- Oral dosing is initiated on nonpregnant patients with a functioning GI system and no indications of hepatotoxicity. The loading dose is 140 mg/kg followed by 17 doses of 70 mg/kg every 4 hours. It is typically available in a 20% solution (200 mg/mL) and it is diluted to a 5% solution with fruit juice, a carbonated beverage, or water.
- The nurse assesses the patient's GI system to evaluate tolerance of the medication. The solution has a foul "rotten-egg" odor and patients best tolerate the smaller volume of solution in chilled orange juice. Antiemetic therapy is considered for the patient with nausea and vomiting. Ondansetron (Zofran) and metoclopramide (Reglan) are frequently used. If the patient vomits within an hour of the dose, it should be repeated as rapidly as possible.
- IV dosing of NAC is acceptable in all cases of acetaminophen toxicity. It is recommended instead of the oral dosing:
  - When the patient is unable to tolerate oral NAC
  - When the patient's condition contraindicates the administration of oral NAC (e.g., GI bleeding/obstruction)
  - In patients with significant hepatotoxicity
  - In pregnant patients
  - With coingestants requiring ongoing GI contamination
- The IV loading dose is 150 mg/kg infused through a peripheral IV over 1 hour using an in-line 0.2-micron filter. Some sources concur with administering the loading dose over 15 minutes (Burns et al., 2007). The maintenance dose is a continuous IV infusion over the next 20 hours. Usually different doses are infused over the first 4 hours and the remaining 16 hours. Depending on the presence or absence of biochemical evidence of hepatic failure (INR < 2 or > 2) and whether it was a single or repeated chronic ingestion, several different maintenance protocols exist. The nurse should follow facility policy for specific dosing protocols and dilution guidelines.
- The nurse assesses for the response to NAC (Mucomyst) by monitoring patients for any signs or symptoms of hepatotoxicity and following the laboratory studies (PT/INR, creatinine, liver function tests). It must be noted that laboratory evidence of hepatic damage may not be seen for 36 hours. Lastly, if the patient is progressing or is likely to progress to ALF, the patient should be transferred to a liver transplant center.

Side and/or Toxic Effects: The nurse assesses for adverse effects of the IV preparation, including pruritus, flushing, nausea, fever, chill, urticaria, bronchospasms, and anaphylaxis. Non-life-threatening effects are treated by holding the infusion, administering antihistamines, and restarting the infusion at a slower rate. IV NAC should be used with caution in patients with a history of bronchospasms or asthma.

COMMONLY USED MEDICATIONS

ACTIVATED CHARCOAL (ACTIDOSE)

Desired Effect: Activated charcoal (Actidose) 50 grams is administered to all patients if ingestion has been within 4 hours. Activated charcoal is a decontamination agent that prevents absorption of acetaminophen by absorbing the drug in the intestine. For maximum effect, it needs to be administered within 30 minutes after ingestion. There has been some concern with administering the charcoal concurrently with the antidote. The administration of activated charcoal or the antidote should not be delayed. Activated charcoal (Actidose) will absorb some of the antidote but not sufficiently to affect its detoxifying effects or to warrant increased doses of the antidote.

Nursing Responsibilities:
- The nurse should administer activated charcoal (Actidose) as ordered. The nurse must consider the patient's mental status, LOC, and ability to cooperate. Altered mental status, decreased LOC, and uncooperative patients are at risk for aspiration and should have the activated charcoal (Actidose) administered through a nasogastric tube.
- Activated charcoal (Actidose) is a black tasteless gritty solution. Some preparations are available in a cherry flavor. The nurse should follow the manufacturer's instructions and the facility's policy regarding administering the activated charcoal. Some preparations need to be mixed with water and others are available in a ready-to-use suspension. All preparations need to be shaken well. The black solution is not very appealing so to increase compliance, the nurse can put it in an opaque container with an opaque cover and offer a straw.

Side and/or Toxic Effects: The nurse anticipates that the patient may vomit, especially if the solution is administered rapidly. The nurse should be prepared to protect the airway if vomiting occurs. The frequency, quantity, color, and consistency of the stools should be assessed. The activated charcoal (Actidose) will color the stools black.

---

scarring. The gradual destruction, death, and regeneration of functional liver tissue (hepatic parenchyma) have significant consequences for the liver and other organs. The regenerative response to cell injury and death involves nodule formation and replacing dead liver cells with fibrous tissue, which leads to fibrosis (scarring).

Anatomically, such an abnormal pattern of regeneration alters the functional component and the architecture of the sinusoids including the vasculature and bile ducts. Over time, liver function deteriorates secondary to altered bile duct flow and stasis, impaired hepatic venous outflow, and decreased blood flow to and through the liver because of increased resistance.

Portal Hypertension

The normal pressure in the portal system is about 5 to 10 mm Hg and higher values are defined as portal hypertension. Portal pressure is the result of two dynamic factors:

- The amount of blood draining into the portal venous system is controlled by:
  - Vascular tone (vasoconstriction/vasodilation) of the mesenteric arterioles.

- Hyperdynamic circulation: an increase in portal venous flow, which is marked by peripheral and splanchnic vasodilation, reduced mean arterial pressure, and increased cardiac output, is responsible for increasing the inflow of systemic blood into the portal circulation.
- The amount of resistance to the blood flowing out of the portal venous system caused by:
  - Distorted hepatic sinusoids.
  - Intrahepatic vasoconstriction.

Portal hypertension (Figure 11-4) develops over time, is asymptomatic, and is responsible for an array of complications that can markedly reduce patients' life expectancy. The following complications are directly attributable to portal hypertension:

- Ascites
- Variceal hemorrhage
- HE, portosystemic encephalopathy (PSE)
- Hepatorenal syndrome

In the earlier stages, treatment can be directed toward the underlying cause of liver disease in an effort to halt the cirrhosis and preserve whatever function may be left. In the late stages, cirrhosis is progressive and irreversible. In alcoholic cirrhosis, abstinence from alcohol may decrease liver cell injury and improve portal hypertension. Prevention and treatment of complications can increase the quality of life and survival for these patients. For patients with end-stage liver cirrhosis, liver transplantation is the only feasible treatment. Because of the increased prevalence of alcohol dependency, obesity, and hepatitis C in the United States, the incidence of cirrhosis is expected to rise.

The severity of the disease can vary. The modified Child-Pugh classification system is used to classify the severity of the disease, predict the development of complications, and correlate with 1-year survival rates. Based on blood tests and presence of symptoms, the system grades five parameters:

- Degree of ascites
- Bilirubin mg/dL
- Albumin g/dL
- Prothrombin time (seconds over control and INR)
- Degree of encephalopathy

Because of the varied functions of the liver, liver failure affects all body systems. Prognosis depends on the cause, severity, presence of complications, and preexisting comorbidities.

Collaborative Management

The assessment and management of chronic liver failure involves recognizing chronic liver disease, establishing the cause, and treating it. The ultimate goal is to

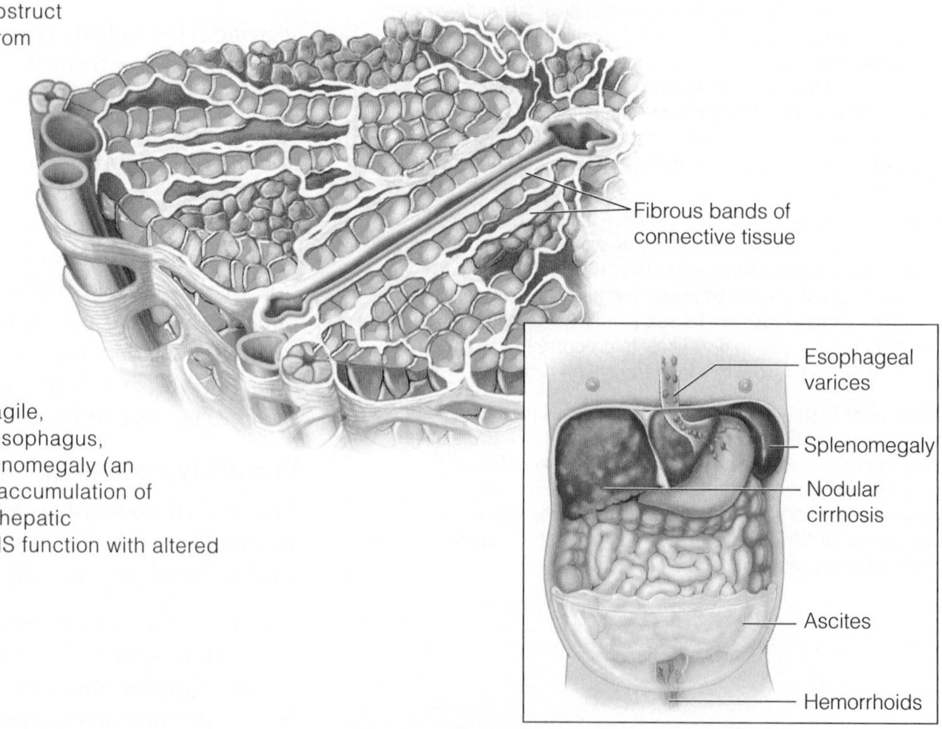
Portal hypertension
Bands of fibrotic scar tissue obstruct the sinusoids and blood flow from the portal vein to the hepatic vein. Pressure in the portal venous system, which drains the gastrointestinal tract, pancreas, and spleen, increases. This increased pressure opens collateral vessels in the esophagus, anterior abdominal wall, and rectum, allowing blood to bypass the obstructed portal vessels. Prolonged portal hypertension leads to the development of (1) varices (fragile, distended veins) in the lower esophagus, stomach, and rectum; (2) splenomegaly (an enlarged spleen); (3) ascites (accumulation of fluid in the abdomen); and (4) hepatic encephalopathy (disrupted CNS function with altered consciousness).
Fibrous bands of connective tissue
Esophageal varices
Splenomegaly
Nodular cirrhosis
Ascites
Hemorrhoids

Figure 11-4 Portal hypertension.

VISUAL MAP Chronic Liver Failure Assessment

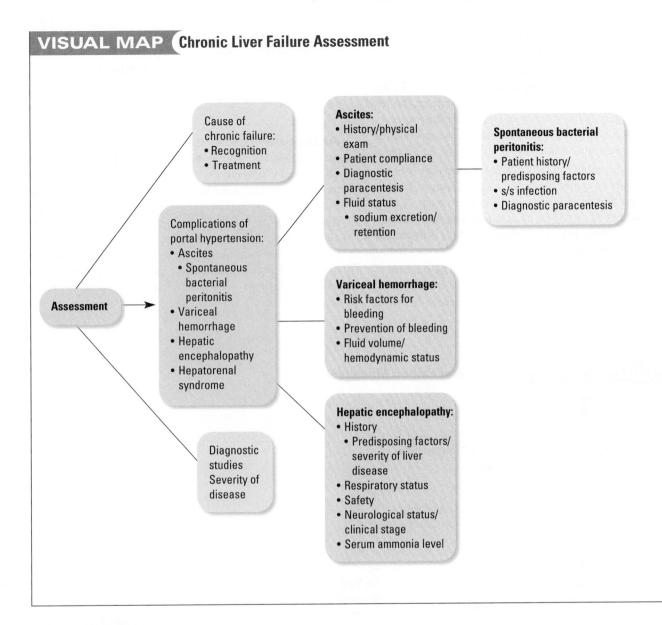

prevent complications, but because cirrhosis is most often progressive and irreversible despite the most appropriate care, many of the patients will still develop complications or decompensated liver disease. Decompensated disease occurs when the liver is so severely damaged it no longer has the capacity to carry out its normal functions and the metabolic functions of the body are affected. This section focuses on decompensated disease, monitoring closely for clinical indications of complications, and prevention and treatment of complications.

Laboratory Studies

The following laboratory studies typically reflect decompensated disease and should be reviewed by the nurse:

- Liver enzymes—In particular aminotransferases (alanine [ALT] and aspirate [AST]) are elevated

related to the increase in the release of enzymes by the damaged liver.

- ALT—Found predominantly in the liver; sensitive and specific for hepatocellular disease.
- AST—Found in the heart, liver, and skeletal muscle. A lesser concentration is found in the kidney and pancreas. Disorders that affect hepatocytes will increase this enzyme.
- Total bilirubin—Reflects the balance between bilirubin production and hepatic clearance. Normally it is metabolized in the liver and excreted in the urine. Total bilirubin is the sum of conjugated (direct) bilirubin and unconjugated (indirect) bilirubin. Elevations cause jaundice. Levels may be normal in well-compensated disease. They rise as liver cell and bile duct damage progresses and can no longer

process the bilirubin. Elevated values reflect a poorer prognosis.

- Serum albumin—Albumin is synthesized in the liver and is a measure of hepatocyte function. Reflecting the synthetic function of the liver, the level will fall as the severity of liver disease progresses. It is also the main determinant of plasma oncotic pressure and is decreased in cirrhosis and ascites.

- Prothrombin time (PT)/INR—Reflects the liver's ability to synthesize blood-clotting factors. It measures how long it takes blood clots to form. A prolonged value will be evident when an estimated 80% of the hepatic synthetic function is impaired. It is a prognostic indicator for declining liver function.

- Complete blood count—Anemia: The patient with cirrhosis typically has anemia from a variety of sources, including acute and chronic blood loss, impaired red blood cell formation, and excess destruction.

Thrombocytopenia: Thrombocytopenia is common in patients with portal hypertension and splenomegaly.

Additional Tests. Additional tests to be reviewed may include abdominal ultrasound and liver biopsy. An abdominal ultrasound shows the appearance of the liver in terms of size and texture as well as blood flow through hepatic and portal veins. Nodularity, irregularity, and atrophy are typical findings in cirrhosis. It can also identify ascites that is less than 100 cc. A liver biopsy is the gold standard to evaluate liver disease and diagnose cirrhosis. It can assist in determining the cause, extent of damage, treatment possibilities, and the long-term prognosis.

VISUAL MAP **Chronic Liver Failure Management**

Nursing Considerations:
- Pain
- Pruritis
- Safety
- Prevention of infection
- Provision of adequate nutrition

Evidence-based interventions for:

Ascites:
- Alcohol abstention
- Sodium restriction
- Diuretic therapy
- Paracentesis (large volume)
- TIPS

Spontaneous Bacterial Peritonitis:
- Diagnostic paracentesis
- Antibiotics

Variceal Bleeding:
- Fluid resuscitation
- Supplemental oxygen
- Octreotide (Sandostatin)
- Endoscopy
- TIPS
- Surgery
- Balloon tamponade
- Beta blockers/ nitrates

Hepatic Encephalopathy:
- Correct precipitating factors
- Lactulose
- Oral antibiotics

Hepatorenal Syndrome:
- Nephrology consult
- Treatments to improve GFR
- TIPS
- Renal replacement therapies
- Patient/family education/ support

End Stage Liver Disease

Transplantation

Collaborative Management

Ascites is the accumulation of a large amount of protein-rich fluid in the peritoneal cavity. Ascites is a marker for severe progression of liver disease. The 2-year survival rate is 50% (Goldberg & Chopra, 2006). Understanding the complex pathogenesis of ascites is critical to understanding management.

The following principles and mechanisms are involved:

- Changes in capillary permeability and the hydrostatic and oncotic pressure gradients due to hypoalbuminemia and low oncotic pressure increase the leakage of plasma from the lymph.
- The release of nitric oxide and other mediators results in splanchnic arterial vasodilation.
- Vasodilation and hyperdynamic circulation cause a marked decrease in systemic vascular resistance (SVR), mean arterial pressure (MAP), and an increase in heart rate and cardiac output.
- Vasodilation activates compensatory mechanisms (such as renin-angiotensin-aldosterone, sympathetic nervous system, and ADH) to restore perfusion pressure and results in sodium and water retention.
- Water retention is related to the increased secretion of ADH. Being unable to excrete water promotes dilutional hyponatremia and hypo-osmolality. The degree of hyponatremia parallels the degree of liver disease.
  - Because of this relationship, the degree of sodium retention and hyponatremia are prognostic predictors.
- Renal blood flow is reduced because of the vasoconstrictors. Initially protective mechanisms maintain perfusion through renal vasodilation but these mechanisms eventually become overpowered. The result is progressive hypoperfusion of the kidneys and a gradual decrease in the glomerular filtration rate.

Assessment: Fluid Status

Ascites is usually one of the early indicators of decompensated disease. The history (chronic liver disease) and physical appearance (large, distended abdomen) are often indicative of the presence of ascites (Figure 11-5).

The nurse questions the patient related to:

- Increased abdominal girth (pants getting tighter)
- Unexplained weight gain
- Alcohol consumption—alcohol-induced injury is the most reversible with abstinence
- Daily dietary pattern and knowledge related to dietary restrictions
- With refractory ascites, ask questions related to:
  - Compliance with the diet restrictions
  - Compliance with medications

The nurse assesses:

- Shifting dullness, abdominal percussion (obese patients often require an ultrasound to detect ascites)
- Presence of peripheral edema (often pitting in the legs and feet)
- Daily weight (fluid loss and weight gain are directly related to sodium balance)
- Abdominal girths (typically inaccurate evaluation of ascites)

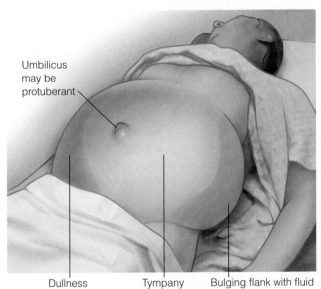

Umbilicus may be protuberant

Dullness   Tympany   Bulging flank with fluid

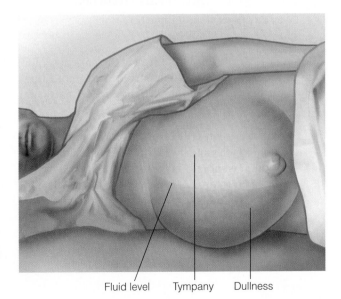

Fluid level   Tympany   Dullness

Figure 11-5 Ascites.

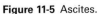

- Difficulty breathing (fluid accumulation and possibly displaced intestines may increase pressure on the diaphragm and decrease lung expansion)
- Lung sounds (decreased especially in the bases. Pleural effusions may develop and threaten respiratory function.)
- Abdominal discomfort/pain using a standardized pain assessment tool
- Skin breakdown or potential risk using a standardized assessment tool (e.g., Braden scale)
- Orthostatic vital signs
- Intake and output

The nurse also anticipates the presence of other signs and symptoms associated with chronic liver disease:

- Nausea, loss of appetite, malnutrition
- Fatigue
- Spider angiomata—dilated blood vessels with a red center and spiderlike branches (number and size often correlated with the severity of the disease)
- Palmar erythema—red area that blanches
- Gynecomastia—endocrine changes related to decreased testosterone in males
- Caput medusae (dilated superficial abdominal blood vessels)
- Splenomegaly—enlarged spleen related to the backup of blood from the portal vein

Hepatomegaly—size may be decreased in more advanced disease

- Jaundice—results from increased serum bilirubin. It is usually not apparent until the bilirubin is greater than 2 to 3 mg/dL; often accompanied by dark-colored urine
- Fetor hepaticus (sweet musty breath odor)
- Asterixis (liver flap, flapping tremor)
- Bleeding tendencies, bruising

Additionally the nurse should review the patient's CBC, clotting studies, and liver functions tests for indications related to the severity of the liver disease. Of particular importance with the patients with ascites is:

- Serum electrolytes: Electrolyte abnormalities are common in chronic liver disease with ascites.
  - Sodium is monitored because diuretic therapy is the main treatment modality for ascites. The degree of sodium retention and hyponatremia are prognostic predictors.
  - Potassium is monitored because of diuretic therapy. Aldosterone-inhibiting diuretics and renal disease can increase potassium, and

potassium-depleting diuretics can decrease potassium.

- Blood urea nitrogen/creatinine are evaluated to assess hydration status and renal function.
- Twenty-four-hour urine for sodium excretion: The sodium content in the urine reflects the balance between dietary sodium and renal excretion of sodium. It is helpful in ascites when weight loss is less than desired. The results can be compared to the patients' dietary sodium restriction and weight loss to determine if patients are compliant with their dietary restrictions.
- Random urine sodium/potassium: A concentration ratio greater than 1 predicts that the patient should be losing weight if a sodium-restricted diet is followed. It is more convenient than a 24-hour urine.
- Abdominal ultrasound can evaluate and confirm ascites in morbid obese patients and may be used to locate an appropriate paracentesis site.
- Abdominal **paracentesis** may be diagnostic or therapeutic. It can confirm the diagnosis or the presence of infection. Fluid relative to portal hypertension can be differentiated from other causes. A therapeutic paracentesis removes larger volumes of fluid in refractory ascites (see Building Technology Skills).
- Ascitic fluid analysis: Cell count with differential, total protein, and albumin concentration is routinely obtained with all paracentesis. If the polymorphonuclear leukocyte count (PMN) is greater than 250 cells/mm³, a specimen for culture should be sent.

Collaborative Management

The nurse works collaboratively with the health care team to promote mobilization of the ascitic fluid. The goal is that the level of sodium excreted is more than the sodium intake, causing a decrease in ascites and peripheral edema because fluid passively follows sodium.

Alcohol Abstention

If there is an alcohol component to the liver injury/disease, it is essential that the patient abstain from all alcohol. The nurse should screen all patients for alcohol abuse and dependency and the risk for AWS. The nurse should provide education to the patient and family related to the serious implications of continued alcohol use. If the patient is unable to abstain from alcohol consumption, appropriate members of the health care team are consulted to evaluate the patient for a treatment program that would best benefit the needs of the individual and family.

Building Technology Skills

Paracentesis

Paracentesis is the removal of fluid from the peritoneal space using a large-bore needle or catheter system. The fluid can be removed by syringe, vacuum bottles, or bags depending on the amount of fluid being removed. A peristaltic pump may be used for therapeutic paracentesis to expedite the fluid removal. The procedure is performed at the bedside as shown in Figure 11-6.

The position of the patient will depend on practitioner preference, acuity of the patient, volume to be removed, and thickness of the abdominal wall. The patient may be positioned sitting on the side of the bed, but, typically, the patient is placed in a semi-Fowler's position. Mild ascites may require a left lateral decubitus position. The midline is the preferred site but tends to have a thicker abdominal wall. Typically, the lower abdominal quadrants are used with the left lower quadrant being preferred. The right lower quadrant is more likely to have scars and an increased chance that the cecum is distended. Surgical scar areas are avoided because of the likelihood that the needle may enter the bowel. Patients with obesity and/or multiple scars may require ultrasound guidance.

The procedure is performed utilizing sterile technique and a topical anesthetic. Commercial paracentesis kits are available with the necessary equipment for the insertion of the needle/catheter. Once the needle/catheter is inserted, specimens are obtained and the needle/catheter will be stabilized if more fluid is to be removed.

Purpose

The purpose of a paracentesis can be diagnostic or therapeutic. Diagnostic procedures withdraw the appropriate amount of fluid for analysis. Therapeutic procedures commonly withdraw large volumes of fluid to relieve pressure to promote patient comfort, increase mobility, decrease pressure on the bladder, and improve respiratory status.

Indications and Expected Outcomes

Indications for a diagnostic paracentesis and fluid analysis are to:

- Confirm the diagnosis of ascites.
- Diagnose the cause of ascites—approximately 15% of the patients may have a cause other than liver disease and some patients have a dual cause.
- Diagnose infection.
- It may be performed in patients without ascites to evaluate for bleeding following trauma or a perforated viscus.

Indications for a therapeutic paracentesis are:

- Initial treatment of tense ascites
- Refractory ascites

The results of a diagnostic paracentesis will determine the patient's overall management. By confirming the diagnosis and establishing the cause, treatment can be specific to the cause. Identification and treatment of infection are critical to survival. After a therapeutic paracentesis that removes larger volumes of fluid, the patient will be temporarily more comfortable, have greater mobility, less urinary frequency, and improved respiratory status.

Technological Requirements

This procedure is generally performed by a physician or a specifically trained physician's assistant or advanced practice nurse. Ultrasonography should be available for patients with difficult site access.

Nursing Responsibilities

The critical care nurse will have pre-, intra-, and postprocedure responsibilities. The critical care patient requiring a paracentesis will require more intense monitoring depending on the acuity, overall hemodynamic status, and volume to be removed.

Preprocedure responsibilities:

- Verifies informed consent
- Provides patient/family teaching
- Reviews the patient's coagulation studies (abnormal studies are common but are not typically a contraindication)
- Reviews allergy history (especially topical anesthetics, novacaine, lidocaine)

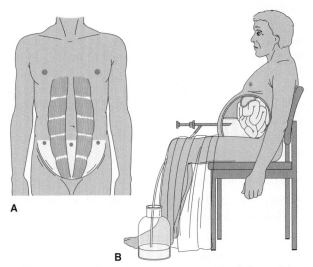

Figure 11-6 Sites and position for paracentesis. *A,* Potential sites of needle or trocar insertion to avoid abdominal organ damage. *B,* The client sits comfortably; in this position, the intestines float back and away from the insertion site.

- If no indwelling catheter, ensures that the patient voids to avoid puncturing a distended bladder
- Measures baseline vital signs, weight
- Ensures proper positioning and appropriate draping

Intraprocedure responsibilities:

- Universal protocol: participates in a "time out" to verify patient identification, procedure, and site marking immediately before the procedure
- Reassures the patient
- Maintains a sterile field and assists the practitioner with obtaining specimens, repositioning, fluid withdrawal, site dressing
- Monitors hemodynamic status for evidence of hypovolemia (drainage can be slowed or stopped for hemodynamic instability)
- Infuses albumin as ordered

Postprocedure responsibilities:

- Monitors hemodynamic status
- Assesses abdominal pain
- Maintains accurate intake and output (amount of fluid removed, colloid/crystalloid infusion)
- Assesses characteristics of fluid withdrawn (color, viscosity, odor)
- Processes specimens per facility protocols
- Monitors dressing for persistent leakage
- Repositions the patient for comfort
- Monitors for signs and symptoms of the following complications:
  - Hemorrhage
  - Perforation of bowel
  - Hypovolemia/shock
  - Infection

Sodium Restriction

Routine daily dietary sodium restriction is 88 mmol/day (2,000 mg). The goal of this intervention is to increase urinary excretion to greater than 78 mmol/L; 10 mmol/L is considered nonurinary losses. Only 10% to 15% of patients attain this excretion goal spontaneously (Such & Runyon, 2006a). Further restriction is possible but often results in noncompliance related to a tasteless diet. A patient on an 88 mmol/L restriction of sodium who is excreting 78 mmol/L should be losing weight. If this is not happening, it is likely that the patient has not been compliant with her diet. In advanced disease, sodium excretion falls to less than 10 mmol/L a day.

Diuretic Therapy

Initial therapy is an oral dose of spironolactone (Aldactone) 100 mg daily. Spironolactone blocks the action of aldosterone and slowly promotes sodium loss and potassium retention (potassium-sparing diuretic). A patient with minimal fluid overload may be managed with monotherapy spironolactone; however, it can be complicated by hyperkalemia and gynecomastia.

Furosemide (Lasix) 40 mg daily, a diuretic that promotes potassium loss as well as fluid loss, is often used in combination with spironolactone to maintain normal potassium and increase fluid loss. If diuresis, as evidenced by weight loss, urine output, and decreased abdominal girth, is insufficient, the doses of the two medications are typically increased simultaneously to help maintain normokalemia. Maximum doses are 160 mg/day for furosemide (Lasix) and 400 mg/day for spironolactone. Dietary sodium restriction and dual diuretic therapy has been successful in achieving acceptable fluid reduction in approximately 90% of patients.

Because of the long half-life (typically 24 hours, prolonged in cirrhosis) of spironolactone, the nurse should be aware that it takes several days after the start for the onset of action to be apparent. It may take up to 2 weeks to a month for a steady state to be achieved. The physician will likely titrate the doses every 3 to 5 days to determine the optimal dose for the patient. If the patient has concurrent renal disease, patient tolerance of spironolactone may be decreased secondary to hyperkalemia. If the patient is managed with dual therapy, furosemide (Lasix) can be held temporally if hypokalemia should occur.

The nurse expects that when ascites is associated with peripheral edema there is no limit to the daily weight loss. In the absence of peripheral edema, the nurse should expect no more that a 0.3 to 0.5 kg/day weight loss. One liter of fluid weighs approximately 1 kilogram or 2.2 pounds. If the desired weight loss is not accomplished, a measurement of the urine sodium excretion may be ordered.

Failure of Diuretic Therapy. Failure of diuretic therapy would be evident by minimal to no weight loss with urine sodium excretion (less than 78 mmol/day) and/or the occurrence of clinically important complications, such as encephalopathy, hyperkalemia, elevated creatinine, or hyponatremia.

The nurse anticipates that diuretic(s) may be discontinued if the following occur:

- Encephalopathy
- Serum sodium less than 120 mmol/L regardless of fluid restriction compliance
- Hyperkalemia (potassium greater than 5.3 mEq/L)
- Metabolic acidosis
- Increased creatinine greater than 2.0 mg/DL

IV administration of a diuretic in patients with cirrhosis and ascites should be avoided because it can cause an acute decrease in glomerular filtration rate.

Fluid Restriction

Fluid restriction is not indicated unless the serum sodium is less than 120 mmol/L, which implies that the kidneys are not excreting free water. As previously noted, cirrhotic patients do not usually develop symptoms unless sodium is less than 110 mmol/L. If not truly warranted, fluid restrictions tend to alienate patients from their health care team. Additionally, it can cause hypernatremia (sodium greater than 145 mEq/L).

Evidence-Based Interventions for the Management of Tense Ascites

Large-volume paracentesis: A paracentesis may be performed on patients presenting with tense ascites and clinically significant symptoms such as shortness of breath, difficulty breathing, and marked decrease in mobility. This does not rectify the underlying problem and it is not recommended as first-line therapy.

In most patients, 4 to 6 liters is removed without causing hemodynamic problems. Albumin infusion can be considered to prevent or decrease intravascular hypovolemia and promote renal perfusion. However, the benefit of the practice is questioned and not all sources are advocates of this practice. Albumin is generally administered 8 to 10 grams per liter removed; usually 50 to 75 grams of a 20% albumin is administered per session. Diuretic therapy and dietary sodium restriction should be initiated and/or adjusted. In patients who have not sought medical attention until their breathing was compromised, large-volume paracentesis can be urgent and greater than 20 liters can be removed safely.

Evidence-Based Interventions for Refractory Ascites

Refractory ascites occurs when fluid mobilization is resistant to sodium restriction and maximal diuretic therapy or if the patient cannot tolerate diuretic therapy. It is managed with routine large-volume paracentesis (Such & Runyon, 2006b). Typically, between 6 and 10 liters of fluid are removed in a patient with no urinary sodium excretion and a dietary restriction of 88 mmol/L. Albumin infusion to avoid hemodynamic difficulties, though controversial as discussed, can be considered when volume removed is expected to be greater than 6 liters. Again, removing the fluid does not alter any mechanisms to decrease ascites; the fluid quickly reorganizes and the patient usually requires a large-volume paracentesis every 2 weeks. This treatment is reserved for patients who truly fail diuretic modalities.

Ascites unresponsive to medical therapy is associated with a 50% 6-month survival and approximately 75% die within a year (Runyon, 2004). Transplant referral should not be delayed in these patients. Mortality rates are higher in patients with alcoholic liver disease.

Surgical Portosystemic Shunts

As described with transjugular intrahepatic portosystemic shunt (TIPS), the placement of these shunts can significantly decrease portal pressure and ascites. Surgical placement has a high morbidity and mortality rate and thus has limited use in patients with ascites. Peritoneovenous shunting, which drains ascitic fluid into the vascular system, is limited to unusual circumstances. This treatment has an increased incidence of complications coupled with no demonstrated survival advantage. It may be considered in a rare patient who is not a candidate for paracentesis, TIPS, or transplant.

Spontaneous Bacterial Peritonitis

Spontaneous bacterial peritonitis (SBP) is an infection in the ascitic fluid without indication of another intra-abdominal source such as a perforated viscus. It is a frequent occurrence in end-stage liver disease. Without early recognition and treatment, mortality is high.

The nurse would review the patient's history for the following predisposing factors:

Elevated serum bilirubin level

Abnormal PT/INR

Child-Pugh classification B or C

GI hemorrhage

Urinary tract infection

Because it is very common for patients with ascites to have SBP on admission, the nurse assesses all appropriate patients for signs and symptoms of SBP. Though the majority of the patients with SBP are symptomatic, the signs and symptoms are often very subtle. Some patients are asymptomatic and only have minor abnormalities in laboratory studies. The nurse assesses for abdominal pain and tenderness; fever; mental status (an infection can exacerbate HE/PSE and sometimes just a minor change in mental status is present); appearance of ascitic fluid.

The nurse would review the following studies for evidence of infection:

- Complete blood count—Elevated white blood cells (WBCs).
- Ascitic fluid PMN leukocyte count—Greater than or equal to 250 cells/mm³. It is rapidly available and it is often sent with culture on hold.
- Ascitic fluid bacterial culture—If PMN is elevated the culture is processed. Typically gram-negative organisms are isolated.

Collaborative Management

The nurse works collaboratively with the health care team to recognize signs and symptoms of SBP, confirm and treat the diagnosis, and prevent future episodes of SBP. The goal is to recognize, successfully treat, and prevent future episodes. Survivors of SBP are evaluated for transplant because they have a poor long-term prognosis.

Diagnostic Paracentesis

As discussed, it is recommended that a diagnostic paracentesis be done on all patients admitted with cirrhosis and ascites. An ascitic fluid analysis should include a cell count with differential, total protein, and albumin concentration and a culture and sensitivity. A clinical diagnosis of SBP without a paracentesis and fluid analysis is not recommended.

Empiric Antibiotic Treatment

Patients with signs and symptoms of SBP, a strong suspicion of SBP, or a PMN count greater than or equal to 250 cells/mm^3 are treated aggressively with empiric therapy. All antibiotic regimens should be reevaluated based on the culture and sensitivity results. Broad-spectrum antibiotics are initially ordered and a narrow-spectrum antibiotic can usually be substituted according to sensitivity results. For certain patients, albumin may be ordered. This is shown to reduce the risk of renal failure and improve survival. Once a patient has had an episode of SBP, the patient should receive long-term antibiotic prophylaxis.

The nurse needs to review allergy history and administer the first dose immediately. Many practitioners will actually write the first dose as a stat order. A typical response to the antibiotic treatment will be evident by the reduction of signs and symptoms, fever, pain, and tenderness within 48 hours. In addition, laboratory studies indicative of infection will return to normal.

The nurse also monitors for hypersensitivity reactions and renal function studies. A repeat paracentesis and fluid analysis is only recommended if within 48 hours there is an atypical response to treatment.

Assessment of Complications of Portal Hypertension

Variceal bleeding is a life-threatening emergency and one of the most significant complications resulting from portal hypertension and cirrhosis. Each episode of active bleeding has a 30% chance of mortality and survivors have a 70% chance of rebleeding (Sanyal, 2006b). More than 50% of the patients awaiting transplant will have a variceal bleed prior to transplant (Gordon, 2007). The portal vein receives blood from the spleen and the intestines. The increased pressure in the portal system causes a backup of blood throughout the digestive vasculature. Additionally, the hyperdynamic circulation resulting from vasodilation increases portal flow. Blood seeks alternate routes and the path of least resistance, which results in the formation of collateral blood vessels in the GI system. The most common locations for these collateral vessels are the esophagus, stomach, and rectum. These vessels, which are intended for low volume and low pressure, become distended, tortuous, and fragile as shown in Figure 11-7.

The high pressure frequently causes the esophageal and/or gastric varicies to rupture and bleed. The most common site for a variceal bleed is the submucosa of the distal end of the esophagus. Gastric varices are less common yet more problematic to manage. It is imperative that the source of bleeding be confirmed. Esophageal variceal bleeding is usually massive related to the high pressure and high volume. Risk factors for bleeding include:

- Decreased clotting factor synthesis, increased platelet destruction by an enlarged spleen, and impaired vitamin K absorption and storage
- The severity of liver disease; the higher the modified Child-Pugh score, the greater the risk of bleeding
- Previous bleed
- Increasing varix size and diameter
- Continued alcohol consumption

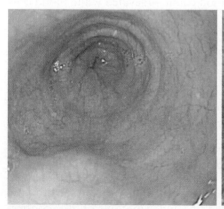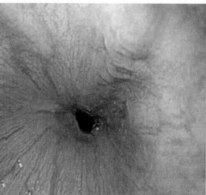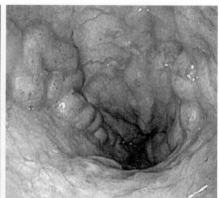

Figure 11-7 Varices increase in diameter progressively.

Collaborative Management

A patient presenting with a suspected variceal bleed is potentially critically ill and may suffer many consequences as a result of the bleed. Variceal bleeding can be massive and management can be complicated by the degree of liver dysfunction, and the presence or absence of coagulopathy, ascites, encephalopathy, and renal involvement. Other complications include aspiration pneumonia, SBP, and sepsis.

Initial assessment and management is the same as for nonvariceal bleeds (see Chapter 11). ∞ The nurse focuses on hemodynamic status, which will direct resuscitation and stabilization efforts. A concurrent history and physical exam needs to focus on the source and severity of the bleed. A team of specialists, including a gastroenterologist/endoscopist, hepatologist, interventional radiologist, and surgeon, must be available for consultation. Differential diagnosis as described under nonvariceal bleeding in Chapter 12 ∞ must be considered, because peptic ulcer disease is more frequent in cirrhotic patients.

For management and evidence-based interventions for the various locations and etiologies of GI bleeds, see Chapter 10. ∞

The goal is to maintain hemodynamic stability, identify the source, implement interventions to stop the bleeding, prevent recurrent bleeding, and prevent and treat complications. In the event that varices are discovered prior to bleeding, the goal is to evaluate them and the degree of liver disease and implement prophylaxis to prevent an initial bleeding event. Additional interventions besides those discussed under Nonvariceal Bleeding for Management of a Variceal Bleed are discussed next.

Assessment of Fluid Volume

Assessment of fluid volume status in the patient with liver disease is discussed earlier in this chapter. The nurse works collaboratively with the health care team to identify and treat hypovolemia. The goal of resuscitation is to restore intravascular volume, maintain the oxygen-carrying capacity of the blood, maintain cardiac output, restore red blood cells, and prevent complications of red blood cell loss such as pulmonary, neurological, cardiac, or renal injury.

Evidence-Based Interventions for Maximizing the Oxygen-Carrying Capacity of the Blood

The nurse protects the patient's airway and supports breathing with supplemental oxygen to maximize the oxygen-carrying capacity of the blood. The oxygen-carrying capacity is decreased by an increased cardiac workload and decreased cardiac output. The nurse will continuously evaluate pulse oximetry and report values less than 92%. With esophageal variceal bleeding, special attention must be directed toward maintaining airway integrity. There is an increased risk of aspiration because bleeding is often brisk with hematemesis, and neurological status may be impaired related to the potential for HE/PSE. Respiratory status is continually assessed, and best practice is to electively intubate and ventilate, avoiding an emergent situation.

Evidence-Based Interventions for Restoration of Normovolemia

Interventions for restoration of normovolemia parallel that which is outlined in the discussion of GI bleeding (see Chapter 12). ∞ Half of the patients with a variceal bleed spontaneously stop bleeding, resulting from hypovolemia triggering splenic vasoconstriction and a decrease in portal pressure. If the patient is hemodynamically stable, caution is taken to avoid fluid overload, which can trigger a rebound increase in portal pressure and increased risk of early rebleeding. Because coagulopathy is commonly present in patients with cirrhosis, patients frequently require aggressive treatment with platelets, fresh frozen plasma (FFP), and vitamin K (Mephyton).

Pharmacological Therapy. Somatostatin is a hormone that has an inhibitory effect on the secretion of several vasodilator hormones (glucagon and vasoactive intestine peptide) that are responsible for splanchnic vasodilation stimulated by blood in the intestines. This, in turn, causes splanchnic vasoconstriction and decreases portal pressure. Octreotide (Sandostatin) is a longer-acting (half-life 80 to 120 minutes) synthetic somatostatin analogue with similar properties. Octreotide (Sandostatin) has an excellent safety profile, even for cardiac patients, and its administration is not limited to ICUs. It may be started when a variceal bleed is highly suspected.

Octreotide is effective in temporarily stopping the bleeding in approximately 80% of the patients. The nurse can expect to administer:

- Octreotide 100 to 150 micrograms IV bolus over 3 minutes
- Followed by 50 micrograms/hour continuous infusion for 3 to 5 days
- Standard dilution is 500 micrograms/250 mL D_5W or normal saline

Higher doses of octreotide may increase systemic venous pressure and do not increase the portal hypotensive effects. To evaluate response to the octreotide (Sandostatin) infusion, the nurse would continue to monitor the patient's hemodynamic status and expect to see the patient's vital signs return to normal, urine output increase, and a decrease in overt bleeding: hematemesis, melena, and hematochezia. Serial hematocrits should be evaluated.

Vasopressin is a potent vasoconstrictor that can decrease portal pressure by directly constricting the mesenteric arterioles. This drug also causes significant systemic vasoconstriction, resulting in myocardial, cerebral, bowel, and limb ischemia. Because of these serious adverse effects, it is generally administered concurrently with a nitroglycerin infusion to try to avoid the systemic vasoconstriction effects. Octreotide (Sandostatin) is the preferred vasoactive agent because of its efficacy and safety profile.

Endoscopic Therapy. Endoscopic sclerotherapy involves injecting a sclerosing (hardening) solution into the varix to stop the bleeding by causing a thrombosis and obliteration of the vein. The nurse should monitor for complications including chest discomfort, sclerosant-induced esophageal ulcers, strictures, and perforations. Esophageal variceal ligation (EVL) involves suctioning the varix into the scope cylinder and deploying a band around the varix. The band strangulates the varix, causing thrombosis and obliteration. Both are effective therapeutic modalities in stopping the bleeding in the majority of the patients. Esophageal band ligation is considered the primary endoscopic therapy and is shown in Figure 11-8. It has fewer complications than sclerotherapy. However, in situations where there is severe active bleeding and poor visibility, banding may be more difficult. The use of endoscopic therapy in combination with a vasoactive agent (octreotide) is more successful than either therapy alone. EVL may be performed every 2 to 4 weeks until the varicies have been eliminated. Repeated surveillance after eradication is recommended every 6 to 12 months.

Ulcer development after banding is common and a small percentage of patients (2% to 5%) will experience bleeding from these ulcers. To decrease bleeding from both the ulcers and the varix, it is also reasonable to administer a daily protein pump inhibitor to prevent ulcer formation and/or promote healing. Proton pump in-

hibitors have a high safety profile, are simple to administer, and are very well tolerated.

See Building Technology Skills in Chapter 12 ∞ for more detailed information about the nursing management of the patient undergoing endoscopic therapy.

Transjugular Intrahepatic Portosystemic Shunt (TIPS)

TIPS is indicated in active variceal bleeding when the patient is refractory to medical therapy.

Building Technology Skills

Transjugular Intrahepatic Portosystemic Shunt (TIPS)

TIPS is a minimally invasive radiological procedure performed with moderate sedation. General anesthesia may be appropriate for hemodynamically unstable patients. It is performed under fluoroscopy to monitor the location of the guidewires and catheters. The jugular vein is accessed with an IV-like catheter called an introducer sheath. All of the work will take place through this sheath.

A guidewire is introduced and advanced through the heart to the hepatic vein. A catheter with a needle is directed by the guidewire and is passed through the wall of the hepatic vein through the body of the liver into the portal vein. This creates a narrow pathway between the branch of the portal vein and the hepatic vein. A catheter with a deflated balloon is advanced over the guidewire to the tunneled area. Once in position, the balloon is inflated to dilate the area and widen the track between the branch of the portal vein and the hepatic vein.

An expandable metal mesh stent (tube), loaded onto another specialized catheter, is advanced over the guidewire to the tunneled area connecting the portal venous system with the hepatic venous system. The stent is then deployed or left in place.

Purpose

The purpose is to manage complications of portal hypertension. The stent creates a passage between the high-pressure portal vein and the low-pressure hepatic vein. It decompresses the portal venous system and reduces elevated portal pressure to decrease rebleeding from varices and stop or reduce the formation of ascites. It allows blood to flow in the normal direction through the liver or from the portal system to the hepatic vein (bypassing the liver) to the vena cava. It does not have any effect on liver function (Boyer & Hasal, 2005).

Indications and Expected Outcomes

The primary indications for TIPS are:

* Acute variceal bleeding uncontrolled by pharmacological and endoscopic therapy

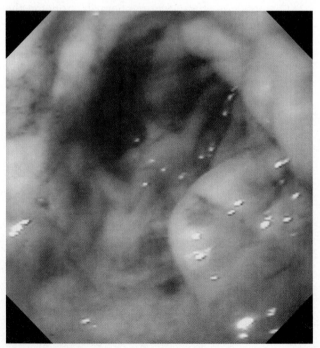

Figure 11-8 Endoscopic banding of esophageal varices.

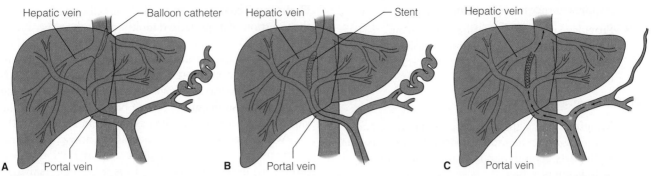

Figure 11-9 Transjugular intrahepatic portosystemic shunt (TIPS). *A*, Guided by angiography, a balloon catheter inserted via the jugular vein is advanced to the hepatic veins and through the substance of the liver to create a portacaval (portal vein-to-vein cava) channel. *B*, A metal stent is positioned into the channel and expanded by inflating the balloon. *C*, The stent remains in place after the catheter is removed, creating a shunt for blood to flow directly from the portal vein into the hepatic vein.

- Recurrent variceal bleeding that is refractory or intolerant to secondary prophylaxis treatments
- Refractory ascites that are intolerant to repeated large-volume paracentesis that may require a transplant

Prior to a TIPS procedure, the patient undergoes an extensive evaluation including liver function tests, coagulation studies, kidney function tests, and imaging to access portal venous system patency and to exclude any liver masses. If the patient has a cardiac history, additional tests may be ordered to rule out heart failure. Absolute contraindications include:

- Severe pulmonary hypertension
- Congestive heart failure
- Systemic infection sepsis (uncontrolled)
- Unrelieved biliary obstruction
- Primary prophylaxis for variceal bleed
- Multiple hepatic cysts

A multidisciplinary approach including the transplant team must look at the risks of the procedure in high-risk patients and address the probability of whether the patient will survive long enough after the procedure to receive a liver transplant.

The expected outcome is that portal pressure will be reduced. In the case of variceal bleeds the hope is to lower the portal pressure, therefore decreasing the pressure in the varices to control the acute bleeding and prevent a recurrent bleed. In refractory ascites, the goals are to decrease production of ascites, eliminate the need for serial paracentesis, and increase the efficacy of other interventions. Because more blood is now bypassing the liver and not being exposed to liver cells that detoxify toxins, more toxins are going directly to the systemic circulation. Hepatic encephalopathy, an anticipated complication of portal hypertension, often appears or worsens after TIPS.

Technological Requirements

Technology requirements include a medical facility that has the radiology equipment, an interventional radiologist, and a support team with expertise in performing such a complex advanced procedure. TIPS avoids the risks of major surgery and, in most cases, that of general anesthesia. However, there are complications associated with the insertion of TIPS:

- Potential reaction to sedation medication/anesthesia
- Cardiac arrhythmias as the catheter is being passed through the heart
- Complications related to creation of the intrahepatic shunt, portal vein manipulation, and stent placement

Nursing Responsibilities

The critical care nurse has both pre- and postprocedural responsibilities.

Preprocedural responsibilities:

- Maintains NPO status for 6 to 8 hours prior to the procedure
- Monitors baseline vital signs including temperature and oxygen saturation
- Evaluates neurological status, LOC, presence of HE/PSE
- Ensures that performed consent has been obtained
- Provides patient/family education
- Determines allergies, especially to contrast solution/topical anesthetics
- Reviews the patient's platelet count and PT/INR. The recommendation is to have a platelet count greater than 60,000 and an INR less than 1.4; however, this is not absolute. The nurse can anticipate the administration of clotting factors or platelets to patients with significant coagulopathy.

- Inquires about antibiotic administration
- Provides Situational Briefing Assessment Record (SBAR) report to interventional radiology nurse/anesthesiologist on transfer (see Chapter 1) ∞

Postprocedural responsibilities:

- Monitors vital signs including temperature and oxygen saturation and compares them to baseline
  - Reports hemodynamic changes, which may indicate bleeding
  - Assesses and treats pain (patients often complain of muscle stiffness)
  - Monitors the insertion site for bruising
  - Monitors for fever or other signs and symptoms of infection
  - Monitors for potential complications related to the portosystemic shunting

To detect HE/PSE—(the incidence is about 30%) (Sanyal, 2006a), the nurse reviews the patient's history for risk factors, including advanced disease, older age, prior history of HE/PSE, and evaluates the patient's neurological status paying attention to the new onset or worsening of symptoms of HE/PSE. The nurse can anticipate initiating standard therapy to those patients who are symptomatic.

The nurse provides education to patient/family because HE/PSE may not appear until 2 to 3 weeks after the procedure. If HE/PSE appears after 6 weeks, patients should notify the physician because the cause is often GI bleeding.

The nurse assesses for the development of additional complications such as Hemolytic anemia—(may present in 7 to 10 days after the TIPS procedure), severe hyperbilirubinemia, and vegetative infections.

The nurse monitors for the development of stent occlusion since the likelihood of stent stenosis has been high (especially in the first year). Coated stents are now being used and studies have been favorable for decreasing the incidence of stenosis.

The nurse educates the patient and family about the signs and symptoms of recurring portal hypertension evident by the reoccurrence of the initial problem(s) (GI bleeding, returning ascites) and the importance of scheduled follow-up visits for evaluation of stent patency (usually at 3- to 6-month intervals).

Surgery

Improvements in endoscopic therapeutic technologies have decreased the need for surgical intervention. There are several surgical options available; however, the 30-day mortality rate nears 80% (Zaman & Chalasani, 2005). In the event of an acute bleeding episode, surgery is limited to those patients who fail medical therapy and where TIPS is not available.

Balloon Tamponade. Balloon tamponade involves the insertion of a specialized multilumen tube either orally or nasally. The tube may have a gastric balloon or, more commonly, a gastric and esophageal balloon. Once inflated, the balloons exert direct pressure (a tamponade effect) on the gastric esophageal junction and the bleeding areas of the esophagus to reduce blood flow through the varix and control the bleeding as shown in Figure 11-10.

With increased use and success of endoscopic therapeutic interventions and the placement of TIPS, this procedure is used infrequently. It is a rescue (salvage) procedure to achieve stabilization when the patient has been unresponsive to medical therapy. It is considered short term to be used as a bridge for a more definitive procedure. It can be successful in accomplishing short-term hemostasis; however, serious complications can occur and there is a high rate of rebleeding once the balloon is deflated. The most common tubes are the Sengstaken-Blakemore tube (three lumens, gastric and esophageal balloon), the Minnesota tube (four lumens, gastric and esophageal balloon), and Linton-Nachlas tube (three lumens, gastric balloon only).

The tube is inserted by a physician according to the manufacturer's instructions. Placement is confirmed by chest radiography. The patient is likely to be critically ill with hemodynamic instability requiring resuscitation. Caring for a patient with one of these tubes requires very specific nursing interventions. The nurse will continuously monitor the patient's respiratory and hemodynamic status. It is recommended that the patient be intubated and sedated prior to insertion to secure airway integrity and prevent aspiration. If the patient is not inubated, the biggest concern is the migration of the

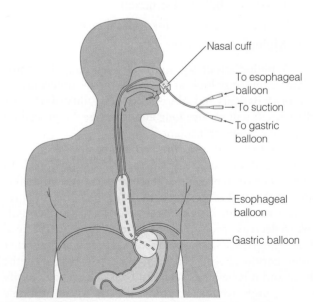

Figure 11-10 Triple-lumen nasogastric tube (Sengstaken-Blakemore) used to control bleeding esophageal varices.

esophageal balloon over the airway. Because of this potential complication, scissors are taped to the bedside and travel with the patient for emergency removal of the tamponade tube. Migration is commonly caused by inadvertent deflation of the gastric balloon. Balloon pressures and traction are monitored at regular intervals. There may be an order to routinely deflate the esophageal balloon for a short period (e.g., 5 minutes every 4 to 6 hours) to avoid pressure injury to the mucosa.

Esophageal and gastric aspirate are assessed for color and amount. Gastric lavage may be ordered. Evidence that the balloon tamponade has been successful in causing hemostasis would be confirmed by clear gastric and esophageal aspirate, stabilization of vital signs, and increase in urine output. The patient requires frequent mouth care and skin assessments around the insertion site. The patient may require continued sedation. Chest pain is a frequent complaint that must be thoroughly investigated. Potential complications include:

- Aspiration
- Tissue injury: ulceration/necrosis
- Perforated esophagus
- Airway compromise
- Tracheal rupture/fistula

Though bleeding stops in 90% of the patients, the majority of the patients rebleed. Once the balloons are deflated, the patients need to be monitored for rebleeding and scheduled for additional treatment modalities.

Prevention of Initial and Recurrent Bleeding from Esophageal Varices

Assessment and management of esophageal varices involves identifying patients with probable progressive liver disease. Once the diagnosis of progressive liver disease is suspected or confirmed, the main goal is to identify the presence of varices and to prevent the first variceal bleeding. Once the patient has bled, secondary prophylaxis is initiated to eradicate the varices and prevent a rebleed. The nurse should be aware that the greatest risk for rebleeding is within 48 to 72 hours and that 50% of all early rebleeding occurs within the first 10 days (Sanyal, 2005b). Because of this high risk, secondary prophylaxis treatment is typically started shortly after the first bleeding episode.

Nonselective beta-blocker therapy is the treatment of choice for primary prophylaxis. Studies have shown that beta blockers decrease the risk of an initial bleed by 45% to 50% (Sanyal, 2007). They are also indicated for secondary prophylaxis following a bleed.

If the patient who has a variceal bleed was not receiving beta-blocker therapy as discussed it may be instituted after a bleeding episode. If the patient has bled despite the use of beta blockers, the addition of a long-acting nitrate, specifically isosorbide mononitrate

---

▎ COMMONLY USED MEDICATIONS

BETA BLOCKERS

Action: Beta blockers decrease cardiac output and block mesenteric arteriole vasodilation, promoting vasoconstriction and a subsequent decrease in portal venous flow. The goal of treatment is to decrease portal and variceal pressure.

Nursing Responsibilities: Either propranolol (Inderal) or nadolol (Corgard) are recommended for primary prophylaxis. The dosage should be titrated to reduce the patient's heart rate by 25%. Some practitioners prefer nadolol because it can be administered once a day, it is excreted in the kidneys, and it has a lower risk of CNS side effects:

- Typical starting dose of nadolol (Corgard) is 40 mg daily (40 to 160 mg orally daily).
- Typical starting dose of propranolol (Inderal) is 40 mg two times a day (40 to 80 mg two times a day).
- Response to the beta blockade is determined by monitoring the patient's heart rate. The goal is to achieve a heart rate of 50 to 60 beats per minute.
- If patients receive high doses without a decrease in pulse rate, individual noncompliance should be considered. Higher doses cause more side effects.
- Nadolol is excreted by the kidneys; thus, renal function must be considered and monitored. Doses may need to be adjusted according to renal insufficiency.

Side and/or Toxic Effects: Because there are numerous side effects associated with beta blockers, they may be contraindicated or not tolerated. Often intolerance is related to headaches, and noncompliance is related to sexual dysfunction and impotence. Clinically significant adverse effects for a patient with cirrhosis include:

- Heart failure
- Bronchoconstriction
- Hypotension—if the patient has a significant systemic hypotension to begin with (MAP less than 85 mm Hg), a lower dose (nadolol 20 mg daily) can be tried

The nurse must monitor the patients for adverse effects of the medication such as heart rate less than targeted rate, hypotension, orthostatic symptoms, respiratory distress, and headache. In an acute bleed, the nurse must be aware that beta blockers can mask the compensatory tachycardia needed to maintain cardiac output. The nurse also needs to educate the patient related to the importance of the medication, the significance of noncompliance, and stopping the medication abruptly.

(Imdur), to the beta-blocker regime can further reduce the rate of recurrent bleeding (Zaman & Chalasani, 2005). Nitrates cause dilation in the venous bed, decreasing portal venous blood flow, thus portal pressure. After a bleed or when beta-blocker therapy is not getting a therapeutic response, isosorbide mononitrate (Imdur) can be added. Because of severe hypotension and headaches, patients usually do not tolerate this course of therapy.

Complication of Portal Hypertension: Hepatic Encephalopathy

HE, also known as PSE, is a condition characterized by a wide range of potentially reversible neuropsychiatric manifestations that occurs in patients with advanced liver disease and portal hypertension. It may be a single event or a frequent occurrence. These manifestations result from a disturbance in the CNS because of impaired liver function. The manifestations can be subtle and intermittent, or progressive with overt confusion and coma. As the encephalopathy progresses, the manifestations become more noticeable. The degree of neurological and intellectual dysfunction of HE is often referred to in clinical stages ranging from I to IV. Because coma may be impending, some practitioners will transition to the Glasgow Coma Scale (see Chapter 9). ∞

The pathogenesis is complex, it is not clearly defined, and it is beyond the scope of this chapter. In cirrhosis, ammonia is a significant factor in the pathogenesis of HE because elevated ammonia levels are present and interventions to decrease ammonia improve HE.

- Ammonia, produced primarily by the GI tract, enters the circulation via the portal vein to the liver.
- The functioning liver detoxifies ammonia before it can reach the systemic circulation. Through a series of enzymatic reactions, ammonia is converted to glutamine, a nontoxic substance, and urea for secretion by the kidneys.
- In advanced liver disease, detoxification is inefficient, resulting in ammonia entering the systemic circulation and consequently the CNS.
- Ammonia is neurotoxic and can interfere with cerebral function and neurotransmission, resulting in changes in consciousness and behavior.
- Portal systemic shunting from the development of collaterals is also responsible for substances absorbed by the gut, bypassing the liver into the systemic circulation without being detoxified.
- Muscle is also a site for ammonia clearance; many patients with advanced liver disease have severe muscle atrophy that may also contribute to an increase in ammonia.

Precipitating factors for HE include:

- GI hemorrhage (metabolism of blood protein in the gut)
- Azotemia/uremia (retention of blood nitrogenous substances by the kidney)
- Electrolyte abnormalities (especially hypokalemia, which increases ammonia production by the kidneys, and hypokalemia and alkalosis, which promote cellular uptake of ammonia)
- Constipation (increases ammonia related to bacterial action on the feces)
- Excessive dietary protein
- Dehydration (vomiting, diarrhea, hemorrhage, diuretics, large-volume paracentesis)

- Blood bypassing the liver and entering the systemic circulation following surgical or radiological shunting procedures)
- Infections
- Medications such as benzodiazepines, narcotics, other sedatives

The majority of the patients with chronic HE have a precipitating cause rather than a progression of hepatocyte dysfunction.

Assessment of the Patient with Hepatic Encephalopathy

Critical care monitoring of a patient with HE involves reviewing the patient's history for severity of liver disease, previous episodes of HE, precipitating factors as discussed, and possible differential diagnoses causing neurological impairment. Medications should also be evaluated as a causative agent. The nurse should routinely assess:

- Respiratory status: airway maintenance and oxygenation
- Safety related to decreased LOC and confusion: fall and aspiration precautions
- Neurological status: for signs and symptoms of impaired personality/behavior, consciousness, and intellectual and neuromuscular functioning. Manifestations are on a progressive continuum and referenced in four stages from mild impairment to coma. Variations in the literature exist related to the exact manifestations in each stage.
  - Stage I—Impaired/shortened attention, lack of awareness, euphoria or depression, inversion of sleep pattern, slight tremor
  - Stage II—Lethargy, memory problems, behavioral changes, slurred speech, tremor progresses to asterixis, apraxia, ataxia
  - Stage III—Somnolence, marked confusion, disorientation, amnesia, asterixis, abusive, violent
  - Stage IV—Coma
  - Glasgow Coma Scale (see Chapter 9) ∞

It is imperative that the nurse identify rapid deterioration promptly and report changes immediately. Rapid changes could be resulting from an acute event.

The nurse anticipates that an array of routine laboratory and imaging tests may be performed to screen for precipitating factors and differential diagnoses or causes of cerebral dysfunction. Tests may include, but are not limited to, CBC, electrolytes, BUN, creatinine, arterial blood gases, glucose, toxic screen, head CT, or EEG. Of particular interest is the blood ammonia level because an elevated ammonia is associated with HE. Because of other neurotoxic substances, a normal ammonia does not exclude the diagnosis.

Collaborative Management

The goal of management is to provide supportive care (airway maintenance, safety [aspiration precautions/fall prevention], adequate nutrition), identify and treat precipitating factors, reduce nitrogenous waste from the gut, and evaluate the need for long-term treatment interventions.

Identification and Correction of Precipitating Factors

All precipitating factors should be aggressively investigated. Determination of specific causes should direct immediate corrective actions. For example, if the patient is hypokalemic, potassium supplementation should be provided. If corrective actions are taken, the nurse anticipates an improvement in neurological status. The time frames for improvement depend on the cause and treatment.

Evidence-Based Interventions for Reduction of Nitrogenous Waste from the Gut

The goal of treatment is to reduce ammonia production and/or increase its removal and lower elevated ammonia levels. This may occur by a variety of methods. One of the simplest is bowel cleansing. Because nitrogenous wastes are produced primarily in the gut, bowel cleansing can reduce colonic bacteria responsible for synthesizing ammonia and thus decrease the amount of ammonia reaching the systemic circulation.

However, lactulose (Cephulac) is the cornerstone of treatment of HE.

Oral antibiotics administration is typically limited to patients who are intolerant or unresponsive to nonabsorbable disaccharides. They work mostly by decreasing the number of colonic bacteria, resulting in decreased enzyme activity responsible for producing ammonia. Neomycin was used for years but because of its nephrotoxicity and ototoxicity, it has limited long-term use and should be avoided (Ferenci, 2006). Alternative antibiotics may be used, but clinical data are lacking. The potential to cause diarrhea, malabsorption, and bacterial overgrowth syndromes must be considered. Chronic use requires meticulous monitoring including renal and neurological status.

Collaborative Management

Hepatorenal syndrome (HRS) is a progressive reversible form of functional renal failure in a patient who has advanced liver disease and ascites. It is characteristic of a progressive sequence of vasoactive circulatory derangements that occur in advanced liver disease, causing a decrease in renal perfusion and glomerular filtration rate. The pathophysiology is complex, but, ultimately, there is profound renal vasoconstriction and prevailing peripheral vasodilation. In this syndrome, the kidneys

COMMONLY USED MEDICATIONS

LACTULOSE

Action: The result of lactulose (Cephulac) and its catabolism by the bacteria flora is a lowering of the colon pH to about 5.0. This causes the formation of a nonabsorbable form of ammonia and trapping it in the colon. Because it is a cathartic, it speeds up transit through the colon, increasing the excretion of nitrogen. Most studies have found that lactulose has successfully decreased ammonia levels and improved encephalopathy in 80% of the cases. The nurse continues to monitor neurological status and expects to see an improvement in severe HE. It can take up to 48 to 72 hours to see a response.

Nursing Responsibilities:
- Lactulose may be administered in a variety of routes and schedules. In an acute situation to induce a rapid drop in serum ammonia, lactulose 45 mL may be ordered orally every hour until a bowel movement occurs.
- A sweet, syrupy liquid, it may be administered orally or through a nasogastric tube (NGT) for comatose patients or for patients with a decreased level of consciousness.
- If the patient cannot tolerate oral or gastric feeding, it may be administered as a retention enema. Then, lactulose (Cephulac) 200 g (300 mL) is diluted in 700 mL to 1 liter of water and ideally retained for an hour. It may be administered with a balloon (Foley) catheter to facilitate retention.
- It may be repeated every 4 to 6 hours as necessary. As a maintenance dose to prevent HE, lactulose 20 to 30 g (30 to 45 mL) may be administered three or four times a day, titrated to achieve two to four soft, controllable bowel movements per day.

Side and/or Toxic Effects: The nurse anticipates that the patient may experience mild side effects such as bloating, flatulence, and cramps. The nurse should evaluate the patient for the development of tolerance to the side effects. Severe side effects such as diarrhea, dehydration, and acidosis need to be addressed. Diarrhea may indicate overdosage and usually responds to dose reduction. The nurse anticipates a dose adjustment or stopping the medication temporarily or permanently if tolerance does not improve.

have no intrinsic renal disease and are histologically normal. A nephrology consult is mandatory.

The diagnosis is one of exclusion and it is important to distinguish HRS from prerenal azotemia and acute tubular necrosis. Manifestations include a decrease in urine output and difficulty managing ascites. The patient may also experience nausea, drowsiness, and thirst that is often indistinguishable from the way the patient typically feels. Eventually, manifestations include hemodynamic instability, oliguria, and coma.

There are two types of HRS. Type I is more serious with acute deterioration and a mortality rate of 80% in 2 weeks (Wadei, Mai, Ahsan, & Gonwa, 2006). Often there is an acute precipitating event such as GI bleeding, bacterial infection, or large-volume paracentesis. Type II is less severe with a gradual progression, subtle onset, and a medium survival of 6 months (Wadei et al., 2006). There is typically no precipitating factor other than worsening of the liver disease. The mortality of patients with ALF who develop HRS is significantly worse. Outcomes of patients with HRS depend on improving or reversing hepatic failure. In the setting of end-stage liver disease, transplantation is the only cure for appropriate candidates.

Assessment and management focuses on prevention, prompt recognition, and treatments to improve glomerular filtration rate (GFR). Prevention stresses meticulous management of ascites, especially diuretics, to avoid overdosing and prevention of precipitating factors. Pharmacological therapy and albumin infusion can be considered in an attempt to manipulate renal and systemic hemodynamics to prolong survival until the patient can undergo a transplant. Appropriate patients may benefit from a TIPS procedure that may also prolong survival to receive a transplant. TIPS has been associated with a gradual improvement in GFR. Renal replacement therapy is also a consideration but often controversial in the setting of end-stage liver disease. Appropriate patients may be selected for dialysis as a bridge to transplantation. The risks of dialysis in this patient population are significant. Liver transplantation early in the course of HRS will most likely reestablish kidney function. Later in the course of the disease, patients may need a liver and kidney transplant. Recognizing that the patients/families are facing a grave situation, the nurse needs to evaluate their understanding and assess the need for the appropriate support services.

Nursing Care

Nursing care of the patient with chronic liver disease can be challenging. The nurse must provide for the patient's comfort while ensuring the patient's safety. It is also the responsibility of the nurse to ensure that the patient is adequately nourished to prevent the problems associated with protein calorie malnutrition.

Pain

Pain should be assessed and treated using a standardized scale, and the facility's pain management protocols should be followed. Patients with liver disease can have both acute and chronic pain from a variety of causes unrelated to their liver disease. Patients with ascites often complain of abdominal pain and low back pain, and patients with gynecomastia often have breast pain.

Patients with mild disease usually have no analgesic medication restrictions. As liver disease worsens, consideration must be given to both the choice of drug as well as the dose (Hamilton, Goldberg, & Chopra, 2005). However, there is no exact criteria or cutoff for modifying drugs and dosages. Generally, patients with cirrhosis, especially those with evidence of portal hypertension, should have their analgesic medications modified. Patients requiring long-term analgesia should be referred to a pain management program. General consid-

erations related to analgesic medications and cirrhosis include the following:

- Nonsteroidal anti-inflammatory drugs should be avoided. They are associated with an increase in the risk of variceal bleeding, impaired renal function, and the development of refractory ascites.
- Opioids should be used with caution and are typically prescribed in reduced doses with prolonged intervals between doses related to decreased clearance and increased bioavailability.
- For patients who are not drinking alcohol, acetaminophen when used in low doses is a safe analgesia. Between 2 and 4 grams per day is suggested.

Pruritus

Itching can be a major source of discomfort for patients. It is caused by the accumulation of bile acids under the skin. It can be treated with medications that bind with the bile acids and prevent them from accumulating under the skin. Common medications are cholestyramine, colestipol, and colesevelam. Additionally, diphenhydramine may be prescribed at night for relief of symptoms and sedative effect. The nurse should caution the patient if a sedative effect is an issue. It is also helpful to keep the patient's nails short and to provide distractions.

Safety

All patients need to be assessed for risk of falls. Patients with advanced liver disease often have ascites and peripheral edema, which restrict their mobility and make ambulation very difficult. Patients experiencing HE may have varying degrees of confusion and disorientation. Fall assessments and prevention protocols should be appropriately implemented.

Patients with altered mental status and decreased level of consciousness are also at risk for aspiration, especially during a variceal bleeding with hematemesis. The nurse should assess the patient's risk and implement aspiration precautions as necessary.

Skin integrity is a concern for critically ill patients who are likely confined to bed related to ascites, peripheral edema, and immobility. Additionally, the patient with advanced liver disease is often malnourished, which is also a major risk factor for skin breakdown. The nurse should assess the patient's risk for skin breakdown by using an objective numerical assessment tool (e.g., Braden Scale). Depending on the risk, prevention measures according to hospital protocol or the guidelines published by the Agency for Health Care Policy and Research (AHCPR) should be implemented.

Provision of Adequate Nutrition

In cirrhosis, protein calorie malnutrition (PCM) is prevalent and often considered a complication, increasing the rate of variceal bleeding, infection, and HE, and influencing both morbidity and mortality. PCM is a diet deficient in calories and proteins that results in body wasting. Additionally, PCM has considerable consequences for patients who may be awaiting transplantation since it may lead to increased complications and postoperative mortality (Henkel & Buchman, 2006).

Patients with HE should be managed with medications and should not have a protein restriction. They actually have an increased need for protein, and limiting it will accelerate PCM. Limiting protein can result in a negative nitrogen balance, weight loss, weakness, malnutrition, and an increased chance of infection. If a patient is awaiting transplant, these factors can significantly influence post-transplant outcomes.

In an acute HE episode, protein may be withdrawn for a day or so, followed by increasing intake according to clinical tolerance. A nutritional consult should be completed to design an individual diet for the patient, evaluate adequate nitrogen intake, and discuss the feasibility of substituting vegetable protein for other sources of protein. Vegetable proteins are preferred over animal sources because they have a higher calorie-to-nitrogen ratio and are less likely to cause HE.

An increase in protein intake and tolerance may also be accomplished by combining other therapies. It is recommended that the restriction of dietary protein be reserved for patients with HE that cannot be controlled in any other way (Blei & Cordoba, 2001). In these cases, a 70 g protein restriction is recommended. Overall, it is recommended that chronic liver disease patients receive 35 to 40 cal/kg/day of nonprotein energy and 1.5 g/kg/day as protein (Sargent, 2006). The nurse may be required to document protein calorie intake and monitor weight. Continued monitoring of neurological status is necessary to evaluate therapeutic effect.

FACTORS THAT INTERFERE WITH ADEQUATE NUTRITION

The nurse needs to be aware of the following factors that interfere with eating, causing insufficient intake in the patient with cirrhosis:

- Anorexia, nausea, and vomiting
- Early satiety (fullness) (increased pressure and compression from ascites)
- Bloating, abdominal distention, constipation, or diarrhea
- Alterations in taste and smell (possibly related to vitamin A and/or zinc deficiency)
- Unpleasant, tasteless diets (low sodium, other restrictions as discussed)
- Fatigue, lack of activity
- Encephalopathy (altered mental status)
- Alcohol

Other factors contributing to PCM include disturbances in carbohydrate, protein and lipid metabolism, malabsorption and vitamin deficiencies, increased energy expenditure, decreased motility, and the increased use of fat stores rather than carbohydrates for fuel.

Nutritional Assessment and Chronic Liver Disease

All patients with chronic liver disease should have a nutritional assessment and interventional plan for nursing to promote. Most likely, patients with compensated disease will be prescribed a normal, balanced, healthy diet with adequate calories, proteins, fats, and carbohydrates. Depending on the cause of the liver disease, vitamins and minerals may be prescribed, but megadoses should be avoided because these may also cause hepatotoxicity. All herbal supplements and nontraditional herbal remedies should be discussed with the physician and nutritionist. The goal is to follow these patients closely to recognize disease progression and implement therapy to prevent PCM.

As the liver disease progresses, the patient's nutritional status is often a challenge and needs close intervention and monitoring. Many of the markers that are typically used for assessment are no longer effective. With ascites and edema, the nurse recognizes that weight is not an accurate measure and that laboratory studies, especially albumin, are also unreliable. The nutritionist can employ several other assessment techniques to evaluate the patient's nutritional status. The goals for nutritional interventions are to prevent PCM, improve existing PCM, and correct nutrient deficiencies.

Prevention of Infection

Twenty percent of the patients with cirrhosis who are admitted with an active bleed have a bacterial infection present on admission, and another 50% of the patients are likely to develop an infection while in the hospital (Sanyal, 2005a). Urinary tract infections, SBP, and respiratory and primary bacteremia are the most common sources of infection. Acute bleeds are often associated with gut translocation and motility issues causing bacterial infections. Infected cirrhotic patients also have a higher rebleeding rate. Therefore, it is imperative that the nurse utilize all appropriate methods to prevent infection. This includes hand washing, implementing the central line bundle, preventing catheter associated urinary tract infections (CAUTI), providing adequate nutrition by the enteral route when possible, and instituting the ventilator bundle (if appropriate). See Chapter 17 for details. ∞

The presence of infection in this population also increases mortality, and studies have shown that the administration of antibiotics may significantly reduce mortality and recurrent bleeding (Sanyal, 2005a). The benefit of antibiotics is likely greater in patients with advanced liver disease. Reasonable practice is to treat all patients with an active bleed with prophylactic antibiotics.

The nurse anticipates the administration of prophylactic antibiotics. If an infection is suspected on admission, appropriate cultures may be ordered. However, in the presence of a massive hemorrhage, cultures will not be a priority and antibiotics will be administered. The nurse must review the patient's allergy history and administer according to facility protocol. Patients need to be monitored for hypersensitivity reactions, evidence of infection/sepsis, and renal function throughout the course of therapy. Antibiotics known to cause nephrotoxicity should be avoided.

ALCOHOL WITHDRAWAL/LIVER FAILURE SUMMARY

Alcohol abuse and dependency can affect an individual's personal, social, and vocational relationships as well as having acute and chronic effects on all physiological systems. Prompt identification and treatment of patients at risk for or who are experiencing AWS, prevention and treatment of complications, and provision of the appropriate level of care directed by clinical assessments are fundamental to positive patient outcomes.

Liver failure is very complex and presents many challenges to the health care team. Though the time frames and durations differ, both acute and chronic liver failure have serious life-threatening complications and implications for transplantation. Acute liver failure is a medical emergency requiring prompt diagnosis, identification, and treatment of the cause and determination of candidacy for liver transplantation. The prognosis of end-stage liver disease or cirrhosis is variable and does not always have end-of-life implications. The health care team may encounter patients experiencing either compensated or decompensated disease. No matter what stage, the nurse's role as an educator and advocate is instrumental in engaging the patient and family to actively participate in their care. It is imperative that patients and families understand the effects of cirrhosis on all body systems and the importance of vigilant compliance with treatment.

CASE STUDY

Barbara Ramsey is a 39-year-old woman admitted to the ICU from the emergency department (ED). On arrival in the ED, her blood pressure was 60 systolic. She says she vomited bright red blood with large clots three times at home then fainted. She just vomited approximately 250 mL on admission to the ICU. On admission to the ED, her hematocrit was 24, her hemoglobin was 8, her systolic blood pressure was 62 mm Hg, and her pulse rate was 146 bpm. She has received a liter of normal saline and two units of blood already. Her blood pressure is now 82 systolic.

Barbara is known to the facility. She was discharged a week earlier after being admitted for bleeding esophageal varices and ascites. In the past, she stated that she drank a pint of vodka with crème de menthe chasers daily. She is scheduled for an immediate endoscopy with possible banding of esophageal varices.

1. What should be the first priority in Barbara's care?

2. What additional information would the nurse want to obtain?

3. What factors are contributing to the severity of Barbara's bleeding?

4. What factors contributed to the likelihood that Barbara would rebleed from her varices?

5. What should the nurse do to prepare Barbara for endoscopy and possible banding?

6. What alternatives are there to banding to control bleeding from esophageal varices?

7. Should the nurse be concerned that Barbara might undergo AWS during this hospitalization?

A day later, Barbara no longer responds to her name. She is disoriented but arousable in the afternoon, but her speech is incomprehensible. By the evening, she is no longer arousable.

8. How should the nurse respond to the change in Barbara's mental status?

9. What is probably happening to Barbara? What is the most likely collaborative management?

Because Barbara has had repeated esophageal bleeding and multiple episodes of ascites, she might be considered for TIPS.

10. Would Barbara be a good candidate for TIPS? Why or why not?

See answers to Case Studies in the Answer Section at the back of the book.

CRITICAL THINKING QUESTIONS

1. What is the relationship between the pharmacological effects of alcohol and the cause of withdrawal?

2. What are the essential components of a focused assessment to screen for alcohol abuse and dependency and the risk for AWS?

3. What is the role of the CIWA-Ar scale in the collaborative management of AWS?

4. What is the clinical significance of a patient developing the DTs?

5. What is the clinical distinction between alcohol hallucinosis and the DTs?

6. What are the safety concerns in the nursing management of AWS?

7. Why are benzodiazepines the drug of choice for the management of AWS? What are the nursing considerations in the administration of benzodiazepines?

8. What is the clinical significance of AWS developing in a critical care patient?

9. Explain the differences between acute liver failure and chronic liver failure.

10. Why is acetaminophen overdose dangerous?

11. When and how is acetylcysteine utilized as an antidote for acetaminophen overdose?

12. What is the relationship between portal hypertension and the development of decompensated liver disease?

13. What are the essential assessments that the nurse should perform for the patient with decompensated liver disease?

14. What are the nursing responsibilities for the patient with ascites or hepatic encephalopathy?

See answers to Critical Thinking Questions in the Answer Section at the back of the book.

EXPLORE MEDIALINK
http://www.prenhall.com/perrin

Additional interactive resources for this chapter can be found on the Web site at http://www.prenhall.com/perrin. Click on "Chapter 11" to select activities for this chapter.

Case Study: Alcohol Withdrawal

Nursing Care Plan

NCLEX Review Questions

MediaLinks:
- Al-Anon Family Group Headquarters Inc.
- Al-Anon World Service Office
- Al-Anon/Alateen
- Alcoholics Anonymous
- American Association for the Study of Liver Disease (AASLD)
- American Gastroenterological Association (AGA)
- American Society for Gastroenterology (ASGE)
- American Liver Foundation

- American Society for Nutrition
- National Institute on Alcohol Abuse and Alcoholism (NIAAA)
- Rational Recovery
- Substance Abuse and Mental Health Services Administration
- SAMHSA's National Clearinghouse for Alcohol and Drug Information
- The National Institute of Diabetes and Digestive and Kidney Diseases
- The Society of Gastroenterology Nurses and Associated (SGNA)
- UpToDate Patient Information

MediaLink Applications

REFERENCES

Al-Sanouri, I., Dikin, M., & Soubani, A. (2005). Critical care aspects of alcohol abuse. *South Medicine Journal, 98*(3), 372–381.

American Psychiatric Association. (2000). *Diagnostic and statistical manual of mental disorders* (4th ed., Text Revision). Washington, DC: Author.

Blei, A., & Cordoba, J. (2001). Practice guidelines: Hepatic encephalopathy. *The American Journal of Gastroenterology, 96*(7), 1968–1976.

Boyer, T., & Hasal, Z. (2005). ASSLD practice guideline: The role of transjugular intrahepatic portosystemic shunt in the management of portal hypertension. *Hepatology, 41*(2), 1–15.

Burns, M., Friedman, S., & Larson, A. (2007). Acetaminophen (paracetamol) intoxication in adults. *UpToDate.* Retrieved July 2, 2007, from http://www.utol.com/utd/content/topic/.do?topicKey=ad_tox/5914&view=print

Ewing, J. A. (1984). Detecting alcoholism. The CAGE questionnaire. *Journal of the American Medical Association, 252*(14), 1905–1907.

Farrell, S. (2006). Acetaminophen toxicity. *eMedicine.* Retrieved June 27, 2007, from http://www.emedicine.com/emerg/topic819.htm

Ferenci, P. (2006). Pathogenesis of hepatic encephalopathy. *UpToDate.* Retrieved February 19, 2007, from http://www.utol.com/utd/content/topic/.do?topicKey=cirrhosi/7310&view=print

Fontana, R. (2006). Acute liver failure. In M. Feldman, L. Friedman, & L. Brandt, *Sleisenger and Fortram's gastrointestinal and liver diseases pathophysiology/diagnosis/management* (8th ed., pp. 1993–2005). Philadelphia: Saunders Elsevier.

Gold, M., & Aronson, M. (2006). Screening for and diagnosis of patients with alcohol problems. *UpToDate.* Retrieved January 27, 2007, from http://www.utol.com/utd/content/topic/.do?topicKey=genr_med/8664&view=textt

Goldberg, E., & Chopra, S. (2005). Fulminant hepatic failure: Definition; etiology; and prognostic indicators. *UpToDate.* Retrieved February 14, 2007, from http://www.utol.com/utd/content/topic/.do?topicKey=hep_dis/14112&view=print

Goldberg, E., & Chopra, S. (2006). Overview of the complications, prognosis and management of cirrhosis. *UpToDate.* Retrieved January 23, 2007, from http://www.utol.com/utd/content/topic/.do?topicKey=cirrhosi/9247&view=print

Gordon, F. (2007). *100 questions and answers about liver transplantation: A Lahey Clinic Guide.* Sudury, MA: Jones and Bartlett.

Gossman, W. (2005). Delirium tremens. *eMedicine.* Retrieved April 24, 2007, from http://www.emedicine.com/EMERG/topic123.htm

Hamilton, J., Goldberg, E., & Chopra, S. (2005). Management of pain in patients with cirrhosis. *UpToDate.* Retrieved January 23, 2007, from http://www.utol.com/utd/content/topic/.do?=cirrhosi/11256&view=print

Henkel, A., & Buchman, A. (2006). Nutritional support in chronic liver disease. *National Clinical Practice of Gastroenterology and Hepatology, 3*(4), 202–209.

Kee, J. L. (2005). *Laboratory and diagnostic tests with nursing implications* (7th ed.). Upper Saddle River, NJ: Pearson Prentice Hall.

Kennedy, M. (2004). Benzodiazepines, barbiturates, and nursing interventions: Dealing with delirium tremens. *American Journal of Nursing, 104*(10), 21.

Mayo-Smith, M., Beecher, L., Fisher, T., Gorelick, D., Guillaume, J., Hill, A., et al. (2004). Management of alcohol withdrawal delirium: An evidence-based practice guideline. *Archives of Internal Medicine, 164*(7), 1405–1412.

McKay, A., Koranda, A., & Axen, D. (2004). Using a symptom triggered approach to manage patients in acute alcohol withdrawal. *Medsurg Nursing, 13*(1), 15–20.

McKinley, M. (2005). Alcohol withdrawal syndrome: Overlooked and mismanaged. *Critical Care Nurse, 25*(3), 40–49.

National Institute on Alcohol Abuse and Alcoholism (NIAAA) Publication. (2005). *Alcohol Alert: Screening for alcohol use and alcohol related problems.* Retrieved April 15, 2007, from http://pubs.niaaa.nih.gov/publications/aa65/AA65.htm

National Institute on Alcohol Abuse and Alcoholism (NIAAA) Publication. (2005). *A pocket guide for alcohol screening and brief intervention.* Retrieved November 24, 2007, from http://pubs.niaaa.nih.gov/publications/Practitioner/pocketguide/pocket_guide2.htm

Polson, J., & Lee, W. (2005). AASLD position paper: The management of acute liver failure. American Association for the Study of Liver Diseases. *Hepatology, 41*(5), 1179–1197.

Puz, C., & Stokes, S. (2005). Alcohol withdrawal syndrome: Assessment and treatment with the use of the Clinical Institute Withdrawal Assessment for Alcohol-Revised. *Critical Care Nursing Clinics of North America, 17,* 297–304.

Runyon, B. (2004). AASLD practice guideline: Management of adult patients with ascites due to cirrhosis. *Hepatology, 39*(3), 1–16

Sanyal, A. (2005a). General principles of the management of variceal hemorrhage. *UpToDate.* Retrieved January 27, 2007, from http://www.utol.com/utd/content/topic/.do?topicKey=cirrhosi/6248&view=text

Sanyal, A. (2005b). Indications and contraindications to the use of transjugular intrahepatic portosystemic shunts. *UpToDate.* Retrieved July 16, 2007, from http://www.utol.com/

utd/content/topic/.do?topicKey=cirrhosi/8755&view=print

Sanyal, A. (2006a). Complications of transjugular intrahepatic portosystemic shunts. *UpToDate.* Retrieved July 16, 2007, from http://www.utol.com/utd/content/topic/.do?topicKey=cirrhosi/573&view=text

Sanyal, A. (2006b). Prediction of variceal hemorrhage in patients with cirrhosis. *UpToDate.* Retrieved January 27, 2007, from http://www.utol.com/utd/content/topic/.do?topicKey=cirrhosi/2191&view=text

Sanyal, A. (2007). Primary prophylaxis against variceal hemorrhage in patients with cirrhosis. *UpToDate.* Retrieved July 6, 2007, from http://www.utol.com/utd/content/topic/.do?topicKey=cirrhosi/2523&view=print

Sargent, S. (2006). Management of patients with advanced liver disease. *Nursing Standard, 21*(11), 48–56.

Such, J., & Runyon, B. (2006a). Initial therapy of ascites in patients with cirrhosis. *UpToDate.* Retrieved July 2, 2007, from http://www.utol.com/utd/content/topic/.do?topicKey=cirrhosi/6767&view=print

Such, J., & Runyon, B. (2006b). Pathogenesis of ascites in patients with cirrhosis. *UpToDate.* Retrieved July 2, 2007, from http://www.utol.com/utd/content/topic/.do?topicKey=cirrhosi/7934&view=print

Wadei, H., Mai, M., Ahsan, N., & Gonwa, T. (2006). Hepatorenal syndrome: Pathophysiology and management. *Clinical Journal of the American Society of Nephrology, 1,* 1066–1079.

Weinhouse, G., & Manaker, S. (2006). Alcohol withdrawal syndromes. *UpToDate.* Retrieved April 9, 2007, from http://www.utol.com/utd/content/topic/.do?topicKey=ad_tox/4456&view=print

Zaman, A., & Chalasani, N. (2005). Bleeding caused by portal hypertension. *Gastrointestinal Clinics of North America, 34*(4), 623–642.

Care of the Patient with an Acute Gastrointestinal Bleed or Pancreatitis

June Kasper, MSN, RN, CGRN

Learning Outcomes

Upon completion of this chapter, the learner will be able to:

1. List common risk factors and causes of gastrointestinal bleeding.

2. Describe clinical manifestations of gastrointestinal bleeding.

3. Compare and contrast upper and lower gastrointestinal bleeding.

4. Explain the significance of hemodynamic status relative to blood loss.

5. Describe collaborative management and nursing responsibilities for a patient with a gastrointestinal bleed.

6. Discuss the importance of endoscopy in the care of the patient with gastrointestinal bleeding.

7. List the predisposing factors for pancreatitis.

8. Explain why the predisposing factors may result in pancreatitis.

9. Differentiate between the manifestations of mild and severe pancreatitis.

10. Describe collaborative management and nursing responsibilities when caring for the patient with severe pancreatitis.

chapter 12

Abbreviations

EGD	Esophagogastroduodenoscopy
FFP	Fresh Frozen Plasma
FNA	Fine Needle Aspiration
LGI	Lower Gastrointestinal
MSOF	Multisystem Organ Failure
PPIs	Proton Pump Inhibitors
SIRS	Systemic Inflammatory Response Syndrome
UGI	Upper Gastrointestinal

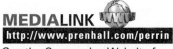

MEDIALINK
http://www.prenhall.com/perrin

See the Companion Website for chapter-specific resources at www.prenhall.com/perrin.

VISUAL MAP (Gastrointestinal Bleeding Overview

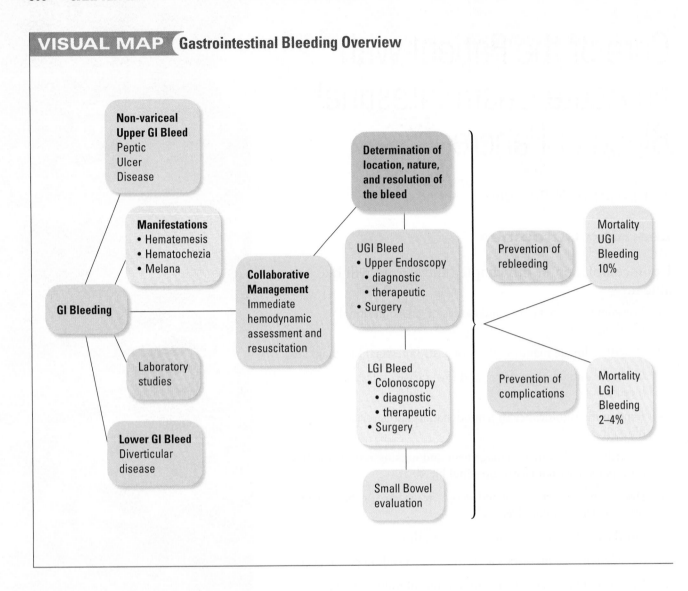

Gastrointestinal (GI) bleeding is a common medical condition accounting for 300,000 hospital admissions each year in the United States (Rockey, 2005). Bleeding can occur from numerous types of lesions anywhere in the GI tract. Upper gastrointestinal (UGI) bleeding originates proximal to the ligament of Treitz. It is five times more common than lower gastrointestinal (LGI) bleeding, which is bleeding distal to the ligament of Treitz. The overall mortality rate is approximately 10% (Ferguson & Mitchell, 2005) for UGI bleeds and 2% to 4% (Bounds & Friedman, 2003) for LGI bleeds.

Best practice is a multidisciplinary team approach. Management focuses on immediate assessment, hemodynamic stabilization, identifying the source, and stopping and treating the bleeding. Patients admitted to the hospital for another medical condition who develop GI bleeding while in the hospital have poorer outcomes (Ferguson & Mitchell, 2005).

Acute **pancreatitis** is a sudden inflammatory process of the pancreas responsible for 210,000 admissions per year in the United States (Banks & Freeman, 2006). The clinical course ranges from a mild interstitial self-limiting illness to a severe life-threatening disorder. Initial treatment is directed at identifying and correcting the cause. Gallstone disease and excessive alcohol use are the most common causes of acute pancreatitis, accounting for an estimated 80%. Management is supportive and emphasizes aggressive fluid management to prevent complications, most notably hypovolemia and hypoxemia. Pancreatic necrosis and the presence, timing, and duration of organ failure influence morbidity and mortality. The majority of the patients with severe pancreatitis without organ failure survive, whereas those with multisystem organ failure (MSOF) have a median mortality of 47% (Banks & Freeman, 2006).

Anatomy and Physiology Review

The GI tract begins at the oral cavity and ends at the anus (Figure 12-1). The structures of the GI tract have overlapping function yet each has an area of specialization and distinct histological characteristics. The major functions of the GI tract include:

* Ingestion
* Mechanical processing
* Digestion
* Secretion
* Absorption
* Excretion

The Gastrointestinal Tract

The structures of the GI tract include the esophagus, stomach, small intestine, ileocecal valve, and large intestine.

The esophagus is a hollow muscular tube, approximately 10 inches long and 1 inch wide, that carries solids and liquids from the pharynx to the stomach. The stomach is a J-shaped organ located below the diaphragm between the esophagus and the small intestine. Functions include storage of food, mechanical breakdown of food, production of gastric secretions (pH 1.0–4.0), and intrinsic factor. The small intestine is a tubular structure, approximately 20 to 25 feet long and $1\frac{1}{2}$ inches wide, responsible for most of the important digestive and absorptive functions. It consists of three sections: the duodenum is 10 inches long with the

Figure 12-1 Organs of the alimentary canal and related accessory organs.

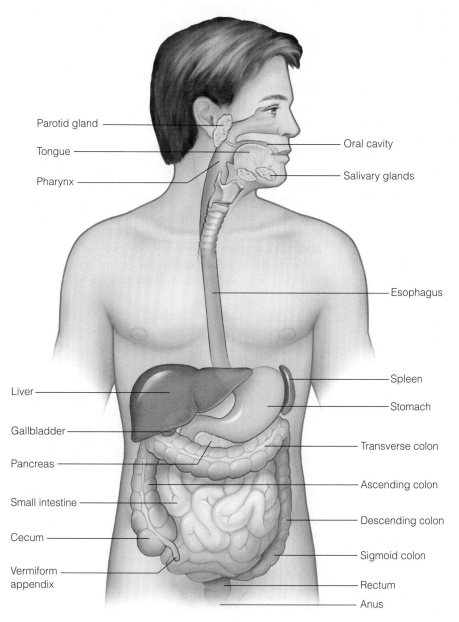

Parotid gland

Tongue

Pharynx

Oral cavity

Salivary glands

Esophagus

Liver

Gallbladder

Pancreas

Small intestine

Cecum

Vermiform appendix

Spleen

Stomach

Transverse colon

Ascending colon

Descending colon

Sigmoid colon

Rectum

Anus

terminal landmark, the "Ligament of Treitz"; the jejunum is 8 feet long; and the ileum is 12 feet long. The distal end of the ileum connects to the large intestine. The ileocecal valve marks the transition between the small and the large intestines. The large intestine is a tubular structure, approximately 5 to 6 feet long and 1 to 2 inches wide. It consists of five sections: cecum/ascending colon, transverse colon, descending colon, sigmoid colon, and rectum. It functions to eliminate wastes and absorb water and electrolytes.

The Pancreas

The pancreas is an elongated, lobulated gland that lies behind the stomach in the retroperitoneal space and extends from the duodenum to the spleen (Figure 12-2). It is an accessory organ to the GI tract with both exocrine and endocrine functions. In addition, the pancreas has both a cellular and a ductal system.

The pancreas is divided into three segments: the head, which lies over the vena cava in the C-shaped curve of the duodenum; the body, which lies behind the duodenum and extends across the abdomen behind the stomach and across the spine; and the tail, which is situated under the spleen.

Cellular Systems of the Pancreas

Exocrine cells make up 98% to 99% of the pancreatic tissue and are responsible for the production of pancreatic juices and digestive enzymes that assist with the breakdown of nutrients in the intestines to facilitate absorption.

Acini cells—the functional cells of the exocrine pancreas responsible for producing pancreatic enzymes.

Pancreatic juices—made up of water and bicarbonate, which neutralizes the acidic chyme, thus protecting the intestines from acid damage.

Pancreatic enzymes.

The major types of pancreatic enzymes are:

Amylase—responsible for breaking down certain starches.

Lipase—responsible for breaking down certain complex fats.

Proteases—responsible for breaking down proteins. These enzymes are stored within the pancreas as proenzymes (inactive enzymes).

Proenzymes serve to protect the pancreatic cells and tissues from the destructive effects of their own products. Trypsinogen, a protease and precursor of trypsin, is activated in the duodenum and is a catalyst for activating other enzymes. Trypsin inhibitor is produced by the pancreas to prevent enzymes from being activated before they reach the duodenum. Should these enzymes become activated prior to reaching the duodenum, autodigestion of the pancreatic tissue can occur.

Endocrine cells make up 1% to 2% of the pancreatic tissue. They are found mostly in the tail of the pancreas in an area known as the islets of Langerhans. They secrete hormones directly into the bloodstream.

Pancreatic Ductal System

The main pancreatic duct, the "Duct of Wirsung," runs the whole length of the pancreas from left to right. It joins the common bile duct at an area known as the ampulla of Vater. The papilla of Vater is a nipple-like protrusion where the common bile duct and the pancreatic duct penetrate the duodenum. At the point where the common bile duct opens into the duodenum is the sphincter of Oddi, a circular muscle constricting the opening. This

Figure 12-2 The pancreas. The gross anatomy of the pancreas. The head of the pancreas is tucked into a C-shaped curve of the duodenum that begins at the pylorus of the stomach.

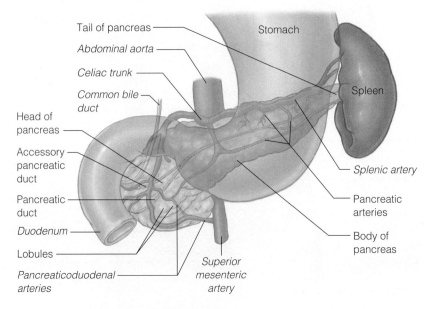

Tail of pancreas
Abdominal aorta
Celiac trunk
Common bile duct
Head of pancreas
Accessory pancreatic duct
Pancreatic duct
Duodenum
Lobules
Pancreaticoduodenal arteries
Stomach
Spleen
Splenic artery
Pancreatic arteries
Body of pancreas
Superior mesenteric artery

sphincter relaxes to promote drainage and constricts to prevent reflux.

Gastrointestinal Hemorrhage

GI bleeding is one of the most common reasons for a patient to be admitted to an intensive care unit (ICU). In addition, approximately 25% of critically ill patients develop a GI bleed during their hospitalization. In most of these instances, the bleeding is self-limited. However, in some patients, it may be life threatening.

Predisposing Factors and Causes of Gastrointestinal Hemorrhage

UGI bleeding is classified as variceal (see Chapter 11) ∞ or nonvariceal. Peptic ulcer disease accounts for approximately 55% (Jutabha & Jensen, 2006a) of the nonvariceal UGI bleeds, and diverticular disease accounts for approximately 20% to 50% (Strate, 2005) of LGI bleeds. LGI bleeds often present with less severity than UGI bleeds. Patients with LGI bleeds are less likely to manifest orthostasis or shock or require blood transfusions.

Peptic Ulcer Disease

Peptic ulcer disease typically refers to ulcers in the stomach and the first part of the duodenum. However, some sources also include esophageal ulcers. The difference between ulcers and erosions is the depth of penetration. Erosions are superficial and do not involve the smooth muscle layer. Figure 12-3 displays a peptic ulcer with an adherent clot.

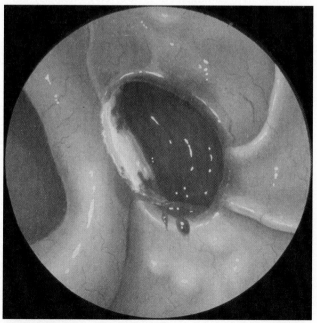

Figure 12-3 Peptic ulcer disease.

The major risk factors for peptic ulcer disease (Jutabha & Jensen, 2006b) are:

- **Helicobacter pylori**—a highly mobile bacterium that avoids acid by burring underneath the mucosa. It causes the mucosa to be more susceptible to peptic acid damage and provokes an inflammatory response, which results in further epithelial injury.
- Nonsteroidal anti-inflammatory drugs (NSAIDs)—cause local and systemic effects that promote mucosal damage.
- Stress ulcers—develop in hospitalized patients with serious illnesses. GI bleeding secondary to these lesions is associated with a fivefold increase in mortality (Weinhouse & Manaker, 2006). The cause may relate to a disproportion in the production of gastric acid and mechanisms to protect the mucosa. Mucosal ischemia may also be a contributing factor. Common risk factors include mechanical ventilation (greater than 48 hours) and coagulopathy.
- Gastric acid and pepsin are co-contributors to the above etiologies. Because of the mucosal impairment, there is increased permeability of acid. In rare occasions, hyperactivity of these secretions can cause ulcers.

Other less frequent causes include:

- Mallory-Weis tear—mucosal lacerations at the gastroesophageal junctions or the cardia of the stomach associated with wrenching and vomiting
- Erosive esophagitis, gastritis, or duodenitis
- Benign or malignant tumors
- Vascular abnormalities

Other contributing factors include smoking and alcohol abuse. Smoking is thought to increase the risk of developing ulcers and impair their healing. Alcohol abuse is also thought to interfere with the healing process.

Clinical risk assessment and prediction of patient outcomes is based on clinical, laboratory, and endoscopic data. Endoscopy within 24 hours of admission has reduced the hospital length of stay and may reduce the incidence of rebleeding and the need for surgical intervention (Ferguson & Mitchell, 2005). Clinical factors linked to poorer outcomes include:

- Hemodynamic instability
- Multiple blood transfusions
- Presence of bright red blood in emesis or stool
- Age greater than 60
- Concurrent illnesses
- Coagulopathy

- Continued bleeding or rebleeding (especially within 72 hours of initial bleed)
- Hospitalized for other problems
- Emergent surgical intervention

Diverticular Disease

Diverticular disease results from weak points on the intestinal wall that herniate to form a saclike projection called diverticula (Figure 12-4). They are most often found in the descending and sigmoid colon, but they can be found throughout the colon. Despite the prevalence in the left side, bleeding is frequently proximal to the splenic flexure.

Bleeding results from rupture of submucosal arterial vessels (vasa rectae) either on the dome or from the neck of the diverticulum. Clinical presentation is usually acute, painless passage of bright red blood. Such bleeding has not been correlated with inflammation (diverticulitis). Age is a very important factor for suspected LGI bleeds because advanced age is the most significant risk factor for the development of diverticula. As the incidence of LGI bleeds increases with age, comorbidities have a significant impact on mortality.

Other less common causes include:

- Ischemic colitis
- Vascular ectasis (angiodysplasia, angioectasis)
- Anorectal disease (hemorrhoids, anal fissures)
- Neoplasms (small intestine/large intestine)
- Postpolypectomy bleed
- NSAID usage

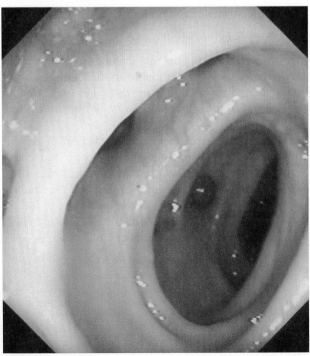

Figure 12-4 Diverticular disease.

Manifestations of Gastrointestinal Bleeding

The most common manifestations of GI bleeding are hematemesis, hematochezia, and melena. **Hematemesis** is vomiting of blood that is either bright red or has a coffee grounds appearance, indicating UGI bleeding. Coffee grounds appearance is caused when blood is mixed with digestive juices. Usually the bleeding has slowed or stopped. **Hematochezia** is the passage of bright red blood from the rectum. It may or may not be mixed with stool. Hematochezia suggests an LGI bleed; however, it can originate from many different sites including the UGI tract. Generally, the higher the site, the more significant the bleed. **Melena** is the passage of black tarry colored stool. It has a very characteristic foul odor. Melena can result from as little as 50 to 100 mL of blood in the stomach. It reflects the action of intestinal contents on the blood. Generally, it suggests a UGI bleed, but the source can also arise from the small bowel or ascending colon.

Typically, the patient with a UGI bleed presents with hematemesis and/or melena, whereas an LGI bleed is suspected in patients with hematochezia. Though helpful in evaluating the source, stool color is not absolute. Both UGI and LGI bleeders can have melena, and a patient with a massive UGI bleed can have hematochezia.

Collaborative Management

Initial assessment focuses on hemodynamic status with a concurrent history and physical focusing on the source and the severity of the bleeding. Historical elements and manifestations may distinguish a UGI bleed from an LGI bleed. Further assessments focus on rebleeding.

Immediate management is directed by hemodynamics and may involve immediate resuscitation and stabilization. A team of specialists including an endoscopist/gastroenterologist and a surgeon should be available for consultation. The goal is to identify the source, stop and treat the bleeding, prevent recurrent bleeding, and prevent and treat complications. A prompt and accurate diagnosis and the severity of the bleeding will direct therapeutic interventions and decrease mortality and complications. Severe bleeds will require ICU monitoring, which has been shown to promote positive outcomes and decrease mortality.

Assessment of Fluid Volume Status

The critical care nurse will evaluate for the extent of blood loss by immediately assessing the patient's hemodynamic status. Assessment of vital signs is the best way to evaluate stability, amount of blood loss, and suddenness of the loss and the extent of cardiac and vascular compensation. They can also provide prognostic information. The nurse assesses for mani-

VISUAL MAP Gastrointestinal Bleeding Assessment

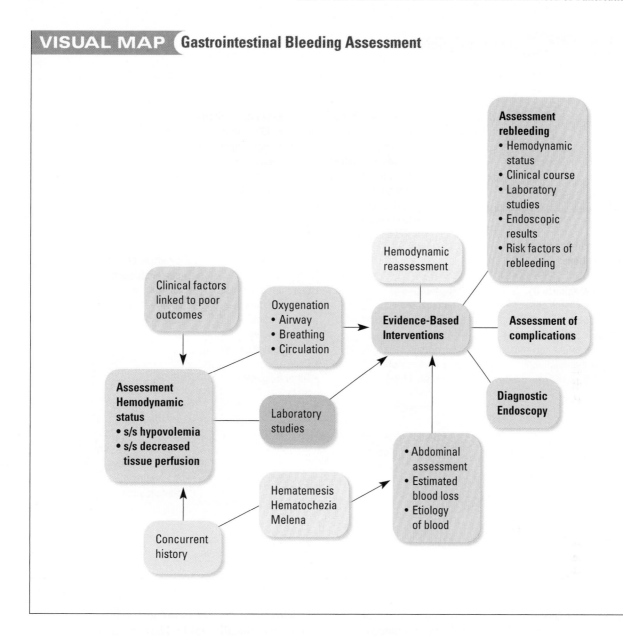

festations of hypovolemia and poor tissue perfusion, including:

- Hypotension (systolic blood pressure less than 90 and mean arterial pressure less than 60 mm Hg).
- Narrowed pulse pressure.
- Orthostatic hypotension—if the patient is not hypotensive, orthostatic signs can pick up smaller volume depletions. Blood pressure (BP) greater than 10 mm Hg decrease or greater than 20 mm Hg increase in heart rate indicates loss of at least 15%.
- Tachycardia (heart rate greater than 100).
- Electrocardiogram (ECG) changes, dysrhythmias, and ST changes in response to ischemia. Advanced age and a history of cardiac disease can increase risk of ischemia.

- Chest pain.
- Capillary refill greater than 3 seconds with cold clammy skin and weak peripheral pulses.
- Dry mucous membranes, poor skin turgor, and flat jugular veins.
- Decreased urine output (less than 30 cc/hour).
- Mental status changes.

Significant comorbidities or hemodynamic instability may necessitate more invasive monitoring, thus the patient may have an indwelling urinary catheter, a central venous pressure (CVP) line, or a pulmonary artery (PA) line (see Chapter 5). ∞ The nurse will assess the characteristics of overt blood loss from hematemesis, melena, and/or hematochezia.

VISUAL MAP GI Bleeding Collaborative Management

Evaluative criteria:
- Pulse oximetry >92%
- Effective breathing patterns
- ABG's prn

Evaluative criteria:
- Hemodynamic stability
- Increased/stable hematocrit
- Adequate tissue perfusion
- Urine output >30 cc/hour

Evaluative criteria:
- NGT aspirate
- Endoscopic evaluation/ treatment
- Hemodynamic stability

Evidenced-based interventions

Maximize O₂ carrying capacity of the blood:
- Supplemental O₂
- Intubation and ventilation

Restoration of normovolemia:
- Fluid resuscitation
  - Crystalloid normal saline
  - Transfusions
    - Red blood cells
    - Platelets
    - FFP
  - Blood warming
- Serial hematocrits

Determining location, nature, and resolution of the bleeding:
- NGT placement
- Endoscopy
- Other diagnostic tests
- Octreotide
- Surgical consult

Prevention of recurrent bleeding:
- Gastric acid suppression

Nursing considerations:
- Maintenance of breathing patterns
- Provision of comfort and safety
- Lessen anxiety
- Prevention of complications

Calculation of blood loss relative to the amount of measured melena or hematochezia is difficult and inaccurate related to being mixed with stool. The nurse recognizes the significance of the patient's hemodynamic vital signs relative to estimated blood loss (see Chapter 8). ∞ The nurse should remember that the sickest patients are the easiest to diagnose. It is the patients with less than 30% blood loss who are more difficult to recognize. Although it is important not to underestimate blood loss, the rate of blood loss is often more critical than the volume.

Laboratory Studies

Additionally the nurse reviews the following laboratory studies:

- Hematocrit—The initial hematocrit may not reflect the degree of blood loss, because there is a delay in intravascular equilibrium that will not immediately reflect blood loss. Patients with chronic slow bleeding may have a very low

baseline hematocrit but are generally hemodynamically stable. Hematocrit is evaluated in perspective with the clinical picture.

- Platelets—A low platelet count may indicate a preexisting thrombocytopenia that needs to be treated.

- Electrolytes—May be abnormal related to vomiting and diarrhea.

- Blood Urea Nitrogen (BUN)/Creatinine—These are evaluated to assess hydration status and renal function. A rise in the BUN may be seen from digested blood proteins being broken down by intestinal bacteria to urea. Typically, there is not a proportional rise in creatinine. A BUN-to-creatinine ratio of 36 or greater suggests UGI bleed in patients without renal insufficiency.

- Prothrombin Time (PT)/International Normalization Ratio (INR)—May indicate preexisting coagulopathy that needs to be treated. It may also be a marker for liver disease.

- Liver Function Tests—Liver function is evaluated to assess for the presence of liver disease.
- Type and Cross-match—Needs to be procured and processed immediately on all patients suspected of a GI bleed to determine blood type.

Collaborative Management

The nurse works collaboratively with the health care team to identify and treat hypovolemia. The goal of resuscitation is to restore intravascular volume, maintain cardiac output, restore blood cells, and prevent complications of red blood cell loss such as pulmonary, neurological, cardiac, and renal injury.

Evidence-Based Interventions to Maximize Oxygen-Carrying Capacity of the Blood Oxygen

The nurse protects the patient's airway and supports his breathing with supplemental oxygen to maximize oxygen-carrying capacity of the blood. The nurse will continuously evaluate pulse oximetry and report values less than 92%. In the event of a massive UGI bleed and/or hemodynamic instability, the need for intubation and ventilation should be evaluated.

Evidence-Based Interventions for Restoration of Normovolemia

Early aggressive resuscitation has been shown to improve patient outcomes. The patient should have two large-bore intravenous catheters placed immediately. The initial resuscitation protocol for hemodynamic instability is the rapid administration of a crystalloid solution, generally normal saline (lactated Ringer's may be preferred by some clinicians), to replace intravascular volume and prevent shock. The crystalloid solution provides adequate circulation for the remaining erythrocytes until the type and cross-matched blood is obtained.

Total fluid deficit cannot be accurately predicted, and fluid resuscitation should remain rapid rate as long as the BP remains low. Other clinical parameters guiding resuscitation are vital signs, urine output, mental status, and peripheral perfusion. The nurse anticipates that the patient's vital signs shall begin to normalize and the urine output will increase within 15 to 20 minutes of the challenge. However, if severe bleeding continues, the vital signs may continue to deteriorate and the patient may experience shock (see Chapter 6). ∞

The nurse closely monitors the patient's cardiovascular and respiratory status for tolerance of rapid infusion rates. Patients with a history of heart failure, valvular disease, pulmonary disease, and other comorbidities may need a PA line to minimize risk for fluid overload. The nurse looks for clinical indications of fluid overload, including:

- Abnormal lung sounds
- Tachypnea/shortness of breath
- Peripheral edema and neck vein distention
- Weight gain
- Chest pain
- Tachycardia
- Oxygen desaturation

Blood Transfusions

The decision to transfuse the patient with blood is based on the patient's clinical picture. There is no single hematocrit value that justifies a transfusion. A patient with chronic anemia and a low hematocrit may receive alternate therapies, whereas a patient with an acute GI bleed may be transfused. Even in the presence of an acute GI bleed, the decision to transfuse will be individualized. Generally, the hematocrit should be kept greater than 20% for young, previously healthy individuals and greater than 30% for elderly or patients with severe comorbid illnesses (Rockey, 2005). However, these values will vary with different practitioners.

The following variables must be considered:

- Hemodynamic status/unstable vital signs
- Age
- Estimated blood loss/severity
- Evidence of active bleeding/rate of bleeding/risk for rebleeding
- Comorbidities, especially cardiovascular/pulmonary disease
- Hematocrit

Packed Red Blood Cells. The nurse anticipates the infusion of packed red blood cells (RBCs) primarily to prevent or alleviate signs and symptoms of inadequate oxygen tissue delivery. The number of units infused and the rate of infusion will again depend on multiple individual variables as discussed. Typically, patients with hemodynamic instability have had considerable blood loss and will require a blood transfusion. Patients with evidence of continued bleeding, poor tissue oxygenation, unresolved hemodynamic instability, and repeatedly low hematocrits will require aggressive transfusion therapy (Rockey, 2005). In rare emergent situations, whole blood may be ordered while awaiting cross-matched blood.

The nurse follows facility protocols for administering blood and blood products and will monitor the patient closely for transfusion reactions. The nurse anticipates that serial hematocrits will be monitored after initial crystalloid resuscitation, the plasma volume may be overexpanded, and an immediate post-transfusion hematocrit may underestimate the final value. Generally, a 300-mL unit of packed RBCs will raise the hematocrit approximately 3%. Given adequate time to equilibrate, an absence of an increased or a decreased hematocrit should cause concern. For additional information on blood transfusions, see Chapter 8. ∞ Hematocrits should not be a replacement for continuing clinical assessment.

If the patient receives multiple transfusions, blood is delivered through a blood warmer to prevent a decrease in body temperature (hypothermia).

Platelets/Fresh Frozen Plasma (FFP)/ Cryoprecipiate (Factor VIII). Preexisting coagulopathy (PT greater than 13 seconds/INR greater than 1.5) or thrombocytopenia (platelets less than 50,000/ul) necessitates the infusion of fresh frozen plasma (FFP) or platelets, respectively. These products are also administered if the patient receives multiple units of RBCs, because the platelets and clotting factors become diluted. Generally, platelets are administered after 10 units of RBCs and FFP after 8 units of RBCs.

Patient Positioning

If a patient's BP is less than 90 mm Hg systolic, the nurse should consider positioning the patient supine with legs elevated to facilitate venous blood return to the right atrium. As the BP returns to normal, the patient's legs can be gradually lowered while the nurse monitors carefully for BP changes.

Nursing Management

Soon after the emergent assessment and resuscitation efforts, the nurse needs to review the patient's clinical history and perform a more focused physical exam. Patient's history must be reviewed for significant risk factors and clues to the etiology and severity of the bleed. The physical examination, including clinical presentation and emesis/stool characteristics, are essential for evaluation of site and acuity.

Key historical elements include:

- Demographics—common disorders according to age
- Previous or current GI disease
- Prior surgery
- Aspirin/NSAID ingestion
- Alcohol abuse/dependence
- Liver disease
- Anticoagulants/clotting disorders
- Pain
- Vomiting/retching, weight loss, anorexia, change in bowel habits
- Non-GI disorders (pulmonary/nasopharyngeal)

The physical exam should focus on abdominal assessment; evidence of liver disease; and quantity, frequency, and characteristics of emesis/stool as shown in Table 12–1.

- Hematochezia or melena is indicative of active bleeding.
- Brown stool is unlikely to have active bleeding.
- Infrequent stools are not likely to have active bleeding.
- Coffee grounds emesis may indicate slowed or stopped bleeding.

Collaborative Management

The nurse works collaboratively with the health care team to identify the etiology of the bleeding and patients at high risk for continued or rebleeding and to resolve continued active bleeding. The etiology of the bleed, risk for rebleeding, and the presence of continued active bleeding will direct further decisions and interventions. The goal is to identify the source, stop the bleeding, and predict risk for rebleeding (ASGE, 2001b). The nurse will assist with modalities to identify the source of the GI bleeding so that it can be appropriately managed.

Nasogastric Tube Placement

There is controversy related to the value of nasogastric tube (NGT) placement. NGT insertion should be considered in certain patients because the results can be of prognostic value (Barkun, Bardou, & Marshall, 2003). Nasogastric aspirate can help to validate UGI bleeding, but it does not provide information about the specific cause of the bleeding. Insertion of an NGT solely for information related to bleeding activity/acuity is not recommended. It should be inserted in hemodynamically unstable patients with hematochezia when there is uncertainty related to location. Approximately 10% to 15% of the patients presenting with severe hematochezia have a UGI source and a significant bleed.

If the aspirate is positive or there is a strong suspicion of a UGI source despite a negative aspirate, the nurse can anticipate that the patient will be scheduled for an emergent upper endoscopy. There is no evidence that NGT insertion affects the overall outcomes (Rockey, 2005).

Gastric lavage may be ordered prior to endoscopy to evacuate blood, clots, and gastric contents that would impair visualization. This may be performed in the critical care unit through an NGT, or if there are large clots through a large-bore oral gastric tube. Most often it is performed during the endoscopic procedure and it is not always successful in providing adequate visualization.

Erythromycin Administration

Patients with severe bleeding are likely to have a stomach full of blood that can be problematic for accurate en-

TABLE 12-1

Interpretation of NGT Aspirate

NGT ASPIRATE	INTERPRETATION
Bright red blood	Validates active UGI bleeding.
Coffee grounds material	Validates UGI bleeding; likely not active bleeding; may also be caused by some foods.
No blood, no bile	Suggests site other than UGI tract; may be a false negative related to a closed pylorus; can still have a UGI site below the pylorus.
Bile, no blood	Suggests no active bleeding, but does not absolutely exclude a UGI bleed site. Approximately 25% of UGI bleeds have a negative aspirate (Rockey, 2005).

doscopic evaluation and intervention related to poor visualization. Because erythromycin can promote gastric emptying, the nurse can anticipate a single dose of intravenous erythromycin 3 mg/kg might be ordered over 20 to 30 minutes approximately 30 to 90 minutes before endoscopy.

Bowel Preparation

A bowel preparation is recommended prior to a colonoscopy. Although the procedure may be performed without a preparation, because blood is considered a cathartic, a cleansed colon allows for a safer procedure and better chance at visualization. There is an increased chance of perforation with an unprepared colon secondary to decreased visibility. If the source of bleeding is strongly suspected to be from the rectal-sigmoid area, a sigmoidoscopy without a preparation is reasonable.

The nurse anticipates that a rapid preparation with a balanced electrolyte solution will be administered to cleanse the colon.

Collaborative Management

Endoscopy is a procedure that uses a flexible fiber-optic endoscope to directly visualize the inside of a hollow organ or cavity. An upper endoscopy, sigmoidoscopy, colonoscopy, and push enteroscopy are all examples of endoscopic procedures that inspect the lumens of the GI tract. The difference is in the specific area to be examined and the intubation orifice. Endoscopy can provide real-time images that are viewed as a video on the monitor in the procedure room. Still photos of areas can also be taken. These procedures can be diagnostic, prognostic, and therapeutic.

Ideally, patients should be resuscitated and stabilized prior to endoscopy. However, urgent endoscopy may be considered for patients experiencing ongoing bleeding and hemodynamic compromise. Such patients will need cardiovascular and respiratory support.

COMMONLY USED MEDICATIONS

POLYETHYLENE GLYCOL SOLUTION (MIRALAX)

Desired Effect: It is an osmotically balanced electrolyte solution that passes through the bowel without significant absorption or secretion, thus avoiding significant fluid and electrolyte shifts.

Nursing Responsibilities:
- It can be administered orally or if the patient's condition necessitates, it can also be administered through an NGT or nasal jejunum tube.
- The nurse can anticipate administering the preparation at a rate of approximately 1 liter every 30 to 45 minutes. The nurse should administer cautiously in patients who are high risk for aspiration and/or fluid overload.
- It has been safely used in patients with liver disease, renal failure, heart failure, and electrolyte imbalances.

Side and/or Toxic Effects: The disadvantage is that relatively large volumes must be given to get a cathartic effect. Patient intolerance evidenced by nausea and vomiting are common side effects.

METOCLOPRAMIDE (REGLAN)

Desired Effect: Metoclopramide is a dopamine antagonist gastroprokinetic. It increases the amplitude of gastric contraction and peristalsis of the duodenum and jejunum. This can be an adjunct to a polyethylene glycol solution (MiraLAX) to help reduce nausea, vomiting, and bloating and promote overall tolerance of the preparation. However, it does not improve colonic cleansing and some studies indicate no improvement in patient tolerance.

Nursing Responsibilities: Metoclopramide (Reglan) 10 mg IV may be administered at the start of the prep.

Patients triaged to intensive care will likely have the procedure performed in the ICU.

Upper Gastrointestinal Endoscopy

An upper GI endoscopy (**esophagogastroduodenoscopy [EGD]**) involves the oral intubation with a flexible endoscope to visualize the esophagus, stomach, and proximal duodenum. A push enteroscopy is similar to an upper endoscopy except a longer scope is introduced and pushed so that the distal duodenum and proximal portion of the jejunum is visualized. Early upper endoscopy, within 24 hours for high-risk patients, is associated with improved outcomes, reduced resource utilization, and best practice in terms of allowing for safe and timely discharge (Barkun et al., 2003).

Colonoscopy

A colonoscopy involves the insertion of the endoscope into the anus to examine the colon or large intestine from the rectum to the ileocecal valve. It is also possible to view the distal portion of the ileum. The bowel wall can be observed for bleeding sites, tumors, and lesions during the insertion and withdrawal. During the procedure, air is introduced into the colon through the endoscope to expand the lumen to facilitate visualization and navigation.

Sigmoidoscopy

A sigmoidoscopy involves only the inspection and visualization of the rectal-sigmoid area of the colon. If bleeding is highly suspected to be coming from the rectum or sigmoid area, an unprepped sigmoidoscopy can be performed. If the source is not revealed, the patient will commonly be prepped for a colonoscopy.

Purpose. The purpose of an endoscopy in patients with an acute GI bleed is to establish the site and etiology of the bleed, allow for endoscopic assessment to determine whether the site has high-risk characteristics for rebleeding (risk stratification/endoscopic stigmata), and to perform therapeutic interventions to resolve active bleeding and prevent rebleeding.

Once the site and source have been determined, there are multiple therapeutic interventions that can be implemented to achieve hemostasis (stoppage of bleeding). The choice is influenced by the endoscopist's preference and experience and the location and characteristics of the bleeding lesion. The interventions, which are performed by either an endoscopy nurse or technician, can be employed as monotherapy or in combination depending on the nature of the bleed.

Categories of Therapeutic Interventions

There are three main categories of therapeutic interventions: injection therapy, thermal coagulation, and mechanical techniques.

Injection Therapy. While directly visualizing the site with an endoscope, an injection needle is used to inject a solution into the desired location. The site may be injected with a variety of agents. The agents may sclerose (harden), vasoconstrict, or cause a tamponade effect. The most commonly used agent is epinephrine. Dilute epinephrine (1-10,000) is injected to create a combination of vasoconstriction and vascular tamponade. Because rebleeding rates are high with injection therapy as a single intervention, this method is typically combined with thermal or mechanical therapy.

Thermal Coagulation. There are multiple types of thermal therapy. Some work by coming in physical contact with the bleeder and applying pressure followed by thermal coagulation of the vessel (bipolar electrocoagulation and heater probes). These are typically used in acute bleeds. No one single method has been found to be superior.

Others work by noncontact thermal energy. Examples would be argon plasma coagulation (APC) and laser therapy. These noncontact methods are not usually used in an acute bleed situation.

Mechanical Techniques. Endoclips (Hemoclips) involve the application and deployment of a clip that achieves hemostasis by compressing the tissue together. Its action is similar to that of a surgical stitch. Depending on the situation, multiple clips may be applied. Frequently this method is combined with an epinephrine injection. Another technique that may be used for variceal bleeding is band ligation (see the discussion on variceal bleeds in Chapter 11). ∞

Indications and Expected Outcomes

An EGD is indicated for any patient with the diagnosis or suspected diagnosis of UGI bleed. The timing of the procedure is critical, depending on the significance of the bleed and the patient's hemodynamic status. Patients considered high risk based on clinical criteria should have an endoscopy within 24 hours. Low-risk patients may have an endoscopy scheduled as an outpatient.

An urgent colonoscopy is the initial treatment of choice for locating and treating an LGI bleed. "Urgent" generally means within 8 to 24 hours after admission following an adequate preparation as discussed. The detection rate for finding an active or recently bleeding diverticular lesion is low. A reduced length of hospital stay is also correlated with early colonoscopy. A colonoscopy is contraindicated in patients in shock or if there is suspicion of an obstruction or perforation. Abdominal x-rays are obtained to rule out these complications prior to the colonoscopy (ASGE, 2005).

The expected outcome of endoscopy is that the bleeding site will be located and treated appropriately to prevent rebleeding. If blood obscures the lining, it may be impossible to determine the site and etiology.

The nurse should expect to see no signs or symptoms of rebleeding evidenced by:

- Normal and stable vital signs
- Adequate urine output (at least 30 mL/hour)
- Negative orthostatic signs
- Stabilization of hematocrit
- Baseline mental status

Nursing Management

If the patient is managed in the ICU, the endoscopy team will likely perform the procedure in the unit. The critical care nurse will have pre-, intra-, and postprocedural responsibilities. The majority of the procedures are performed with moderate/procedural sedation administered by the endoscopy nurse. In the critical care setting, especially if the patient is intubated on a ventilator, the patient may already be receiving sedation. In this situation, the critical care nurse may be accountable for continued sedation. It is essential that the endoscopy nurse and the critical care nurse have ongoing communication related to the patient's condition and their roles and responsibilities.

Preprocedural nursing responsibilities of the critical care nurse:

- Maintains NPO status ideally for 6 to 8 hours prior to the procedure (depending on urgency, this may not be possible)

- Ensures informed consent
- Removes dentures for EGD patients
- Monitors baseline vital signs including temperature and oxygen saturation
- Provides patient/family education
- Performs gastric lavage if ordered to clear the stomach of blood for better visualization (this may be performed during the procedure)
- If the patient is being mechanically ventilated, consults the endoscopist and respiratory therapy related to temporarily adjusting the ventilator setting to maximize oxygenation during sedation

Intraprocedural nursing responsibilities of the critical care nurse:

- May be responsible for administering continued sedation
- Continues interventions to maintain hemodynamic stability
- Participates in a universal protocol "time out," which will verify the correct patient and procedure immediately prior to the procedure
- Assists the endoscopy team as needed

Postprocedural nursing responsibilities of the critical care nurse:

- If the patient is not intubated, maintains recovery position (left lateral decubitus) to protect the airway until the patient is fully awake:
  - EGD patients may have a topical anesthetic sprayed to the throat area, which may impair swallowing.
  - In addition to airway protection, colonoscopy patients benefit from the left lateral decubitus position because it facilitates the passage of air that was inserted during the procedure.
- Monitors vital signs, including temperature and oxygen saturation and level of pain and consciousness, until the patient returns to baseline (typically every 10 to 15 minutes for 30 minutes to an hour, then per ICU protocol, or more frequently depending on acuity).
  - Colonoscopy patients require abdominal assessments for distention. The air that is purposely introduced commonly causes distention. In most cases, this distention is resolved by having the patient bear down and push in an effort to pass gas.
- Monitors for potential complications:
  - Gastrointestinal blood loss (rebleeding)
  - Perforation
  - Aspiration
  - Adverse reaction to procedural sedation medications. Patients are typically given an intravenous (IV) narcotic and a short-acting benzodiazepine.

Other Diagnostic Tests

In the event that colonoscopy cannot be performed or does not yield a bleeding site, other diagnostic options can assist in locating the LGI site, including angiography, radionuclide imaging, and a helical computer tomography scan (Green & Rockey, 2005). A colonoscopy is recommended prior to radionuclide imaging and angiography because of its ability to more accurately diagnose and its ability to treat. Angiography is reserved for patients who cannot have a colonoscopy because of massive ongoing bleeding or when colonoscopy has failed to reveal a source. If both the colonoscopy and upper endoscopy are negative, patients who are hemodynamically stable should have a capsule endoscopy to evaluate the small bowel.

Surgical Consult

The role of surgery in the emergent management of UGI bleeding has diminished; however, it is the most definitive and may be the final option for some bleeding lesions. The majority of patients with UGI bleeding related to peptic ulcer disease (PUD) are managed with resuscitation, medical, and endoscopic interventions. Patients must be evaluated very carefully for surgical management, especially those with severe comorbidities that will affect surgical outcomes. Because surgery has a high morbidity and mortality, it is generally reserved for patients whose bleeding is not controlled by endoscopic treatment or where massive bleeding prevents visualization and treatment (Ferzoco & Ashley, 2006). A second attempt at endoscopic therapy is recommended prior to surgical consideration. Surgical consults should be considered early for critical patients at high risk for a failed endoscopic therapy.

In extreme cases where the source of bleeding cannot be established, a laparotomy may be indicated. Surgical intervention for a bleeding peptic ulcer may involve ligation of the vessel and closure of the ulcer.

Approximately 10% of the patients with a LGI bleed require emergency surgery (Cagir & Cirincirone, 2005). Patients with a significant continuing bleed requiring more than 6 units of RBCs in a 24-hour period, or if bleeding reoccurs, should be considered for surgery (ASGE, 2001a). Depending on the acuity of the patient, every effort should be made to accurately localize the bleeding site prior to surgery. If the bleeding is localized, a segmental resection can be performed as opposed to a subtotal colectomy for patients with continued bleeding and undiagnosed site. A subtotal colectomy is associated with higher morbidity than a segmental colectomy. Whenever possible, it is better to stabilize the patient and perform surgery on an elective basis. Emergent surgery is associated with more complications.

Identification and Prevention of Recurrent Bleeding

The majority of patients with UGI bleeds caused by PUD and LGI bleeds secondary to colonic diverticula will not rebleed during the hospitalization. However, certain patients with an initial severe bleed are at high risk for rebleeding. Determining risk for rebleeding can guide triaging the patient to the appropriate level of care. The absence of these high-risk characteristics can identify patients who can be safely discharged as opposed to those who need further assessment and management.

Risks for Recurrent Gastrointestinal Bleeding

The nurse reviews the patient's clinical course, laboratory studies, and endoscopic results to identify risk factors for rebleeding:

- Older age
- Comorbid disease states
- Hemodynamic instability
- Coagulopathy/anticoagulants
- Endoscopic diagnosis/stigmata (active arterial bleeding, visible vessel, adherent clot)

The patients who are identified as high risk for rebleeding will require continued close nursing assessment for rebleeding, including:

- Hemodynamic/fluid volume status
- Mental status/restlessness
- Pain/discomfort
- Presence of hematemesis, melena, hematochezia
- Serial hematocrits, renal function tests

▌Collaborative Management

The nurse works collaboratively with the health care team to prevent rebleeding. Management efforts should be directed at healing the ulcer/lesion and eliminating precipitating factors.

Acid Suppression: Proton Pump Inhibitors

Proton pump inhibitors (PPIs) cross the parietal cell membrane, resulting in irreversible inhibition of gastric secretion by the proton pump. Their gastric suppression is superior to that of histamine H_2-receptor blockers. They have minimal side effects and few significant drug interactions. Evidence has shown that high-dose PPIs administered intravenously significantly reduce the rebleeding rate in patients with an acute UGI bleed. Additionally, PPI administration in patients with high-risk ulcers receiving therapeutic endoscopy results in a decrease in hospital length of stay, rebleeding rate, and

---

COMMONLY USED MEDICATIONS

PANTOPRAZOLE (PROTONIX)— A PROTON PUMP INHIBITOR

Desired Effect: Pantoprazole acts at the secretory surface of the gastric parietal cell to suppress gastric acid production. Half-life is approximately 1 hour and duration of effect is longer than 24 hours (Soll, 2006).

Nursing Responsibilities:
- Typically dosed as an 80-mg bolus followed by an 8-mg/hour drip. Administration through a dedicated line is preferred but a Y site may be used. The line should be flushed before and after administration of intermittent or bolus doses of pantoprazole.
- Protonix is used with caution in patients with severe hepatic disease.
- The nurse reviews evaluative criteria: a stable hematocrit, absence of signs and symptoms indicating a rebleed, and evidence of a healed ulcer if follow-up endoscopy is performed.

Side and/or Toxic Effects: Protonix has a high safety profile. The nurse monitors the patient for hypersensitivity reactions, headache, diarrhea, abdominal pain, and nausea.

---

need for blood transfusions. Besides their acid suppression action that can keep the gastric pH above 6.0, PPIs can also protect a clot from fibrinolysis (decomposition). The nurse anticipates administrating a PPI, most often pantoprazole (Protonix), initially on presentation and continued until a definite cause can be established. Once the cause, the presence of active bleeding, and other high-risk stigmata have been established, further treatment with PPIs will be determined.

Elimination of Precipitating Factors

To prevent recurrent bleeding, it is essential that patients be assisted to eliminate the precipitating factors. Patients whose GI bleeding has been attributed to the use of NSAIDs should be advised to discontinue these medications. Counseling related to safer alternative medications should be provided. If the NSAIDs need to be continued, a maintenance dose of PPI should be continued to decrease risk.

All patients presenting with a UGI bleed should be tested for *Helicobacter pylori (H. pylori)* and if positive should receive eradication therapy. Additionally *H. pylori* infection and NSAID ingestion act synergistically to cause ulcers. There is evidence that eliminating *H. pylori* is associated with higher healing rates and decreases ulcer reoccurrence and bleeding complications. There are a variety of eradication treatment regimens. Antimicrobial agent(s) are typically administered with a PPI. It is not clear if any one treatment regimen is superior. Cost, side effects, and simplicity of administration are considered. Patient compliance significantly influences outcome. Therapy can be started immediately or during a follow-up visit. The goal is to promote compliance by educating the patient related to the medication action and administration regimen, the importance of the treatment, and to prevent further complications.

Nursing Care

The nurse is responsible for ensuring the patency of the patient's airway, providing adequate nutritional intake when appropriate, maintaining patient comfort and safety, and relieving patient and family anxiety.

Maintenance of Airway/Breathing Patterns

Airway, breathing, and circulation are the immediate nursing priorities during the initial assessment and resuscitation management. Respiratory compromise can occur in patients with both a UGI and LGI bleed related to significant blood loss, potential or actual hemorrhagic shock resulting in decreased oxygen delivery to all vital organs, and changes in mental status. In addition, hemorrhage can worsen preexisting pulmonary disease.

Patients presenting with a UGI bleed with significant blood loss, potential mental status changes, and hematemesis may have difficulty protecting their airway and are at an increased risk for aspiration. Aspiration is an avoidable complication that significantly affects morbidity and patient outcomes. With vigilant nursing assessment and monitoring, these high-risk patients should be readily recognized and electively, rather than emergently, intubated in a controlled setting. The nurse will frequently monitor patients':

- Respiratory status: ability to protect the airway, continuous oxygen saturation, breathing patterns, arterial blood gases, adventitious lung sound associated with pulmonary edema
- Hemodynamic status: stability of vital signs
- Level of consciousness: mental status, ability to follow commands, lethargy
- Hematemesis: presence, frequency, amount

The nurse will:

- Implement aspiration precautions (head of bed elevated; if unable, left lateral decubitus position)
- Confirm the presence of necessary resuscitation/suctioning equipment
- Administer oxygen using the appropriate delivery system and flow rate to maintain pulse oximetry 95% or greater

The expected outcomes for all patients presenting with a GI bleed is that the airway will be protected and adequate breathing patterns will be maintained.

Provision of Adequate Nutrition

The patient experiencing a UGI bleed will typically remain NPO until he undergoes the necessary diagnostic tests, most often an upper endoscopy. NPO status is maintained for visualization and safety. The patient will receive procedural sedation and possibly a topical anesthetic to the pharynx. After endoscopic evaluation, patients considered low risk for rebleeding may be fed immediately. Studies have shown that the timing of feeding for this low-risk group does not influence the hospital course. Patients scheduled for a colonoscopy will be NPO with the exception of the laxative that must be ingested to purge the colon for visualization.

The decision to feed patients with LGI bleeding or patients not in the low risk for UGI rebleeding category will be made according to the individual patient's clinical status, evidence that bleeding has subsided, and the potential for repeated endoscopy or other procedures or surgery. Patients likely to remain unable to take or tolerate oral feeding for an extended period should have a nutritional consult and be evaluated for enteral or parenteral nutrition.

Provision of Comfort and Safety

The majority of upper and lower GI bleeding is painless. The nurse will routinely assess and treat pain per pain management protocol. However, patients are likely to experience discomfort related to invasive monitoring devices, NGT insertion, and diagnostic tests. The discomfort associated with tests and invasive monitoring can often be lessened by basic nursing care through assisting with patient positioning, hygiene (mouth, nares care, bathing, back care), and patient education. It is important for patients to be aware of the rationale for invasive monitoring devices and any discomfort associated with the procedures. Often the discomfort is short term, and preparing the patient can help the patient better deal with the discomfort.

If nursing care interventions are not successful in easing the discomfort, the nurse should collaborate with the physician related to the nature of the discomfort and the possibility of medications or other interventions that may help with management.

Patients should also be routinely assessed for fall risk, utilizing a standardized risk assessment tool. Certain medications, unstable vital signs, positive orthostatic signs, syncope, and altered mental status commonly occur with GI bleeding and will increase a patient's fall risk potential. Fall risk protocols should be implemented.

As discussed, patients with altered mental status who are vomiting must have aspiration precautions implemented.

Anxiety of Patient and Family

The patient/family often experience different degrees of anxiety related to the stress of experiencing an acute crisis that may be life threatening; has totally disrupted their roles and responsibilities; has put them in an unfamiliar environment with a loss of control; has potentially caused pain and discomfort related to invasive procedures and therapeutic treatments; and has created fear, especially of the unknown: diagnosis, prognosis, treatments.

The critical care nurse must be sensitive to the patient/family's fears, needs, and coping skills and implement interventions to decrease anxiety. The nurse should empower the patient/family to take an active role in the patient's care. In addition to compassionate care and realistic hopefulness, the nurse should encourage questions and participation in decision making.

All members of the health care team should provide education and consistent information related to the diagnosis, treatments, and overall plan of care based on the patient/family's readiness and willingness to learn. Barriers to learning (cognitive development, language, culture, etc.) should be addressed appropriately. The patient/family should be evaluated for appropriate referrals: pastoral care, social services, and the like. The nurse should routinely assess for evidence of decreased anxiety by verbal and nonverbal communication and evaluating physical, behavioral, emotional, and cognitive signs and symptoms.

Prevention of Complications

Prevention of complications is essential for promoting positive patient outcomes. Acute GI bleeding needs to be systematically assessed and treated. Aggressive resuscitation and stabilization, identifying the source, stopping and treating the bleeding, and preventing recurrent bleeding are the fundamentals of care. Depending on the rate of bleeding and the patient's response to treatment, hypotension and potential shock states can result from acute blood loss. Vigilant assessment, interventions, and evaluation of the patient's response to the interventions are critical in preventing shock and the consequences of shock. The nurse must monitor for evidence of:

Myocardial ischemia/infarction

Cerebral ischemia/thrombosis

Respiratory insufficiency/failure

Acute renal failure

Hepatic failure

Disseminated intravascular coagulation

Sepsis

MSOF

Invasive monitoring devices and procedures, the hospital environment, surgery, and immobility increase the patient's risk for developing infections. Essential nursing interventions to minimize the development of infections are implemented (see Chapter 17 ∞ for the discussion on sespis).

Patients who have had surgery need meticulous postoperative care and monitoring. Patients with lower GI surgery are especially prone to complications. During the recovery period the nurse must closely observe for the following common early postoperative complications:

- Bleeding
- Mechanical small bowel obstruction

Nursing Diagnoses

GASTROINTESTINAL BLEEDING

- Deficient fluid volume related to active blood loss
- Acute pain related to mucosal irritation
- Nausea related to gastrointestinal bleeding
- Anxiety related to health status

PANCREATITIS

- Acute pain related to edema of the pancreas
- Deficient fluid volume related to severe fluid shift
- Imbalanced nutrition less than body requirements related to inability to ingest and digest foods

- Ileus
- Intra-abdominal sepsis
- Localized/generalized peritonitis
- Wound infection or disruption
- Thrombophlebitis

Pancreatitis

Patients with severe pancreatitis are usually critically ill. For optimum patient outcomes, they require care by a multidisciplinary team familiar with the essential elements of care for the patient with pancreatitis as well as the potential complications of the disease.

Predisposing Factors and Causes of Acute Pancreatitis

The most common risk factors for acute pancreatitis include gallstone disease and excessive alcohol use. Other less common risk factors include infections, medications, toxins, developmental abnormalities, hypertriglyceridemia, hypercalcemia, trauma, heredity, and vascular abnormalities. Determination of the cause is critical for decision making and directing immediate interventions (Gardner, Berk, & Yakshe, 2006). An example of a causal event needing prompt intervention is the presence of common bile duct stones. Such patients are evaluated for stone removal within the first 24 hours and a possible gallbladder removal in the near future.

The exact mechanism as to how the different predisposing factors induce pancreatitis is uncertain. General consensus regarding pathogenesis is autodigestion. The acinar cells are damaged, causing inappropriate activation of trypsinogen to trypsin. Trypsin activates a cascade of other enzymes that begin digestive functions in the pancreas, resulting in inflammation and tissue damage. The normal defense and inhibitory mechanisms are overwhelmed by the large amounts of activated enzymes.

VISUAL MAP Acute Pancreatitis Overview

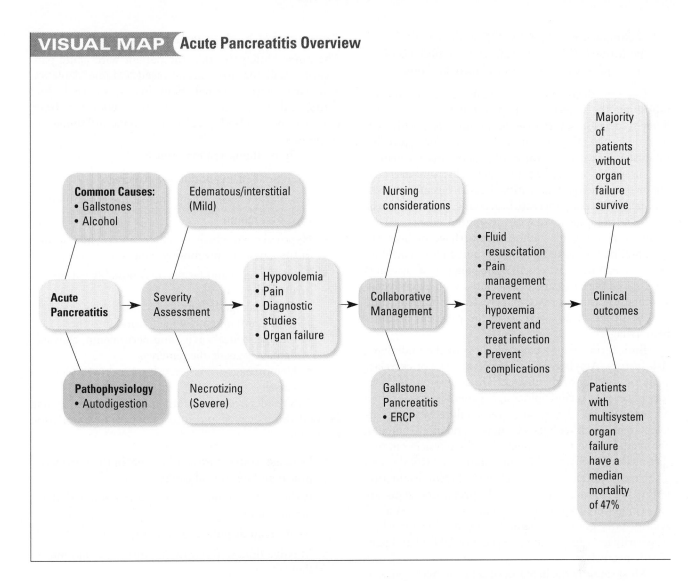

The release of inflammatory mediators causes increased vascular permeability with varying degrees of edema, hemorrhage, and necrosis. For the majority of the patients, the inflammatory response is self-limiting. However, 10% to 20% of the patients will experience increased local inflammation, resulting in toxic enzymes and mediators entering the systemic circulation. The inflammatory response goes beyond the pancreas to a systemic inflammatory response syndrome (SIRS), which can also contribute to pancreatic necrosis and result in multisystem organ dysfunction (see Chapter 17). ∞

Determination of the Severity of Pancreatitis

The diagnosis of acute pancreatitis is based on careful consideration of medical history, differential diagnoses, clinical assessment, and laboratory and radiographic imaging studies. Once the diagnosis is made, further studies may be conducted to find a cause and assess for complications. Early diagnosis is essential for halting the disease progression and preventing complications. According to Vege and Chari (2006a), the diagnosis requires two of the following:

- Characteristic abdominal pain.
- Serum amylase and/or lipase greater than or equal to three times the upper limit of normal.
  - Serum amylase: rises within 6 to 12 hours and is typically elevated for 3 to 5 days. It is a nonspecific test because other disorders can also cause an elevation, though they typically do not elevate to such levels. It has no correlation with severity or patient outcomes.
  - Serum lipase: rises within 24 to 48 hours and is typically elevated for 14 days. It is a more specific and sensitive test than amylase because it will stay normal in some nonpancreatic disorders that would increase the amylase. Because it rises later and stays elevated longer, it is a good marker for those who linger at home and present later.
- If the enzyme limits are below three times the upper limit and doubt exists about the diagnosis,

a computer tomography (CT) scan may be performed to look for characteristic findings of acute pancreatitis (Banks & Freeman, 2006).

Once the diagnosis of acute pancreatitis is made, establishing the severity and identifying those patients likely to develop severe disease is critical to positive patient outcomes (Vege & Chari, 2004). The literature distinguishes between two forms of pancreatitis: edematous and interstitial or mild acute pancreatitis, and necrotizing or severe acute pancreatitis. Edematous and interstitial or mild acute pancreatitis accounts for 80% of the cases and is associated with interstitial edema, an inflammatory infiltrate without hemorrhage or necrosis, with minimal or no organ damage and an uneventful recovery. Necrotizing or severe acute pancreatitis accounts for 20% of the cases and is associated with extensive inflammation and necrosis, pancreatic dysfunction, and MSOF. In the most severe cases the pancreas becomes hemorrhagic.

Both forms may occur regardless of the underlying risk factors. Amylase and lipase levels do not correlate with the severity of the disease. On admission, risk factors of severity include older age (generally greater than 55 years of age), obesity, and organ failure. Several scoring systems, each with its advantages and disadvantages, are available and may be helpful to the physician in predicting the severity, thus distinguishing mild from severe. The acute physiology and chronic health evaluation (APACHE II) and Ranson's early prognostic signs are two commonly used systems. In addition, there is a CT scan severity grading system. The most critical markers of severity are organ failure (especially MSOF) and pancreatic necrosis.

Most recently the hematocrit is being investigated as a possible prognostic marker for the presence of necrotizing pancreatitis. It is thought that a normal hematocrit on admission as opposed to a hemoconcentrated hematocrit (greater than 44%) predicts an absence of necrosis and a mild clinical course (Whitcomb, 2006).

Collaborative Management

The critical care patient is likely to be experiencing moderate to severe acute disease. Assessments focus on hemodynamic stability, pain, electrolyte balances, safety, and preventing and recognizing complications. Management involves correcting the underlying cause and aggressive supportive care, including fluid resuscitation, pain relief, restoring electrolyte balance, and nutritional support. Local and/or systemic complications create many clinical challenges that will determine further priorities and interventions. Additionally, if alcohol is thought to be a predisposing factor, the risks and complications of alcohol withdrawal must be considered concurrently with acute treatment (see Chapter 11). ∞

Assessment of Hypovolemia

The nurse anticipates that the patient with acute pancreatitis will manifest pronounced volume depletion associated with external fluid losses, internal fluid shifts, and third spacing secondary to vomiting, fever, diaphoresis, and both local and systemic inflammatory responses.

Local inflammation may cause:

- Interstitial edema within the pancreas
- Vascular damage causing increased permeability
- Loss of albumin
- Hypovolemia, which affects the microcirculation of the pancreas, promoting pancreatic necrosis
- Tissue damage and fat necrosis possibly eating through the pancreas
  - Fluid leakage (albumin, activated enzymes, toxins, inflammatory mediators) into the retroperitoneal cavity and peritoneum, causing damage outside the pancreas
  - Hemorrhage from necrosis or ruptured blood vessels

SIRS results from the inflammatory mediators going beyond the pancreas and into the systemic circulation may cause:

- Damage to structures and organs in the retroperitoneal and peritoneal cavity
- Peripheral (systemic) vasodilatation and vascular permeability
- Vital organ dysfunction and failure
- Massive fluid sequestrations (third spacing) into the:
  - Retroperitoneal space
  - Intraperitoneal cavity
  - Gut
  - Pleural space
- Hypovolemic, septic, cardiogenic shock

The nurse reviews the patient's past and current history for predisposing factors, risk factors associated with severity, and evidence of systemic involvement and pancreatic necrosis. The nurse assesses for the signs and symptoms of hypovolemia described earlier in the chapter, including: thirst; poor skin turgor with dry mucous membranes; cool, clammy skin; flat jugular veins; hypotension or orthostatic hypotension with dizziness; narrowed pulse pressure; tachycardia; decreased capillary refill; decreased urine output; and mental status changes. Significant comorbidities or hemodynamic instability may necessitate more invasive monitoring, thus the patient may have an indwelling urinary catheter, a central venous pressure line, or a PA line.

Low central venous pressure (CVP)

Low pulmonary artery wedge pressure (PAWP)

VISUAL MAP Acute Pancreatitis Assessment and Management

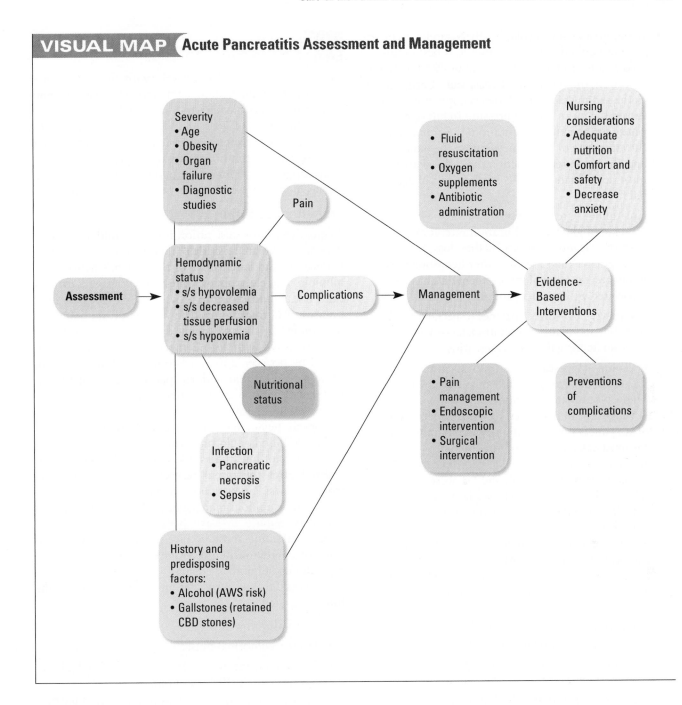

In addition, the nurse observes for two infrequent but classic signs associated with severe necrotizing pancreatitis: Cullen's sign and Grey-Turner's sign. Cullen's sign is a bluish discoloration around the umbilicus from the escape of blood into the peritoneum. Grey-Turner's sign is a bluish brown discoloration around the flanks from blood in the retroperitoneal space.

The nurse also reviews the following laboratory tests to identify the patient's volume status and the severity of the disease:

- Hematocrit—A hematocrit greater than 44 on admission is consistent with hemoconcentration, evidence of volume depletion, and an apparent risk

factor for pancreatic necrosis (Whitcomb, 2006). An excessively low hematocrit would be indicative of bleeding. A normal hematocrit on admission suggests an uneventful clinical course. Serial hematocrits may be followed at 12 and 24 hours and used as severity and evaluative criteria.

- Leukocytes—The degree of elevation is an indicator of severity.

- Serum electrolytes—Sodium, chloride, potassium, and magnesium are evaluated and replaced as needed. The values can influence the type of crystalloid solutions infused.

- Blood urea nitrogen (BUN)—BUN can be useful in evaluating fluid volume status and is best evaluated relative to the serum creatinine. With volume depletion, the BUN will increase out of proportion to the serum creatinine. However, if hypovolemia causes the mean arterial pressure to fall significantly for an extended duration, the glomerular filtration rate of the kidneys cannot be maintained and change in renal function can occur. Patients must be evaluated for the development of acute renal failure.

- Creatinine—Creatinine provides the most accurate estimate of glomerular filtration rate. It may rise with significant intravascular fluid loss, but a value greater than 2 mg/dL after hydration may be suggestive of renal involvement and has been associated with greater mortality.

- Liver enzymes—Liver enzymes (especially total bilirubin and alanine aminotransferase) are used to evaluate for gallstone pancreatitis.

- Calcium—Hypercalcemia (total calcium greater than 11 mg/dL) may be a causal factor. Hypocalcemia (total serum Ca^{++} less than 8.5 mg/dL) can be caused by multiple factors in acute pancreatitis, including hypoalbuminemia (as most calcium is bound to albumin), hypomagnesemia (especially where excessive alcohol use is implicated), and fat necrosis. The breakdown of fats releases fatty acids. Ionic calcium combines with the fatty acids to form soaps. Calcium values less than 8 are considered in evaluating for severity. Routine monitoring and replacement is necessary to prevent neuromuscular and cardiac dysfunction. It may be evaluated concurrently with magnesium.

- Glucose—Hyperglycemia on admission is a consideration in predicting severity and may indicate pancreatic endocrine dysfunction.

- Abdominal ultrasound—This is performed on admission to assess for gallstone etiology.

- CT scan—CT scan usually is not required in mild pancreatitis cases. It may be indicated as mentioned for differential diagnosis situations on admission, or days after admission when the patient's clinical status supports increasing severity. It can confirm the presence and extent of necrosis. There is also a severity grading system based on CT scan results. Later scans may be performed for suspected infected necrosis to guide fine needle aspiration for staining and culture or to identify other complications. Patient's renal and hydration status must be considered prior to IV contrast. If performed too early (less than 48 hours) after onset, tissue damage may not have reached its maximum extent.

Collaborative Management

The nurse works collaboratively with the health care team to maintain hemodynamic stability, restore and maintain normovolemia, and, ultimately, maintain tissue perfusion. The goal of therapy is to avoid hypovolemia not only to prevent systemic complications, but because early restoration is instrumental in resolving existing organ involvement. In addition, aggressive fluid replacement can prevent or limit pancreatic necrosis.

Fluid Resuscitation

Aggressive fluid resuscitation for both mild and severe disease is the most critical therapeutic intervention. Choice of fluid is reflective of the patient's hematocrit, albumin, and electrolytes. Unless hemorrhage is evident the nurse should expect to provide the patient with fluid boluses of normal saline. The volume of the boluses is determined by the assessment data. It is not unusual to initially bolus with 1 to 2 liters of saline rapidly followed by between 250 and 500 mL per hour for 24 to 48 hours. Fluid that is third spaced is difficult to estimate and hypovolemia is frequently underestimated (Nathens et al., 2004).

Severe hemorrhagic pancreatitis may require transfusions of blood or clotting factors, depending on hematocrit and clotting studies. Electrolyte solutions may be ordered after the initial resuscitation based on electrolyte values. Patients with existing cardiovascular disease need scrupulous management of their infusion rates and may require invasive hemodynamic monitoring. Careful attention must be given to clinical manifestations of overhydration, especially respiratory compromise and/or pulmonary edema.

Successful fluid resuscitation will be evident by the following changes:

- Normalization of BP.
- Decreased/normal pulse.
- Increased urine output greater than 0.5 cc/kg/hour, approximately 30 cc per hour.
- Increased CVP to 8 to 12 and/or increased PAWP.
- If the hematocrit was initially hemoconcentrated, adequate fluid resuscitation would result in decreasing the hematocrit.
- Normal capillary refill with warm, dry skin.

Strict cardiovascular and respiratory monitoring is warranted and subtle changes must not be overlooked. It is imperative to recognize either deterioration or improvement. If the patient's fluid status does not improve or worsens, consider hypovolemic shock or other complications. Dopamine may be used if there is continuing hypotension. It does not damage the pancreatic microcirculation like other vasoconstrictors (Steinberg, 2006).

SAFETY INITIATIVES — Implement Multidisciplinary Rounds

PURPOSE: Enhance the communication among members of the health care team, improve the flow of patients through the ICU, increase satisfaction among members of the health care team, and improve patient outcomes

RATIONALE: "Multidisciplinary rounds (MDR) enable all members of the team caring for critically ill patients to come together and offer expertise in patient care" (IHI). When nursing, pharmacy, nutrition, respiratory therapy, social work, patients, families, and physicians from other specialties caring for a patient contribute their expertise to identify patient goals and develop a plan of care, patient outcomes are better.

HIGHLIGHTS OF RECOMMENDATIONS:

1. Convene a multidisciplinary rounds conference preferably at the patient's bedside daily if possible but hopefully at least 2 or 3 times a week
2. Invite: Intensivists, generalists, ICU nurses, pharmacists, respiratory therapists, nutritionists, social workers, case managers, family members

3. Discuss:
   Patient's goals and preferences
   Patient's care needs
   Acuity assessment and discharge planning
4. Tips:
   Agree to one person who writes orders based on the recommendations made by the group
   Agree that team members will present issues to the person in charge during multidisciplinary rounds
   Expect the person in charge to request and rely upon information from other team members
   Carefully monitor patient progress by assessing whether goals are met
   Adhere to protocols
   Prepare for patient discharge and assure follow-up services are available

Source: Institute for Healthcare Improvement

 Available: http://www.ihi.org/IHI/Topics/CriticalCare/IntensiveCare/Changes/ImplementMultidisciplinary Rounds.htm

Assessment and Management of Pain

Pain is the characteristic diagnostic sign of acute pancreatitis. It results from irritation and edema of the inflamed pancreas and, in severe cases, the release of pancreatic enzymes into the surrounding tissues.

The nurse needs to conduct a thorough GI evaluation and pain assessment, using an appropriate standardized pain scale. Because manifestations may vary depending on severity, the nurse can expect that the patient will display many of the following characteristics:

- Sudden, severe epigastrium pain often peaking within 30 to 60 minutes and lasting hours to days.
- Deep, visceral, steady pain
- Poorly localized pain often radiating to the back, chest, lower abdomen, and flanks.
- Abdominal guarding, rebound tenderness.
- Increased intensity supine, somewhat decreased with sitting, trunk flexed forward.
- Frequently accompanied by nausea and vomiting. Vomiting does not relieve the pain and might make it worse.
- Associated diminished or absent bowel sounds, paralytic ileus.
- May display physiological signs: tachycardia, hypertension, tachypnea, splinting.
- Patient appears acutely distressed, anxious, and inconsolable.

Collaborative Management

The nurse works collaboratively with the health care team to provide the patient with adequate pain relief. Adequate pain relief is a critical goal because the pain is severe, it increases the patient's anxiety level, and unrelieved pain may indicate disease progression.

Because the pain of acute pancreatitis is generally severe and the patient is unable to take anything by mouth, adequate pain control requires IV administration of medications related to rapid onset and ease of titration.

Depending on the severity of the pain, medications may be ordered on a set schedule, as necessary, as a continuous infusion, or as patient-controlled analgesia (PCA). If the patient is cognitively and physically able, PCA is preferred because it maintains patient control and provides more effective pain management. If the pain is unrelieved with IV opioid administration, epidural analgesic may be considered. Epidural analgesia requires expert consultation and not all patients qualify.

There is no evidence that any one medication has the advantage in acute pancreatitis (Banks & Freeman, 2006). Generally, severe pain requires opiates; milder cases may be managed with nonsteroidal anti-inflammatory medications such as ketorolac tramethamine (Toradol). Past literature recommended meperidine (Demerol) as the narcotic of choice, because it was presumed that morphine and other opioids increased sphincter of Oddi spasms, thus worsening the disease. Current recommendations discourage the use of meperidine (Demerol) related to:

- Short duration.
- Repeated doses produce an accumulation of a toxic metabolite that causes increased central nervous system irritability and toxicity.

Because there is no evidence that sphincter of Oddi spasms affect the outcome of the disease, morphine is the preferred opioid medication related to longer duration (Lankisch & Lerch, 2006).

The nurse should anticipate, because of the severity of the pain, that the patient may require high doses of analgesia. It is imperative that the patient is monitored for pain and hemodynamic responses. The nurse should assess the patient's pain response frequently, using the initial assessment tool. Expected outcomes are that the patient verbalizes decreased pain less than 4 on a scale of 0 to 10, and visible behavioral clues such as body movement and facial expressions of pain. If the patient has received the maximal dose and the pain is still severe, the nurse must realize that the analgesia treatment is not working and therefore confer with the physician. The nurse must consider that unsuccessful analgesia may indicate that the disease is progressing. A pain management consult may also be considered. Further, vital signs including oxygen saturation must be monitored frequently by the nurse and evaluated concurrently with the patient's overall hemodynamic status.

The nurse would expect to see the following:

- BP would decrease because of decreased pain and the vasodilator effects of the opioids. If a decrease in pain is not attained, the BP may stay the same or increase.
- Pulse would decrease related to decreased pain, anxiety, and release of catecholamines or stay elevated if pain intensity continues.
- Respirations may increase or decrease. Pain relief may allow the patient to breathe easier; however, the depressant effects of the opioids may cause respiratory depression.
- Oxygen saturation may increase related to comfort or decrease related to respiratory depression.

Nalaxone (Narcan) in small doses may reverse the respiratory depressant effects without affecting the analgesia. However, the decision to support the patient's respiratory status with intubation and ventilation must be considered.

Nursing Management

Often, impaired respiratory function is the first sign of MSOF (Papachristou & Whitcomb, 2004). Therefore, the nurse is especially attentive to the assessment and management of hypoxemia in the patient with pancreatitis.

Assessment

The nurse must frequently assess the patient's respiratory status. Factors influencing the risk of developing hypoxemia include:

- Potential/actual hypovolemia and decreased tissue perfusion
- Depressant effects of opioid administration
- Abdominal pain resulting in:
  - Hypoventilation, decreased lung expansion, vital capacity, and alveolar ventilation
  - Increased catecholamine release, tachycardia, hypertension, increased metabolic rate, increased cardiac workload, and oxygen demand/consumption
- Overhydration related to massive fluid resuscitation, pulmonary edema
- Release of toxins from the pancreas resulting in increased incidence of pleural effusion (especially on the left), pneumonia, and adult respiratory distress syndrome (ARDS). ARDS can develop rapidly.

Indications of Hypoxemia. To identify hypoxemia, the nurse assesses for the following clinical indicators:

- Decreased oxygen saturation/pulse oximetry (less than 92%)
- Increased or decreased respiratory rate
- Labored breathing, shortness of breath
- Abnormal lung sounds: crackles, wheezes, or decreased lung sounds (may indicate a pleural effusion)
- Restlessness, anxiety, or decreased level of consciousness
- Cardiac dysrhythmias
- Respiratory insufficiency/failure necessitating intubation ventilation (PaO_2 less than 60 despite increased oxygen concentrations is a criterion for intubation/ventilation)

The nurse should also review the arterial blood gases, which are ordered initially as part of the severity evaluation criteria and as necessary when the patient exhibits decreased oxygen saturations with or without other symptoms. Particular attention should be on the PaO_2 and the pH. The nurse also reviews the chest x-ray, which is routinely part of the initial evaluation. Particular attention is given to the presence of pleural effusions or infiltrates on admission or within 24 hours. Such findings are risk factors correlated with increased severity of pancreatitis.

Collaborative Management

The nurse works collaboratively with the health care team to maintain oxygenation and prevent hypoxemia.

The goal of therapy is to maintain oxygen tissue delivery, which can minimize pancreatic necrosis and prevent and sometimes resolve organ dysfunction. As discussed aggressive fluid resuscitation is necessary to prevent hypovolemia and maintain tissue perfusion.

Supplemental Oxygen

Supplemental oxygen is administered usually for the first 24 to 48 hours or until there is no threat of hypoxemia. Oxygen percentage and delivery system should be appropriate to maintain the patient's oxygen saturation 92% or greater. Mild self-limiting cases are managed with nasal cannula at 1 to 4 liters. Progressive desaturation should be treated aggressively as respiratory insufficiency/failure, and the patient should be intubated and ventilated (see Chapter 3). ∞

The nurse continues to monitor the patient's respiratory status, assessing for signs and symptoms of hypoxemia concurrently with the patient's hemodynamic status. Pain relief interventions, as discussed, may help or hinder the patient's respiratory efforts. The nurse also positions the patient for maximal comfort.

Assessment and Management of Infection

Infection is a constant threat to the patient with severe necrotizing pancreatitis related to both local and systemic complications. It is a significant contributing cause of late death (after 2 weeks). Because of SIRS and MSOF, the patient is at risk for all types of infections and sepsis. In necrotizing pancreatitis, the necrotic tissue is categorized as sterile (absence of bacteria) or infected (presence of bacteria). The probability that the necrotic tissue may become infected is greater than 40% and usually occurs between 7 and 14 days after the onset of the illness (Papachristou & Whitcomb, 2004).

Assessment of Infection

The nurse assesses for the signs and symptoms of infection and sepsis. However, because the patient with pancreatitis without infected necrosis is likely to have a systemic inflammatory response, he may have fever and leukocytosis from SIRS. This can make it difficult to distinguish when sepsis has developed in the necrotic tissue.

Infected necrosis is suspected if the patient fails to improve or deteriorates rapidly and unexpectedly, presents with new progressive or persistent signs and symptoms of infection, and has a CT revealing greater than 30% necrosis.

▌Collaborative Management

The nurse works collaboratively with the health care team to prevent, recognize, and appropriately treat infected pancreatic necrosis. It is crucial to distinguish be-

tween sterile and infected necrosis. Sterile necrosis is usually less extensive and can be managed conservatively, whereas infected necrosis needs aggressive management and is associated with poorer outcomes.

Evidence-Based Interventions

Evidence-based interventions for the prevention and treatment of infected pancreatic necrosis include:

- Fluid resuscitation, avoidance of hypovolemia and hypoxemia, and the maintenance of tissue perfusion, as previously discussed, can prevent or limit pancreatic necrosis.

- Early enteral nutritional support helps to preserve the functioning of the gut's mucosal barrier and decrease bacterial translocations (movement of bacteria across the intestinal wall), resulting in decreased infectious complications. Organisms from the GI tract are typically the cause of infected necrosis.

- There is consensus that prophylactic antibiotics are not justified in interstitial pancreatitis secondary to an increased rate of secondary, superimposed bacterial and fungal infections. The role of prophylactic antibiotics in severe necrotizing pancreatitis remains unclear. The current practice guidelines do not recommend the use of prophylactic antibiotics to prevent infected necrosis. The patient's individual clinical picture will influence the decision to begin antibiotics. Some sources believe that greater than 30% necrosis warrants a trial of antibiotics for a limited duration of 7 to 10 days (Vege & Chari, 2006b). Other sources advocate for starting antibiotics while the source is actively being investigated. Deteriorating conditions suggesting infection or sepsis and the presence and degree of organ dysfunction are also clinical indicators justifying antibiotics.

The nurse anticipates that the patient will have blood, urine, sputum, and other appropriate cultures as ordered. In some cases a CT scan with a fine needle aspiration (FNA) and culture of the necrotic tissue will be performed by the interventional radiologist. If appropriate cultures and the FNA are negative, antibiotics should be discontinued. Pending positive cultures and sensitivities, the choice of antibiotics will vary. Initially a broad-spectrum antibiotic that can penetrate the pancreatic tissue will be ordered. Not all antibiotics have the ability to penetrate pancreatic tissue and achieve therapeutic levels. Some practitioners may also consider an antifungal agent, though this practice has not been validated.

The nurse would continue to monitor for signs and symptoms of infection and improvement of overall clinical status for indications that treatment is working, including decreasing white blood cell count, stable vital signs with normal temperature, decreasing pain, and overall clinical improvement.

Radiological and Surgical Interventions

Sterile necrosis is managed medically for the first 2 to 3 weeks. Surgery may be required if there is persistent pain, nausea, and vomiting. The standard of care for infected necrosis is surgical debridement, depending on the patient's clinical status. Timing is critical to patient survival (Besselink et al., 2007). Improved survival rates have been observed when surgical debridement is delayed up to 30 days. Delayed treatment enables the patient's clinical status to optimize and allows demarcation between the viable tissue and the unviable tissue to occur (Whitcomb, 2006). Ultimately the surgeon makes the determination about timing and extent of surgery. Surgical necrosectomy is the resection of the necrotic tissue. The goal is to remove all of the necrotic tissue and preserve the viable tissue. Less-invasive alternatives may be appropriate for certain patients. Choice is relative to the individual clinical picture, a diffuse (spread or scattered) versus localized collection of necrotic tissue, and the available expertise. Less-invasive procedures include percutaneous retroperitoneal necrosectomy, laparoscopic necrosectomy, percutaneous catheter drainage, and endoscopic drainage.

Post procedure or surgery, the nurse will monitor the patient's vital signs and pain level and be alert for evidence of bleeding. Typically the patient will return with an array of drains and irrigating tubes. The nurse is responsible for monitoring, promoting drainage, and maintaining patency of the tubes as prescribed.

Nursing Care

The nursing care of the patient with acute pancreatitis is focused on maintaining adequate nutrition for healing, promoting comfort and safety, and relieving anxiety.

Provision of Adequate Nutrition

Because of pain and associated GI symptoms (nausea, vomiting, distention, ileus) all patients are initially kept NPO. The patient with a mild pancreatitis is NPO on average for 2 to 7 days. There is usually no impact on nutritional status. However, the nurse must also consider the patient's pre-illness nutritional status, especially if alcohol is the predisposing factor. This population is at high risk for malnutrition and vitamin deficiencies. If the patient fails to start and/or tolerate eating after 7 days, enteral feeding should be initiated.

In mild pancreatitis clear liquids are initiated when the abdominal pain subsides enough so that the patient no longer requires opiates, anorexia resolves, the patient's appetite returns, bowel sounds are present, and GI symptoms resolve.

If clear liquids are tolerated for 24 hours (no increase in pain, nausea, or vomiting), the diet as well as the caloric content is advanced from a liquid to soft then solid diet over the next couple of days. The recommended diet is greater than 50% carbohydrates with moderate amounts of protein and fat.

The patient with moderate to severe pancreatitis has an increased metabolic demand and increased resting energy expenditure related to severe pain, hemodynamic status, and inflammation. He may also have a negative nitrogen balance up to 40 grams/day. As with all critically ill patients, early nutritional support positively affects outcomes. In these cases, enteral nutrition is preferred over total parenteral nutrition (TPN) (Meier et al., 2006). The advantages of enteral nutrition include:

- Maintenance of the intestinal barrier, thus prevention of translocation of intestinal bacteria, reducing septic complications (Vege & Chari, 2006b)
- Elimination of the many complications encountered with parenteral nutrition (including sepsis and metabolic abnormalities)
- Decreased rates of infection, resulting in decreased need for surgical intervention (Whitcomb, 2006)
- May modify the stress response (McClave, Chang, Dhaliwal, & Heyland, 2006)
- Fewer overall complications
- Decreased hospital lengths of stay

Postpyloric jejunal feedings should be started early in the course of severe disease. The advantage in acute pancreatitis is that by avoiding the mouth, stomach, and duodenum, pancreatic stimulation is decreased. In addition, the chance of aspiration is minimized when proper tube positioning is maintained. The tube should be in the distal duodenum or jejunum beyond the ligament of Treitz. In severe cases, enteral feeding may be required for weeks while inflammation decreases and necrotic areas have been debrided or drained. The disadvantages of jejunal feedings are the difficulty with placement of the tubes, maintaining proper position, and patency. The tube's small diameter often causes clogging.

The patient should have an early nutritional consult to evaluate enteral caloric requirements based on energy expenditure and formula selection. The patient's pancreatic endocrine function related to glucose metabolism, acid-base balance, and electrolyte balance must also be considered. Recommended energy requirements can fluctuate between 25 and 30 kcal/kg/day. Nutritional support should also integrate vitamins and trace elements, especially vitamins A, C, and E and zinc (Cano, 2004).

There are studies looking at the feasibility of initiating gastric feedings in patients with severe pancreatitis. The likelihood of gastric feedings being tolerated by a specific patient is unknown because individual patients will have a wide range of tolerance based on the different degrees of severity of the disease. In addition, tolerance can be influenced by the level of infusion, the specific formula, the stress response, and the mode of infusion. If gastric feedings are initiated and not tolerated, the jejunal route should be tried. Changing the level of the feeding further down the GI tract should improve tolerance.

TOTAL PARENTERAL NUTRITION TPN is appropriate when enteral feedings cannot be tolerated and may be used in combination with enteral feedings when caloric requirements cannot be met (see Chapter 2 ∞ for a more detailed discussion of nutrition).

The nurse assesses the patient for indications of adequate nutrition:

- Intake and output.
- Weight—because of the potential for massive fluid sequestration and the aggressive fluid resuscitation, weight may not be initially reliable.
- Tolerance of the feedings.
- Laboratory studies: electrolytes and glucose.

The nurse also assesses the patient for potential complications of feeding, most importantly, the increase or return of pain; nausea, vomiting, cramping; aspiration; tube obstruction; hyperglycemia; diarrhea/constipation.

Provision of Comfort and Safety

The patient will often experience nausea and vomiting. If the nausea and vomiting are persistent, the patient may be treated with an antiemetic medication. Once administered the patient must be reevaluated for relief. The patient may also have an NGT inserted to relieve persistent nausea, vomiting, and gastric distention. This is not a routine intervention and is only performed to promote comfort when nausea and vomiting continue despite medication. Such decompression has not been shown to affect outcomes. While the patient may get relief, the NGT is uncomfortable and the patient must receive meticulous nasal and oral care.

The patient should be positioned for optimal comfort, often sitting with the trunk flexed forward.

Relief of Anxiety

Whether patients have mild or severe forms of the disease, they are usually extremely anxious related to the severe pain, sudden onset of the illness, and the lack of knowledge regarding the disease. As discussed, pain management is a necessity. Patients and families should be instructed about the disease, the rationale for the interventions, and expected outcomes. Because anxiety often impairs patients' and families' readiness and ability to learn, simple, consistent, and repetitive information needs to be given by all members of the health care team. Comprehension of the information should be consistently evaluated. Consistent staff and family visitation often promotes comfort and trust and decreases anxiety.

Prevention of Complications

The development of complications clearly affects the patient's clinical course and patient outcomes. The nurse recognizes that the severity of acute pancreatitis often cannot be predicted early in the course of the disease. Crucial to preventing complications is prompt diagnosis, identification and treatment of the cause, and management according to evidence-based guidelines. All patients should receive aggressive fluid resuscitation and supplemental oxygen until the severity of the disease is established. In general, the mortality rate is 5% for interstitial pancreatitis and 17% for necrotizing pancreatitis. Early deaths, usually within 2 weeks, are caused by organ failure; later deaths are attributed to infections and sepsis related to pancreatic necrosis. As mentioned, the majority of the patients with severe pancreatitis without organ failure survive, whereas those with MSOF have a median mortality of 47% (Banks & Freeman, 2006).

All routine evidence-based interventions for protecting the patient from injury must be implemented, including hand washing and strict aseptic technique, fall, and immobility protocols. The two most important clinical parameters that precipitate both systemic and local complications are hypovolemia and tissue hypoxia. Third spacing of massive amounts of fluid is easily underestimated. Nurses need to be vigilant in monitoring the patient's hemodynamic and respiratory status. It is imperative that the nurse evaluates the adequacy of fluid resuscitation, oxygenation efforts, and overall tissue perfusion. The nurse realizes the significance of assessment and management in preventing and recognizing complications. Effective communication with the health care team is essential. The nurse must assess for and implement measures to prevent the following:

- Respiratory failure, ARDS (see Chapter 3) ∞
- Cardiovascular collapse: hypovolemic shock (see Chapter 6) ∞
- Renal failure, acute tubular necrosis (see Chapter 14) ∞
- Decreased cerebral perfusion/neurological dysfunction
- Metabolic abnormalities (electrolyte and acid-base imbalances, hyperglycemia)
- GI bleeding
- Disseminated intravascular coagulation (see Chapter 17) ∞
- Sepsis/septic shock (see Chapter 17) ∞

Other local complications include pancreatic pseudocysts and abscesses. A pancreatic pseudocyst is a collection of debris, tissue, fluid, and pancreatic juices that is enclosed by a nonepithelialized wall. Pseudocysts are generally sterile and they can take up to 4 weeks after a severe episode of acute pancreatitis to develop. Some resolve on their own, whereas others may become infected or rupture. An infected pseudocyst is a pancreatic abscess. Treatment depends on the size and the presence of symptoms. Pseudocysts can produce persistent pain, the inability to eat, and, depending on the size, an abdominal mass may be palpated. Drainage of a pseudocyst can be performed surgically, endoscopically, or percutaneously.

Building Technology Skills
Endoscopic Retrograde Cholangiopancreatography (ERCP)

ERCP is an invasive, endoscopic, and radiological procedure that involves oral intubation with a flexible fiber-optic endoscope and advancing it into the duodenum to directly view the ampulla/papilla of Vater. Once the papilla is identified, a small cannula is advanced into the orifice of the ampulla. It can then be manipulated to enter either the common bile duct or the pancreatic duct. Direct visualization of the ducts is accomplished by injecting radiographic contrast medium and taking a series of x-ray films. An example of directly visualizing a stone in the biliary tract is shown in Figure 12-5.

Purpose

The goal of a prompt ERCP is to remove the obstruction, create a passageway for sludge and other stones,

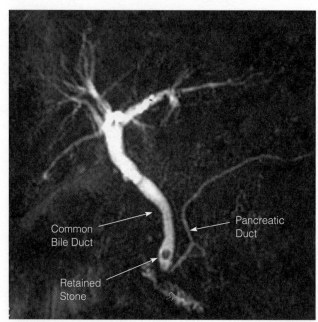

Figure 12-5 MRCP stone.
(Courtesy Lahey Clinic Medical Center, Burlington, MA)

improve pancreatitis, and prevent cholangitis. ERCP is a therapeutic intervention in this setting and has no diagnostic role. Most gallstones causing acute pancreatitis pass spontaneously through the ampulla of Vater to the duodenum. Because the gallbladder ERCP shares a duct, gallstones that become lodged in the duct can prevent the flow of pancreatic enzymes, thus triggering acute pancreatitis. Lodged stones can also cause cholangitis, a rare bacterial infection of the common bile duct that may progress to sepsis, further complicating the patient's condition. Both persistent obstruction and cholangitis contribute to severity and mortality.

The x-ray films can show the configuration of the ducts and identify strictures and obstructions. To remove an impacted stone, the endoscopist performs a sphincterotomy (also called papillotomy) that involves electrosurgical cutting of the papilla of Vater and the muscle fibers of the sphincter of Oddi. The goal of the sphincterotomy is to split tissue and fiber that may be hindering the passage of stones and bile. The endoscopist then manipulates a variety of instruments to remove the stone, thus relieving the obstruction. If there is a stricture, a stent can be placed to facilitate drainage through the stricture. If an impacted stone is not found, a sphincterotomy will most likely be performed to prevent further impactions until a cholecystectomy can be performed.

Indications and Expected Outcomes

Urgent ERCP within 24 to 72 hours (preferably 24 hours from admission) should be considered in any patient with acute gallstone pancreatitis complicated by:

- Obstructive jaundice
- Concomitant cholangitis/biliary sepsis
- Severe pancreatitis (organ failure) with high suspicion of retained common bile duct stones

There is a higher mortality associated with gallstone-induced pancreatitis compared to alcohol-induced pancreatitis. The expected outcome after removing the biliary obstruction is that the patient's clinical picture will improve. Indications of improvement include:

- Decreased pain
- Resolution of the signs and symptoms of infection/sepsis
- Resolution of jaundice
- Decreased nausea, vomiting, gastric distention

Technological Requirements

Technology requirements include a medical facility that has the endoscopic and radiological equipment to perform an ERCP. It is of utmost importance to have an endoscopist and supportive staff with the expertise to perform such an advanced procedure.

Nursing Responsibilities

The critical care nurse has both pre- and postprocedure responsibilities. The majority of the procedures are performed with moderate/procedural sedation administered by a specially trained registered nurse (RN). However, in the case of a critically ill patient who may be unstable, anesthesia may be required.

Preprocedural Responsibilities Include

- Maintains NPO status for 6 to 8 hours prior to the procedure
- Removes dentures
- Monitors baseline vital signs, including temperature and oxygen saturation
- Determines any allergies to contrast material
- Ensures that informed consent has been obtained
- Situation-background-assessment-recommendation (SBAR) communication (see Chapter 1) ∞

Postprocedural Responsibilities Include

- Maintains recovery position until the patient is fully awake (throat is typically sprayed with a topical anesthetic)
- Monitors vital signs including temperature, oxygen saturation, and level of pain and consciousness until the patient returns to baseline
- Monitors for an adverse response to medications
- Monitors for potential complications: worsening pancreatitis, perforation, bleeding
  - Worsening of pain
  - Nausea and vomiting
  - Fever and chills
  - Unstable vital signs

Once that patient has stabilized, a cholesectomy should be performed because too long of a delay in surgery could put the patient at risk for a recurrent attack.

ACUTE GASTROINTESTINAL BLEED AND PANCREATITIS SUMMARY

Gastrointestinal bleeding remains a common clinical problem with cost, morbidity, and mortality implications. The clinical situations are very diverse, depending on the source of bleeding, type of lesion, and rate of bleeding. Positive patient outcomes rely on the nurses' thorough monitoring, comprehension of the patients' hemodynamic status, and effective communication with the health care team. Advances in gastrointestinal endoscopy have become instrumental for diagnosing and treating the bleeding lesions as well as predicting the risk for rebleeding. The success of interventional endoscopy has decreased the need for surgical intervention, which continues to have a high morbidity and mortality. Diagnosis of an initial bleed affords the opportunity for the health care team to not only treat the bleed but also provide secondary prevention. The nurse must provide patients and families the necessary knowledge to understand the risks factors and causes associated with the bleeding and the importance of medication compliance. Decreasing or eliminating alcohol consumption and NSAID usage are often two common lifestyle changes that will decrease the risk of future bleeding.

Patients who are critically ill with pancreatitis require comprehensive medical and, possibly, surgical care coupled with extensive nursing care. Fluid resuscitation is key to preventing continuing pancreatic destruction as well as to limiting organ failure. Initial treatment is directed at identifying and correcting the cause, for example, relieving a gallstone obstruction.

The nurse must be vigilant in monitoring the patient's fluid balance, managing the patient's pain, and assessing for the early signs of complications, most notably hypovolemia and hypoxemia. Pancreatic necrosis and the presence, timing, and duration of organ failure influence morbidity and mortality.

Gerontological Considerations

Forty-five percent of all admissions for GI bleeding are in older adults.

More than 20% of patients admitted to hospitals for bleeding GI ulcers are older adults who were taking NSAIDs for osteoarthritis. Adults over the age of 60 are four times more likely to die from GI bleeding due to NSAIDs than younger persons.

GI bleeding in the older adult may present with signs of dehydration and abdominal cramping.

More than 50% of adults over the age of 50 have radiologic evidence of diverticulitis, which is believed to contribute to the incidence of lower GI bleeding in the older adult.

In older adults, pancreatitis is rarely due to alcohol use and often presents with subtle symptoms rather than acute pain, making the diagnosis more difficult.

Acute pancreatitis is responsible for between 5% and 7% of abdominal pain in older adults.

CASE STUDY

George Jenson is a 57-year-old male admitted to the ICU for acute pancreatitis. His mother died 4 months ago, and shortly after that he lost his job. Recently, he has been drinking a gallon of vodka a day. In addition, he has a history of diabetes mellitus. He was brought to the ED by ambulance when his brother found him unresponsive at home.

He was intubated in the ambulance on the way to the ED and remains intubated and ventilated due to hypoxia. In the ED, his serum hematocrit was 45%, his WBC 21,000 ul (mm³), BUN 35 mg/dL, creatinine 1.4 mg/dL, blood glucose 425, and serum amylase 1,250 SI units. If he awakens, he writhes in pain. He is currently receiving 5 mg of midazolam an hour, 200 mcg of fentanyl an hour, and 8 units of insulin per hour. Since arrival in the ED 2 hours ago, he has received 4 liters of normal saline and is currently receiving 500 mL NS/hour. His blood pressure is currently 92/65 mm Hg, heart rate 124 bpm, and cvp 8 mm Hg.

1. What do his laboratory studies tell you about his hydration status?

2. Is that information confirmed by his vital signs? Why or why not?

3. What is the most likely reason why he developed pancreatitis?

4. How severe is Mr. Jenson's pancreatitis? Why do you believe that?

5. Why is he experiencing such pain?

6. What are the two most essential collaborative interventions for Mr. Jenson?

7. What is the most important nursing diagnosis for him?

See answers to Case Studies in the Answer Section at the back of the book.

CRITICAL THINKING QUESTIONS

1. What is the most frequent cause of gastrointestinal bleeding in the older adult? Why is it a common cause of GI bleeding?

2. What are the differences between the manifestations of upper GI bleeding in the middle-aged and older adult?

3. How do the manifestations of upper GI bleeding differ from the signs and symptoms of a lower GI bleed?

4. How can a nurse identify when a patient who is GI bleeding has received adequate fluid and blood replacement?

5. What are the important components of discharge teaching for the patient with a GI bleed?

6. What are the essential nursing interventions when caring for a patient who has just had an endoscopy for upper gastrointestinal bleeding?

7. How do alcohol misuse and gallstones result in pancreatitis?

8. What manifestations should suggest that the patient was developing severe pancreatitis?

9. What are the two priorities of care for the patient with severe pancreatitis?

See answers to Critical Thinking Questions in the Answer Section at the back of the book.

EXPLORE MEDIALINK
http://www.prenhall.com/perrin

Additional interactive resources for this chapter can be found on the Web site at http://www.prenhall.com/perrin. Click on "Chapter 12" to select activities for this chapter.

Case Study: Acute Pancreatitis

Nursing Care Plan

NCLEX Review Questions

MediaLinks:
- The National Pancreas Foundation
- The American Pancreatic Association
- American Gastroenterological Association (AGA)

- American Society for Gastroenterology (ASGE)
- The National Institute of Diabetes and Digestive and Kidney Diseases
- The Society of Gastroenterology Nurses and Associated (SGNA)
- UpToDate Patient Information

MediaLink Applications

REFERENCES

ASGE. (2001a). An annotated algorithmic approach to lower gastrointestinal bleeding. *Gastrointestinal Endoscopy, 53*(7), 859–863.

ASGE. (2001b). An annotated algorithmic approach to upper gastrointestinal bleeding. *Gastrointestinal Endoscopy, 53*(7), 853–858.

ASGE. (2005). ASGE guideline: The role of endoscopy in the patient with lower GI bleeding. *Gastrointestinal Endoscopy, 62*(5) 656–660.

Banks, P., & Freeman, M. (2006). Practice guidelines in acute pancreatitis. *American Journal of Gastroenterology, 101*(10) 2379–2400.

Barkun, A., Bardou, M., & Marshall, J. (2003). Consensus recommendations for managing patients with nonvariceal upper gastrointestinal bleeding. *Annals of Internal Medicine, 139*(10), 843–857.

Besselink, M., Verwer, T., Schoenmaeckers, E., Buskers, E., Ridwan, B., Visser, M. et al. (2007). Timing of surgical intervention in necrotizing pancreatitis. *Archives of Surgery, 142*(2), 1194–1201.

Bounds, B., & Friedman, L. (2003). Lower gastrointestinal bleeding. *Gastroenterology Clinics of North America, 32*, 1107–1125.

Cagir, B., & Cirincirone, E. (2005). Lower gastrointestinal bleeding: Surgical perspective. *eMedicine.* Retrieved May16, 2007, from http://www.emedicine.com/med/topic2818.htm

Cano, J. (2004). Nutrition in acute pancreatitis. *Critical Care and Shock, 7*(20), 69–76.

Ferguson, C., & Michell, R. (2005). Nonvariceal upper gastrointestinal bleeding: Standard and new treatment. *Gastroenterology Clinics of North America, 34*(4), 607–621.

Ferzoco, S., & Ashley, S. (2006). Surgical management of complications of peptic ulcer disease. *UpToDate.* Retrieved

June 1, 2007, from http://www.utol.com/utd/content/topic/.do?topicKey=acidpep/2489&view=print

Gardner, T., Berk, B., & Yakshe, P. (2006). Acute pancreatitis. *eMedicine.* Retrieved January 2, 2007, from http://www.emedicine.com/med/topic1720.htm

Green, B., & Rockey, D. (2005). Lower gastrointestinal bleeding—management. *Gastroenterology Clinics of North America, 34*(4), 665–678.

Jutabha, R., & Jensen, D. (2006a). Major causes of upper gastrointestinal bleeding in adults. *UpToDate.* Retrieved January 23, 2007, from http://www.utol.com/utd/content/topic/.do?topicKey=gi_dis/9702&view=text

Jutabha, R., & Jensen, D. (2006b). Treatment of bleeding peptic ulcers. *UpToDate.* Retrieved January 2, 2007, from http://www.utol.com/utd/content/topic/.do?topicKey=gi_dis/10994&view=print

Lankisch, P., & Lerch, M. (2006). Pharmacological prevention and treatment of acute pancreatitis: Where are we now? *Digestive Diseases, 24*(1-2), 148–159.

McClave, S., Chang, W., Dhaliwal, R., & Heyland, D. (2006). Nutrition support in acute pancreatitis: A systematic review of the literature. *Journal of Parenteral and Enteral Nutrition, 30*(2), 143–156.

Meier, R., Ockenga, J., Pertliewicz, A., Milinic, N., & MacFie, J. (2006). ESPEN guidelines on enteral nutrition: Pancreas. *Clinical Nutrition, 25*, 275–284.

Nathens, A., Curtis, J., Beale, R., Cook, D., Moreno, R., Romand, J., et al. (2004). Management of the critically ill patient with severe acute pancreatitis. *Critical Care Medicine, 32*(12), 2524–2536.

Papachristou, G., & Whitcomb, D. (2004). Predictors of severity and necrosis in acute pancreatitis. *Gastroenterology Clinics of North America, 33*(4), 871–890.

Rockey, D. (2005). Gastrointestinal bleeding. *Gastroenterology Clinics of North America, 34*(4), 581–588.

Soll, A. (2006). Pharmacology of antiulcer medications. *UpToDate.* Retrieved February 14, 2007, from http://www.utol.com/utd/content/topic/.do?topicKey=acidpep/8883&view=print

Steinberg, W. M. (2006). Acute pancreatitis. In M. Feldman, L. Friedman, & L. Brandt (Eds.), *Sleisenger and Fortram's gastrointestinal and liver diseases pathophysiology/diagnosis/management* (8th ed., pp. 1241–1267). Philadelphia: Saunders Elsevier.

Strate, L. (2005). Lower GI bleeding: Epidemiology and diagnosis. *Gastroenterology Clinics of North America, 34*(4), 643–663.

Vege, S., & Chari, S. (2004). Predicting the severity of acute pancreatitis. *UpToDate.* Retrieved January 27, 2007, from http://www.utdol.com/utd/content/topic.do?topicKey=pancdis/2975&view=text

Vege, S., & Chari, S. (2006a). Clinical manifestations and diagnosis of acute pancreatitis. *UpToDate.* Retrieved January 27, 2007, from http://www.utdol.com/utd/content/topic.do?topicKey=pancdis/7667&view=text

Vege, S., & Chari, S. (2006b). Treatment of acute pancreatitis. *UpToDate.* Retrieved March 31, 2007, from http://www.utdol.com/utd/content/topic.do?topicKey=pancdis/11212&view=print

Weinhouse, G., & Manaker, S. (2006). Stress ulcer prophylaxis in the intensive care unit. *UpToDate.* Retrieved February 14, 2007, from http://www.utol.com/utd/content/topic/.do?topicKey=acidpep/16176&view=print

Whitcomb, D. (2006). Acute pancreatitis. *New England Journal of Medicine, 354*(20), 2142–2149.

Care of the Patient with Endocrine Disorders

Betsy Swinny, MSN, RN, CCRN Pending

Learning Outcomes

Upon completion of this chapter, the learner will be able to:

1. Describe the pathophysiology associated with diabetic ketoacidosis (DKA) and hyperglycemic hyperosmolar nonketotic syndrome (HHNS).

2. Identify five precipitating factors associated with DKA and HHNS.

3. List six essential elements of a focused assessment for a client with DKA and HHNS.

4. Define two differences in assessment between DKA and HHNS.

5. Explain five important considerations related to the administration of insulin.

6. Describe five complications that may occur during the management of DKA or HHNS.

7. Define 10 elements of diabetic teaching that are important to assess in order to assist the client in the prevention of another episode of DKA or HHNS.

8. List five risk factors associated with metabolic syndrome.

9. Explain the pathophysiology associated with hyperglycemia during critical illness.

10. Differentiate short-term complications from long-term complications associated with hyperglycemia.

11. Describe three essential elements to teach a client who has experienced hyperglycemia during a critical illness.

Abbreviations

ADA	American Diabetes Association
CDE	Certified Diabetic Educator
CSS	Corrected Serum Sodium
DKA	Diabetic Ketoacidosis
HHNS	Hyperglycemic Hyperosmolar Nonketotic Syndrome
JDRF	Juvenile Diabetes Research Foundation International

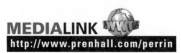

MEDIALINK
http://www.prenhall.com/perrin

See the Companion Website for chapter-specific resources at www.prenhall.com/perrin.

VISUAL MAP Diabetic Ketoacidosis

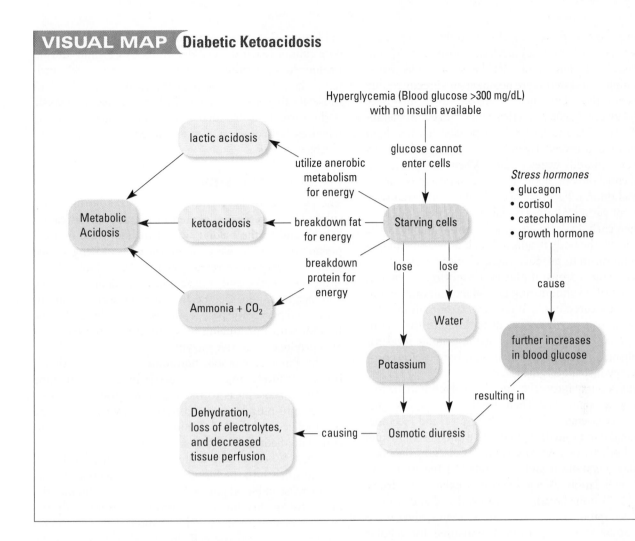

Anatomy and Physiology Review

In order to understand the pathophysiology of diabetic ketoacidosis and hyperglycemic hyperosmolar nonketotic syndrome (HHNS), it is important to first review the normal process of food metabolism. Foods are composed of carbohydrates, fats, and proteins. Each of these components is metabolized into a different set of end products during the process of digestion and absorption.

Carbohydrate Metabolism

Carbohydrates are composed of carbon, hydrogen, and oxygen. They are catagorized as monosaccharides, disaccharides, or polysaccharides depending on the number of sugars they contain. Carbohydrates are broken down into simple sugars such as glucose, galactose, and fructose during the process of digestion. Once digested, these simple sugars enter the bloodstream through the intestinal mucosa. These simple sugars are taken into the cell with insulin, and they are a direct source of fuel for the body. Sugars are used by cells during the process of metabolism to produce energy. Carbohydrates produce 4 kilocalories per gram (kcal/g). Extra hydrogen ions are excreted through the kidneys in the urine. Carbon and oxygen combine to form carbon dioxide, which is excreted through the lungs (Wardlaw & Kessel, 2002).

If more carbohydrates are consumed than are needed for immediate metabolism, the body stores the excess digested sugars as glycogen in the liver and muscle. **Glycogenesis** is the conversion of excess glucose to glycogen. In addition to storing sugars as glycogen, the body may convert excess sugars to fat and store it in adipose tissues. Conversely, when the body needs glucose for metabolism and none is available, glycogen (stored in the liver) is broken down into glucose. **Glycogenolysis** is the conversion of glycogen to glucose. If glycogen stores are used up or carbohydrate intake is limited, the body begins to create glucose from fats and amino acids.

Fat Metabolism

Fats or lipid particles are also composed of carbon, hydrogen, and oxygen. Fats come from the diet in the forms of saturated fats and unsaturated fats. Saturated fats include animal products such as butter, milk, and cheese. Unsaturated fats include monounsaturated fats such as olive oil and polyunsaturated fats such as vegetable oils (e.g., corn oil) and fish.

Fats are digested and absorbed into the bloodstream as glycerides (such as triglycerides), phospholipids, and sterols (such as cholesterol). Unlike sugars, glycerides, phospholipids, and sterols are not taken up directly by any cell. Instead, these fats must be broken down into fatty acids and glycerol, which can then enter the cell for metabolism. Fatty acids and glycerol are produced when lipid particles are hydrolyzed. **Hydrolysis** is a process that splits the bonds and adds water to fats. When fatty acids and glycerol enter the cell, lipolysis (fat breakdown) occurs in the mitochondria. Fats produce 9 kcal/g, compared with 4 kcal/g for carbohydrates (Wardlaw & Kessel, 2002).

When carbohydrate (glucose) is not available at the cellular level, the body begins to break down fats for cellular metabolism to produce energy. This process occurs for three main reasons: if glucose cannot reach the cell due to lack of insulin; during prolonged starvation; and when fats are eaten in the absence of carbohydrates, for example, in carbohydrate-free diets. In all of these situations, glucose is not available at the cellular level for metabolism, so fatty acids and glycerol are used to produce energy instead of glucose.

Breakdown of fatty acids and glycerol result in the formation of ketone bodies. There are three types of ketone bodies: acetoacetate, ß-hydroxybutyrate, and acetone. Acetoacetate and ß-hydroxybutyrate can be used for fuel by most body tissues. Acetone cannot be used by the body in cellular metabolism and is excreted in the urine and through exhalation. When acetone is exhaled a "fruity breath" or "ketone breath" odor is produced and is a recognized symptom of ketosis. Ketosis occurs when more ketone bodies are being formed than used for cellular metabolism, resulting in extra ketones in the bloodstream.

Protein Metabolism

Proteins contain carbon, hydrogen, oxygen, and nitrogen. Nitrogen is an essential component of protein because it is important to the formation of amino acids. Both animal and vegetable proteins form amino acids when they are digested. Animal proteins include various meats. Vegetable proteins include beans and legumes. Once digested, most amino acids are converted to glucose in the liver. The glucose derived from amino acids can then be transported to the cellular level with insulin and used for cellular metabolism. The end products of protein metabolism include adenosine triphosphate (ATP), carbon dioxide, water, urea, and ammonia. ATP is used at the cellular level to produce energy (Wardlaw & Kessel, 2002). Proteins, like carbohydrates, produce 4 kcal/g. Water and carbon dioxide are excreted through the lungs and kidneys. Urea and ammonia are also excreted in the urine through the kidneys.

If more proteins are eaten than are needed, they are converted to glycogen and stored in the liver, or converted to fat and stored in adipose tissues. Conversely, proteins are broken down to be used in cellular metabolism to produce energy when dietary intake of carbohydrates is inadequate. Use of proteins for energy occurs when glucose cannot reach the cell due to lack of insulin, during prolonged starvation, and when the diet is solely protein. The proteins in the liver are used in preference to those of other tissues such as the brain. **Gluconeogenesis** is the formation of glucose from amino acids and fats when carbohydrate intake is limited and there are no glycogen stores.

Function of Insulin

The pancreas is the organ that makes the hormone insulin. The pancreas is located in the abdominal cavity behind and to the medial side of the stomach. A small portion of the pancreas contains the islets of Langerhans. Four hormones are secreted from the islets of Langerhans. Alpha cells make and secrete glucagon. Beta cells make and secrete insulin. Delta cells make and secrete somatostatin, and pancreatic polypeptide is secreted by the F cells. In addition to producing these hormones, the pancreas also produces digestive enzymes.

Insulin is an **anabolic hormone**, which means that it becomes more complex as glucose binds onto it. One function of insulin is to move glucose from the bloodstream into muscle, fat, and liver cells, where it can be metabolized into fuel. A second function of insulin is to stimulate the liver to store excess glucose in the form of glycogen. When carbohydrate (glucose) is absorbed from the intestines into the bloodstream, the pancreas detects the increase in blood glucose and releases insulin into the bloodstream. Insulin travels into the various body tissues (in the muscle, fat, and liver) and binds to insulin receptor sites within the cell. Insulin then facilitates the transport of glucose from the bloodstream into the cell. Once glucose is inside the cell, it can be used by the cell to create energy or be stored by the liver. If glucose cannot be transported into the cell because there is a lack of insulin, then the cells will starve. Even though there may be too much glucose in the bloodstream, without insulin the glucose cannot reach the cellular level to be converted into energy, and the cells cannot produce the energy needed for normal cellular metabolism.

Pathophysiology of Diabetes

Diabetes is a very common condition with increasing prevalence in the United States. According to the Centers for Disease Control and Prevention (2005), National Diabetes Fact Sheet, it is estimated that 13 million people are currently diagnosed with diabetes. Another 5.2 million people may have diabetes but have not yet been diagnosed. People with diabetes constitute over 6% of the population of the United States. There are different types of diabetes with various pathophysiologies. Some people with diabetes do not produce enough insulin. Others produce insulin, but insulin resistance is present. All diabetics have high blood glucose as a result of altered production or function of insulin.

Type 1 Diabetes

The defining characteristic of type 1 diabetics is that the beta cells produce negligible or no insulin. Without insulin, glucose builds up in the bloodstream but cannot enter the cells. The type 1 diabetic needs to take insulin in order to maintain normal cellular glucose uptake and metabolism.

Type 1 diabetes is usually diagnosed in childhood. Adults diagnosed with the disease are usually less than age 30. Type 1 diabetes is caused by a hereditary autoimmune process where the beta cells of the islets of Langerhans are targeted and destroyed. The trigger for the destruction of the beta cells is still under investigation. Some feel that the trigger is a virus, others think it is an environmental trigger, and others feel that the autoimmune trigger occurs as a result of an internal trigger based on genetics (Travis, 1997a, b). Within 5 to 10 years after diagnosis, the insulin-producing beta cells of the pancreas are completely destroyed, and therefore no more insulin is produced. The onset of symptoms in type 1 diabetes is severe and usually occurs rapidly. Because of the rapid onset of type 1 diabetes, people are often in diabetic ketoacidosis at the time of diagnosis.

Type 2 Diabetes

The prevalence of type 2 diabetes is far more common than the prevalence of type 1 diabetes, making up 90% or more of all cases of diabetes. In the past, most people with type 2 diabetes were diagnosed in adulthood, though the disease is now much more common in younger adults and children as more people have common risk factors associated with type 2 diabetes. Common risk factors associated with the disease include genetic predisposition or family history plus obesity, failure to exercise, and poor dietary habits. In addition, older people are at risk for type 2 diabetes and the prevelance of diabetes is increasing as the population of older Americans increases (Table 13–1).

TABLE 13–1

Risk Factors for Type 2 Diabetes

Family history of diabetes
Race/ethnicity (the following all have high rates of diabetes) • African Americans • Hispanic Americans, and • Native Americans
Obesity
Identified impaired glucose tolerance
High blood pressure
High cholesterol • HDL cholesterol of less than 35 mg/dL • Triglyceride level of greater than 250 mg/dL
Gestational diabetes or delivering a baby weighing more than 9 pounds
Age greater than 45 years

Type 2 diabetes is characterized by insulin resistance. The insulin produced by the pancreas is unable to bind to the insulin receptor sites inside the cell. Therefore, glucose is unable to move into the cell, and cells are unable to produce energy. Because the cells are not getting the glucose they need, the pancreas produces more and more insulin. The insulin resistance, lack of functioning insulin, causes abnormally high levels of glucose to build up in the blood (hyperglycemia). People with type 2 diabetes have hyperglycemia and high blood insulin levels (hyperinsulinemia) at the same time.

The onset of type 2 diabetes usually occurs over a period of years as insulin resistance increases. Most people with the disease are overweight. People who are overweight have a higher risk of insulin resistance, because fat interferes with the body's ability to use insulin. Because of its gradual onset people with type 2 diabetes are often not aware that they have the disease at the time of diagnosis. The chronic complications of diabetes such as heart disease, stroke, vascular disease, renal disease, retinopathy, and neuropathy may have already occurred prior to diagnosis. For this reason, the American Diabetes Association recommends that all adults be screened for diabetes at a minimum of every 3 years. Those at high risk should be screened more often.

Gerontological Considerations

The prevalence of type 2 diabetes increases with age and affects 18% to 20% of people over age 65 in the United States (with as many as half of these people being undiagnosed).

The diagnosis of diabetes in the older person is problematic because the older patient with diabetes may not present with the classic symptoms. Typical symptoms of hyperglycemia such as polyuria, polydipsia, and polyphagia may be masked. Because increased thirst can be absent, the initial presentation among older patients may be dehydration with dry eyes, dry mouth, and confusion.

Both diabetic ketoacidosis (DKA) and hyperglycemic hyperosmolar nonketotic syndrome (HHNS) occur in older adults. However, DKA is rare and its features and management do not differ from those in younger diabetics, but its mortality is greater primarily because of associated cardiovascular disease.

HHNS almost always occurs in older people and half the time it is the initial manifestation of diabetes. The ready development of HHNS in the older adult can be explained by a combination of factors, including reduced thirst perception. Acute infection is the most frequent predisposing factor of HHNS, with pneumonia being the most common infection.

The risk of hypoglycemia associated with insulin increases with age. In older adults, symptoms of hypoglycemia might not appear until the blood sugar is less than 50 mg/dL.

Pathophysiology of Diabetic Ketoacidosis

DKA is caused primarily by insulin deficiency. It was traditionally thought that DKA occurred in type 1 diabetics, though DKA can also occur in type 2 diabetics. In DKA, no insulin is present in the bloodstream to facilitate the transport of glucose from the bloodstream into the cells. Hyperglycemia is present (usually higher than 300 mg/dL) because glucose continues to be absorbed from the intestines into the bloodstream, and the liver continues to produce glucose through the processes of gluconeogenesis and glycogenolysis. However, the glucose is not transported into the cells because of the lack of insulin. The lack of cellular glucose causes the cells to "starve." Because the cells are starving, stress hormones are released to induce more glucose production. Stress hormones include glucagon, cortisol, catecholamines such as epinephrine, and growth hormone. These stress hormones induce even more hyperglycemia. Catecholamines also reduce glucose absorption in skeletal muscles (Carroll & Schade, 2001).

In the presence of hyperglycemia osmotic diuresis occurs. The increased levels of glucose result in increased osmolarity of the blood. As a result, water is absorbed into the vascular space from the interstitial spaces and even from cellular tissues such as the brain and other organs to decrease serum osmolarity (dilute the glucose). Glucose and water are diuresed from the vascular space through the kidneys. Severe diuresis in hyperglycemia results in loss of water, sodium, potassium, magnesium, and phosphates. Osmotic diuresis causes severe dehydration, including cellular dehydration, as well as loss of electrolytes.

Severe dehydration also causes several other complications. The viscosity of the blood increases as blood volume decreases and results in increased probability of platelet aggregation and thromboembolism. Decreased organ perfusion results from dehydration and can rapidly progress to hypovolemic shock with accompanied organ dysfunction. Perfusion to all vital organs and tissues is decreased, causing organ dysfunction and potential acute organ failure. As a result of decreased perfusion, cells will begin anaerobic metabolism. This in turn results in the production and buildup of lactic acid and contributes to metabolic acidosis.

Because there is a lack of glucose at the cellular level, the body begins to break down fats and proteins for use as cellular fuels. The breakdown of fatty acids results in the formation of three ketone bodies: acetoacetate, ß-hydroxybutyrate, and acetone. Brain cells cannot use the by-products of fatty acids. Brain cells use only glucose and oxygen for metabolism. Acetoacetate and ß-hydroxybutyrate are used for fuel within the cells of organs (other than the brain). Acetone cannot be used in cellular metabolism and is excreted through the kidneys and lungs. When acetone is exhaled a "fruity breath" or "ketone breath" odor is produced and is a recognized symptom of ketosis. **Ketoacidosis** occurs as a result of buildup of fatty acids. Ketoacidosis causes metabolic acidosis. Both lactic acid from anaerobic cellular metabolism as well as ketoacidosis contribute to metabolic acidosis.

Proteins are also metabolized to create cellular energy during cellular starvation. High levels of circulating cortisol increase protein lysis. The end products of protein metabolism include ATP, carbon dioxide, water, urea, and ammonia. ATP is used for fuel at the cellular level. Water and carbon dioxide are excreted through the lungs and kidneys. Urea and ammonia are also excreted through the kidneys in the urine.

Because organ function is decreased due to decreased perfusion, by-products of glucose, fat, and protein metabolism often build up in the bloodstream. Decreased kidney function results in additional acidosis caused by the buildup of hydrogen ions and ketones, which are normally excreted through the kidneys. Brain function is also impaired. The severe dehydration caused by osmotic diuresis contributes to the loss of cellular fluid in the brain cells. Glucose and oxygen, both vital to brain function, cannot reach brain cells due to lack of insulin and decreased perfusion. All organs are affected by cellular dehydration, lack of perfusion, and lack of glucose. Overall mortality from DKA is 2% to 10%.

Pathophysiology of Hyperglycemic Hyperosmolar Nonketotic Syndrome

HHNS is common in the patient with type 2 diabetes. It is similar to DKA in that hyperglycemia is present. However, hyperglycemia is often more severe (usually greater than 600 mg/dL). The severe hyperglycemia results in the same physiological results described in DKA. The increased levels of glucose result in increased osmolarity of the blood. In the presence of hyperglycemia osmotic diuresis occurs. As a result, water is absorbed into the vascular space from the interstitial spaces and even from cellular tissues such as the brain and other organs to decrease vascular serum osmolarity (dilute the glucose). Glucose and water are diuresed from the vascular space through the kidneys. Severe diuresis in hyperglycemia results in loss of water, sodium, potassium, magnesium, and phosphates. Osmotic diuresis causes severe dehydration, including cellular dehydration, as well as loss of electrolytes.

Severe dehydration causes the same complications as seen in DKA. The viscosity of the blood increases as blood volume decreases. Cellular, interstitial, and vascular dehydration as well as loss of electrolytes is often more severe in HHNS than in DKA and is proportional to the levels of vascular glucose. Increased blood viscosity results in increased probability of platelet aggregation and thromboembolism. Decreased organ perfusion results from dehydration and can rapidly progress to hypovolemic shock with accompanied organ dysfunction

VISUAL MAP Hyperglycemic Hyperosmolar Nonketotic Syndrome

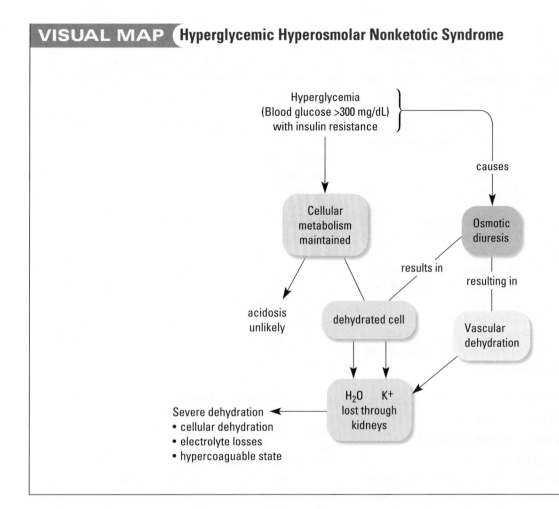

(see the section "Focused Assessment of a Client with Diabetic Ketoacidosis and Hyperglycemic Hyperosmolar Nonketotic Syndrome"). Perfusion to all vital organs and tissues is decreased. As a result of decreased perfusion, cells will begin anaerobic metabolism. This in turn results in the production and buildup of lactic acid and contributes to metabolic acidosis.

A main difference between DKA and HHNS is that in HHNS insulin is present. Insulin facilitates the transport of enough glucose into the cells that the breakdown of fatty acids for cellular energy is minimal. As a result the cells do not starve and often there is no ketosis, or if present ketosis is mild. Metabolic acidosis, if present, is often mild. However, the overall mortality of HHNS is higher (12% to 46%) and is related to the severe dehydration and associated complications that result from osmotic diuresis.

Precipitating Factors of Diabetic Ketoacidosis and Hyperglycemic Hyperosmolar Nonketotic Syndrome

The most common cause of DKA and HHNS is infection. Of all clients presenting with DKA and HHNS, Chiasson et al. (2003) report that as many as 20% to 25% are precipitated by infection. An infection causes a physio-

Nursing Diagnoses

DIABETIC KETOACIDOSIS AND HYPERGLYCEMIC HYPEROSMOLAR NONKETOTOTIC SYNDROME

- Deficient fluid volume related to active fluid loss (increased urine output)
- Imbalanced nutrition less than body requirements related to inability to utilize glucose
- Ineffective tissue perfusion related to hypovolemia and interruption in peripheral blood flow
- Risk for ineffective management of the therapeutic regimen related to complexity of the medical regimen
- Risk for injury related to abnormal blood glucose
- Risk for infection related to abnormal blood glucose and interruption in peripheral blood flow

logical stress reaction, which precipitates hyperglycemia. Failure of a type 1 diabetic to take adequate insulin during the physiological stress of illness increases the body's insulin demand even more and often starts the cascade to DKA. Because infection is a common cause of DKA and HHNS, it is important to evaluate for its presence when a client with DKA or HHNS presents to the hospital.

There are also several other common causes of DKA and HHNS. Clients presenting for the first time with type 1 diabetes are often in DKA at the time of presentation. Due to the insulin production in HHNS, this condition is most commonly seen in type 2 diabetics. Type 2 diabetics presenting for the first time with type 2 diabetes may have HHNS at the time of presentation. HHNS may also develop slowly and chronically in type 2 diabetics with poor compliance.

Conditions that induce stress such as heart attack, cerebral vascular accident, trauma, or surgery also can lead to DKA and HHNS. Pregnancy causes metabolic strain and can induce DKA or HHNS. Medications such as glucocorticoids, thiazide diuretics, calcium channel blockers, propranolol, phenytoin, sympathomimetics, and total parenteral nutrition (TPN) increase the blood glucose and can complicate or precipitate DKA and HHNS. Alcohol and cocaine use are also associated with the development of DKA or HHNS. In addition to the effects of cocaine or alcohol, clients who use these substances are at risk for poor nutrition and poor compliance with the treatment of their diabetes (Table 13–2).

Focused Assessment of a Client with Diabetic Ketoacidosis and Hyperglycemic Hyperosmolar Nonketotic Syndrome

Some of the symptoms that the client with DKA or HHNS presents with are similar. All clients will present with some degree of dehydration. The following assessment findings indicate dehydration: poor skin turgor, sunken appearance of the eyes, dry mouth and mucous membranes, tachycardia, orthostatic drop in blood pressures, and low urine output. Urine output may be an inaccurate method to measure the degree of dehydration because the client may continue to have high urine output even in the presence of dehydration as a result of osmotic diuresis. All clients also present with hyperglycemia. The hallmark symptoms that indicate hyperglycemia include thirst and frequent urination. Clients with both DKA and HHNS should be assessed for presence of infection. Increased temperature and increased white blood cell (WBC) count are signs of infection. The source of infection should be identified. Common sources of infection include urinary tract infections, pneumonia, and even tooth abscesses. The skin should also be inspected for signs of a wound or skin infection. Culture and sensitivity of the source of infection (e.g., sputum cultures, urine cultures, or wound cultures) will help identify the type of infection and aid in identifying effective antibiotics. Blood cultures may also be completed to assess for sepsis. Clients with high blood glucose are at increased risk for sepsis, or sepsis may be a precipitating factor of DKA and HHNS. Change in level of consciousness and changes in mental status are important assessments that correlate with the degree of hyperosmolarity. Assessment for deep vein thrombosis and other thromboses is important because of the increased blood viscosity. Clients with fluid and electrolyte imbalances may exhibit leg cramps and ECG changes.

The presentation of the client with DKA may differ slightly from the presentation of the client with HHNS (Langdon & Shriver, 2004). The client with type 1 diabetes often presents in metabolic acidosis. Signs and symptoms that need to be assessed for include gastrointestinal symptoms such as loss of appetite, abdominal pain, and nausea and vomiting. These symptoms sometimes make the client appear to have an acutely inflamed abdomen. The cause of these symptoms is actually related to decreased perfusion of the mesentery. **Kussmaul respirations** are also present in metabolic acidosis. These deep and rapid respirations decrease carbon dioxide in order to compensate for metabolic acidosis. Ketosis is also a sign of DKA. Positive assessment findings for ketosis include acetone or fruity odor of the breath and positive urine ketones.

The client in HHNS should be assessed for visual disturbances, blurred vision, and weight loss. These are signs of severe dehydration complicated by high blood osmolarity and high blood glucose.

The client with DKA or HHNS may present with mild, moderate, or severe symptoms. Some clients will be ambulatory and able to give an accurate history. Others will be comatose, in shock, and close to death. The client may present in either hypovolemic or septic shock. General signs of shock include tachycardia and low blood pressure. Shock also includes decreased perfusion of organs and is

TABLE 13–2
Precipitating Factors for DKA and HHNS
Infection • May be complicated by the client failing to take adequate insulin
New onset of diabetes • DKA results from new onset of type 1 diabetes • HHNS results from new onset of type 2 diabetes
Conditions that induce a stress reaction • Heart attack • Stroke • Trauma • Surgery • Pregnancy
Commonly prescribed medications • Calcium channel blockers • Propanolol (Inderal) • Thiazide diuretics (hydrochlorothiazide[HCTZ]) • Sympathomimetics (dopamine, dobutamine, epinephrine, norepinephrine, albuterol, and phenylephrine) • Phenytoin (Dilantin) • Glucocorticoids (hydrocortisone, prednisone, dexamethasone) • Total parenteral nutrition (TPN)
Other toxins • Alcohol • Cocaine

reflected through organ failure. Assessments include function of each organ and laboratory findings indicating failure. For instance renal failure is evidenced through urine output less than 0.5 cc/kg/hr, decreased glomerular filtration rate, and increased creatinine. Table 13–3 differentiates the symptoms of DKA and HHNS.

Diagnostic Criteria

Laboratory criteria that are important in the diagnosis of DKA include blood glucose higher than 300 mg/dL but often over 500 mg/dL. In HHNS the blood glucose is often higher than 600 mg/dL and can be 1,000 mg/dL or higher. The serum osmolarity will be increased and is proportional to the amount of blood glucose.

Serum osmolarity is equal to $(2 \times sodium) +$ (serum glucose/18) + (BUN/2.8). Normal serum osmolarity is 280 to 300 mmol/L. In DKA and HHNS, clients typically have a serum osmolarity over 300 mmol/L. In HHNS serum osmolarity is often higher than in DKA as a result of increased serum glucose. Table 13–4 illustrates how serum osmolarity becomes more critical as serum glucose rises. The first calculation is based on normal laboratory values and the serum osmolarity is

normal. The second calculation represents laboratory values typically seen in DKA. The third example, typical of a client with HHNS, illustrates how critical osmolarity can become.

Both the anion gap and arterial blood gases will show the presence of acidosis. Metabolic acidosis is profound in DKA and can be life threatening, though there is often little to no acidosis in HHNS. The anion gap is calculated to show the presence of metabolic acidosis in DKA. The normal anion gap is 10 to 17 mEq/L and is found using the following equation: (Sodium + potassium) − (chloride + bicarbonate). An anion gap that is higher than normal is evidence of metabolic acidosis (Kee, 2005). Arterial blood gases will also show the presence of metabolic acidosis. Serum pH will be lower than 7.35, showing acidity. The pO_2 may be normal or low if the client is comatose and breathing shallowly. The pCO_2 will be low as the client attempts to blow off carbon dioxide (CO_2) to compensate for acidosis. Bicarbonate is also often low because the client has used up bicarbonate stores in an attempt to correct acidosis (Table 13–5).

Other laboratory findings that are significant include electrolytes, a complete blood count (CBC), cultures, urine

TABLE 13–3

Differentiating the Symptoms of DKA and HHNS

ASSESSMENTS INDICATING DKA	ASSESSMENTS INDICATING HHNS
• Dehydration: poor skin turgor, sunken appearance of the eyes, dry mouth and mucous membranes, tachycardia, orthostatic drop in blood pressures, and low urine output • Hyperglycemia: thirst and frequent urination • Presence of infection: fever, increased WBC • Ketosis: fruity odor to the breath, positive urine ketones • Metabolic acidosis: loss of appetite, abdominal pain, nausea and vomiting, and rapid deep respirations (Kussmaul respirations) • High osmolarity and dehydration: mental status changes, loss of consciousness, increased blood viscosity • Fluid and electrolyte abnormalities: abnormal labs, leg cramps, and ECG changes • Shock: tachycardia, low blood pressure, and signs of organ failure	• Dehydration: poor skin turgor, sunken appearance of the eyes, dry mouth and mucous membranes, tachycardia, orthostatic drop in blood pressures, and low urine output • Hyperglycemia: thirst and frequent urination • Presence of infection: fever, increased WBC • High osmolarity and dehydration: visual disturbances, blurred vision, weight loss, mental status changes, loss of consciousness, and increased blood viscosity • Fluid and electrolyte abnormalities: abnormal labs, leg cramps, and ECG changes • Shock: tachycardia, low blood pressure, and signs of organ failure

TABLE 13–4

Calculating Serum Osmolarity

1. Na$^+$ 140	K$^+$ 3.8	Glucose 90	BUN 15	$(2 \times 140) + (90/18) + (15/2.8) = (280) + (5) + (5.36) = 290.36$ mmol/liter (normal)
2. Na$^+$ 130	K$^+$ 6.2	Glucose 604	BUN 36	$(2 \times 130) + (604/18) + (36/2.8) = (260) + (33.5) + (12.8) = 306$ mmol/liter (elevated)
3. Na$^+$ 128	K$^+$ 4.5	Glucose 990	BUN 40	$(2 \times 128) + (990/18) + (40/2.8) = (256) + (55) + (14.29) = 325$ mmol/liter (very elevated)

TABLE 13–5

Calculating Anion Gap

1. Na$^+$ 140	K$^+$ 3.8	CL 102	Bicarb 30	$(140 + 3.8) − (102 + 30) (143.8) − (132) = 11.8$ mEq/L (normal)
2. Na$^+$ 132	K$^+$ 4.4	CL 100	Bicarb 17	$(132 + 4.4) − (100 + 17) (136.4) − (117) = 19.4$ mEq/L (metabolic acidosis)

studies, and clotting studies. Initial electrolyte findings often reveal high potassium even though intracellular potassium is often depleted. Once the client is treated with insulin, potassium moves rapidly toward the intracellular space, and serum potassium is often very low (Kee, 2005). The sodium, magnesium, phosphorus, and calcium are also often low due to osmotic diuresis. Electrolytes are repeated often until they are within normal limits. A CBC will show high WBCs if infection is present and also can be used to determine the extent of dehydration. Blood cultures should be anticipated if the client is febrile to rule out sepsis. Urine is collected and tested for **glycosuria** and **ketonuria**. Urine cultures will detect the presence of urinary tract infection. Sputum cultures may be done if the client has signs of pneumonia. If pulmonary congestion is heard on auscultation, a chest x-ray should be anticipated to rule out pneumonia or other signs of infection. If wounds are present, wound cultures should also be completed prior to the initiation of antibiotics. Clotting studies such as a prothrombin time (PT), partial thromboplastin time (PTT), and a D-Dimer are accomplished to detect increased potential of blood clots.

Kidney function is evaluated through the findings of glomerular filtration, serum creatinine, and BUN. In renal failure both BUN and creatinine will be elevated. Glomerular filtration is being used more routinely in clinical practice because it is a good measure of early renal failure or of a renal insult due to low perfusion. If glomerular filtration is decreased the findings indicate a renal insult or renal failure. Liver function is also analyzed through analysis of liver enzymes. Aspartate aminotransferase (AST), also known as SGOT, and alanine aminotransferase (ALT), also known as SGPT, will be elevated in liver failure (Kee, 2005). Lactate dehydrogenase (LDH) will be more elevated in DKA, not only as a result of liver dysfunction but also as a result of lactic acid production seen in anaerobic metabolism.

Additional laboratory studies are aimed specifically at identifying the precipitating cause of DKA or HHNS. Cardiac enzymes are completed to rule out acute myocardial infarction. A computerized tomography (CT) scan of the head may be done to rule out a stroke. A pregnancy test should be completed on any premenopausal female. As previously mentioned, cultures should be completed to identify infections. A toxic screen should be anticipated to identify presence of illegal drugs or alcohol. Levels of prescribed medications, especially those that precipitate DKA and HHNS, are also analyzed.

Monitoring the heart rhythm using ECG is also an essential diagnostic tool. Findings from ECG monitoring can help to identify cardiovascular dysfunction as a result of electrolyte imbalances. Sodium, potassium, calcium, and magnesium all participate in cardiovascular function. A sign of elevated serum potassium is high, peaked T waves. A sign of hypokalemia is U waves. If the client has been prescribed calcium channel blockers or beta blockers they will be unable to clear the circulation due to decreased perfusion to the liver and kidney, resulting in toxicity. A low heart rate and potential heart blocks may result.

Collaborative Management

Both DKA and HHNS are life-threatening emergencies. Initial therapies are aimed at correcting conditions that are a threat to life. Collaborative management includes fluid therapy, insulin therapy, correction of electrolytes, correction of acidosis, and treatment of the precipitating cause. When the client is stable, collaborative management changes to focus on maintaining a stable state, preventing another episode, and teaching the client how to manage diabetes as well as complications that arise. Although DKA is complicated by metabolic acidosis, the treatment for both DKA and HHNS are similar.

Fluid Therapy

Fluid therapy is an important first step to correct vascular volume as well as interstitial and cellular fluid deficits. Perfusion to vital organs as well as cells is increased as fluid volume increases. As a result of increased perfusion, all organs will function more effectively. The kidneys need to function well to clear metabolites such as ketone bodies. Hydration also improves the effectiveness of insulin and decreases blood viscosity.

In severe dehydration or hypovolemic shock, Farhat (2001) recommends replacing one half of the total body water deficits in the first 8 hours of therapy, and replacing the remaining total body water deficit during the following 16 hours. A common calculation used to estimate fluid loss is 100 mL/kg of weight. Table 13–6 presents an

TABLE 13–6	
Example of Fluid Replacement in Severe Dehydration	
Client weight = 165 pounds (75 kg)	Fluid replacement — 100 mL/kg, equals 7,500 mL in the first 24 hours
First hour: IV rate = 1,000 mL/hr	Total: 1,000 mL
Hours 2–8 (7 hours): IV rate = 500 mL/hr	+ 3,500 mL = total: 4,500 mL
Hours 9–24 (16 hours): IV rate = 200 mL/hr	+ 3,200 mL = total 7,700 mL

example of fluid replacement based on estimated losses in severe dehydration. It should be noted that following 8 hours of therapy, the client has received approximately one half of the total fluid replacement. The second half of the volume is given in the remaining 16 hours.

Normal saline (0.9%) is the intravenous (IV) fluid used most often when a client is in shock because it is retained in the intravascular space, and it replaces severe sodium losses. Once the blood pressure returns to normal, and minimum urine output is 0.5 mL/kg/hr, then the IV fluid is often changed to half-normal saline (0.45% NS). Another method to determine whether to use normal saline (0.9% NS) or half-normal saline (0.45% NS) is to calculate the corrected serum sodium (CSS). The CSS = Serum Na^+ + {[(Serum glucose (mg/dL) – 100)/100] × 1.6}. The determination of which IV fluid to use is based on the corrected serum sodium result. Normal serum sodium is 135 to 145 mEq/L. If the CSS is high or normal then half-normal saline (0.45% NS) is used. If the CSS is low then normal saline (0.9% NS) will help to correct sodium losses. Table 13–7 presents two examples of the calculation of CSS.

In addition to replacing total body water deficits, hourly fluid losses due to osmotic diuresis need to be considered. If hourly urine output is extremely high, then the client will continue to lose fluid even though IV fluid is being administered. The volume lost each hour in urine may be measured, and the hourly IV fluid rate is calculated to add volume lost in urine output. Osmotic diuresis will decrease as the serum glucose decreases. Dextrose (5%) is added to the IV fluid to help prevent hypoglycemia when the serum glucose drops below 250 mg/dL to 300 mg/dL.

The example of fluid volume replacement (above) may also be more volume than some clients need or could tolerate. It should be noted that the example in Table 13-7 illustrates that the client weighing 165 pounds (75 kg) would receive 7,500 mL of fluid in the first 24 hours of therapy. Clients present with varying degrees of dehydration, and fluid therapy needs to be tailored to the level of dehydration. Rapid administration of IV fluid can cause rapid fluid shifts and can result in edema in vital organs such as the brain and the lungs. In addition, preexisting medical conditions such as renal failure, heart failure, and pulmonary disease also need to be considered prior to instituting large amounts of IV fluids.

Hemodynamic monitoring may be indicated to measure central venous pressure (CVP), pulmonary artery pressure (PAP), pulmonary capillary wedge pressure (PCWP), cardiac output (CO), cardiac index (CI), mixed venous oxygen saturation (SVO_2), and systemic vascular resistance (SVR). The data collected can help determine the rate of fluid volume tolerated for the client with preexisting renal, heart, or pulmonary disease. The nurse should be vigilant to the signs of fluid volume overload such as pulmonary congestion, neck vein distention, increasing CVP and PCWP, and generalized edema.

In addition to hemodynamic monitoring, assessment of the outcome of fluid replacement includes frequent vital signs. Vital signs are done every hour at the minimum, though they may be much more frequent until the client is initially stabilized. Strict intake and output is also essential. Daily weights will accurately measure fluid volume increases or losses over a 24-hour period. Neurological assessments are also important. Decreasing level of consciousness and headache may be signs of cerebral edema.

Insulin Therapy

Insulin therapy facilitates the transport of glucose in the cells. The glucose promotes normal cellular metabolism. When glucose is present, fat and protein breakdown for the production of cellular energy will stop. Toxic metabolites, such as ketoacids, and lactic acids will also stop being produced.

COMMONLY USED MEDICATIONS

INSULIN

REGULAR INSULIN Regular insulin, also known as Humulin R, Novolin R, Velosulin, Velosulin BR, and Velsulin Human, is a hormone. It is a short-acting insulin that travels into the various body tissues (in the muscle, fat, and liver) binding to insulin receptor sites within the cell.

It lowers blood glucose by transporting glucose from the bloodstream into the cell and is metabolized primarily in the liver.

Dose and Desired Effect: Given by IV route in critically ill patients, usually as a bolus infusion of 0.15 Units/Kg followed by an infusion of 0.1 Units/Kg/hour, the insulin should have an onset of effect within 15 to 30 minutes and a peak of 2 to 3 hours. It should decrease the serum glucose by 50 to 70 mg/dL/hour.

Nursing Responsibilities: Always use an insulin syringe to measure insulin doses.

- Bolus may be administered undiluted, up to 20 units over 1 minute.

- Note that the insulin infusion should be diluted in 0.45% NS or 0.9% NS.

- Prior to initiating the IV infusion waste 25–50 mL through the new IV tubing because insulin adheres to the IV tubing.

- Measure the blood glucose hourly during IV insulin infusions.

- When the blood glucose reaches 250–300 mg/dL then the rate of administration of insulin is either stopped and transitioned to SQ insulin or decreased by half to 0.05 unit/kg/hr until signs of acidosis have resolved.

Potential Side and/or Toxic Effects: Adverse effects include hypoglycemia, which is common, and anaphylaxis, which is rare (Wilson, Shannon, Shields, & Stang, 2007).

TABLE 13–7

Calculating Corrected Serum Sodium

1. Na^+ 128 Glucose 400	128 + {[(400 − 100)/100] × 1.6} = 128 + {[300/100] ×1.6} = 128 + {3 ×1.6} = 128 + 4.8 = 132.8	IV Fluid Choice: Normal saline (0.9% NS)
2. Na^+ 128 Glucose 990	128 + {[(990 − 100)/100] ×1.6} = 128 + {[890/100] ×1.6} = 128 + {8.9 ×1.6} = 128 + 14.24 = 142.24	IV Fluid Choice: Half-normal saline (0.45% NS)

The standard of care is to administer regular insulin IV until blood glucose returns close to normal limits. Subcutaneous (SQ) insulin therapies, including insulin pumps, are stopped until the blood glucose is stabilized. Prior to administering insulin, it is important to identify and correct hypokalemia to prevent an unsafe serum potassium level. It is also essential to know renal function to manage fluid and electrolyte replacement. A bolus of IV insulin is common prior to starting an insulin infusion. A common bolus dose is equal to 0.15 unit/kg. Insulin infusions are often started at 0.1 unit/kg/hr. Using these calculations, an adult weighing 176 pounds, or 80 kg, would require a bolus dose of 12 units of insulin and an initial infusion starting at 8 units per hour.

Regular insulin is most commonly used for IV infusions. An important consideration when starting an insulin infusion is to waste 25 to 50 mL through the new IV tubing prior to initiating the IV infusion because insulin adheres to the IV tubing. After the first hour and each hour thereafter, the rate of infusion is adjusted based on hourly bedside blood glucose measurements. The goal is to decrease serum glucose by 50 to 70 mg/dL/hr. Complications result if insulin is infused too rapidly. Quick drops in blood glucose may result in hypoglycemia as well as a rapid shift in potassium from the serum into the intracellular compartment. This rapid electrolyte shift can cause hypokalemia and result in life-threatening cardiac arrhythmias. Conversely, if serum glucose does not decrease by 50 to 70 mg/dL in the first hour, insulin doses are doubled or additional bolus doses of IV insulin may be administered. Complications result if insulin is infused too rapidly. Quick drops in blood glucose may result in hypoglycemia as well as a rapid shift in potassium from the serum into the intracellular compartment. This rapid electrolyte shift can cause hypokalemia and result in life-threatening cardiac arrhythmias.

Once the serum glucose reaches 250 to 300 mg/dL then the insulin infusion is either transitioned to the SQ route or decreased by half to 0.05 unit/kg/hr. If there is little to no acidosis present, then IV insulin may be transitioned to SQ insulin. IV insulin is normally discontinued 1 to 2 hours after the initial dose of SQ insulin. This transition prevents hypoglycemia or hyperglycemia. If acidosis is present, then IV insulin is continued until acidosis is beginning to resolve, which is defined by bicarbonate greater than 18 mEq/L, venous pH greater than 7.3, normal anion gap, and no ketones in the urine.

Correction of Electrolytes and Acidosis

Fluid therapy corrects dehydration and increases perfusion to vital organs. Insulin therapy corrects hyperglycemia and ketosis. Acidosis is beginning to resolve. The next step is correction of abnormal electrolytes to prevent life-threatening cardiac arrhythmias, promote cellular metabolism, improve smooth and skeletal muscle function, and maintain endocrine function. Although fluid therapy, insulin therapy, and correction of electrolytes are discussed separately and in detail, it is important to mention that treatment is rapid and often concurrent in the clinical setting.

Serum potassium may be high, normal, or low in the client presenting with DKA or HHNS. High serum osmolarity pulls potassium into the vascular space, making serum potassium high. Once in the vascular space potassium is lost through the urine due to osmotic diuresis, making serum potassium normal or low. It is important to remember that clients who present with normal or even slightly elevated serum potassium have intracellular potassium deficits.

SAFETY INITIATIVES   **Prevent Harm from High-Alert Medication: Insulin**

PURPOSE: To prevent harm from high-alert medications by implementing the changes in care recommended in the Institute for Healthcare Improvement (IHI) guide. High-alert (or high-hazard) medications are medications that are likely to cause significant harm to the patient even when used as intended.

RATIONALE: Insulin has resulted in improved quality and length of life for diabetics. However, mismanagement can result in hyperglycemia or hypoglycemia, both of which are harmful to the patient. Hypoglycemia is the most common complication of any insulin therapy in a hopspital; one study reported 56 occurrences of hypoglycemia in 100 treatment days.

HIGHLIGHTS OF RECOMMENDATIONS: Changes designed to ensure standardization, such as eliminating the use of sliding insulin dosage scales or standardizing the scale through the use of a preprinted protocol that clearly designates the specific increments of insulin coverage and using a single concentration of IV infusion insulin which is prepared in the pharmacy. Requires an independent double-check of the drug, concentration, dose, pump settings, route of administration, and patient identity before administering all IV insulin.

Changes designed to ensure better partnering with patients and families, such as encouraging patient self-management and patient questions about doses and timing of insulin administration. It is even better to have patients manage their own insulin and coordinate meal and insulin times during hospitalization if they are capable.

Source: Institute for Healthcare Improvement

 Available: http://www.ihi.org/IHI/Programs/ Campaign/HighAlertMedications.htm

COMMONLY USED MEDICATIONS

POTASSIUM

Potassium Chloride and Potassium Phosphate are electrolyte replacements. Potassium, an intracellular electrolyte, is essential for nerve conduction, muscle contraction (cardiac, skeletal, and smooth), maintenance of normal kidney function, and maintenance of normal enzyme action. Potassium also plays a role in acid-base balance.

Dose and Desired Effect: Given intravenously as a usual dose of 10 mEq/hr or a high dose of 20–40 mEq/hr and diluted to 10–20 mEq per 100 mL of solution, The desired effect is a slow increase in serum potassium. The goal is to keep serum potassium levels between 4 and 5 mEq/L.

Nursing Responsibilities:
- NEVER give potassium IV push or in any concentrated form. Rapid infusion may cause fatal arrhythmias.

- Always use an IV infusion pump to administer potassium.

- Never add potassium to an IV that is infusing. After adding potassium to an IV bag invert it several times to ensure even distribution of potassium in solution.

- If possible infuse into a central vein to prevent pain at the IV site and phlebitis.

- Assess renal function prior to administration of potassium because impaired renal function may cause severe hyperkalemia

- Monitor the ECG of patients receiving infusions exceeding 10 mEq/hr.

- Monitor serum electrolytes frequently (Wilson, Shannon, Shields, & Stang, 2007).

Potential Side and/or Toxic Effects: Adverse effects include: hyperkalemia, respiratory distress, cardiac depression, arrythmias, cardiac arrest, flaccid paralysis

In DKA the additional problems of anaerobic cellular metabolism and acidosis cause potassium to shift from intracellular to extracellular (vascular and interstitial) spaces. Replacement of potassium will depend on initial potassium levels. In addition, renal function must be adequate prior to administering potassium. Serum potassium often drops rapidly with fluid administration and insulin therapy as potassium shifts back into the intracellular compartment. The goal is to keep serum potassium levels between 4 and 5 mEq/L. Potassium is never given IV push or in any concentrated form. Rapid infusion may cause fatal cardiac arrhythmias. An IV infusion pump must always be used to administer potassium. Potassium is normally administered at 10 to 20 mEq/hr. It is common to give as much as 100 to 200 mEq of potassium over the first 24 hours to treat intracellular deficits.

In addition to potassium, serum sodium, calcium, and magnesium are also low in the client presenting with DKA or HHNS as a result of losses due to osmotic diuresis. Sodium losses are replaced using the calculated corrected sodium as discussed previously. It is also important to replace calcium and magnesium if levels are very low. All of these electrolytes (sodium, potassium, calcium, and magnesium) are important to cellular function and uptake of glucose, skeletal and smooth muscle function, CNS function, and endocrine function.

Low phosphate can contribute to respiratory depression, muscle weakness, and cardiac arrhythmias. However, recent literature does not recommend phosphate replacement. Giving too much phosphate can cause low serum calcium. In addition, research has not demonstrated a clinical benefit to the routine administration of phosphate. However, because phosphate is expected to be low, some authors still recommend giving one third of potassium replacement as potassium phosphate. The other two-thirds potassium replacement is administered as potassium chloride (Coursin & Murray, 2003).

Bicarbonate therapy is reserved for those clients with severe acidosis (those clients with DKA). Giving too much bicarbonate can cause rebound alkalosis, hypokalemia, hypernatremia, elevated lactate, paradoxical cellular acidosis, and slowed improvement of ketosis. In addition, there has not been a researched improvement in morbidity and mortality by administering bicarbonate to clients with pH as low as 6.9 to 7.1. On the other hand, treating severe acidosis is helpful because it promotes insulin absorption, improves hemodynamic functioning, raises the threshold for ventricular fibrillation, improves CNS functioning, and improves organ function. Therefore, treatment of acidosis with bicarbonate is typically reserved for those clients with a pH less than 7.0. It is recommended that bicarbonate be mixed in an IV solution of water or hypotonic saline (0.45% NS) so that it is isotonic. Bicarbonate is then administered slowly, over an hour.

Electrolytes and arterial or venous blood gases are typically measured every hour or two initially. Neurological assessments, strength, orientation, and mentation should all be assessed hourly. If sodium levels are low, seizure precautions are appropriate. Frequent monitoring is essential because levels change rapidly as fluids and insulin are administered. Acidosis will resolve as metabolism returns to normal. Maintaining adequate electrolyte levels is important to cellular metabolism, organ function, neuromuscular function, and endocrine function.

Treatment of the Precipitating Cause

Treatment of the initial precipitating cause is essential. Failure to recognize and treat underlying medical conditions such as myocardial infarction, drug toxicity, or sepsis can be life threatening (Langdon & Shriver, 2004). Other precipitating factors can cause serious complications. A careful admission history is paramount to determine if the client has signs of infection or is not aware of having diabetes, such as a newly diagnosed diabetic. Because infection is a common precipitating factor to the development of DKA or HHNS, it is important to start appropriate treatment immediately. If infection is suspected broad-spectrum antibiotics, including antibacterials, and antifungal agents are often started. The culture and sensitivity results will be available 24 to 72 hours after the initial culture.

Cardiovascular disease (myocardial infarction and heart failure) is the leading cause of death in the United

States, and diabetics who have experienced hyperglycemia are at increased risk for cardiovascular diseases. In addition to myocardial infarction and heart failure, this includes stroke, deep vein thromboses, and other thromboembolisms, as well as decreased arterial perfusion to organs. One common result of decreased arterial perfusion to the kidneys is partial or total renal failure. The admission history should be focused to assess for potential cardiovascular disease and any history of organ failure. All precipitating causes of DKA and HHNS are treated in the usual ways. However, as a result of the presence of DKA or HHNS plus other comorbiditites, morbidity and mortality rates are increased.

Commonly prescribed medications such as calcium channel blockers, propranolol, thiazide diuretics, symathomimetics, phenytoin, and steroids may be used during the treatment or may have been used prior to admission for DKA or HHNS. Calcium channel blockers and propranolol are used to treat hypertension. Thiazide diuretics are used to treat preexisting heart failure. Sympathomimetics such as dopamine, dobutamine, epinephrine, or norepinephrine may be used to improve blood pressure and CO in the critically ill. Albuterol is often used as an inhalant in clients with asthma, and phenylephrine is an ingredient in some over-the-counter cold medications. Phenytoin is a medication used to prevent seizures. Glucocorticoids such as hydrocortisone, prednisone, or dexamethasone may be topical for skin disorders, inhaled for treatment of inflammatory pulmonary conditions, or taken orally to decrease a variety of inflammatory responses. All of the medications listed complicate the treatment of DKA and HHNS because they raise the blood glucose. If they are given concurrently during treatment more insulin may be needed to achieve expected decreases in serum glucose levels. It is important to have an accurate list of preadmission medications, including prescribed medications as well as over-the-counter medications, vitamins, and herbals.

Nursing Management

When the client is no longer critically ill, collaborative management changes focus to maintaining stability, preventing another episode, and teaching the client how to manage diabetes as well as complications that arise. Although it is important to begin teaching as soon as the client is ready, it is even more important to wait until the client is no longer critically ill. An assessment of knowledge needs to be completed because each client has different levels of knowledge and different teaching needs. In order to individualize the teaching plan knowledge of the following topics needs to be assessed:

- Basic knowledge about diabetes
- Monitoring blood glucose
- Recognition and treatment of hypoglycemia and hyperglycemia
- Diet, including adjustments during high and low blood sugars
- Exercise, including adjustments during high and low blood sugars
- Awareness of all aspects of medications used to treat diabetes
- Proficiency in insulin administration
- Insight into diabetes complications and how to prevent them
- Knowledge of how to manage diabetes during illnesses
- Awareness of the specific precipitating factor that caused the present DKA or HHNS episode and a plan to prevent future occurrences

Because infection is the most common precipitating cause of DKA and HHNS (20% to 25%), it is important to understand diabetes care during acute illness. Table 13–8 presents guidelines recommended by the American Diabetes Association (ADA) for diabetes management at home during acute illness (2003a, b).

In addition to passing on knowledge, it is important to positively reinforce or strengthen desirable behaviors, while coaching to improve undesirable habits. In order to determine the success of past compliance, the hemoglobin A_{1C} is used. This blood test determines the amount of glucose in the bloodstream over the life span of the red blood cell, which is the preceding 100 to 120 days. In other words, the hemoglobin A_{1C} is an accurate measure of blood glucose over the preceding 3 to 4 months! Normal hemoglobin A_{1C} is 2% to 5%. The most recent recommendations by Ryden et al. (2007) advise that clients with diabetes keep their hemoglobin A_{1C} less than 6.5%. Additionally, diabetics should keep their blood glucose levels as close to normal as possible, within 90 to 130 mg/dL, and peak blood glucose results should not exceed 180 mg/dL. These recommendations are based on many well-conducted research studies. Research has shown that clients with lower blood glucose and hemoglobin A_{1C} levels are healthier and have fewer complications. Even the cost of diabetes care is less for those with better glucose control. Table 13–9 correlates the results of hemoglobin A_{1C} with serum blood glucose results.

The certified diabetic educator (CDE) is a valuable resource to assess knowledge, provide in-depth information based on individual needs, and coach diabetic clients. There are many outpatient resources available to diabetics, such as classes, community support groups, and even camps for children. Many companies offer low-cost or free glucose meters to those who need them. Medicare, as well as many private insurance providers, covers the cost of diabetes supplies (meter strips, syringes, insulin, etc.).

TABLE 13-8

Diabetes Management During Acute Illness

1. Increase frequency of blood glucose checks. At the minimum glucose should be checked every 3-4 hours, though checks may be more frequent.
2. Take your medications.
   * Continue to take oral medications if blood sugar is high.
   * If you take insulin, continue taking it. The dose or type of insulin may be adjusted. For instance, some individuals may switch to using only short-acting insulin on a sliding scale. This scale is prescribed by the doctor.
3. Check urine for ketones every 4 hours.
4. Eat!
   * If you are vomiting, you still need to eat 15 grams of carbohydrates every hour. There are many examples of foods that contain 15 grams of carbohydrate available from the ADA.
   * If blood glucose is high, drink fluids with no calories.
5. Watch over-the-counter medications. Many contain sugar or other ingredients that raise your blood sugar. Others, such as aspirin, may lower your blood sugar. Recommendations regarding over-the-counter medications should come from your doctor.
6. Make a "sick day" bag. Include a blood glucose chart, a urine ketone chart, sliding scale insulin recommendations, a list of foods that contain 15 grams of carbohydrates, and the name and phone number of your physician(s).

When to call the doctor:
1. Unusually high blood glucose readings, over 240
2. Vomiting or diarrhea for more than 6 hours
3. High fever that keeps rising, or that lasts for more than one day
4. Moderate or high urine ketones or ketones in the urine for more than 12 hours
5. Signs of dehydration, abdominal pains, chest pains, or any other symptom that is new or bothersome

TABLE 13-9

Correlation of Hemoglobin A$_{1C}$ to Blood Glucose

HEMOGLOBIN A$_{1C}$	BLOOD GLUCOSE MG/DL	BLOOD GLUCOSE MMOL/L
6%	135	7.5
7%	170	9.5
8%	205	11.5
9%	240	13.5
10%	275	15.5
11%	310	17.5
12%	345	19.5

The ADA and the Juvenile Diabetes Research Foundation International (JDRF) offer lots of information, are a resource for current research studies and research findings, and encourage communities to develop support and fundraising groups. Individuals who are interested in these resources can learn about them through the CDE, their doctor, or directly on the Internet. Contact information for these organizations and others is found at the end of the chapter.

Prevention and Detection of Common or Life-Threatening Complications

Complications that can result from DKA or HHNS or its treatment include hypokalemia, hypoglycemia, fluid volume overload, heart failure, cerebral edema, adult respiratory distress syndrome (ARDS), hyperchloremic metabolic acidosis, and thrombosis. Prevention of these complications is an important aspect of care. However, sometimes prevention is not possible. In those cases, early detection and management will improve health care outcomes.

Hypokalemia

Hypokalemia is caused by rapid shifts of potassium into the cell as fluid and insulin are administered. Careful monitoring of potassium is important to prevent life-threatening deficits. Continuous ECG monitoring is helpful. Subtle rhythm changes, such as U waves, indicate potassium deficits. Often potassium supplementation is started when levels are normal because intracellular deficits and rapid fluid shifts are anticipated.

Hypoglycemia

Hypoglycemia is defined as a blood glucose level less than 70 mg/dL. During treatment of hyperglycemia, the goal is to decrease serum glucose by 50 to 70 mg/dL/hr. In order to prevent hypoglycemia the following strategies are used. Bedside blood glucose monitoring is performed every hour during IV insulin administration. Once the serum glucose reaches 250 to 300 mg/dL, 5% dextrose is added to the IV solution in order to prevent hypoglycemia. In addition, the rate of IV insulin is either decreased by half or changed to SQ administration depending on the presence of metabolic acidosis.

The signs and symptoms of hypoglycemia vary based on the severity of the episode (Table 13–10). In addition, those with hypoglycemic unawareness may have a very severe hypoglycemic episode with few warning signs. People with diabetes lose the ability to release

TABLE 13–10

Signs of Hypoglycemia

Early signs: shakiness, dizziness, sweating, hunger, and tachycardia
As hypoglycemia progresses: headache, pale skin color, tingling sensations around the mouth, sudden moodiness or behavior changes, loss of coordination, and difficulty paying attention
Late signs: confusion, loss of consciousness, and seizures

glucagon in response to hypoglycemia. As a result, those with diabetes rely on the release of epinephrine to raise the blood sugar. Early signs of hypoglycemia include shakiness, dizziness, sweating, hunger, and tachycardia. These signs are caused by the release of epinephrine. As hypoglycemia progresses signs include headache, pale skin color, tingling sensations around the mouth, sudden moodiness or behavior changes, loss of coordination, and difficulty paying attention. Neurological signs are related to the lack of glucose in the brain. Late signs or signs of severe hypoglycemia include confusion, loss of consciousness, and seizures. When a diabetic has hypoglycemic unawareness he or she does not have an epinephrine surge and therefore does not have the typical early warning signs of hypoglycemia. The first warning signs of hypoglycemia in those with hypoglycemic unawareness are often lethargy and confusion, followed quickly by loss of consciousness and seizures. Hypoglycemic unawareness occurs more in the following populations: type 1 diabetics, those who have frequent hypoglycemic episodes, those who are on beta blockers (which block the effects of epinephrine), older diabetics, and those with autonomic neuropathy.

Hypoglycemia is treated by giving oral carbohydrates if the client is alert and able to take oral fluids. If the client is unable to safely take oral fluids, glucagon may be given via the SQ or intramuscular (IM) routes. Glucagon is a hormone that promotes rapid conversion of glycogen to glucose. Though this injectable hormone is often prescribed to diabetics at home, it is rarely used in the critical care setting. In the critical care setting, 50% dextrose administered via the IV route is a more common therapy. This concentrated sugar rapidly raises the blood sugar.

Fluid Volume Overload and Heart Failure

Fluid volume overload and heart failure are complications that are caused by administering fluids more rapidly than the client can tolerate. Those with comorbidities such as heart failure or renal insufficiency are at very high risk for fluid volume overload and should be monitored very closely. Hemodynamic monitoring gives the health care team additional information that helps to prevent fluid overload in clients with existing heart disease, pulmonary disease, or renal failure. Signs of fluid volume overload include pulmonary congestion evidenced by new or worsening rales or rhonchi on auscultation, neck vein distention evidenced by full neck veins with the head of bed elevated 30 degrees, increasing CVP, PAP, and PCWP, and generalized edema. Although fluid volume overload and heart failure cannot always be prevented, prevention strategies include precise management of intake and output. This includes accurate measurements of intake and output and accurate administration of fluids. Management of fluid volume overload includes maintaining normal oxygenation, diuretics (if indicated), and/or decreasing the rate of fluid administration. Medications to improve heart contractility and CO are also commonly used in the presence of heart failure.

Cerebral Edema and Adult Respiratory Distress Syndrome

Cerebral edema and ARDS are both caused by rapid intracellular fluid shifts during administration of fluids. Those with higher serum osmolarity are at highest risk for both of these complications.

Early signs of cerebral edema include headache, lethargy, confusion, and irritability. A CT scan can help to identify cerebral edema. Prevention of rapid fluid shifts by decreasing serum glucose slowly and slow replacement of sodium are indicated to prevent cerebral edema. The serum osmolarity should be decreased gradually. Treatment of this complication includes the use of mannitol and may include short-term hyperventilation to decrease intracranial pressure. A neurosurgeon should be consulted. Mortality of those with cerebral edema is high.

Symptoms of ARDS include scattered rhonchi, decreased oxygenation, and decreased lung compliance. Chest x-ray will show scattered infiltrates throughout lung fields. Treatment includes slow rehydration with gradual decrease in serum osmolarity. Mechanical ventilation is used to improve oxygenation. Medications to improve lung compliance are also commonly prescribed. Both of these complications contribute to the high mortality rates seen in clients with DKA and HHNS.

Vascular Thrombosis

Clients experiencing DKA and HHNS are at higher risk for a variety of thromboembolic complications such as myocardial infarction, stroke, deep vein thrombosis, and pulmonary embolism. Various factors are responsible for this increased risk. Dehydration causes increased viscosity of the blood. In addition, many clients are predisposed for this risk due to the presence of atherosclerosis. Early hydration decreases the viscosity of the blood. Low molecular weight heparin may also be used. Focused assessment to detect these complications is important. If detected, thromboembolisms are treated rapidly because they can be life threatening.

Hyperchloremic Metabolic Acidosis

Hyperchloremic metabolic acidosis is mainly a complication of DKA. It occurs as a result of several altered metabolic processes. Bicarbonate cannot be regenerated through the kidneys because of the lack of ketoanions. Bicarbonate that is regenerated moves rapidly to the intracellular space. Additionally, the chloride in IV solution contributes to hyperchloremic metabolic acidosis. This complication causes metabolic acidosis to continue longer than expected. However, with fluid therapy, insulin therapy, and correction of electrolytes, it is usually self-limiting, correcting itself within 24 to 48 hours.

Pathophysiology of Hyperglycemia in Critical Illness

Critical illness causes a physiological stress response that causes the body to enter a hypermetabolic state in an attempt to heal. The physiological stress response can be caused by a variety of critical illnesses including acute myocardial infarction, trauma, severe infections, postsurgical healing, burns, or other conditions in which the body has a stress response. Two main processes cause hyperglycemia. First, the reaction to counterregulatory hormones has a direct hormonal effect to produce

VISUAL MAP **Hyperglycemia During Critical Illness**

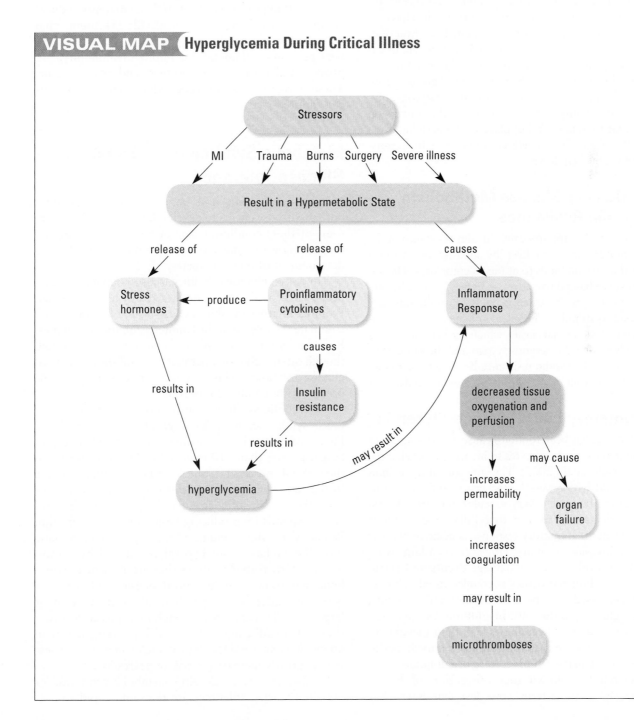

hyperglycemia. Second, proinflammatory factors cause insulin resistance, which also leads to hyperglycemia. In addition, new research findings show that the inflammatory results of hyperglycemia cause decreased vascular flow to cellular tissues and to organs.

Stress Hormones

During the hypermetabolic state the body releases a variety of counterregulatory hormones including catecholamines (epinephrine, norepinephrine, and dopamine), cortisol, growth hormones, and glucagon. These counterregulatory hormones contribute to hyperglycemia through the following processes. Catecholamines specifically inhibit insulin secretion from the beta cells and also have an anti-insulin effect. Glycogenesis is inhibited; the liver does not convert excess glucose to be stored as glycogen. In addition, glycogenolysis, the conversion of glycogen to glucose, and gluconeogenesis, the formation of glucose from amino acids and fats, are both accelerated. Glycogenolysis also occurs in muscle tissue. Lipolysis, the conversion of stored fat to glucose, takes place in the peripheral tissues. Later, as metabolic needs continue to be high, muscle protein is broken down.

Alterations in Glucose Metabolism and Insulin Resistance

Proinflammatory cytokines cause insulin resistance in the skeletal muscle, fat, and liver by altering biochemical markers that insulin binds to at the receptor sites. This insulin resistance has a direct effect on hyperglycemia by preventing glucose from entering cells. Proinflammatory cytokines also stimulate the release of the counterregulatory hormones described earlier, which further contributes to hyperglycemia. The nervous system and the blood cells are affected less by insulin resistance because these tissues do not rely on insulin to transport glucose into cells.

Inflammatory Effect of Hyperglycemia

Hyperglycemia has been found to cause an inflammatory response that causes leukocytes to invade endothelial tissue (Langouche et al., 2005). The endothelial tissue lines the blood and lymph vessels, the heart, and the serous cavities of the body. It is very vascular and provides essential nutrients and oxygen to cellular tissues. On a small scale an inflammatory response is positive because it heals an invasion or injury. However, on a large scale significant endothelial tissue damage occurs and perfusion of the endothelial tissues is compromised. This results in decreased transport of oxygen and nutrients, including glucose, to the cells. In addition, vascular permeability increases and capillaries leak fluids, leading to increased coagulation. Microthromboses impede perfusion, and cell damage can proceed to organ failure.

Research has shown that prevention of hyperglycemia, even short-term episodes, can have very positive results on health and healing. Van den Berghe (2003) reports findings from a large randomized study in Leuven, Belgium, of 1,548 surgical intensive care unit (ICU) patients. When blood glucose levels were kept within normal ranges, between 80 and 110 mg/dL, there were 30% to 40% improvements in mortality, 46% reduced risk of severe infections, and reduced use of antibiotics. Those receiving standard treatment during the study (those not in the control group) had blood glucose levels averaging 153 mg/dL. These participants had much worse outcomes. The study was terminated a year early because results were so conclusive that maintaining blood glucose in normal ranges (80 to 110 mg/dL) saves lives and significantly reduces complications. Langouche et al. (2005) found that maintaining normal blood glucose during critical illness prevents inflammation, improves immunity, improves lipid profiles, and protects endothelial tissue. These outcomes also prevent cellular damage and organ failure.

Metabolic Syndrome and Impaired Glucose Tolerance

Metabolic syndrome and impaired glucose tolerance both predispose clients to develop hyperglycemia. Symptoms of these conditions cannot be separated because they cross over in many areas and both often lead to the development of type 2 diabetes.

Impaired glucose tolerance is also known as prediabetes. This condition is characterized by hyperglycemia. Proinflammatory cytokines cause insulin resistance and stimulate the release of the counterregulatory hormones. Random blood glucose readings are sometimes normal, though often a glucose tolerance test will show impaired glucose tolerance. This condition may or may not be present with metabolic syndrome.

Metabolic syndrome, also known as insulin resistance syndrome, includes a group of abnormalities. First, insulin levels are elevated and fasting blood glucose is greater than 110 mg/dL. Insulin receptor sites in the skeletal muscle, fat, and liver become unresponsive to the action of insulin. As this occurs, glucose cannot enter the cells in sufficient quantities. Initially, the pancreas responds by producing larger amounts of insulin. People with this condition are often asymptomatic though they have both hyperglycemia and hyperinsulinemia. Other abnormalities that are present in metabolic syndrome include central obesity, defined as a waist circumference larger than 40 inches in men or larger than 35 inches in women; high triglyceride levels, over 150 mg/dL; high LDL; and low HDL, less than 40 mg/dL in men and less than 50 mg/dL in women. These factors greatly increase the risk of heart disease.

Those at risk to develop metabolic syndrome or impaired glucose tolerance are the same population as those predisposed to type 2 diabetes (see Table 13–1). In fact, those who have metabolic syndrome or impaired glucose tolerance usually do develop type 2 diabetes, though the development can be delayed through weight loss and exercise. Metabolic syndrome affects a huge percentage of the population. Estimates indicate that 23.7% of the population of the United States are affected, which equals almost one in four people! Ryden et al. (2007) estimate that up to 50% of those with diabetes have not been diagnosed with the disease because they have no symptoms. They theorize that those diagnosed with diabetes would greatly increase through mass screening.

Focused Assessment of a Client with the Disorder

An assessment of risk factors related to metabolic syndrome should be accomplished. Table 13–11 summarizes risk factors related to metabolic syndrome.

An assessment should also include identification of other factors that frequently increase or decrease serum blood glucose. Table 13–12 summarizes a list of factors to take into account that may increase or decrease serum blood glucose.

Clients may become hyperglycemic due to the physiological stress of critical illness. Many of the clients with hyperglycemia resulting from critical illness initially have no signs and symptoms. The typical and easy-to-recognize clinical signs of thirst and frequent urination that accompany hyperosmolarity have not yet occurred. When blood glucose is less than 200 mg/dL it does not cause osmotic diuresis.

Diagnostic Criteria

It is recommended that all clients in the ICU be screened every 4 to 6 hours for hyperglycemia. Normal fasting blood glucose ranges from 70 to 110 mg/dL. Though any result over 110 mg/dL meets the definition of hyperglycemia, most protocols recommend waiting until two or three consecutive readings are over 130 mg/dL before initiating therapy.

Both the hemoglobin A_{1C} and the glucose tolerance tests are tests that help diagnose diabetes. The hemoglobin A_{1C} determines the amount of glucose in the bloodstream over the life span of the red blood cell, the preceding 100 to 120 days. In other words, it is an accurate measure of blood glucose over the preceding 3 to 4 months. The normal hemoglobin A_{1C} in the nondiabetic adult is 2% to 5%. The glucose tolerance test measures serum blood glucose levels at prescribed intervals following a large dose of oral glucose solution. Normally, blood glucose should not exceed 200 mg/dL during the test, though the prescribed dose of glucose solution varies. Pediatric doses are 1.75 grams per kilogram, pregnant women usually receive 50 grams of glucose solution, and nonpregnant adults usually receive 75 to 100 grams. The time of the test also varies from 2 to 6 hours. Table 13–13 gives an example of normal results of a 4-hour glucose tolerance test (Kee, 2005).

TABLE 13–11

Risk Factors Related to Metabolic Syndrome

1. Central obesity
   - Waist circumference larger than 40 inches in men
   - Waist circumference larger than 35 inches in women
2. Abnormal lipid panel
   - Triglyceride levels over 150 mg/dL
   - High LDL
   - HDL less than 40 mg/dL in men
   - HDL less than 50 mg/dL in women
3. Fasting blood glucose is greater than 110 mg/dL
4. Hyperinsulinemia

TABLE 13–12

Factors That Increase or Decrease Serum Blood Glucose

FACTORS THAT MAY INCREASE SERUM GLUCOSE	FACTORS THAT MAY DECREASE SERUM GLUCOSE
1. Commonly prescribed medications • Calcium channel blockers • Propranolol (Inderal) • Thiazide diuretics (hydrochlorothiazide/HCTZ) • Sympathomimetics (dopamine, dobutamine, epinephrine, norepinephrine, albuterol, and phenylephrine) • Phenytoin (Dilantin) • Glucocorticoids (hydrocortisone, prednisone, dexamethasone) 2. Feedings • Total parenteral nutrition (TPN) • Enteral/tube feedings • Oral intake of foods and fluids 3. Change in dialysis or continuous renal replacement therapy (CRRT) schedule 4. Change in clinical condition	1. Advanced age 2. Malnutrition 3. Change in dialysis or CRRT schedule 4. Gastrointestinal malabsorption syndromes • Inflammatory bowel disease 5. Septic shock 6. Burns 7. Alcoholism

TABLE 13–13

Normal Results of a Four-Hour Glucose Tolerance Test

TIME	SERUM GLUCOSE MG/DL	SERUM GLUCOSE MMOL/L
First glucose value—Fasting	70–110 mg/dL	Less than 6.4 mmol/L
30 minutes	Less than 200 mg/dL	Less than 11.1 mmol/L
1 hour	Less than 200 mg/dL	Less than 11.1 mmol/L
2 hours	Less than 140 mg/dL	Less than 7.8 mmol/L
3 hours	70–110 mg/dL	Less than 6.4 mmol/L
4 hours	70–110 mg/dL	Less than 6.4 mmol/L

Collaborative Management

It used to be considered standard to allow moderate hyperglycemia, 110 to 180 mg/dL during critical illness. Prior beliefs were that some hyperglycemia during critical illness must be helpful and even necessary to heal because the stress response caused hyperglycemia in nondiabetic populations. However, recent research, including findings from the Leuven Study in 2001 summarized by Van den Berghe (2003), and Langouche et al. (2005), find that even moderate hyperglycemia is damaging to cellular tissues, causing increased complications and increased rates of death.

Insulin Protocols

Current evidence supports the use of IV insulin infusions rather than SQ sliding scale insulin. Blood glucose levels are controlled best and hypoglycemic episodes are avoided when insulin protocols are used. Protocols should be developed through collaboration of a multidisciplinary team. Physicians, nurses, and pharmacists all need to provide input into new insulin protocols. Protocols should be thought out so that they are easy to use and decisions to change insulin infusion rates can be made quickly and accurately. Rapid decisions regarding titration are important because these decisions will be made each hour. Tools that are user friendly will help to reduce errors in medication calculations and ensure that hyperglycemia is precisely controlled. Outcomes of the use of insulin protocols should be studied to ensure that the intent of providing an easy, rapid, and accurate tool has occurred.

Goldberg et al. (2004) present the use of the Yale Insulin Infusion Protocol, shown in Table 13–14, as a safe and effective way to manage hyperglycemia during critical illness. This protocol is unique in that it was developed through the collaboration of a multidisciplinary team and has been revised based on clinical research findings. The intent of its use is for those experiencing hyperglycemia during critical illness. It is not intended for use during diabetic emergencies such as DKA and HHNS.

Prevention and Detection of Common or Life-Threatening Complications

Both short- and long-term complications may result from hyperglycemia. Short-term complications of hyperglycemia include higher mortality, increased risk for infection such as sternal wound infections and sepsis, increased risk of acute organ failure, and longer lengths of stay in the ICU. The Diabetes and Insulin Glucose Infusion in Acute Myocardial Infarction (DIGAMI) study (Malmberg, Norhammer, Wedel, & Ryden, 1999) as well as Finney, Zekveld, Elia, and Evans (2003) found that mortality was significantly lower in patients receiving intensive IV insulin infusions to keep glucose close to normal ranges. Van den Berghe (2003) found decreased risk of sepsis, anemia, and acute renal failure when intensive insulin therapy was used. Langouche et al. (2005) additionally found decreased length of stay in ICU and decreased length of mechanical ventilation related to prevention of hyperglycemia with intensive insulin therapy.

Though long-term complications are not immediately recognizable, more research shows that even short-term episodes of hyperglycemia cause undesirable cellular changes and vascular damage. These changes led to long-term complications, such as peripheral and autonomic neuropathies, retinopathy, renal dysfunction, and vascular changes, over a period of years. Because it is not yet known how long it takes to cause permanent damage related to hyperglycemia, it is important to maintain normal blood glucose levels during critical illness.

Following an episode of hyperglycemia during a critical illness, follow-up and teaching are important. Follow-up should focus on aggressive management of risk factors associated with metabolic syndrome. Tests to detect the presence of type 2 diabetes should be performed, and if diabetes is present early management is important. Client teaching should focus on risk factors for the development of diabetes and how to prevent or delay its onset.

Nursing Management

Nursing management includes maintaining fluid, electrolyte, and acid-base balance.

Fluid Volume Deficit

Goals: To improve vascular fluid volume to increase perfusion of essential organs and to replace interstitial and cellular fluid losses.

Interventions:

- Assess level of dehydration: physical appearance, neurological assessments, initial blood glucose, vital signs, urine output, and serum osmolarity.
- Calculate corrected serum sodium.
- Administer fluids to correct fluid deficits.
- Review laboratory results for signs of organ failure and report abnormalities to the physician.

TABLE 13-14

Yale Insulin Infusion Protocol

INITIATING AN INSULIN INFUSION

1. INSULIN INFUSION: Mix 1 unit of regular human insulin per 1 mL of 0.9% NaCl. Administer via infusion pump (in increments of 0.5 unit/hour).
2. PRIMING: Flush 50 mL of infusion through all IV tubing before insulin begins (to saturate the insulin binding sites in the tubing).
3. TARGET BLOOD GLUCOSE (BG) LEVELS: 100–139 mg/dL
4. BOLUS & INITIAL INSULIN INFUSION RATE: Divide initial BG level by 100, then round to nearest 0.5 unit for bolus AND initial infusion rate.

Examples:
1. Initial BG = 325 mg/dL; 325 ÷ 100 = 3.25, round ↑ to 3.5; IV bolus 3.5 units + start infusion @ 3.5 units/hour.
2. Initial BG = 174 mg/dL; 174 ÷ 100 = 1.74, round ↓ to 1.5; IV bolus 1.5 units + start infusion @ 1.5 units/hour.

BLOOD GLUCOSE MONITORING

1. Check BG hourly until stable (three consecutive values within target range). In hypotensive patients, capillary blood glucose (i.e., fingersticks) may be inaccurate and obtaining the blood sample from an indwelling vascular catheter is acceptable.
2. Then check BG every 2 hours; once stable × 12–24 hours BG can then be spaced to every 4 hours IF:
   a. no significant change in clinical situation AND
   b. no significant change in nutritional intake.
3. If any of the following occurs, consider the temporary resumption of hourly BG monitoring until BG is again stable (two to three consecutive values within target range):
   a. Any change in insulin infusion rate (i.e., BG out of target range)
   b. Significant changes in clinical condition
   c. Initiation or cessation of pressor or steroid therapy
   d. Initiation or cessation of renal replacement therapy (hemodialysis, CVVH, etc.)
   e. Initiation, cessation, or rate change of nutritional support (TPN, PPN, tube feedings, etc.)

CHANGING THE INSULIN INFUSION RATE

If BG < 50 mg/dL: D/C INSULIN INFUSION	Give 1 amp (25 g) D50 IV; recheck BG every 15 minutes. → When BG ≥ 100 mg/dL, wait 1 hour, then restart insulin infusion at 50% of original rate.
If BG 50–74 mg/dL: D/C INSULIN INFUSION	If *symptomatic* (or unable to assess), give 1 amp (25 g) D50 IV; recheck BG every 15 minutes. If *asymptomatic*, give 1/2 amp (12.5 g) D50 IV or 8 oz. juice; recheck BG every 15–30 minutes. → When BG ≥ 100 mg/dL, wait 1 hour, then restart insulin infusion at 75% of original rate.

If BG > 75 mg/dL:

STEP 1: Determine the *CURRENT BG LEVEL*—identifies a *COLUMN* in the table

BG 75–99 MG/DL	BG 100–139 MG/DL	BG 140–199 MG/DL	BG > 200 MG/DL

STEP 2: Determine the *RATE OF CHANGE* from the prior BG level—identifies a *CELL* in the table—then move right for INSTRUCTIONS:
[Note: if the last BG was measured 2–4 hours before the current BG, calculate the hourly rate of change. Example: if the BG at 2 P.M. was 150 mg/dL, and the BG at 4 P.M. is now 120 mg/dL, the total change over 2 hours is 30 mg/dL; however, the hourly change is 30 mg/dL ÷ 2 hours = 15 mg/dL/hr.]

BG 75–99 MG/DL	BG 100–139 MG/DL	BG 140–199 MG/DL	BG > 200 MG/DL	INSTRUCTIONS*
		BG ↑ >50 mg/dL/hr	BG ↓	↑ INFUSION by "2Δ"
	BG ↑ >25 mg/dL/hr	BG ↑ by 150 mg/dL/hr, OR BG UNCHANGED	BG UNCHANGED OR BG ↓ by 1–25 mg/dL/hr	↑ INFUSION by "Δ"
BG ↑	BG ↑ by 1–25 mg/dL/hr, BG UNCHANGED OR BG ↓ by 1–25 mg/dL/hr	BG ↓ by 1–50 mg/dL/hr	BG ↓ by 26–75 mg/dL/hr	NO INFUSION CHANGE
BG UNCHANGED OR BG ↓ 1–25 mg/dL/hr	BG ↓ by 26–50 mg/dL/hr	BG ↓ by 51–75 mg/dL/hr	BG ↓ by 76–100 mg/dL/hr	↓ INFUSION by "Δ"
BG ↓ >25 mg/dL/hr See below^	BG ↓ by >50 mg/dL/hr	BG ↓ by >75 mg/dL/hr	BG ↓ by >100 mg/dL/hr	HOLD × 30 min, then ↓ INFUSION by "2Δ"

^ D/C INSULIN INFUSION: Check BG every 30 min; when BG > 100 mg/dL restart infusion @ 75% of most recent rate

*<u>CHANGES IN INFUSION RATE</u> ("Δ") are determined by the current rate:

CURRENT RATE (UNITS/HOUR)	Δ = RATE CHANGE (UNITS/HOUR)	2Δ = 2X RATE CHANGE (UNITS/HOUR)
< 3.0	0.5	1
3.0–6.0	1	2
6.5–9.5	1.5	3
10–14.5	2	4
15–19.5	3	6
20–24.5	4	8
≥ 25	≥ 5	10 (consult MD)

Source: Courtesy Yale University School of Medicine, New Haven, Connecticut.

- Continue assessment of fluid balance: physical appearance, neurological assessments, lung sounds, strict intake and output, vital signs, hemodynamic monitoring, review current laboratory findings, and daily weights.

Altered Electrolyte Balance

Goals: To prevent life-threatening cardiac arrhythmias, improve cellular metabolism, improve smooth and skeletal muscle function, and maintain essential endocrine function.

Interventions:

- Determine initial electrolyte values, and perform frequent reevaluation during therapies.
- Determine renal function by laboratory values.
- Perform continuous ECG monitoring.
- Perform frequent neurological assessments.
- Replace electrolytes as necessary.

Altered Acid-Base Balance

Goal: Transport of glucose into the cell, resulting in normal cellular metabolism evidenced by bicarbonate greater than 18 mEq/L, venous pH greater than 7.3, normal anion gap, and no ketones in the urine.

Interventions:

- Assess arterial blood gas results.
- Determine anion gap and recalculate when current laboratory results available.
- Provide insulin therapy.
- Measure urine ketones.

Identify Precipitating Factor

Goal: To identify and treat precipitating cause and prevent further complications.

Interventions:

- Assess for presence of infection.
- Culture any sites of infection to identify type of organisms.
- Assess for presence of deep vein thromboses, signs of acute myocardial infarction, and signs of stroke.
- Assess toxic screen (if completed).
- Assess for presence of pregnancy (women of childbearing age).

Risk for Injury

Goal: To provide safety measures during critical illness.
Interventions:

- Assess skin integrity and risk for skin breakdown on admission.

- Consult the dietitian in regard to providing adequate nutrition during critical illness.
- Provide basic hygiene: Keep the skin clean and dry, provide adequate oral hygiene, and, if immobile, reposition every 2 hours.
- Safety measures: Implement fall precautions, secure lines, cords, and equipment, and prevent the patient from dislodging lines and equipment.

Knowledge Deficit Related to Management of Diabetes and/or Acute Illness

Goals: To improve knowledge of precipitating factors of DKA and HHNS and improve knowledge of management of sick days and when to seek medical advice.

Interventions:

- Assess current knowledge level of the client and significant others.
- Provide information regarding diabetes management.
- Consult the CDE if available.

Potential Noncompliance Diabetes Management

Goals: To encourage compliance of diabetes management, ensure that hemoglobin A_{1C} is less than 6.5%, and encourage healthy lifestyle.

Interventions:

- Assess the results of the last hemoglobin A_{1C}.
- Provide positive reinforcement of application of knowledge to the client and significant others.
- Coach the client and significant others to help overcome barriers to healthy management of diabetes.

High Risk for Infection Related to the Effects of Hyperglycemia

Goal: To maintain blood glucose within normal ranges throughout the majority of the time during a critical illness.

Interventions:

- Perform bedside blood glucose monitoring.
- Assess concurrent treatments that increase or decrease the serum glucose (see Table 13–14).
- Provide insulin therapy and adjust it based on blood glucose monitoring results.

Risk for Injury Related to Immobility

Goal: To provide safety measures during critical illness.
Interventions:

- Assess skin integrity and risk for skin breakdown on admission.
- Implement measures to prevent skin breakdown such as frequent repositioning, providing adequate nutrition during critical illness, and providing basic hygiene measures (keeping the skin clean and dry and providing adequate oral hygiene).

Potential Knowledge Deficit Related to Maintenance of Health

Goals: To improve knowledge of factors that lead to the development of type 2 diabetes and how to delay or prevent the onset of the disease.
Interventions:

- Assess for risk factors related to metabolic syndrome.
- Provide education related to diet and nutrition, exercise, and weight management.
- Consult the dietitian.

Building Technology Skills for Diabetics

Insulin is commonly given via the IV or SQ routes while in the critical care setting. However, a client may be admitted to the critical care area using various insulin therapies such as insulin pens, injection aids, a continuous insulin pump, or inhaled insulin. The following is a short discussion of various insulin therapies that are available to clients. More information on these therapies can be found at manufacturer Web sites such as those that are listed on the companion Web site.

Insulin Pens

Many clients use insulin pens. They are easy to use, are inexpensive, allow for consistent measurement of insulin, are portable, and the user does not need as much manual dexterity as is required for the traditional vial and syringe. In addition, insulin pens are available in many of the premixed insulin preparations, preventing the client from having to mix two types of insulin into one syringe. Insulin pens look like a writing pen. There are two types of pens: nondisposable and disposable. When using the nondisposable pens, a disposable cartridge of insulin is replaced when empty. In contrast, the disposable pens are discarded when the insulin cartridge in the pen is empty. The needle is disposed of and replaced after each injection. To use the pen the client simply dials in an insulin dose and gives the injection SQ. There are three important considerations that the nurse should know about insulin pens in order to

teach or reinforce teaching. First, the client should detach the needle after each injection and use a new needle for each new injection. In addition to preventing infection, this step prevents leakage of the pen. Second, the client should dial the dose into the pen slowly to ensure accuracy of the dose. This is especially true when higher doses are used. Third, the client should leave the needle in place 5 to 6 seconds after injecting the insulin. This is done to ensure that the correct dose is administered from the pen.

Injection Aids

Injection aids help clients give insulin safely and accurately. Some of the aids available include syringe magnifiers, devices for clients who cannot see, needle guides and vial stabilizers, and devices to simplify injections (Austin, Boucher, & Peragallo-Dittko, 2006). Syringe magnifiers attach to the insulin syringe and magnify the syringe so that users can accurately draw up a dose or see air in the syringe. A product for those who cannot see called Count-A-Dose makes an audible click as each unit of insulin is drawn into the syringe. Needle guides and vial stabilizers hold the insulin syringe and the vial together. These devices prevent the needle from coming out of the vial while the diabetic fills the syringe and are helpful for those with limited dexterity. Devices used to simplify the process of giving an injection include spring-loaded syringe holders. The filled syringe is loaded into the device. Some models hide the needle from view. The needle inserts into the skin when a button is pushed, or some devices even insert the needle when pressure is put against the skin. Once the needle is in the skin, some devices inject the insulin automatically, whereas others require the diabetic to push the plunger. Many spring-loaded syringe holders accommodate prefilled insulin pens. These devices are optimal for those who have a fear of injecting insulin as well as those who do not have the dexterity to administer an injection.

Insulin Pump

A continuous SQ insulin infusion pump closely imitates the physiological secretion of insulin by delivering a basal rate of insulin. The basal rate can be programmed to automatically change based on the time of day, and the diabetic can also deliver boluses of insulin for meals. Insulin doses are accurate, the pump is small and discrete, and programming can be changed as needed. It also eliminates the need for frequent insulin injections. The pump enables the diabetic to have a more flexible lifestyle. The insulin pump is worn externally with a catheter that is inserted into the SQ tissue. The catheter is changed every 2 to 3 days. The pump includes an insulin reservoir and a computerized control mechanism. Many newer pumps have programs that can be downloaded to a computer or a PDA, and some can even be programmed wirelessly. The insulin pump is powered by a battery and has alarms that alert the user if the catheter is occluded or the insulin reservoir is low. The reservoir is usually filled with 300 units of rapid-acting insulin. The insulin pump would not be the optimal tool for those who are not willing to monitor blood glucose frequently and make frequent dose adjustments. The pump requires a user who is knowledgeable, motivated, and able to do simple calculations. Because the pump uses rapid-acting insulin, if it does not deliver insulin for several hours, diabetic ketoacidosis can result. The pump is also more expensive than other products. Though the insulin pump may be the best option for some diabetics, it may not be the optimal method of insulin delivery for others. The nurse should encourage the diabetic to keep insulin and syringes on hand in case the insulin pump malfunctions.

Inhaled Insulin

Inhalation is a newer method of insulin delivery. Inhaled insulin is as beneficial as SQ injected insulin in measurements of reduction of the hemoglobin A_{1C}. Inhaled insulin is administered with a handheld nebulizer. Once it is inhaled, the insulin has a large surface area within the lungs to be absorbed. The onset of action of inhaled insulin is within 15 to 30 minutes, and it lasts 2 to 4 hours.

A big advantage is that it does not require injection, though there are disadvantages to its use. Because the long-term effects of inhaled powder on pulmonary function is not well understood, those with lung disease should not use inhaled insulin. It also is not recommended for those who smoke. There is no information on the effects of inhaled insulin in children and pregnant women. Inhaled insulin is a new form of insulin delivery, and more information will be forthcoming.

New Technologies

Several new methods of insulin delivery are still being researched. Alternative sites of insulin delivery such as oral, buccal, ocular, and transdermal routes are being studied. New technologies, including implantable insulin pumps, are under investigation. Islet cell transplantation is also being researched. For many years insulin was available only in a vial and was drawn up and administered for each injection using a traditional syringe. Diabetics had to deal with the inconvenience of storage and fear or social stigma related to using a needle and syringe. Currently there are many new technologies to help diabetics administer insulin safely, more discreetly, and with more convenience.

ENDOCRINE DISORDERS SUMMARY

Because diabetes is a very common condition with increasing prevalence in the United States, it is important for the nurse to know how to manage common diabetic emergencies such as DKA and HHNS. In addition to managing the critical events associated with DKA and HHNS, glucose control is an important aspect of nursing care. Short-term glucose control is important to prevent the creation of proinflammatory cytokines that cause insulin resistance and stimulate the release of counterregulatory hormones. Long-term glucose control is important to prevent the long-term complications of diabetes such as systemic vascular disease, renal failure, neuropathies, and retinopathy. Once the critically ill patient is stable it is important to focus on helping the patient to maintain glucose control at home by providing knowledge and coaching the patient to make lifestyle changes.

 CASE STUDY 1

Type 1 Diabetes with Diabetic Ketoacidosis

Mrs. D is a 27-year-old accountant who comes to the emergency department with complaints of fever and extreme fatigue. She states that she has had the "flu" for 2 days and is also diabetic. The triage nurse notes that Mrs. D appears dehydrated and lethargic and that her breath has a fruity odor. The following rapid history and assessment is obtained in the emergency department.

Her vital signs are: blood pressure 96/70, pulse 104, respiratory rate 28, oral temperature 100.8, and pulse oximeter reading 99%. Mrs. D states that she has some abdominal pain, which is not localized to a specific area, but has no other pain. Her height is 68 inches and her weight is 155 pounds. She has no allergies.

- Her medications include:
  - Lantus 30 units every a.m., client did not take this medication today.
  - Humalog 5 units with meals, client took 2 units of Humalog 2 hours ago and 4 hours ago.
  - Prinivil 5 mg every a.m., client did not take this medication today.
  - No vitamins, no herbals.
  - Pulse oximeter reading 99%
- Past Health History:
  - Type 1 diabetes since age 11 (16 years)
  - Denies any other medical problems
  - Last hemoglobin A_{1C} was 6.2 (2 months ago)

1. Name five interventions that would be important to initiate.

2. Based on the following laboratory findings, calculate the serum osmolarity.
   - Na^+ 132, K^+ 6.2, Chloride 100, Glucose 644, creatinine 1.4, BUN 31, Bicarbonate 17

3. What is your assessment of the serum osmolarity? What physiological changes, if any, will result?

4. Calculate the anion gap based on the laboratory findings from question #2.

5. What is your assessment of the anion gap? What do you anticipate the findings of arterial blood gases to show?

6. Calculate the corrected serum sodium based on the laboratory findings from question #2.

7. Based on the results of the corrected serum sodium, what intervention would you expect to implement?

8. Calculate the 24-hour fluid replacement based on severe fluid losses of 100 mL/kg of weight. How would the total fluid replacement be administered?

9. Answer the following questions regarding insulin administration.
   a. What type of insulin would you anticipate giving Mrs. D?
   b. What route would you expect insulin to be administered?
   c. Calculate an initial bolus dose and an initial hourly dose.
   d. When would this dose be adjusted?
   e. What should you assess prior to giving insulin?

10. Once Mrs. D recovers, what topics would be important to focus on during diabetic teaching?

See answers to Case Studies in the Answer Section at the back of the book.

CASE STUDY 2

Type 2 Diabetes with Hyperglycemic Hyperosmolar Nonketotic Syndrome

Mr. S is a 67-year-old retired professional who comes to the emergency department with complaints of shortness of breath, extreme fatigue, and headache. He states that he has had a cold for the past 2 weeks. He also has diabetes and heart failure. The triage nurse notes that Mr. S appears weak with fever. He also has a cough with production of tan, yellow sputum. Diagnostic findings include the following: Na^+ 128, K^+ 5.7, chloride 95, glucose 1074, creatinine 2.4, BUN 62, and bicarbonate 21. During his stabilization in the emergency department Mr. S experiences respiratory failure, is intubated, and placed on mechanical ventilation. Mr. S is diagnosed with HHNS, pneumonia, and heart failure and is admitted to the ICU. Fluid replacement and insulin therapy are started.

1. In addition to HHNS, pneumonia, and heart failure, what other problem is evident based on Mr. S's lab values. How will this affect the care that you provide? What additional intervention might be anticipated?

2. Mr. S has been prescribed albuterol and dexamethasone to treat his pneumonia. How do these medications specifically help Mr. S's pneumonia? What would you anticipate as a result of these medications?

3. Upon review of the history and physical you note that the last outpatient hemoglobin A_{1C} was 10.5. What was Mr. S's average blood sugar based on this result? What is the significance of this finding? What action would be appropriate based on this finding?

4. What three complications is Mr. S at high risk to develop? Why? What assessments or diagnostics would point to the development of these complications?

See answers to Case Studies in the Answer Section at the back of the book.

CRITICAL THINKING QUESTIONS

1. What are the most common precipitating factors for ketoacidosis (DKA) and hyperosmolar nonketotic syndrome (HHNS)?

2. What are two differences in the assessment findings between patients with DKA and HHNS?

3. What intervention(s) are critical prior to the administration of insulin to the patient with DKA?

4. What medications can increase insulin resistance and the blood sugar in patient's with type 2 diabetes?

5. What are the most common complications that may occur during management of DKA or HHNS?

6. What are the risk factors associated with metabolic syndrome?

7. Why is treatment of hyperglycemia during critical illnesses important?

See answers to Critical Thinking Questions in the Answer Section at the back of the book.

EXPLORE MEDIALINK

http://www.prenhall.com/perrin

Additional interactive resources for this chapter can be found on the Web site at http://www.prenhall.com/perrin. Click on "Chapter 13 " to select activities for this chapter.

Case Study: Type 1 Diabetes with DKA

Nursing Care Plan

NCLEX Review Questions

MediaLinks:

- American Association of Diabetes Educators
- American Diabetes Association
- Eli Lilly and Company
- Juvenile Diabetes Research Foundation International

- National Diabetes Information Clearinghouse (NDIC)
- National Institute of Diabetes and Digestive and Kidney Diseases (NIDDK) National Institute of Health (NIH)
- Novo Nordisk Inc.
- Owen Mumford Inc.
- Sanofi-Aventis US
- U.S. Food and Drug Administration Department of Health and Human Services

MediaLink Applications

REFERENCES

American Diabetes Association. (2003a). *Surviving sick days*. Retrieved December 8, 2003, from http://www.diabetes.org/uedocuments/SurvivingSickDays.pdf

American Diabetes Association. (2003b). *When you're sick*. Retrieved December 8, 2003, from http://www.diabetes.org/Type-2-diabetes/sick.jsp

Austin, R., Boucher, J., & Peragallo-Dittko, V. (2006). *Insulin delivery systems and their role in the treatment of diabetes*. Hopewell, NJ: Sherer Clinical Communications.

Carroll, M., & Schade, D. (2001). Ten pivotal questions about diabetic ketoacidosis. *Postgraduate Medicine, 110*(5), 89–94.

Centers for Disease Control and Prevention (CDC). (2005). *National Center for Chronic Disease Prevention and Health Promotion, national diabetes fact sheet*. Retrieved October 9, 2006, from http://www.cdc.gov/diabetes/pubs/estimates.htm

Chiasson, J., Aris-Jilwan, N., Bélanger, R., Bertrand, S., Beauregard, H., Ékoé, J., et al. (2003). Diagnosis and treatment of diabetic ketoacidosis and the hyperglycemic hyperosmolar state. *CMAJ: Canadian Medical Association Journal, 168*(7), 859–867.

Coursin, D. B., & Murray, M. J. (2003). How sweet is euglycemia in critically ill patients? *Mayo Clinic Proceedings, 78*(12), 1460–1462.

Farhat, D. (2001). Disorders of glucose. *Topics in Emergency Medicine, 23*(4), 27–44.

Finney, S. J., Zekveld, C., Elia, A., & Evans, T. W. (2003). Glucose control and mortality in critically ill patients. *Journal of the American Medical Association (JAMA), 290*(15), 2041–2047.

Goldberg, P., Siegel, M., Sherwin, R., Halickman, J., Lee, M., Bailey, V., et al. (2004). Implementation of a safe and effective insulin infusion protocol in a medical intensive care unit. *Diabetes Care, 27*(2), 461–467.

Kee, J. L. (2005). *Laboratory and diagnostic tests with nursing implications* (7th ed.). Upper Saddle River, NJ: Pearson-Prentice Hall.

Langdon, C. D., & Shriver, R. L. (2004). Clinical issues in the care of critically ill diabetic patients. *Critical Care Nursing Quarterly, 27*(2), 162–171.

Langouche, L., Vanhorebeek, I., Vlasselaers, D., Perre, S. V., Wouters, P. J., Skogstrand, K., et al. (2005). Intensive insulin therapy protects the endothelium of critically ill patients. *Journal of Clinical Investigation, 115*(8), 2277–2286.

Malmberg, K., Norhammer, A., Wedel, H., & Ryden, L. (1999). Glycometabolic state at

admission: Important risk maker of mortality in conventionally treated patients with diabetes mellitus and acute myocardial infarction: long term results from the diabetes and insulin glucose infusion in acute myocardial infarction (DIGAMI) study. *Circulation, 99*(20), 266–32.

Ryden, L., Standl, E., Bartnik, M., Van den Berghe, G., Beteridge, J., deBoer, M., et al. (2007). Guidelines on diabetes, pre-diabetes and cardiovascular diseases: executive summary. *European Heart Journal* (28), 88–136.

Travis, J. (1997a, February 1). Diabetes results from suicidal cells. *Science News, 151*(1), 72.

Travis, J. (1997b, October 4). Hidden virus suspected in diabetes. *Science News, 152*(1), 218.

Van den Berghe, G. (2003). Intensive insulin therapy in the ICU. *Indian Journal of Critical Care Medicine, 7*(2), 106–111.

Wardlaw, G. M., & Kessel, M. (2002). *Perspectives in nutrition* (5th ed.). Boston: McGraw-Hill.

Wilson, B., Shannon, M., Shields, K., & Stang, C. (2007). *Nurse's drug guide 2007*. Upper Saddle River, NJ: Pearson-Prentice Hall.

Care of the Patient with Acute Renal Failure

Kathleen Perrin, PhD, RN, CCRN

Learning Outcomes

Upon completion of this chapter, the learner will be able to:

1. Differentiate between prerenal, intrinsic renal, and postrenal causes of acute renal failure.

2. Explain the lab tests that may be used to differentiate between prerenal failure and intrinsic renal failure.

3. Discuss ways to restore renal perfusion in prerenal dysfunction.

4. Explain measures the critical care nurse may use to prevent further renal injury to the patient in renal failure.

5. Discuss collaborative management of the electrolyte imbalances commonly seen in acute renal failure.

6. Describe fluid volume management in acute renal failure.

7. Explain why peritoneal dialysis is of limited use in patients with acute renal failure.

8. Discuss the advantages and disadvantages of hemodialysis and continuous renal replacement therapies in acute renal failure.

9. Describe nursing management of the patient requiring hemodialysis or continuous renal replacement therapy.

Abbreviations

ATN	Acute Tubular Necrosis
CRRT	Continuous Renal Replacement Therapy
CVVH	Continuous Venovenous Hemofiltration
CVVHD	Continuous Venovenous Hemodialysis
CVVHDF	Continuous Venovenous Hemodiafiltration
IHD	Intermittent Hemodialysis
PD	Peritoneal Dialysis
RRT	Renal Replacement Therapy
SCUF	Slow Continuous Ultrafiltration

Acute renal failure (ARF) occurring in approximately 20% of intensive care unit (ICU) admissions is the sudden onset of at least a 50% reduction in glomerularfiltration rate. Causes of ARF are classified as prerenal (due to decreased renal blood flow), intrarenal (due to disturbances within the glomerulus or renal tubules), or postrenal (due to obstruction of urinary outflow). ARF results in retention of nitrogenous wastes along with disruptions in serum and urinary electrolytes. It may be oliguric, with the patient having a daily urine output of less than 400 mL per day, or nonoliguric. Management is based on

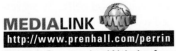

MEDIALINK
http://www.prenhall.com/perrin

See the Companion Website for chapter-specific resources at www.prenhall.com/perrin.

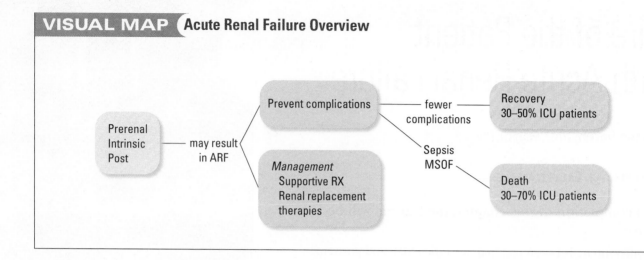

VISUAL MAP (**Acute Renal Failure Overview**

supportive treatment, prevention of complications, and, possibly, renal replacement therapy (RRT). Of patients who develop ARF, 50% to 70% die, usually after developing sepsis or multisystem organ failure (MSOF). The majority of patients who survive regain renal function.

Anatomy and Physiology Review

The kidneys are complex organs responsible for multiple metabolic functions, including the regulation of:

Fluid volume status

Acid-base balance

Electrolyte concentrations in the body

They also clear the body of nitrogenous and other wastes.

These functions are performed by the approximately 2 to 3 million nephrons, the functional unit of filtration and reabsorption, in the human kidney (Figure 14-1). Nephrons are composed of a glomerulus, Bowman's capsule, and renal tubules. The glomerulus is a system of tiny capillaries with thin walls. Filtration of particles and wastes occurs as blood passes through the glomerulus. The renal filtrate then enters Bowman's capsule, the structure surrounding the glomerulus, and is channeled into the renal tubules. Most of the water and electrolytes contained in the filtrate are reabsorbed into the blood from the renal tubules. To regulate electrolyte concentration in the body, electrolytes may be actively secreted into the filtrate along the tubules. The filtrate, containing nitrogenous and other wastes as well as the secreted electrolytes, is then excreted as urine.

The glomerulo-filtration rate (GFR) refers to the rate at which the filtrate is formed, approximately 125 mL/min in a healthy adult. The GFR is driven by the pressure gradient between the pressure in the renal capillaries and the pressure within the renal tubules. Factors that decrease pressure within the renal capillar-

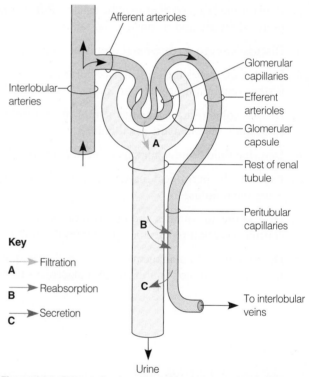

Figure 14-1 Schematic view of the three major mechanisms by which the kidneys adjust to the composition of plasma: *A*, Glomerular filtration. *B*, Tubular reabsorption. *C*, Tubular secretion.

ies or increase pressure within the renal tubules may decrease the GFR. The most accurate measurement of GFR is the creatinine clearance rate (normally 85 to 135 mL/min).

However, the regulation of fluid electrolyte and acid-base balance is not the only essential function the kidneys perform. By producing erythropoietin, the kidneys stimulate production of red blood cells. By secreting renin, which is converted to angiotensin I and II, they have a role in the regulation of blood pressure. In addition, they produce active vitamin D, assisting in the regulation of calcium balance.

Acute Renal Failure

ARF may result from prerenal, intrarenal, or postrenal causes. The critical care nurse assesses the patient in ARF for the development of fluid and electrolyte imbalances, institutes supportive care, and attempts to prevent additional renal injury.

Risk Factors for Development of Acute Renal Failure

Prerenal causes account for 60% of cases of ARF. Although an obstruction in renal blood flow resulting from renal vascular diseases or obstruction of a renal artery may cause prerenal failure, it more commonly results from a pronounced reduction in cardiac output due to severe hypotension, hypovolemia, or severe vasoconstriction. In prerenal dysfunction, the nephrons and glomeruli are structurally and functionally normal and the GFR decreases due to the reduction in renal blood flow.

The patient with a prerenal cause of ARF often is hypotensive and may demonstrate severe vasoconstriction due to a pronounced decrease in cardiac output. The nephrons and glomeruli are still relatively normal so the patient responds to the decreased kidney perfusion by retaining sodium and by producing less than 400 mL/day of concentrated urine. Urinalysis typically shows a concentrated urine with a high osmolality (greater than 500 mOsm/L) and a decreased urine sodium (less than 20 mmol/L). The **fractional excretion of sodium (FENa)**, a test for assessing how well the kidneys can concentrate urine and conserve sodium, is usually less than 1%. There are rarely more than a few casts and/or a little sediment present in the urine.

Intrarenal causes account for 30% to 40% of the cases of ARF. In critically ill patients, it most commonly results from prolonged hypoperfusion of the kidney. If prerenal failure is not treated adequately and promptly, oxygen delivery to the kidneys does not meet the demand. The renal tubules respond to hypoxia with dysfunction, inflammation, and, possibly, necrosis. With the release of inflammatory mediators and death of cells there is further disruption in renal blood flow and damage to the basement membranes and renal tubules. In 30% to 70% of cases, renal tubular epithelial cells are shed in the urine. There is tubular dysfunction with impaired sodium and water reabsorption. Thus, intrinsic renal failure can be differentiated from prerenal dysfunction by urinalysis (Table 14–1). In intrinsic renal failure, urinalysis typically reveals an osmolality less than 350 mOsm/L, an increased urine sodium (greater than 40 mmol/L), and a FENa greater than 1% with granular casts and sediment.

Postrenal causes, accounting for 5% to 10% of cases of ARF in hospitalized patients, are usually obstructions in the urine collection system. The most common reason is the development of benign prostatic

TABLE 14–1

Contrasting Laboratory Findings in Prerenal and Intrinsic Renal Failure

LABORATORY FINDING	PRERENAL	INTRINSIC RENAL
Urine osmolality	>500 mOsm/L	<350 mOsm/L
Urine sodium	<20 mmol/L	>40 mmol/L
FENa	Less than 1%	>1%
Casts and/or sediment	Rare	Present

Gerontological Considerations

Normal aging results in a significant reduction in renal reserves—as much as a 30% reduction between the ages of 30 and 75.

The most common cause of postrenal failure in the older male is the development of benign prostatic hypertrophy.

Adults over the age of 70 may require a higher MAP (perhaps as high as 100 mm Hg) to maintain adequate renal perfusion.

Renal toxins are a significant precipitating factor for the development of intrinsic renal failure in people who already have decreased renal function, such as older adults.

hypertrophy in the older male. Other causes include tubular obstruction from crystals (caused by uric acid or acyclovir), bilateral ureteral obstruction, or other sources of urethral obstruction such as prostatic cancer. Renal failure results when the obstruction causes an increase in the tubular pressure, resulting in a decrease in the GFR. Most commonly it is characterized by the sudden onset of anuria (production of less than 50 mL of urine/day). It may be identified quickly and accurately by renal ultrasound. Postrenal failure usually resolves rapidly with removal of the urinary tract obstruction and the return of renal filtration pressure.

Collaborative Management

Prerenal dysfunction most commonly results from a significant decrease in cardiac output or an obstruction in a renal artery resulting in a decrease in renal perfusion pressure. It is identified when the patient demonstrates signs of decreased cardiac output and oliguria with characteristic changes in urinalysis. Management involves improving the cardiac output, usually by volume administration, or relieving the renal artery obstruction. With prompt return of renal perfusion, most patients regain renal function. If inadequate renal perfusion is prolonged, patients may develop intrinsic renal failure.

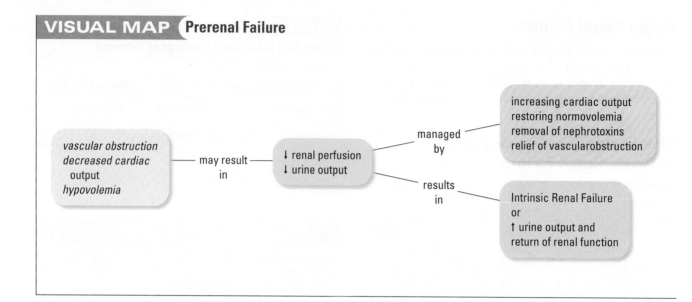

VISUAL MAP (Prerenal Failure)

- *vascular obstruction*
- *decreased cardiac output*
- *hypovolemia*

— may result in —

↓ renal perfusion
↓ urine output

— managed by —

increasing cardiac output
restoring normovolemia
removal of nephrotoxins
relief of vascularobstruction

— results in —

Intrinsic Renal Failure
or
↑ urine output and
return of renal function

Nursing Management

The acutely ill patient may develop a decrease in cardiac output, leading to prerenal dysfunction in a variety of ways. The nurse reviews the patient's history for potential sources of decreased cardiac output. Common causes include:

- Hypovolemia from hemorrhage, trauma, hypovolemic shock, inadequate volume replacement prior to surgery, burns, pancreatitis, or excessive use of diuretics
- Cardiovascular disorders such as heart failure or dysrhythmias
- Vasodilation from sepsis or medications such as antihypertensive agents

The nurse assesses the patient for manifestations of hypovolemia (Figure 14-2), including:

Hypotension or orthostatic hypotension

Tachycardia

Dry mucous membranes

Poor skin turgor

Flat jugular veins

Weight loss

Low central venous pressure (CVP) or pulmonary artery wedge pressure (PAWP)

The nurse looks for indications of increased extracellular fluid that may develop when the decreased renal perfusion is due to vasodilation or cardiovascular disease. These include:

Edema

Ascites

Weight gain

Increased CVP or PAWP

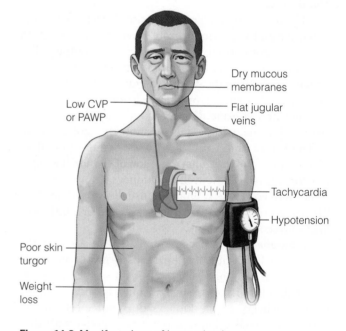

Figure 14-2 Manifestations of hypovolemia.

Additionally, the nurse reviews the following laboratory studies.

1) *Urinalysis:* As described earlier, reviewing the urinalysis helps to differentiate between prerenal and intrinsic renal causes of ARF. To most accurately reflect the patient's situation, urine for evaluation should be obtained prior to the administration of a diuretic.

2) *Serum Blood Urea Nitrogen (BUN):* A normal level is 5 to 25 mg/dL. Urea is filtered freely but its absorption from the tubules is a function of the urine flow rate. When the urine flow rate is reduced, more urea is absorbed. Thus, in prerenal failure, the rise in BUN may be out of proportion to the renal dysfunction.

3) *Serum Creatinine:* Serum creatinine provides a more accurate estimate of renal function than BUN. Normal levels in adults are 0.5 to 1.5 mg/dL. A doubling of serum creatinine normally indicates a 50% reduction in GFRs.

4) *Creatinine Clearance:* Creatinine clearance provides the most accurate estimate of GFR. Normal values range between 85 and 125 mL/min/1.73 m² for adult men and 75 and 115 mL/min/1.73 m² for adult women. Values below normal indicate at least a 50% reduction in the number of functioning nephrons.

5) *BUN-to-Creatinine Ratio:* Because prerenal failure results in increased reabsorption of urea, the serum BUN-to-creatinine ratio may rise to greater than 20:1 in prerenal causes of ARF.

Collaborative Management

The nurse works collaboratively with the physician to identify and then resolve prerenal dysfunction. The goal of therapy is restoration of normal renal perfusion by attaining normovolemia, increasing cardiac output, or relieving the obstruction in the renal artery.

Restoration of Normovolemia

For restoration of normovolemia, protocols suggest normal saline fluid challenges until the patient's CVP reaches 12. However, the fluid of choice may vary depending on the reason for the patient's fluid volume deficit.

- To deliver a fluid challenge, the nurse infuses 250 to 500 mL of normal saline rapidly. Although definitions of rapid administration vary depending on the circumstances, a fluid challenge of 500 mL may be administered over half an hour.

- The nurse anticipates that the patient's blood pressure (BP), heart rate, urine output, and CVP or PAWP will begin to normalize quickly if the challenge has been successful. The urine output usually begins to increase within 10 to 20 minutes following the volume challenge and is maximal at 30 to 45 minutes if hypovolemia was the cause of the decreased urine output.

- The first fluid challenge may be followed by additional fluid challenges if it does not have the anticipated effect.

- When such a protocol is initiated, it is imperative that the nurse observe the patient closely and identify immediately any signs of fluid volume overload that could develop if an excessive amount of fluid was inadvertently administered. Signs of fluid volume overload are discussed in the section titled "Assessment of Fluid Volume Status in the Patient with Acute Renal Failure" and displayed in Figure 14-3.

Restoration of Adequate Renal Perfusion

One of the major determinants of renal perfusion is the mean arterial pressure (MAP). In a middle-aged or younger adult, maintaining the MAP above 70 to 80 mm Hg usually allows for adequate renal perfusion. However, adults over the age of 70 may require a higher MAP (perhaps as high as 100 mm Hg) to maintain adequate renal perfusion. The most effective way to attain a MAP of 70 or greater is with adequate administration of volume. So the nurse should be attentive to the increase in the MAP when administering fluid challenges.

In the past dopamine was used to increase BP with the assumption that a dopamine infusion of 0.5 to 3 mcg/kg/min would increase renal perfusion. Although dopamine does appear to increase renal blood flow in healthy individuals, it does not seem to do so in critically ill patients. In fact, there is some indication that it may create a mismatch between perfusion and oxygen requirements, causing further damage to kidney cells. No studies have indicated that the use of renal dose

---

COMMONLY USED MEDICATIONS

NOREPINEPHRINE

INTRODUCTION
Norepinephrine is a potent a-adrenergic agonist with some b-adrenergic effects.

Dose and Desired Effect: Norepinephrine is administered by continuous intravenous (IV) infusion. Usual maintenance range of the infusion is 2 to 12 mcg/ min. The usual maximum dose is 25 mcg/min. Due to its vasoconstrictive effects, norepinephrine usually results in a significant increase in MAP with little change in heart rate or cardiac output. Initial response should begin 1 to 2 minutes after IV administration is started.

Nursing Responsibilities:
- The nurse monitors the BP every 2 to 5 minutes after beginning a continuous infusion. Norepinephrine may be titrated up or down cautiously to obtain a MAP of 80. The lowest dose possible to attain the MAP should be utilized.

- In addition to monitoring the MAP, the nurse will keep an eye on the heart rate, monitor pattern, CVP, and urine output continuously during administration.

- If at all possible, norepinephrine should be administered through a central venous catheter. If norepinephrine is administered through a peripheral IV line, severe vasoconstriction may result. Veins in the hands, ankles, and legs should be avoided but a large antecubital vein may be acceptable if necessary. Blanching along the vein is an indication of extravasation that can lead to severe tissue necrosis, sloughing, and gangrene. If extravasation does occur, phentolamine (Regitine) 5 to 10 mg diluted in 10 to 15 mL of normal saline is injected liberally throughout the tissue to prevent necrosis.

Potential Side and/or Toxic Effects: Side effects are rare when used as directed. However, previously there was concern that the vasoconstriction that occurs with norepinephrine would result in deterioration in renal functioning. This does not appear to be the case. Instead, by increasing the MAP, norepinephrine appears to increase glomerular filtration and renal function. However, the nurse should be certain to monitor the urine output and serum creatinine of the patient receiving norepinephrine.

dopamine in the patient in renal failure results in a decrease in morbidity or mortality (Friedich, Adhikak, Herridge & Beyene, 2005). Thus, norepinephrine, rather than dopamine, is now indicated to increase the patient's BP when adequate fluid administration does not result in a sufficient increase in MAP (Ievins, 2004).

Management of decreases in cardiac output or dysrhythmias that may result in prerenal ARF are discussed in Chapters 4 and 5. ∞

Nephrology Consult

When patients do not respond to volume repletion and appropriate management of decreased cardiac output with improved urinary output and renal function, a consult to a nephrologist should be suggested. Studies have shown that early referral of patients with ARF to a nephrologist results in better patient outcomes (Mehta, McDonald, & Gabbai, 2002). Patients with ARF who were seen by a nephrologist within 48 hours of ICU admission had shorter stays in the ICU and the hospital as well as lower mortality rates.

Relief of Renal Artery Obstruction

When the patient's decrease in renal function is accompanied by pronounced hypertension, the physician may suspect that the renal failure is caused by an obstruction in renal blood flow rather than hypovolemia or a decreased cardiac output. She may order renal Doppler flow studies or a renal angiogram to rule out such an obstruction. If an obstruction is identified, it may be treated invasively by angioplasty with stent placement or surgically. Usually prompt relief of the vascular obstruction results in return of renal function.

Avoidance of Additional Renal Injury

During the period of decreased renal perfusion and lowered GFR that occurs in prerenal ARF, the kidneys are vulnerable to insults from other sources such as medications, radiocontrast dyes, and toxins. These insults may precipitate the development of intrinsic ARF. Therefore,

- The nurse avoids administering nephrotoxic agents to the patient if possible.
- Drugs that are known to be excreted by the kidneys and potentially harmful to the kidneys are given in reduced doses based on the patient's creatinine clearance.
- The nurse monitors the peak and trough blood levels of medications known to be damaging to the kidney. A trough level is usually drawn 1 hour prior to administration of the next dose of a medication, whereas a peak level is usually drawn immediately following the administration of a drug.
- If contrast dye must be administered, it is given sparingly or the physician may prescribe and the nurse administer acetylcysteine for its renal protective effects.

- The nurse is scrupulous in his use of aseptic technique to prevent the development of an infection because removal of the by-products of infection and excretion of antibiotics may impose additional burdens on the damaged kidneys.

Intrinsic Renal Failure

In critically ill patients, intrinsic or intrarenal failure, sometimes called acute tubular necrosis (ATN), is primarily caused by a prolonged reduction in renal perfusion (prerenal failure) but may also be precipitated by other conditions, including nephrotoxic agents. Intrinsic ARF may be differentiated from prerenal failure by the previously described characteristic findings on urinalysis. Although there are normally four phases to the disease process—onset, oliguric, diuretic, and recovery—not all patients in ARF are oliguric.

Predisposing Conditions

As noted earlier, the most common reason for development of intrinsic renal failure is prerenal failure. Other causes such as inflammatory disorders, infiltrative diseases, and nephrotoxins account for the remaining cases of intrinsic renal failure. Because inflammatory disorders and infiltrative diseases are less likely to be the cause of ARF in critically ill patients, they are not discussed further. Renal toxins are a significant precipitating factor for the development of intrinsic renal failure in people who already have decreased renal function, such as diabetics, older adults, or patients who have decreased renal perfusion. Drugs that have been implicated in the development of renal failure include:

> Nonsteroidal anti-inflammatory agents (NSAIDs)
>
> Antimicrobials such as aminoglycosides, acyclovir, and cephalosporins
>
> Contrast media
>
> Angiotensin-converting enzyme (ACE) inhibitors
>
> Cyclosporine

Conditions that create endogenous toxins capable of causing renal failure are rhabdomyolysis and hypercalcemia. Rhabdomyolysis is the breakdown of muscle fibers, resulting in the release of muscle fiber contents such as myoglobin into the circulation. Myoglobin, an oxygen-binding protein pigment found in the skeletal muscle, is normally filtered out of the bloodstream by the kidneys. When released in large amounts, myoglobin may block the structures of the kidney, causing ARF. The disorder may be caused by any condition that results in damage to skeletal muscle. Risk factors include severe exertion, ischemia or necrosis of muscles, trauma, crush injuries, or seizures. Rhabdomyolysis may account for as much as 25% of the cases of intrinsic renal failure. In

VISUAL MAP Intrinsic Renal Failure

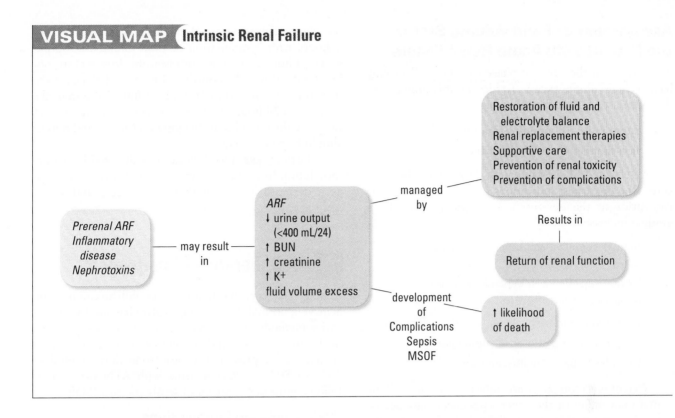

addition to the normal findings of ARF, the patient with rhabdomyolysis may manifest dark-, red-, or cola-colored urine; muscle tenderness; and/or weakness of the affected muscle(s).

Pathophysiology and Manifestations

Intrinsic renal failure usually has four distinct phases, the first of which is the **onset phase**. This phase immediately follows the period of renal injury and lasts approximately 2 to 4 days. During this phase, the patient's urinary output typically decreases to 20% of normal and the BUN and creatinine may begin to increase slightly.

Most patients then enter the second phase of ARF, the **oliguric phase**, during which the patient excretes less than 400 mL of urine/day. During this phase that typically lasts 10 to 14 days, the patient retains fluid, is unable to maintain electrolyte and/or acid-base balance, and cannot excrete sufficient amounts of nitrogenous wastes.

This renal dysfunction is probably the result of cyclical damage to the renal tubules. Decreased renal perfusion begins the process, resulting in decreased glomerular capillary pressure and a reduction in the GFR. There is concurrent ischemic injury to epithelial cells. The renal tubules respond to hypoxia with dysfunction, inflammation, and patchy tubular necrosis that does not correlate with the level of renal dysfunction. With the release of inflammatory mediators and death of cells there is further disruption in renal blood flow and damage to the basement membrane. Persistent vasoconstriction and congestion from white cells and

cell debris lead to ongoing hypoxia and necrosis (Agraharkar, Gupta, & Agraharkar, 2004). In 30% to 70% of cases, renal tubular epithelial cells are shed in the urine; in the past this type of ARF was called ATN.

Some patients in ARF do not develop oliguria; this is termed **nonoliguric ARF**. They still have problems with electrolyte imbalances and uremia but their urine outputs are more than 400 mL/day, usually about 1,000 mL/day. Studies have shown that patients with nonoliguric ARF have a higher mortality rate than patients with oliguric renal failure. The outcomes may be worse for these patients because they are producing "adequate" amounts of urine so their referral to a nephrologist, management of electrolyte imbalances, and subsequent start of RRT are delayed.

As patients begin to regain renal function, they enter the **diuretic phase** of ARF. During this phase, patients usually begin to increase their urinary output, often producing up to 5 liters of urine each day. However, these patients still may not be able to completely excrete wastes and regulate electrolyte or acid-base balance. The BUN and creatinine usually decrease slowly toward normal over a 10-day period.

The final phase of ARF is the **recovery phase**. This phase typically lasts from 6 months to a year. During this phase, most patients' renal function returns to normal. Only 5% to 10% of patients who survive continue to require dialysis. However, patients are thought to be vulnerable to repeated insults to their renal function and are counseled to avoid renal toxins.

Assessment of Fluid Volume Status in the Patient with Acute Renal Failure

The patient in the oliguric phase of ATN will usually have a fluid volume excess. To identify this fluid excess the nurse assesses for the following:

Rapid pulse of bounding quality

Skin that is pale and cool to the touch

An elevated BP, possibly with decreased pulse pressure. One of earliest indications of fluid excess, occurring prior to the development of edema, may be a gradual increase in BP.

Jugular venous distention and/or hepatojugular reflex

Nonpitting edema in dependent areas

Increased CVP or PAWP

Increased respiratory rate with shallow respirations

Dyspnea on exertion or in supine position

Crackles in bases on auscultation

Weight is a more accurate indicator of fluid volume status than many of the other assessment parameters. The nurse determines the patient's "dry" weight (the weight after the patient has been diuresed or had dialysis). Then, the patient should be weighed daily at the same time on the same properly calibrated scale with the same amount of clothing or bed linens. A patient will gain 0.5 kg (1 lb) for each 500 mL of extra fluid intake.

Although intake and output are carefully measured in most critically ill patients, they have been shown to be inaccurate. Still the nurse attempts to maintain as accurate a record as possible. In the patient in ARF, the nurse usually measures sources of intake and output every 1 to 2 hours with a summation of total intake and output every 24 hours. Allowing for insensible loss, a nonventilated patient may be considered to be in balance if she has an intake of 500 to 700 mL of fluid more than she excretes in 24 hours. However, a ventilated patient does not have the same insensible losses so intake and output should be roughly equivalent.

The nurse examines laboratory values to identify hemodilution from fluid volume excess. It may be evident as a decrease in hemoglobin, hematocrit, and serum sodium values.

Collaborative Management

Management is primarily supportive with an emphasis on achieving normal fluid and electrolyte balance by conservative methods or renal replacement therapies, avoiding nephrotoxic agents, and preventing complications. Survival has not improved since the introduction of dialysis—50% to 80% of ICU patients with ATN die, usually following the development of sepsis and/or MSOF.

Evidence-Based Interventions for Fluid Volume Excess

The most effective interventions for fluid volume excess in the ARF patient are fluid restriction and renal replacement therapies. Diuretics, once a mainstay of treatment, are being reconsidered.

Fluid Restriction. Fluid restriction may be instituted in an attempt to prevent worsening fluid volume excess. The physician might prescribe a specific amount of fluid (such as 1,000 mL) per 24 hours or might calculate the intake for each day depending on the patient's previous day urine output plus the estimated insensible loss. For example:

Previous day's urine output (330) + insensible fluid loss estimate (400) = 770 mL. The fluid allotment may be divided over the course of the day. One common example is:

1/2 of calculated fluid may be allotted to days

1/3 for evening

Balance (1/6) at night

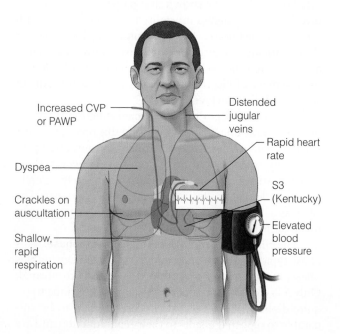

Increased CVP or PAWP

Distended jugular veins

Rapid heart rate

Dyspea

S3 (Kentucky)

Crackles on auscultation

Elevated blood pressure

Shallow, rapid respiration

Figure 14-3 Manifestations of excess fluid volume.

Nursing Diagnoses

PATIENT WITH ACUTE RENAL FAILURE

- Ineffective tissue perfusion: renal related to hypovolemia and reduced arterial blood flow
- Excess fluid volume related to renal failure
- Imbalanced nutrition less than body requirements related to altered metabolic requirements
- Risk for infection related to malnutrition, intubation, and indwelling catheters, drains, or IVs.

For the 770-mL fluid limit calculated, this would mean that the patient would receive 385 mL of fluid on days, 255 mL on evenings, and the balance (130) mL at night.

It can be extremely difficult to maintain a conscious patient on a restricted fluid intake, especially if the patient is receiving IV fluids and/or medications.

Diuretics. In the past, the excess fluid intake and volume overload were often resolved with the use of diuretics. It was believed that the use of diuretics would convert oliguric renal failure to nonoliguric renal failure and make the renal failure easier to treat. After patients had been provided adequate amounts of volume, if their urine outputs did not increase, they were started on a diuretic, often a furosemide (Lasix) infusion at 2 mg/hr. There is growing evidence that this practice not only does not help patients but also may harm them. One study indicated that the use of diuretics would result in a 68% increase in hospital mortality (Mehta, Pascaul, Soroko, & Charlow, 2002). In addition, the use of diuretics in ARF have been implicated in permanent hearing loss and pronounced hyponatremia. Severe fluid volume excesses are now usually dealt with by some method of renal replacement therapy. RRT is discussed later in the chapter under Building Technology Skills: Renal Replacement Therapies.

Nursing Management

The critical care nurse must be prepared to assess her patient in ARF for development of the following electrolyte imbalances. The nurse recognizes that these serious imbalances may require immediate management on discovery.

Dilutional (Hypervolemic) Hyponatremia

The critical care nurse assesses the ARF patient for an abnormally low serum sodium due to fluid overload. Manifestations depend on the serum sodium level and how rapidly the level dropped. The manifestations of hyponatremia are most apparent when serum sodium levels fall from normal levels (135 to 148 mEq/L) to below 120 to 125 mEq/L in less than 12 to 24 hours. However, nearly all patients with serum sodium levels less than 120 mEq/L will demonstrate some symptoms and patients with serum sodium levels less than 110 mEq/L will demonstrate severe symptoms. The nurse assesses the patient with the following serum sodium levels for these potential symptoms:

125 to 135 mEq/L	Generally no manifestations
124 to 111 mEq/L	Headache, lethargy, disorientation
110 to 100 mEq/L	Confusion, hostility, nausea and vomiting, lethargy or violence
Less than 100 mEq/L	Delirium, convulsions, coma, Cheyne-Stokes respirations

Fluid restriction is the most effective method of treatment in asymptomatic patients. It allows for the gradual loss of free water with a subsequent rise in the serum sodium. If the patient is awake, the nurse will need to carefully explain the rationale for the fluid restriction, assist with the allocation of fluid intake as described previously, and carefully monitor the patient's intake.

If fluid restriction is not successful in increasing the serum sodium or if the patient is symptomatic, diuretics may be administered with a saline infusion. This must be done very carefully because the use of diuretics results not only in the loss of fluid but may result in the loss of sodium as well.

For a severely ill patient with a serum sodium less than 110 mEq/L, a loop diuretic may be cautiously administered in conjunction with hypertonic saline (3% or 5%). When administering these agents, the nurse checks urine output along with urine and blood electrolytes hourly.

Hyperkalemia (Serum Potassium Greater Than 5.5 mEq/L)

Hyperkalemia may represent a life-threatening complication. Although some patients complain of nausea or muscle weakness, usually hyperkalemia is identified through a laboratory test or an ECG. The changes that occur in the ECG are described next and shown in Figure 14-4.

K+ = 5.6 to 6.0 mEq/L	tall, peaked Ts
6.0 to 6.5 mEq/L	prolonged PR and QT intervals
6.5 to 7.0 mEq/L	diminished Ps and depressed STs
7.0 to 7.5 mEq/L	bundle branch blocks may develop
7.5 to 8.0 mEq/L	Ps disappear, QRS widens

Death may occur when the potassium exceeds 7.0 mEq/L and is the result either of diastolic arrest caused by block of the distal Purkinje fibers or ventricular fibrillation caused by reentrant circuits.

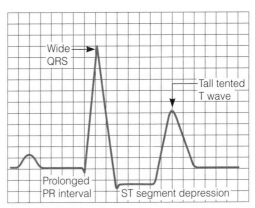

Figure 14-4 ECG in hyperkalemia.

If the serum potassium is less than 6.5 mEq/L and the patient is asymptomatic, the potassium level may be reduced by limiting potassium intake and increasing the potassium loss in the urine through the use of a diuretic. Once the level rises to above 6.5 mEq/L, the following efforts may be made to counteract or rapidly decrease the serum potassium:

A. IV calcium may be administered to patients who are not receiving digitalis to counteract the potassium.

   Dose and Desired Effect: The dose is dependent on whether calcium chloride or calcium gluconate is administered. Ten milliliters of 10% Ca++ gluconate (4.5 mEq) or 5 mL of Ca++ chloride (6.8 mEq) might be administered IV push over 2 minutes. The counteracting effect of IV calcium is short lived; buying time for other types of interventions, the onset of action should be 1 to 3 minutes and the duration of effect 30 to 60 minutes. The nurse may recognize that calcium is having the desired effect by normalization of the ECG on the monitor.

   Nursing Responsibilities: The nurse maintains the patient on a cardiac monitor and observes for bradycardia, stopping the administration of the calcium should bradycardia develop.

B. In an attempt to drive the excess potassium into the cell, three other medications might be utilized. None of the medications lowers the total body concentration of potassium but all temporarily shift the potassium intracellularly, allowing time to institute other interventions that will decrease the total body concentration of potassium. These medications are:

   1. Insulin plus glucose (5 to 10 Units of regular insulin with 50 g of glucose); the onset of action is about 30 minutes and the duration 4 to 6 hours

   2. Sodium bicarbonate (50 to 100 mEq total dose—or 1 mEq/kg); the onset of action is about 5 to 10 minutes with 1- to 2-hour duration of effect.

   3. Inhaled beta agonists such as albuterol (2.5 mg/3 mL saline) may be given by nebulizer every 20 minutes. The dose is problematic because it is so much higher than what is normally used for treatment of reactive airway disease and may result in central nervous system (CNS) and cardiovascular (CV) symptoms. The onset of action is about 30 minutes and the duration 2 to 3 hours.

   When administering medications that either counteract potassium or drive it into the cell, the nurse recognizes that the effect is temporary and definitive management is still required. Still she should observe for the desired effects, an improvement in the ECG waveform, and the cardiac output. If insulin, glucose and sodium bicarbonate, or inhaled β-agonists have been utilized, there should also be a rapid reduction in serum potassium.

C. A cation exchange resin such as sodium polystyrene sulfonate (Kayexelate) might be utilized to decrease total body potassium through gastrointestinal transport.

   Dose and Desired Effect: The usual dose is 15 to 50 g of the resin administered with sorbitol to hasten delivery. It may be administered either orally or rectally by retention enema. Onset is usually within 1 to 2 hours but may be delayed as long as 12 hours with oral administration. Rectal administration results in more rapid reduction in serum potassium because most of the transporters are located in the colon.

   Nursing Responsibilities: Because gastric ulceration may result from its administration, it may be administered either with ginger ale, if given orally, or in 500 to 700 mL of D₅W or saline, if given rectally. The nurse observes for the reduction in serum potassium and monitors the patient until the potassium level has stabilized.

D. Finally, dialysis may be utilized to return the serum potassium to a normal level. This is the most effective method of adequately treating severe hyperkalemia. Care of the patient receiving dialysis is discussed with Building Technology Skills.

Hypocalcemia (Ionized Ca++ Less Than 4.25 mg/dL, Which Is 1.2 mmol/L or Serum Ca++ Less Than 8.5 mg/dL)

Calcium is found in the blood bound to albumin or free in its ionized form. Because only ionized calcium is metabolically active, it is the preferred value for identifying and treating hypocalcemia.

Manifestations of hypocalcemia may develop as soon as 48 hours after the onset of the oliguric phase of ARF because renal tubule disorders often result in excessive loss of calcium.

- With mild hypocalcemia, the patient may complain of some numbness and tingling in the digits or about the mouth.

- As the calcium level continues to drop, contraction of the corner of the patient's eye and mouth may occur when the patient's facial nerve is tapped gently. This represents a positive Chvostek's sign and may indicate hypocalcemia (Figure 14-5). However, the sign is not definitive for hypocalcemia because it occurs normally in response to tapping of the facial nerve in 10% to

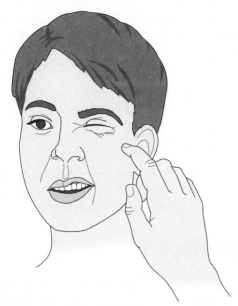

Figure 14-5 Positive Chvostek's sign.

COMMONLY USED MEDICATIONS

CALCIUM FOR SUPPLEMENTATION

INTRODUCTION

Calcium, a therapeutic mineral and electrolyte replacement/supplement, is available as two separate forms of elemental calcium for IV use. It is imperative that the nurse recognize the differences in amounts of elemental calcium found in calcium gluconate and calcium chloride.

- One gram of CA++ gluconate (10% injection) contains 90 mg of elemental calcium or 4.5 mEq.

- One gram of CACl contains 272 mg of elemental calcium or 13.6 mEq.

Dose and Desired Effects: For tetany, a total dose of 4.5 to 16 mEq of calcium might be required for treatment. Often the initial dose is 1 to 2 amps of 10% solution of calcium gluconate (4.5 to 9 mEq) in 50 to 100 mL of D_5W administered IV over 5 to 10 minutes. The nurse should expect to see an improvement in serum calcium values drawn 4 to 6 hours later.

Nursing Responsibilities:
- It is preferable to administer the medication through a central line, although, if necessary, a large peripheral vein is acceptable. If a peripheral vein is utilized the nurse must assess the IV site closely for signs of extravasation and tissue damage.

- The nurse monitors the patient's ECG during the infusion to detect the signs of hypercalcemia, a decreased QT interval, and an inverted T.

Potential Side and/or Toxic Effects: If the infusion is given too rapidly, pronounced hypotension, bradycardia, and cardiac arrest can occur.

12% of the population and it occurs in response to conditions other than hypocalcemia.

- Spasm of the hand and wrist, Trousseau's sign, may become apparent when a BP cuff placed on an arm is inflated to 20 mm Hg above the systolic pressure for at least 3 minutes.

- Serious physiological effects occur when total calcium levels are less than 7.0 and ionized calcium levels are less than 0.8 mmol/L; then the patient may develop tetany or convulsions.

Management of mild hypocalcemia is supportive and may involve oral supplementation, whereas serious hypocalcemia is managed as described next with IV calcium replacement.

Hyperphosphatemia (Serum Level Greater Than 4.5 mg/dL)

In ARF, hyperphosphatemia, an increase in the serum phosphorus, does not usually occur until the GFR has decreased to 10% to 20% of normal. Because serum phosphorus and calcium are usually in an inverse relationship, hyperphosphatemia is usually accompanied by hypocalcemia. Patients experience few symptoms unless problems with hypocalcemia or soft tissue calcifications develop. Treatment includes ensuring adequate hydration, dietary restriction of phosphate (less than 200 mg/day), calcium supplementation, and administration of phosphate binders. Dietary restriction of less than 200 mg of phosphate is difficult for a patient to maintain so elimination of phosphate is required.

Phosphate binders are the primary means for decreasing the serum phosphorus. Historically, aluminum-based antacids were used as phosphate binders. However, when patients began to develop symptoms that were attributable to aluminum toxicity, their use decreased dramatically. Now calcium-containing phosphate binders such as calcium carbonate and calcium citrate are routinely used.

Maintenance of Acid-Base Balance

ARF may lead to metabolic acidosis due to the inability of the renal tubules to secrete hydrogen ions into the renal tubules or to conserve bicarbonate. It may be identified by a pH less than 7.35, a HCO_3 less than 23, with an initially normal pCO_2. If the patient is able to compensate by increasing the rate and depth of respirations resulting in a decrease in the pCO_2, the pH may return toward normal. This is the preferred method of compensation because there are fewer problems. As long as the patient is able to compensate, there is no need for further intervention. However, the nurse assesses the patient for the development of manifestations of metabolic acidosis, including:

- CNS effects such as confusion, hyperactive reflexes, tingling, and, possibly, tetany or seizures

- Effects associated with hyperkalemia such as dysrhythmias

The nurse continues to assess the patient's pH and bicarbonate levels as well. If any of the listed symptoms develop and/or the pH falls below 7.2 with the bicarbonate

COMMONLY USED MEDICATIONS

CALCIUM CARBONATE AND CALCIUM CITRATE PHOSPHATE BINDERS (E.G., CALCIUM CARBONATE)

INTRODUCTION
Calcium carbonate and calcium citrate serve a dual purpose: binding the excess phosphate and providing needed calcium simultaneously.

Dose and Desired Effect: Dosages of the binders are adjusted to bring the serum phosphate level to approximately 4.0 mg/dL.

Nursing Responsibilities: Phosphate binders are provided with meals, if the patient is eating, or down a nasogastric tube otherwise to bind phosphate in the gastrointestinal tract where it will be excreted in the feces rather than absorbed into the blood.

Potential Side and/or Toxic Effects: When binders containing calcium are utilized, soft tissue calcification occasionally develops. Therefore, the nurse assesses the patient for the following indications of soft tissue calcification:

- A papular rash that may be itchy
- Painful deposits in the joints that may limit movement
- Red eyes from calcium deposits in the eyes

  In the event that soft tissue calcifications develop, either sevelamer (Renagel) or lanthanum carbonate (Fosrenal) would be the preferred phosphate binder. Recent studies have indicated that these medications may also limit atherosclerosis in the chronic renal failure patient and therefore may be a better choice as a phosphate binder for the patient in renal failure (Fatica & Dennis, 2002).

---

below 15, sodium bicarbonate might be given. Bicarbonate is given only if necessary because it may result in:

- Hypernatremia
- Hyperosmolality
- A decreased release of oxygen from hemoglobin to the tissues

The base deficit might be calculated by a formula such as the following to guide the total amount of bicarbonate administration:

Deficit = (Desired bicarbonate-measured)
$\times$ weight (kg) $\times$ 0.5

Intractable or severe acidosis in the patient with ARF is treated with dialysis.

Removal of Nitrogenous Wastes

Serum creatinine provides an estimate of GFR. A doubling of serum creatinine normally indicates a 50% reduction in GFRs. Normal levels in adults are 0.5 to 1.5 mg/dL. When there is an abrupt cessation in GFR the serum creatinine will usually rise between 1 and 2 mg/dL each day.

The rise in the BUN is more variable because it is not only dependent on the loss of renal function but can also be affected by a change in the patient's protein intake, tissue catabolism, or gastrointestinal (GI) bleeding. A normal level is 5 to 25 mg/dL. Usually in intrinsic renal failure, the BUN and creatinine increase relatively proportionally and maintain approximately a 10:1 ratio.

Regardless of the source, the presence of excess urea in the blood (uremia) may have consequences for the patient. The nurse assesses the patient for the following potential manifestations:

- Mental status changes
- Anorexia, nausea, and vomiting
- Pruritus
- Pericardial friction rub

Management may be by limiting protein intake (see nutrition later) or, when the BUN reaches approximately 100 and the creatinine about 10, dialysis may be initiated.

Nursing Care

Nursing care of the patient with ARF includes ensuring that the patient receives adequate nutrition and promoting patient comfort.

Provision of Adequate Nutrition

Patients in ARF have increased energy expenditures and their energy requirements range between 25 and 45 kcal/kg/day. They also have disruptions in water, acid-base metabolism, electrolytes, and protein breakdown that must be considered when planning their nutritional intake. Goals for nutritional intervention in the ARF patient include:

Preserving lean body mass

Preventing metabolic alterations

Enhancing renal recovery by limiting uremic toxicity

Nutritionists should be involved early in determining the patient's nutritional requirements and developing appropriate interventions. Two major considerations that affect the provision of nutrition are the patient's protein requirements and whether and what type of RRT the patient is undergoing. Protein requirements can be calculated roughly based on the rise in the patient's BUN in 24 hours, and the amount of protein in the patient's diet can be based on this calculation. The remainder of the calories the patient requires is supplied as carbohydrates or lipids. As the degree of renal failure and the rate of tissue catabolism increases, the provision of appropriate nutrition becomes more complex. A nutritionist is needed to clarify patient needs and to distinguish the most appropriate therapy from among the products created for patients with special nutritional needs.

For most patients in ARF, oral or enteral nutrition is preferred to parenteral. Enteral nutrition has the benefit of helping to maintain the GI mucosal barrier. There are usually fewer problems with volume overload and electrolyte imbalance for patients with ARF when enteral feedings are employed. Parenteral nutrition is usually instituted only after a trial of enteral has failed because it is associated with more problems. Potential problems include infection, worsening of fluid volume and electrolyte problems, or an increase in tissue catabolism. (See Chapter 1 ∞ for a more detailed discussion of enteral and parenteral nutrition in the critically ill patient.)

The nurse assesses the patient for indications that he is being adequately nourished. These include:

- Maintenance of body weight (with no evidence of excessive fluid intake or output)
- Albumin level 3.5 to 4.0 g/dL
- Total protein level 6 to 8 g/dL
- Normalizing serum electrolytes

Promotion of Patient Comfort

Patients who are in renal failure usually have multiple sources of discomfort, one of the most significant of which may be thirst. Other sources include discomfort from turning, itching, pain, and anxiety.

THIRST Patients who are on restricted fluid intakes often complain of thirst. The free water that they are allowed may barely be enough to administer their medications whether orally, by feeding tube, or parenterally. Thus, the nurse will need to allocate the fluid carefully, allowing for small amounts of oral fluids at regular intervals to increase patient comfort. Consistent, thorough mouth care also helps to maintain patient comfort. Although there have been no published studies detailing its use in patients with ARF, artificial saliva, especially if it contains mucin, may be effective in relieving a dry mouth that leads to complaints of thirst. However, the nurse may need to experiment with different varieties of artificial saliva to determine which one provides the most relief and is most palatable for the specific patient.

PRURITUS Pruritus may develop because some urea is excreted through the skin. As renal failure progresses, the skin may take on a yellowish tinge or actually show a "uremic frost." Severe itchiness may be relieved with the onset of dialysis when the BUN decreases. Other methods that may be helpful include:

- Keeping the skin moist and cool by bathing the patient, then applying a thin layer of moisturizer over the damp skin and covering the patient with a superficial covering.
- Bathing the patient with tepid water only. Although hot water will initially be relaxing and may reduce any itching briefly, the itchiness will eventually worsen due to the vasodilation from the heat.
- Applying Steifl Sarna Anti-itching lotion with camphor and menthol. Some nurses report that patients get immediate relief from this over-the-counter reasonably priced lotion.
- Administering an H1 receptor antagonist such as clemastine fumarate (Tavist). The usual dose is 2.68 mg bid.

PAIN Pain is not likely to occur from the ARF itself but may result from the patient's initial insult (e.g., surgery or trauma) or any invasive lines (e.g., dialysis access). The nurse identifies the source of the pain. Appropriate pain management will depend on the source of the pain.

ANXIETY Anxiety is likely to be a concern for any critically ill patient and his or her family. Usually, the patient with ARF has already had a series of problems so the development of this additional one may be especially anxiety provoking for the patient and/or family. The nurse should explain how and why ARF probably developed and ensure that the patient understands the chosen management strategy. When the patient is anxious, this usually means repeated explanations of the same material. It is important that all members of the health care team repeat similar information. It can be very anxiety provoking to the patient and family when they hear contradictory information from health care providers. The amount of information provided should be determined by the patient's readiness to learn. Explaining the equipment is helpful to some patients/families but is more information than others can tolerate.

━━━━━━━━━━●━━━━━━━━━━

Prevention of Complications

Prevention of complications is essential to ensuring good patient outcomes for the patient in ARF. Patients who are septic, whether they developed the ARF in response to the sepsis or the sepsis in response to the ARF, are more likely to die than patients without sepsis (Schroeder et al., 2004). In addition, sepsis is a major contributor to the development of MSOF. Patients with ARF who develop respiratory failure have an eightfold increase in the likelihood of dying, whereas patients with liver failure have a two to three times increase in mortality. Each additional failing organ results in an increase in mortality of 30%.

Nurses need to be vigilant in preventing, identifying, and treating infections in the patient with ARF. Sepsis is discussed in detail in Chapter 17. ∞ However, a few of the evidence-based nursing interventions are listed next. The nurse:

- Ensures that she or he and other members of the health care team wash their hands prior to patient care
- Uses strict aseptic technique when caring for invasive devices
- Limits the use of invasive catheters as much as possible—for example, removes a Foley catheter and utilizes intermittent catheterization if the patient is anuric
- Utilizes "bundling" to prevent ventilator-associated pneumonia
- Monitors the patient's temperature, complete blood count (CBC), and differential to detect indications of infection

- If an infection is suspected, collects specimens from appropriate sites (usually urine, sputum, blood, and wound) to be sent to the lab for cultures and sensitivities prior to the administration of any antibiotic

Building Technology Skills

Renal Replacement Therapies

Choosing the most appropriate method of RRT is a complex decision that is best made after careful consideration of a number of important factors.

Indications

Approximately half of the patients with ARF cannot be managed with conservative treatment alone. In order to prevent or treat potentially life-threatening complications, these patients will require some form of RRT. Development of any of the following signs or symptoms despite ongoing medical therapy usually means RRT is indicated:

- Oliguria with fluid volume overload
- Hyperkalemia (serum K greater than 6.5)
- Hyponatremia (serum sodium less than 115)
- Severe academia (pH less than 7.1)
- Azotemia (BUN greater than 90 to 100)
- Symptoms of uremia such as mental changes, neuropathy, or pericarditis

Principles of Therapy

The principles underlying RRTs are diffusion, osmosis, and ultrafiltration. They are depicted in the following figures and defined as follows.

Diffusion. Solutes move across a semipermeable membrane from a solution where they are in higher concentration (the plasma) to a solution where they are in a lower concentration (the dialysate). Small molecules (such as electrolytes) are able to diffuse easily across the semipermeable membrane, whereas larger molecules (such as bacteria) are not. The amount of solute removal is proportional to the dialysate flow rate and the duration of dialysis (Figure 14-6).

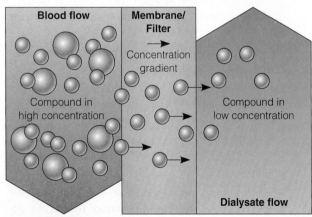

Figure 14-6 Diffusion.

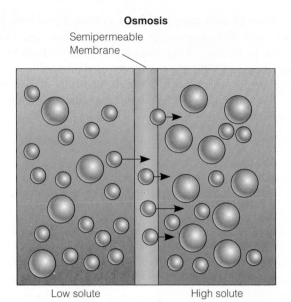

Figure 14-7 Osmosis.

Osmosis. A solution (water) moves from an area of low solute concentration (the plasma) to an area of higher solute concentration (the dialysate). (See Figure 14-7).

Ultrafiltration (Convection). A pressure gradient is created between the sides of the semipermeable membrane. Solute is carried in solution across the semipermeable membrane in response to the pressure gradient, producing an ultrafiltrate. The rate of ultrafiltration depends on the porosity of the membrane and the hydrostatic pressure of the blood (which is dependent on the blood flow). Astle (2005) recommends thinking of convection as a waterfall. A slow gentle waterfall will not pull much material along with it, whereas a rushing waterfall will drag more and larger particles (solutes) with it. Thus, ultrafiltration is able to remove fluid and the midsized solute molecules that are associated with uremia (Figure 14-8).

Methods of Renal Replacement Therapy

There are three forms of renal replacement therapy (RRT): hemodialysis, peritoneal dialysis, and continuous renal replacement therapy (CRRT).

Intermittent Hemodialysis

Intermittent hemodialysis (IHD) utilizes both ultrafiltration and diffusion to rapidly correct electrolyte imbalances, restore fluid balance, adjust acid-base balance, and remove wastes.

Indications and Expected Outcomes

IHD is indicated in patients with:

- Severe fluid overload and electrolyte imbalances
- Acute or chronic renal failure

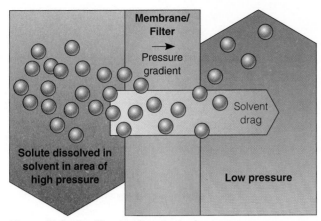

Figure 14-8 Ultrafiltration (convection).

- Certain types of drug overdoses or poisonings
- Transfusion reactions

In the past, IHD for ARF patients was usually provided in 3- to 4-hour sessions that occurred two or three times a week at the ICU patient's bedside. The disadvantage to this approach is that fluid overload, waste accumulation, and electrolyte imbalances develop between each dialysis session. Studies suggest that daily hemodialysis results in a higher rate of return of renal function and

decreased mortality for critically ill patients in ARF (Schiffl, Lang, & Fischer, 2002).

Technological Requirements: Dialysis Machinery

After the blood leaves the patient's body, it travels through a blood pump and an arterial pressure monitor to a dialyzer (filter). In the dialyzer, the blood is separated from the dialysate (deionized water) by a synthetic semipermeable membrane. The dialysate runs countercurrent to the blood flowing on the other side of the semipermeable membrane, allowing diffusion and ultrafiltration to occur. Then the blood travels through venous pressure and air leak detectors before being returned to the patient (Figure 14-9). In hemodialysis, the blood flow rate is maintained between 200 and 400 mL/min and the dialysate rate at 500 mL/hr. This high rate of flow is the reason why hemodialysis is able to correct imbalances so rapidly (Figure 14-10). It is also the reason many critically ill patients have difficulty tolerating IHD.

Hemodialysis Requires Vascular Access.

In ARF, hemodialysis access is usually through a double lumen venous catheter that may be located in the internal jugular, subclavian, or femoral veins. The catheter is normally inserted at the bedside and is available for dialysis

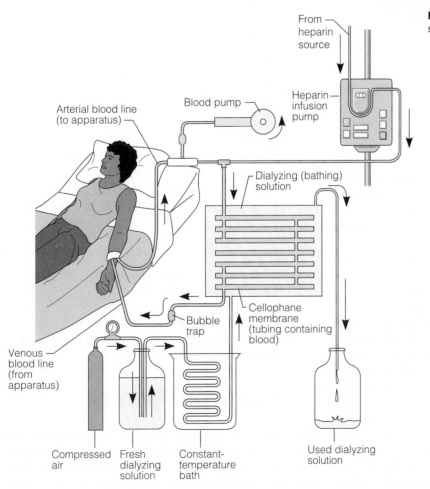

Figure 14-9 Components of a hemodialysis system.

Blood from access port

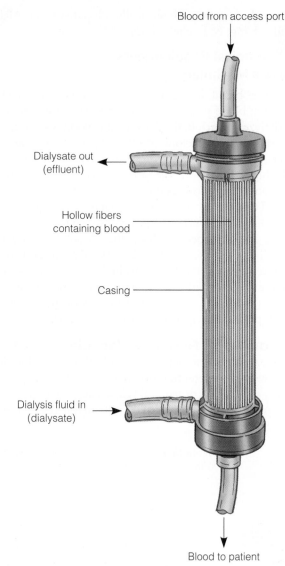

Dialysate out
(effluent)

Hollow fibers
containing blood

Casing

Dialysis fluid in
(dialysate)

Blood to patient

Figure 14-10 Hollow fiber dialyzer.

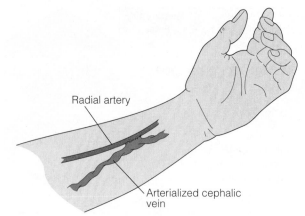

Radial artery

Arterialized cephalic
vein

Figure 14-11 An arteriovenous fistula.

as soon as placement has been verified. The catheter is usually sutured to the skin so that it will not be inadvertently dislodged and may remain in place and be utilized for dialysis for 3 to 4 weeks. There are more permanent versions of dual lumen venous catheters that may be utilized for months. Between dialysis treatments, the catheter is usually filled with a concentrated heparin solution to prevent clotting and dressed aseptically with an occlusive dressing. Maintenance of the catheter and site are normally the responsibility of the dialysis nurse because these catheters are used only in extraordinary circumstances for any purpose other than hemodialysis.

In end-stage renal disease, there are more permanent forms of access for hemodialysis. The most commonly used types are arteriovenous (AV) fistulas and AV grafts. These are surgically created connections between an artery and a vein. The AV fistula is a direct connection, whereas the AV graft uses a graft to connect the artery and vein. These anastamoses create vessels that are capable of tolerating high flow rates. Although AV fistulas

are the preferred access because they are usually more durable than grafts, a disadvantage is that it may take weeks to months for the fistula to mature and be able to tolerate the flow rate needed for dialysis. See the Safety Initiative for a discussion of the Fistula First: National Vascular Access Improvement Initiative. Potential problems with these forms of access include clotting of the access, bleeding, and infection (Figure 14-11).

When caring for a patient with an AV fistula or graft, the nurse assesses and maintains the patency of the access by:

- Palpating for the thrill or auscultating the bruit over the access.
- Checking the CSM in the access extremity.
- Avoiding any obstruction of blood flow in that extremity such as:
  - BP measurement
  - IV placement
  - Phlebotomy
  - Positioning the patient so there is pressure on the access
- Observing and preventing bleeding from the access by ensuring that gentle pressure is placed on the access site at the completion of a hemodialysis session and reviewing laboratory bleeding and clotting studies.
- Preventing infection by ensuring that aseptic technique is employed when the AV fistula or graft is in use. Usually, the nurse limits personnel in the area and wears a mask as well as sterile gloves when accessing the fistula or graft or completing the dialysis procedure.

Nursing Management

Prior to dialysis, the nurse discusses the process with the patient and/or the patient's health care proxy. The nurse clarifies that the patient or proxy understands the benefits, risks, and likely outcomes of undertaking dialysis. By doing so, the nurse ensures that informed consent has been obtained and the patient's wishes are being respected.

Next, the nurse determines if there is a "dry weight" for the patient on record and determines the patient's current weight. The difference identifies the likely amount of fluid overload the patient is experiencing. A goal for the approximate amount of fluid to be removed by dialysis will be made by the nephrologist. Other measurements of fluid balance the nurse should assess before dialysis include BP, skin turgor, intake and output, breath sounds, and CVP or PAWP if available. The nurse also reviews the patient's laboratory results and identifies the goals the nephrologist has established for correction of electrolyte and acid-base abnormalities.

The nurse will hold certain medications prior to hemodialysis. The doses of medications that may cause hypotension such as beta blockers, angiotensin-converting enzyme (ACE) inhibitors, and calcium channel blockers that are due to be administered 2 to 4 hours prior to dialysis are usually held until dialysis has been completed. Medications that are removed from the body by dialysis (a current list is usually available from the dialysis center) are also held until the end of dialysis. Finally, prior to dialysis, the nurse may check the patient's temperature and should assess the patient's access.

Care of the critically ill patient during the dialysis session requires specialized knowledge and experience. Initiation and maintenance of the dialysis session is usually the responsibility of a nurse from a dialysis unit. All hemodialysis is a controlled hypotensive state but BP management is usually even a more significant concern in the patient with ARF. Thus, the patient's BP may be measured as frequently as every 2 to 5 minutes at the start of dialysis but may be taken every 15 to 30 minutes after the patient has stabilized. The entire dialysis session will usually take between 2 and 4 hours.

At the completion of the dialysis session, the nurse determines the patient's weight, ascertains that appropriate laboratory tests have been sent, monitors the patient's BP, assesses the patient's access site, and administers any med-

ications that may have been held prior or during dialysis. Later the nurse reviews the laboratory results, paying particular attention to clotting studies and electrolyte balance.

Potential Complications

Of patients in ARF who undergo IHD 20% to 30% experience rapid shifts in plasma volume that can result in hypotension. An additional 10% to 20% of patients experience sudden changes in electrolyte concentration that may cause dysrhythmias. The dialysis nurse usually manages these problems. The nurse might manage hypotension by administering normal saline boluses, providing volume expanders such as albumin or mannitol, and/or decreasing the rate of ultrafiltration on the dialyzer. Decreasing the rate of fluid removal may help to manage dysrhythmias. These problems also can be limited and even avoided by short periods of daily dialysis for the patient in ARF. Other frequent problems with the utilization of IHD for the patient in ARF include difficulties with vascular access, problems with anticoagulation, and dialysis membrane incompatibility.

Dialysis disequilibrium syndrome may also occur. It is especially common in patients undergoing their first or second dialysis treatment who experience sudden, large decreases in their BUN. The most likely explanation for this syndrome is that the levels of urea do not drop as rapidly in the brain as the plasma because of the blood-brain barrier. The higher levels of urea in the brain result in an osmotic concentration gradient between the brain cells and the plasma. Fluid enters the brain cells by osmosis until the concentration levels equal that of the extracellular fluid, resulting in cerebral edema and the dialysis disequilibrium syndrome. Manifestations of the syndrome include:

- Headache and mental impairment that may progress to confusion, agitation, and seizures
- Nausea that may lead to vomiting

The most effective management strategy is prevention with daily hemodialysis for 1 to 2 hours.

Continuous Renal Replacement Therapy

Continuous renal replacement therapy (CRRT) is an umbrella term for several methods of dialysis that allow for continuous fluid removal from the plasma (known as ultrafiltrate). The modalities differ in the principles, accesses, technology requirements, and nursing interventions.

Indications and Expected Outcomes

CRRT was originally proposed for use with patients who were hemodynamically unstable and could not tolerate the rapid fluid shifts that occur with traditional hemodialysis. With CRRT patients can be dialyzed over a 24-hour period, resulting in a controlled removal of fluid from the plasma. Because the methods differ in whether they utilize convection and/or diffusion, they differ in their abilities to remove different types of solutes and amounts of urea. Numerous articles describe the theoretical advantages of CRRT for the patient in ARF. Yet randomized controlled studies have not demonstrated that CRRT is more likely to result in patients surviving or recovering renal function than IHD (Augustine, Seifert, & Paganni, 2004).

Technological Requirements. Although all types of CRRT remove fluid and some electrolytes and wastes through a filter, they vary in the process(es) they use to remove fluids and electrolytes, the types of access they require, the setup and technology utilized, and whether they require dialysate or replacement fluids. All forms are usually initiated and maintained by the ICU nurse rather than the dialysis nurse. A brief description of some types of CCRT follows.

Slow Continuous Ultrafiltration. Slow continuous ultrafiltration (SCUF) uses ultrafiltration alone to remove 100 to 300 mL of fluid hourly from the patient. It has little ability to remove urea and other midsized molecules so its usefulness for patients in ARF is limited. SCUF utilizes both arterial and venous accesses and therefore does not require a pump but does require a MAP greater than 70. It does not require dialysate or replacement fluid.

Continuous Venovenous Hemofiltration. Continuous venovenous hemofiltration (CVVH) uses convection with replacement fluid flowing through the filter at a fast rate (1,000 to 2,000 mL/hr), creating a "solute drag" that removes fluids and small to midsized molecules. This results in removal of significant amounts of fluid (7 to 30 L/24 hr) and adequate amounts of urea and other midsized molecules. It utilizes venous accesses only and requires a pump as well as replacement fluid.

Continuous Venovenous Hemodialysis. Continuous venovenous hemodialysis (CVVHD) is a continuous process of slow dialysis that works by diffusion. However, because it removes mostly small molecules, its usefulness is somewhat limited. It requires dialysate fluid but does not require replacement fluid.

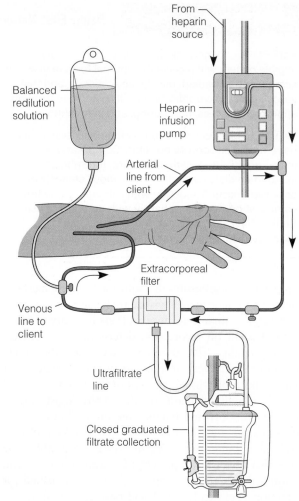

Figure 14-12 Continuous venovenous hemodiafiltration circuit (CAVH).

Continuous Venovenous Hemodiafiltration. Continuous venovenous hemodiafiltration (CVVHDF) is the most popular and efficient mode of CRRT because it is able to remove small and midsized particles and clear urea quickly. It uses both convection and diffusion simultaneously to remove fluids and solutes. It utilizes venous accesses only and requires a pump, dialysate fluid, and replacement fluid. Figure 14-12 displays a CVVHDF circuit.

Nursing Management

Prior to the start of any form of CRRT, the nurse assesses the patient's volume status and discusses initiation of the therapy with the patient and/or health care proxy as she or he would prior to hemodialysis. The nurse then clarifies with the nephrologist the fluid balance goal. Lab studies, including electrolytes, BUN, creatinine, glucose, and activated clotting times or partial thromboplastin time (PTT), are drawn before the procedure is started. The ICU nurse is responsible for priming all lines in the circuit and expelling all air. Sterile technique should be maintained throughout the connection procedure and any time that the circuit is entered (Astle, 2005).

During the process, the nurse:

- Monitors the patient's vital signs and hemodynamic and fluid balance status every half hour.

- Assesses the ultrafiltration rate hourly and administers replacement fluid (if required by the CRRT method). The amount of replacement fluid administered each hour is determined by the hourly fluid balance goal set by the nephrologist. The hourly goal for fluid removal is added to all sources of fluid input in the previous hour. That sum is then subtracted from the sum of all sources of fluid output. The result is the amount of replacement fluid that needs to be provided in the subsequent hour. The type and composition of replacement fluid are prescribed by the physician and determined by the patient's electrolyte and acid-base status. Lab studies to monitor the patient's electrolyte status, BUN, and creatinine are checked at least twice a day but often every 4 to 6 hours.

- Maintains the patency of the system by ensuring adequate blood flow rates, maintaining any heparin infusion, reviewing PTT and clotting studies, and assessing the hemofilter for clotting. PTT and clotting studies may be checked as often as every 1 to 2 hours (Dirkes & Hedge, 2007).

Potential Complications

Frequent complications include hypotension, hypothermia, electrolyte imbalances, coagulation abnormalities or bleeding, and sepsis. Transient hypotension is not uncommon when CRRT is initiated. If this occurs, the nurse might assess the patient for blood loss, decrease the rate of ultrafiltration temporarily then gradually increase it again, increase vasopressor support, and/or notify the physician. The patient may develop hypothermia and experience chills. This may be prevented or alleviated by a warmer on the blood return line to the patient or a warming blanket. Monitoring lab studies every 4 to 6 hours will help to prevent electrolyte imbalances and coagulation abnormalities or bleeding. Keeping all connections securely tightened and all lines visible at all times will help to limit bleeding. Sepsis is the primary cause of death for patients in ARF; to assist in preventing it, all access dressings should be done aseptically and all CRRT lines should be cared for meticulously.

Peritoneal Dialysis

Peritoneal dialysis (PD) uses osmosis and diffusion to produce a steady, gradual restoration of fluid, electrolyte, and acid-base balance while removing nitrogenous and other wastes.

Indications and Expected Outcomes

The gradual restoration of fluid volume and electrolyte balance that results from PD can be an advantage

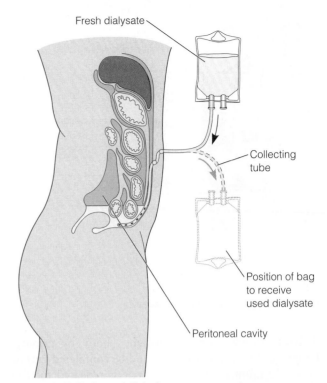

Figure 14-13 Peritoneal dialysis.

because the patients are less likely to experience hypotension, dysrhythmias, or electrolyte imbalances than with hemodialysis (Figure 14-13). However, PD is rarely used in ARF because there are a variety of disadvantages. First, PD is often not speedy or efficient enough to adequately remove the midsized wastes such as urea, which accumulate rapidly in catabolic ARF patients. Second, the volume of fluid that is placed in the peritoneum in PD tends to have a negative impact on respiratory function. Lastly, several studies have demonstrated poorer outcomes for patients who received PD rather than other modalities of treatment for ARF (Daugirdas, 2002).

Technological Requirements. PD may be managed manually or by an automated PD system (cycler). In either case, there are three steps to the process and the critical care nurse is usually responsible for the functioning of the system.

During inflow a specific amount of sterile, body temperature solution (dialysate) is allowed to infuse into the peritoneum over approximately 5 to 10 minutes. After completion of inflow, the dialysis tubing is clamped.

During the dwell stage, the second step in the process, the dialysate dwells in the peritoneum. Diffusion and osmosis occur between the blood and the dialysate across the peritoneal membrane. The duration of the dwell time is determined by the type of PD and prescribed by the nephrologist. In manual or continuously cycling PD the dwell time is often 30 to 40 minutes.

At the completion of the dwell time, either the inflow tubing or tubing leading to a collection system is placed below the patient's body and unclamped so the

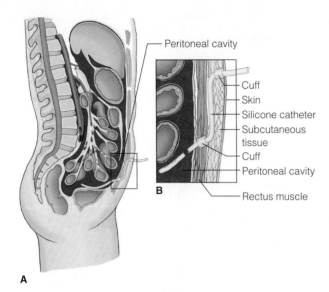

Peritoneal cavity

Cuff
Skin
Silicone catheter
Subcutaneous tissue
Cuff
Peritoneal cavity
Rectus muscle

A
B

Figure 14-14 Peritoneal dialysis access.

dialysate drains from the patient's body by gravity. Drainage should occur rapidly and be completed within about 20 minutes. The entire cycle is repeated for the amount of time or the total number of cycles prescribed by the nephrologist with new dialysate for each cycle. At the completion of the series of dialysis cycles, the patient may be left either with an empty peritoneum or with dialysate dwelling in the peritoneum.

Access. Access to the peritoneum is by tunneled catheter (Figure 14-14). The catheter has several sections, the first outside the body, the next located in the subcutaneous layer and having at least one dacron cuff or flanged collar to anchor the catheter, and a section in the peritoneal cavity with multiple lumens for rapid delivery of fluid. The nurse maintains aseptic technique when caring for the catheter and assesses the access site at least daily. Infections of both the access site and the tunneled catheter may develop. Indications of these infections include redness, swelling, and exudates at the catheter site or along the tunneled tract. If exudates or leakage occurs at the access site, by testing for the presence of glucose, the nurse can determine if the leaking fluid contains dialysate. If the fluid contains dialysate, it will test positive for glucose.

Nursing Management

Prior to the onset of PD, the nurse assesses the patient's volume status as she or he would if the patient were receiving hemodialysis. The nurse also pays specific attention to the patient's temperature and laboratory studies to detect infection or severe electrolyte imbalances. The nurse identifies whether the patient should begin the dialysis process with the inflow step, or whether the patient has had dialysate dwelling in his or her peritoneum and should begin with the drain step.

The nurse is responsible for setting up the PD system, whether it is a manual system or a cycler. First the nurse selects the appropriate concentration of dialysate solution. The nephrologist will have prescribed the concentration of glucose in the dialysate (1.5, 2.5, or 4.5%) based on the amount of fluid to be removed. The nephrologist may also prescribe additives such as antibiotics, potassium, insulin, or heparin for the dialysate, and the nurse ensures that they are present in the appropriate amounts. The dialysate must be warmed to body temperature. If the procedure is being performed manually this is usually done before the dialysate bag is spiked. It should be warmed by an approved device and not in a microwave or ever in a water bath. The connections are then made. At each step in the process, the nurse must ensure that all connections (between dialysate bags, tubings, and patient) are done aseptically according to agency policy.

After the connections are made, PD can begin. If a cycler is being used, it will warm the dialysate prior to inflow and ensure that the inflow, dwell, and drain times are maintained for the entire time of the dialysis. If manual dialysis is occurring, the nurse must time each of the stages and monitor the process. At the completion of each dwell time, the dialysate return must be either measured (by the nurse) or weighed (by the machine) to determine the amount of return. If the dialysate return is less than the amount of dialysate infused, there may be an obstruction. This may be resolved by examining the tubing for a kink or helping the patient change position. If the catheter is starting to clot off, heparin may need to be added to the dialysate.

The nurse also inspects the dialysate return. It should be clear enough to read newspaper print through. Cloudy dialysate is suggestive of infection and should be reported immediately to the nephrologist or dialysis center.

After completion of the entire series of cycles, the tubing should be disconnected aseptically, the patient's access capped, the access site covered with a sterile dressing, and the patient weighed.

Potential Complications

The most significant risk to the patient with PD is the development of peritonitis. It is usually caused by contamination of the system and that is why it is essential that aseptic technique be maintained consistently. The nurse continually observes the patient for signs that peritonitis may be developing. These include an elevated temperature or white blood count, malaise, cloudy dialysate return, and abdominal pain that is most pronounced on inflow. Treatment of peritonitis may involve adding an appropriate antibiotic to the dialysate fluid.

Recovery from Acute Renal Failure

When patients respond to supportive treatment and do not develop complications such as sepsis, they usually regain renal function. As renal function returns, patients enter a diuretic phase when they may fail to concentrate

VISUAL MAP Acute Renal Failure Summary

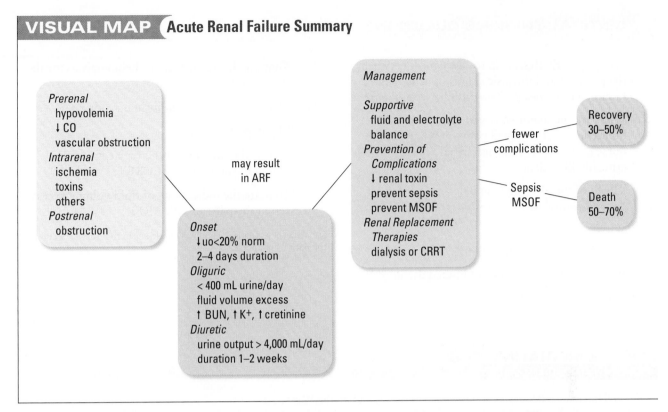

Prerenal
  hypovolemia
  ↓ CO
  vascular obstruction
Intrarenal
  ischemia
  toxins
  others
Postrenal
  obstruction

may result
in ARF

Onset
  ↓uo<20% norm
  2–4 days duration
Oliguric
  < 400 mL urine/day
  fluid volume excess
  ↑ BUN, ↑ K+, ↑ cretinine
Diuretic
  urine output > 4,000 mL/day
  duration 1–2 weeks

Management

Supportive
  fluid and electrolyte
  balance
*Prevention of
Complications*
  ↓ renal toxin
  prevent sepsis
  prevent MSOF
*Renal Replacement
  Therapies*
  dialysis or CRRT

fewer
complications

Sepsis
MSOF

Recovery
30–50%

Death
50–70%

---

urine and produce up to 5 liters of urine each day. In addition, they may not be able to adequately excrete wastes or regulate their electrolyte and acid-base balance. Their serum BUN and creatinine levels usually decrease slowly toward normal over a 10-day period. Patients may continue to need RRT during this phase until their GFR improves sufficiently to clear metabolic wastes. During this phase, the nurse needs to carefully monitor the patient's

BUN, and creatinine,

fluid volume status for a fluid volume deficit,

and serum electrolytes for hyponatremia and hypokalemia that may result from the diuresis.

The final phase of acute renal failure is the **recovery phase**. This phase typically lasts from 6 months to a year. During this phase, most patients' renal function returns to normal. Only 5% to 10% of patients who survive continue to require dialysis. However, patients are thought to be vulnerable to repeated insults to their renal function and are counseled to avoid renal toxins.

● CASE STUDY

A 42-year-old woman who had been found by her neighbor lying in her closet was admitted to the hospital with the diagnosis of ARF and weakness. On admission she was barely verbal but complaining of severe back and leg pain. Her vital signs were stable with a BP of 78/50, pulse 56, respirations 22, and temperature of 102. She was unable to state how long she had been lying in the closet but there were pressure ulcers forming on her right arm and leg. According to her medical record, she had a history of pneumonia with renal failure, hepatitis C, and bipolar disorder. On admission her labs revealed the following:

WBC 21.1, Hg 17.2, and HCT 52.7

In conjunction with her BP, what do these labs imply about her fluid status?

Her BUN was 88, creatinine 5, potassium 6, calcium 8.4, and CK 23,890.

Creatine kinase (CK) levels increase with skeletal and heart muscle breakdown; the normal for women is 26 to 140 U/L.

1. What do these lab studies reveal about her renal status?

2. Why might her CK be so elevated?

3. What are the likely factors contributing to her current renal failure?

4. What should the immediate management strategies be for her ARF?

5. Is renal replacement therapy indicated at this time? Why or why not?

See answers to Case Studies in the Answer Section at the back of the book.

CRITICAL THINKING QUESTIONS

1. Why does urinalysis help to distinguish between the prerenal and intrinsic causes of acute renal failure? How does it distinguish between them?

2. What are the major causes of intrinsic renal failure in the critically ill patient? What can the nurse do to prevent intrinsic renal failure in the critically ill patient?

3. Which of the electrolyte imbalances is the most dangerous in ARF?

   Why?

   How is it managed emergently?

4. Why is peritoneal dialysis of limited use in patients with ARF?

5. What are the advantages of hemodialysis for the patient in ARF?

6. What is dialysis disequilibrium syndrome?

   Why does it occur?

7. What is the function of the replacement fluid utilized in some forms of CRRT?

8. What are the indications of fluid volume excess seen in the patient with ARF?

See answers to Critical Thinking Questions in the Answer Section at the back of the book.

EXPLORE MEDIALINK

http://www.prenhall.com/perrin

Additional interactive resources for this chapter can be found on the Web site at http://www.prenhall.com/perrin. Click on "Chapter 14" to select activities for this chapter.

Case Study: Acute Renal Failure

Nursing Care Plan

NCLEX Review Questions

MediaLinks:
- American Kidney Foundation
- Journal of the American Medical Association Patient Page
- Kidney Dialysis Foundation

- National Kidney foundation
- Medline Plus
- The Nephron Information Center
- Virtual Dialysis
- Fistula First: National Vascular Access Improvement Initiatives

MediaLink Applications

REFERENCES

Agraharkar, M., Gupta, R., & Agraharkar, A. (2004, June 7). Acute renal failure. *eMedicine*. Retrieved March 7, 2005, from http://www.emedicine.com/med/topic1595.htm

Astle, S. M. (2005). CRRT made easy. *Program and Proceedings: AACN 2005 NTI & Critical Care Exposition*, 463–466.

Augustine, J. J., Seifert, T. H., & Paganni, E. P. (2004). A randomized, controlled trial comparing intermittent with continuous dialysis in patients with acute renal failure. *American Journal of Kidney Diseases, 44*(6), 1000–1007.

Daugirdas, J. T. (2002). Peritoneal dialysis in acute renal failure—why the bad outcome? *New England Journal of Medicine, 347*(12), 933–935.

Dirkes S., & Hodge, K. (2007). Continuous renal replacement therapy in the adult intensive care unit: History and current trends. *Critical Care Nurse, 27*(2), 61–77.

Fatica, R. A., & Dennis, V. W. (2002). Cardiovascular mortality in chronic renal failure: Hyperphosphatemia, coronary calcification, and role of phosphate binders. *Cleveland Clinic Journal of Medicine, 69*(Suppl. l3), S21–27.

Friedrich, J. O., Adhikak, N., Herridge, M. S., & Beyene, J. (2005). Meta-analysis: Low dose dopamine increases urine output but does not prevent death. *Annals of Internal Medicine, 144*, 510–521.

Ievins, F. A. (2004). Post-traumatic acute renal failure: Its pathophysiologic basis and treatment. *Trauma, 6*, 111–120.

Mehta, R. L., McDonald, B., & Gabbai, F. (2002). Nephrology consult in acute renal failure: Does timing matter? *American Journal of Medicine, 113*, 456–461.

Mehta, R. L., Pascaul, M. T., Soroko, S., & Charlow, G. M. (2002). Diuretics, mortality, and nonrecovery of renal function in acute renal failure. *Journal of the American Medical Association, 288*(20), 2547–2553.

Schiffl, H., Lang, S., & Fischer, R. (2002). Daily hemodialysis and the outcome of acute renal failure. *New England Journal of Medicine, 346*(5), 305–310.

Schroeder, T. H., Hansen, M., Dinkalaker, K., Krueger, W. A., Nohe, B., Fretscher, R., et al. (2004). Influence of underlying disease on outcome of critically ill patients with acute renal failure. *European Journal of Aneasthesiology, 21*(11), 848–854.

Care of the Organ Donor and Transplant Recipient

Kathleen Perrin, PhD, RN, CCRN

Learning Outcomes

Upon completion of this chapter, the learner will be able to:

1. Describe the criteria used to evaluate living organ donors.

2. Explain the evaluation of a deceased individual for organ donation, including the determination of brain death.

3. Describe collaborative management of the deceased organ donor awaiting organ recovery.

4. Compare and contrast eligibility criteria and evaluation of candidates for kidney, liver, and heart transplants.

5. Explain the role of immunosuppressants in the prevention and management of rejection.

6. Compare and contrast how acute rejection is manifested and detected in patients receiving kidney, liver, or heart transplants.

7. Discuss prevention and management of infection in transplant recipients.

8. Compare and contrast the postoperative collaborative management of patients who have received a transplanted kidney, liver, or heart.

Abbreviations

DGF	Delayed Graft Function
MELD	Model for End-Stage Liver Disease
OPO	Organ Procurement Organization
UNOS	United Network for Organ Sharing

The demand for donated organs in the United States has far outstripped the supply of available organs. This is largely because the patient who receives a donated organ, such as a kidney, usually lives a longer life with better quality at less cost to the health care system. However, to achieve these results, the organ donor and transplant recipient require expert health care. Nurses provide skilled care to patients in all stages of organ donation, from identifying and caring for potential donors to providing information to patients and families making a decision about donation or transplant to caring for the organ recipient.

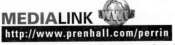

MEDIALINK
http://www.prenhall.com/perrin

See the Companion Website for chapter-specific resources at www.prenhall.com/perrin.

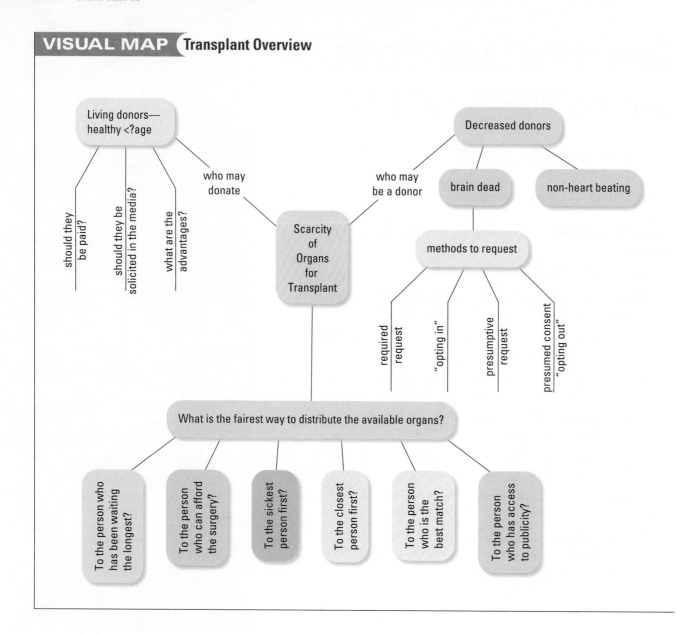

VISUAL MAP Transplant Overview

Living donors—healthy <?age

should they be paid?

should they be solicited in the media?

what are the advantages?

who may donate

Scarcity of Organs for Transplant

who may be a donor

Decreased donors

brain dead

non-heart beating

methods to request

required request

"opting in"

presumptive request

presumed consent "opting out"

What is the fairest way to distribute the available organs?

To the person who has been waiting the longest?

To the person who can afford the surgery?

To the sickest person first?

To the closest person first?

To the person who is the best match?

To the person who has access to publicity?

Anatomy and Physiology Review: Review of Basic Immunology

When the body detects the presence of a foreign substance, the immune system responds in the two overlapping ways that are displayed in Figure 15-1.

Cell-mediated immune response results in the stimulation of T-lymphocyte activity. T lymphocytes recognize foreign antigens then bind to them and produce sensitized clones of the T lymphocyte. These sensitized T lymphocytes migrate throughout the body to locate the antigen, bind with it, and release chemicals that result in lysis of the foreign cells. Cell-mediated responses are usually triggered by antigens such as viral infected cells, cancer cells, and foreign tissue.

Antibody-mediated (humoral) immune response results in the stimulation of B-lymphocyte activity. The B lymphocyte differentiates into a plasma cell that produces antigen-specific antibodies that bind to the antigen

and inactivate it. This initial response is followed by inflammation and phagocytosis. Antibody-mediated responses are usually triggered by bacteria, bacterial toxins, and some viruses. However, a potential organ recipient may have developed antihuman antibodies from a previous blood transfusion, an organ transplant, or during pregnancy.

Antigens are substances that are recognized by the body as foreign or nonself. HLA antigens found on Chromosome 6 help the immune system determine what tissue is foreign and what is self. **Tissue typing** is used to determine how much overlap exists between a potential donor's and the recipient's HLA antigens. Although there may be overlap in HLA antigens between siblings, and parents should each be half similar to their children, complete matches occur only with identical siblings.

A recipient may have antihuman antibodies in his blood that would react with the tissue of a potential donor. The potential recipient cannot receive a transplant from that donor because the antibodies would immediately

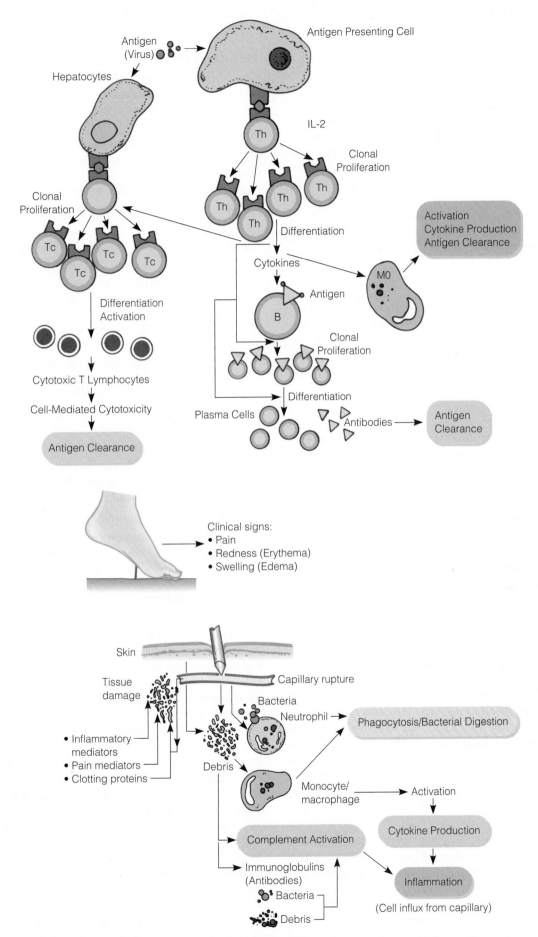

Figure 15-1 Overview of cell and antibody mediated immune response.
(Reprinted with permission from Organ Transplant http://www.medscape.com/viewarticle/436533 © 2002, Medscape)

attack and damage the organ. Called hyperacute rejection, this type of rejection usually results in loss of the transplanted organ.

ABO typing identifies the blood group of a donor and recipient. Unmatched blood or organs that are transplanted across ABO compatibility will cause an immediate immune response. Type AB is considered to be a universal recipient because the person can receive blood or organs from any ABO group. Type O is a universal donor because any other group can accept the blood or organ. However, a person with type O can only receive blood or an organ from another person with type O. Types A and B may receive blood or organs from their own blood group or type O.

Donors

There is a severe shortage of organ donors in the United States. In 2006, there were approximately 95,000 people awaiting organs but only about 15,000 donors (United Network for Organ Sharing [UNOS], 2007). Approximately half of these donors were living individuals and half were deceased donors.

Living Donors

According to the UNOS, living donors accounted for 6,721 of the 14,743 donors in 2006. Most of these living donors donated kidneys, although some donated a portion of their liver or lung.

Receiving an organ from a living donor provides a number of benefits for the recipient. First, living donation decreases the risk of organ **rejection** for the recipient. Because the operation can be scheduled in advance rather than as an emergency, the recipient may begin taking immunosuppressant drugs a day or two before the operation and the organ is less likely to be rejected. Also, when there is a better tissue match between the donor and the recipient, as is often the case in living donation, the recipient is less likely to experience an episode of rejection. In addition, the recipient does not have to be placed on the waiting list and wait for a match. The waiting period for an organ may be several years during which time the recipient's health often declines. However, according to UNOS (2007), "the most important aspect of living donation is the psychological benefit." The recipient often experiences positive feelings knowing that the gift came from a loved one or a caring stranger, and the donor often has the satisfaction of having benefited another human being.

Qualifying as a Living Donor

UNOS (2007) states that the potential kidney donor must be physically fit; in good general health; and free from high blood pressure, diabetes, cancer, kidney disease, heart disease, and a variety of infectious diseases including the human immunodeficiency virus (HIV) and tuberculosis. Individuals considered for living donation are usually between 18 and 60 years of age. Gender and race are not factors in determining a successful match.

Testing to Determine Eligibility for Donation

First, the potential donor's blood type is identified and compared to the recipient's to determine if they are compatible and a donation is possible. If the donor and recipient have compatible blood types, the donor undergoes a medical history review and a complete physical examination. According to UNOS (2007) and Sommerer, Wiesel, Schweitzer-Rothers, Ritz, and Zeier (2003), the following additional tests may be performed:

- *Tissue typing:* The donor's blood is drawn for HLA typing.
- *Crossmatching:* A "crossmatch" is done just before every transplant to prevent hyperacute rejection. In a crossmatch, the lymphocytes of the donor are mixed with the serum of the recipient. If the recipient has antibodies to the white cells of the donor, the cells are destroyed. This is called a "positive" crossmatch and means that the transplant is contraindicated. If there is no reaction between the blood of the donor and the blood of the recipient (called a "negative" crossmatch), then the transplant may proceed.
- *Renal function:* Serum creatinine, urea, electrolytes, urinary sediment, albuminuria, 24-hour proteinuria, creatinine clearance, and glycosuria are evaluated.
- *Renal structure:* This set of tests includes a renal ultrasound and angiogram, allowing visualization of the blood vessels of the organ to be donated.
- 24-hour ambulatory monitoring of blood pressure.
- *Psychiatric and/or psychological evaluation:* The donor and the recipient may undergo a psychiatric and/or psychological evaluation.

The Ethical Issues

Ethical questions arise when a healthy individual is asked to undergo a surgical procedure that removes a body organ solely for the benefit of another. Most agree that such a procedure is ethically acceptable when the patient provides fully informed consent. Informed consent means the living donor must be made aware of the physical and psychological risks before he consents to donate even though the risks are slim. The risk of death is low for kidney and liver donation (0.04%) and the short-term risks, primarily postoperative infections, are uncommon (Steinberg, 2004). If the donor has any concerns preoperatively, he should be encouraged to discuss them with a transplant professional and/or social worker.

Another important element of informed consent is that the donor has made the decision to donate voluntarily and has been offered opportunities to change his mind throughout the process. If the donor does change his mind during the process, the donor's decision and reasons should be kept confidential. This is especially important because "living donors may feel pressured by their families into donating an organ and guilty if they are reluctant to go through with the procedure" (UNOS, 2007).

World Health Organization: Global Knowledge Base on Transplantation (GKT-3)

PURPOSE: To ensure that transplant centers worldwide address their responsibilities to living organ donors

RATIONALE: Because it has demonstrated both cost-effectiveness and enhanced quality of life for recipients, kidney transplantation is by far the most frequently carried out transplantation globally. Although kidney donation by well-selected living donors with good health coverage carries negligible risks, this level of care is not always available worldwide. According to the World Health Organization (WHO), "The welfare of the live kidney donor is largely neglected in schemes where disadvantaged individuals are exploited and encouraged to sell their kidneys. Resolution *WHA57.18.* (2004) acknowledges the risk of exploitation of live kidney donors and urges Member States to protect the poorest and vulnerable groups from transplant tourism and the sale of tissue and organs."

HIGHLIGHTS OF RECOMMENDATIONS:
Therefore, GKT-3 was established to:

Track and report adverse events and reactions incurred by recipients and living donors to enable appropriate decisions on safety measures to be taken.

Provide vigilance, surveillance, and the rapid dissemination of information about the transmission of infectious agents by cell, tissue, and organ transplantation.

Establish links to vigilance and surveillance systems set up by developed countries so that a single portal is available for information on transplant safety.

Source: World Health Organization

 Available: http://www.who.int/transplantation/organ/en/http:// www.who.int/transplantation/gkt/vigilance/en/index.html

Postdonation Care Requirements of Living Donors

Care of the donor following the most common living donor procedure, kidney donation, is discussed because procedures are different and more complex for donation of other organs. In the past, the surgery for living kidney donation was open nephrectomy. This procedure is performed less frequently now because the donor is more likely to experience pain and have a more extensive recovery period.

One of the major concerns for the donor following open nephrectomy is pain. Postoperative nephrectomy pain is usually managed with epidural analgesia. However, even with pain relief, because of the location of the surgery, the donor may splint and limit respiratory effort to diminish her pain. Therefore, the nurse must ensure adequate pain control; routinely assess the donor's pain level; and instruct her to turn, cough, and breathe deeply. Movement is also essential and several hours after the operation, the donor is encouraged to get out of bed and walk around. The donor may remain hospitalized for 4 to 8 days before returning home. Postoperative restrictions include no heavy lifting or rough contact sports until at least 6 weeks after the operation with return to work 4 weeks after surgery.

In recent years, laparoscopy has been used more frequently to recover kidneys from living donors because it involves a smaller incision, less pain, better cosmetic results, and a shorter recovery time. Although donors having laparoscopic surgery recover much more quickly and are usually discharged from the hospital in 1 or 2 days, they indicate they still experience problems with pain and wish they had ongoing contact with a nurse for assistance with post-op care (Rudlow, Charlton, Sanchez, & Chang, 2005). These donors are usually out of work for about a week and need almost 3 months to "feel like themselves again" (Rudlow et al., 2005). In the long term, donors report a positive effect on their lives but state that they continue to experience physical limitations, primarily fatigue and discomfort, at the surgical site.

The majority of donors are satisfied with their decision to donate with only 4% to 10% of living kidney donors regretting they had agreed to donate. Donors are more likely to regret their decision if the recipient encountered problems with poor kidney function and/or an episode of rejection (Rudlow et al., 2005). Regret may also occur when the donation precipitated conflict within the family. Additionally, approximately 5% of donors experience depression, anxiety attacks, or suicidal tendencies after transplantation.

Deceased Donors

Although deceased donors account for only slightly more than half of the total number of organ donors, in 2006 they accounted for more than 75% of the total number of organs recovered. This is because when deceased donors are managed intensively, multiple organs may be transplanted from a single donor. Eligible donors should have been in good health previously and are usually less than 70 years of age. However, age is a relative contraindication and people older than 80 have been organ donors. Absolute contraindications to donation include:

- Uncontrolled sepsis
- Active viral infections (e.g., hepatitis B or C and cytomegalovirus [CMV])
- HIV positive serology
- Any malignancy except a primary intracranial tumor

There are two types of donation from deceased donors: donation after pronouncement of brain death (death by neurological criteria) and donation after cardiac death.

Imminent Death

Since 1998, all acute care hospitals have been required to have a definition of imminent death. In addition, they are required to notify the appropriate Organ Procurement Organization (OPO) of any patient who meets that definition. Guidelines developed by the Center for Medicare and Medicaid Services suggest that the definition of impending death include the following:

- A patient who has had a severe acute brain injury who requires mechanical ventilation and is in an intensive care unit (ICU) or emergency department and
- Has clinical findings on a Glasgow Coma Scale below a threshold established by the agency (e.g., 5) or
- Has had withdrawal of life-sustaining treatment ordered by a physician and a decision is being made by the family or
- Is being evaluated for the diagnosis of brain death (Ehrle, 2006)

Criteria for Brain Death or Death by Neurological Criteria

Brain death is defined by the American Academy of Neurology as the irreversible loss of function of the brain, including the brainstem. Common causes of brain death include severe head trauma, rupture of a cerebral aneurysm, hypoxic-ischemic brain insults, and fulminate hepatic failure. (See Visual Map on page 389.) The criteria for the clinical diagnosis of brain death were established by the American Academy of Neurology in 1994. Subsequent testing and medical opinion have determined that they continue to be valid determinants of brain death in adult patients (Flowers & Patel, 2000; Wijdicks, 2001) when the following conditions are met:

- Evidence of an acute neurological catastrophe that is compatible with the clinical diagnosis of brain death. A computed tomography (CT) scan is often essential for determining the cause of brain death.
- Exclusion of complicating medical conditions that may confound clinical assessment (no severe electrolyte, acid-base, or endocrine disturbance).
- Absence of drug intoxication or poisoning. Screens should be done as appropriate for alcohol, barbiturates, sedatives, and antiepileptic drugs that may affect findings on neurological examination.
- Core temperature 32°C (90°F). Hypothermia suppresses neurological activity. Pupillary response to light is lost at core temperatures of 28°C to 32°C

and brainstem reflexes disappear with core temperatures of less that 28°C. Therefore, the nurse may use thermal blankets and warm inspired air and/or intravenous solutions to treat hypothermia (Henneman & Karras, 2004). A core temperature of greater than 36.5°C (97°F) is required before apnea testing is conducted.

- Normotension (systolic blood pressure [BP] greater than or equal to 90 mm Hg) or euvolemia hypotension may suppress neurological activity and hence preclude the diagnosis of brain death. Hypotension should be corrected with appropriate therapy (usually fluid administration and vasopressors) before the apnea test is conducted.

Three Cardinal Findings in Brain Death

The three cardinal findings in brain death are coma or unresponsiveness, absence of brainstem reflexes, and apnea.

Coma. The first cardinal finding, coma or unresponsiveness, is demonstrated by the absence of cerebral motor response in all extremities in response to noxious stimuli.

- There should be no spontaneous movement, no response to painful stimuli, and no decorticate or decerebrate posturing at any time in a brain dead person.
- Spinal or deep tendon reflexes persist in approximately 13% of patients (Dosemeci, Cengiz, Yilmaz, & Razamoglu, 2004) and may coincide with the diagnosis of brain death because they do not require brain innervation to occur (Henneman & Karras, 2004). These reflexes may be generated by forceful flexion of the neck, body rotation, and respiratory acidosis. They include obvious reflexes like the Babinski or knee jerk but may also include flexion at the waist and arm raising. It is often the role of the critical care nurse to explain the persistence of these movements to a distressed or perplexed family.

Absence of Brainstem Reflexes. The second cardinal finding, absence of brainstem reflexes, is demonstrated by the following:

No pupillary response to light:
- Pupillary reflexes should be assessed in a semi-dark room. A bright light is shone first into one then the other eye. Pupil size is assessed in both eyes each time. Any response to light by either pupil excludes the diagnosis of brain death. Most commonly pupils in brain dead patients are midposition and midsize (4 to 6 mm), but they may be dilated. Nonreactive round, oval, and irregularly shaped pupils are also compatible with brain death.

VISUAL MAP Brain Death

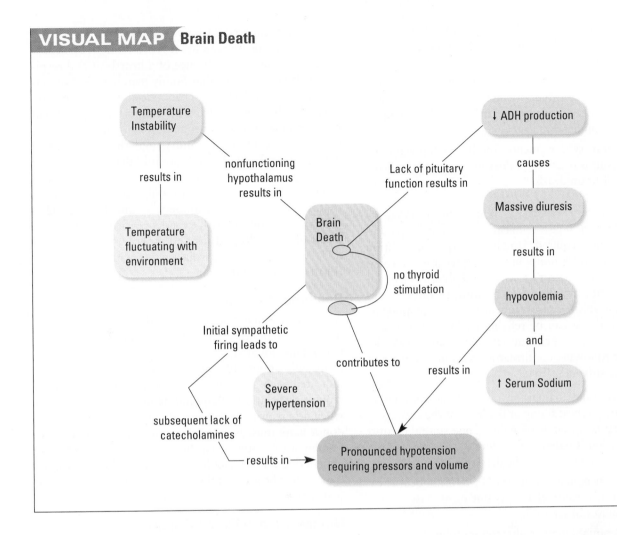

No ocular movement with either the oculo-cephalic or oculovestibular response:

- Oculocephalic reflex testing (doll's eyes testing) is performed only when there is no fracture or instability of the cervical spine. The patient's head is turned to one side and the eyes are examined for movement. Any movement of the eyes indicates that some pathways are intact.
- For oculovestibular testing, the ears must be free of significant wax or clotted blood, which may diminish the response to cold stimulation. The eardrums should be evaluated to determine that they are not perforated. When brain death is present, no deviation of the eyes occurs when either ear is irrigated with 50 mL of lukewarm or cold water. A neurologist normally performs this test and any movement of the eyes indicates that some brain pathways are intact.

Absence of facial sensation and facial motor response as evidenced by the following:

- No corneal reflex to touch with a cotton swab
- No jaw reflex
- No grimacing to noxious stimuli

Absence of pharyngeal and tracheal reflexes:

- No response after stimulation of the posterior pharynx with a tongue blade (Because this may not be adequate stimulus to cough for some patients, suctioning is recommended.)
- No cough response to bronchial suctioning

Apnea. The third cardinal finding, apnea, is demonstrated by apnea testing. Apnea testing must be performed according to specific parameters. As noted previously, the patient should be normotensive and normothermic. In addition the patient should have a normal pCO_2 and a normal pO_2. The patient may be preoxygenated to obtain an arterial PO_2 greater than or equal to 200 mm Hg. The steps in the process according to the American Academy of Neurologists are the following:

- Connect a pulse oximeter and disconnect the ventilator.
- Deliver 100% O_2, 6 L/min, into the trachea. Or place a cannula at the level of the carina.
- Look closely for respiratory movements (abdominal or chest excursions that produce adequate tidal volumes).

- Measure arterial PO$_2$, PCO$_2$, and pH after approximately 8 minutes and reconnect the ventilator.
- If respiratory movements are absent and arterial PCO$_2$ is greater than or equal to 60 mm Hg, the apnea test result is positive; it supports the diagnosis of brain death.
- If respiratory movements are observed, the apnea test result is negative; it does not support the diagnosis of brain death.

Confirmatory Testing. Brain death is a diagnosis for which a repeat clinical evaluation is recommended but not required. Usually the repeat evaluation is performed after 6 hours but this interval is arbitrary. In addition, confirmatory tests are often performed. Although it is not mandatory to perform a confirmatory test, it is desirable because frequently not all components of the clinical test can be reliably performed or evaluated. The American Academy of Neurology (1995) described the following confirmatory tests in the order of the most sensitive test first:

A. Conventional angiography. In brain death, there is no intracerebral filling at the level of the carotid bifurcation or circle of Willis. The external carotid circulation is patent, and filling of the superior longitudinal sinus may be delayed.

B. Electroencephalography (EEG). In brain death there is no electrical activity during at least 30 minutes of recording.

C. Transcranial Doppler ultrasonography.

D. Technetium-99m hexamethylpropyleneamineoxime brain scan. In brain death there is no uptake of isotope in brain parenchyma ("hollow skull phenomenon").

E. Somatosensory evoked potentials.

The EEG is the most commonly used confirmatory test. It is considered to be somewhat unreliable because it assesses only cerebral, not brainstem, function. Additionally, because it is usually performed at the bedside, monitors, infusion pumps, and ventilators may produce artifacts.

Approaches to Obtaining Family Consent for Transplantation of Organs

In the majority of cases, the potential donor has not signed a donor card or indicated intent to donate prior to death. In these cases, the consent of a family member or person with durable power of attorney is obtained before donation.

Declaration of Death First

Before the potential organ donor's family is approached about donation, they should have been informed about and should understand that their family member has died. Death is death whether it is pronounced by neurological criteria or the absence of a heartbeat and respiration. It is important that family members realize that once the patient has been pronounced dead, the person will either be removed from life support or support will be maintained only long enough for organ donation. It may help the family to understand that their family member is truly dead if they are told that even with the ventilator breathing for him, a person who has been pronounced brain dead can only maintain a heart rhythm for a very limited amount of time. In fact, "62% of brain dead donors will experience cardiac arrest as a result of physiological instability within 24 hours and 87% will experience cardiac arrest within 72 hours" (Ehrle, 2006, p. 90).

Required Request

An individual may "opt in" to the donor system by signing an organ donor card, stating that she desires to have her organs donated, if it is possible, after she dies. Because only about 20% of the American population has indicated such a preference, Congress enacted required request legislation. **Required request** stipulates that when a person is imminently dying, the regional organ donor bank must be notified so the organ bank can determine if the patient qualifies as an organ donor. If the patient does qualify but has not signed a donor card, the family must be asked if they are willing to donate the patient's organs.

Nurses' Role in Organ Donations

Within the current system, nurses have a significant role in enhancing donations. Nurses are often the health care providers most intimately involved with the bereaved family. The amount of trust that is established between the family and the health care team during the period just preceding the patient's death is a factor in which families decide to donate organs. Rodrigue, Cornell, and Howard (2006) state that an adequate understanding of brain death is essential for obtaining consent for donation. They found that nearly 20% of families of potential donors believed that it was possible to recover from brain death and 24% believed it was comparable to a coma. The nurse may be the person who repeatedly says to the family that even though the person may still have a heartbeat, he is really dead.

When and how the family is approached about organ donation also affects whether they will donate. Families are more likely to donate organs if:

- They are **not** asked to donate at the same time that they are informed their family member has died
- They perceive that the timing of the request is optimal
- They view the requestor as sensitive to their needs

- They are approached in a quiet, private place where they can consider their options
- An organ procurement specialist from an organ donor bank makes the request

These simple interventions can increase the percentage of families who decide to donate by as much as 20% (Randhawa, 1998; Rodrigue et al., 2006).

Normally, between 30% and 50% of families asked to donate organs refuse. Some of the reasons are lack of time and private space as described previously, but in the absence of a donor card or a discussion with the patient about donation, many families believe they cannot be sure of the patient's wishes. Therefore, they refuse to donate (Rodrigue et al., 2006). Opting in, permitting people to indicate their desire to donate by obtaining a donor card, and required request, requiring health care institutions to request family members donate a dead patient's organs, have not increased the supply of these scarce resources as much as envisioned.

Presumptive Approach. Zink and Wertlieb (2006) recommend changing the request for organ donation from a value neutral to a presumptive consent approach. In this approach, the organ donor requestor approaches the family with the assumption that the family will consent to organ donation. The requestor does not present the pros and cons of donation as would occur in informed consent but focuses on the good the donation will do for the transplant recipients and the pride the donor family will experience from their family member saving multiple lives. The donor's family may be led to the donation without necessarily ever making a specific decision. For example, the statement just before consent for donation might be: "If you don't have any more questions, I will guide you through the process." This shift away from the traditional value neutral approach to a clearly pro-organ donation stance has resulted in an increase in donations by families of deceased patients of about 10% (Zink & Wertlieb).

Nursing Management

The critical care nurse is actively involved in the identification, evaluation, and provision of care to the deceased organ donor. According to Tamburri (2006), it is essential for the critical care nurse to know how to identify a potential donor, to recognize when a patient meets the agency's definition of impending death, and to notify the appropriate OPO promptly. In addition, Tamburri recommends that nurses partner with their OPO, introducing themselves to the OPO coordinators and working with them to establish protocols. She believes that nurses should serve as advocates for their patients and families by honoring the patients' last wishes, upholding the families' right to be offered the option of organ donation, and promoting compassionate communication between the health care team and the potential donors' families.

Communication between family and health care team is essential. Although it is the responsibility of the neurologist to initially offer the explanation of brain death and the certified organ requestor to approach the family about donation, it is the nurse who must reinforce the explanations and ensure the families' understanding. When families have someone with whom they can consistently communicate their concerns and ask their questions, they are more likely to donate their family members' organs.

Care of the Donor's Family

Although the bedside nurse will not be the health care professional who initially explains brain death or requests the donation from the family, there is a great deal that the critical care nurse does to influence the family's decision about donation. First, the nurse will need to be sensitive to what the family is experiencing. Does the family perceive the nurse as being harried or uncaring? Or, does the nurse have time to welcome them, spend time with them, and answer their questions? Are they hearing differing pieces of information and opinions from different health care providers? Or, have the health care providers spoken with each other and does the nurse reaffirm the information that has been given to the family? One of the major issues that family members may need to keep revisiting is: What happened? How did the patient go from being a healthy and productive person to suddenly being brain dead?

When speaking with the family, another of the specific things the nurse may need to explain or reinforce is that the time of death was when the patient was declared dead and not when the patient was taken to the operating room (OR). This reassures the family that donation was not the cause of the patient's death. The family might not understand testing for brain death, particularly apnea testing. The nurse might liken this to when a living person tries to hold his breath for as long as possible. After a minute or so, the person absolutely has to take a breath; he can't hold his breath any longer. However, the brain dead patient did not take a breath. Because he was brain dead, he had no urge to breathe. Family members can also be confused by the occurrence of spinal reflexes and may think that these represent actual patient movement. The nurse may need to explain that they are only reflexes and do not depend on the function of the brain to occur.

Families need privacy and a chance to say goodbye. They benefit from a quiet space with minimal disruption. Most families want time alone with the donor at some time. Some stay in the hospital and say goodbye just before the patient is transported to the OR for organ retrieval. Many ask for some private time to say goodbye after the patient has been declared brain dead and they have signed the consent form for donation. After that, they may leave the hospital, perhaps hours before organ retrieval is scheduled in the OR.

Collaborative Management

The nursing and medical care of the deceased individual awaiting organ recovery is extensive. To maximize the number and viability of transplanted organs, a representative of the OPO is usually responsible for completing the evaluation and managing the care of the prospective donor. The nurse may need to reassure the family that the organ procurement organization and not the family assumes the financial cost of the evaluation and management.

Because nursing care of the deceased donor is complex and time consuming, O'Connor, Wood, and Lord (2006) suggest the nurse recognize that she is providing care not to just a single patient (the donor) but to multiple patients (the recipients). By providing optimal, intensive care to the donor, the nurse is investing in better outcomes for many other patients. During this time, the nurse's focus is on attaining the goals of hemodynamic stability and body homeostasis until the organs are retrieved (Shah & Bhosale, 2006).

Achieving these goals requires intensive care because brain death is a catastrophic event associated with disruption in autonomic and other basic organ functions. Shortly before herniation, a massive sympathetic outflow occurs in response to cerebral ischemia. The donor's BP rises dramatically in an attempt to maintain cerebral perfusion, resulting in an increase in afterload, possible cardiac ischemia, and decreased cardiac output. A neurogenic pulmonary edema may also develop. Concurrently, ischemia and dysfunction of the hypothalamus and pituitary gland result in temperature and endocrine instability. After herniation occurs there is a profound reduction in sympathetic activity, resulting in pronounced vasodilation and a sudden drop in BP.

Management of Hemodynamic Instability

Hypotension develops in over 90% of organ donors (Shah & Bhosale, 2006) and nearly always requires vasoactive medications for management (Salim, 2006). It may be due to the reduction in sympathetic tone described previously, or it may result from hypovolemia, decreased cardiac output due to left heart failure, and/or endocrine instability. According to O'Connor et al. (2006), the goal of therapy is to maintain patient stability as evidenced by:

- Mean arterial pressure (MAP) greater than or equal to 60
- Urine output greater than or equal to 1 mL/kg/hr
- Ejection fraction greater than or equal to 45%
- Vasoactive drug requirement at a minimum (usually dopamine less than 10 mcg/kg/min)

Because hypovolemia occurs frequently in the organ donor, invasive monitoring techniques are often used to guide fluid administration. Central venous pressures (CVPs) may not accurately reflect actual pulmonary artery (PA) pressures in brain dead patients. Therefore, if the patient is unstable, or the ejection fraction is less than 45%, PA lines are usually inserted and wedge pressures (pulmonary capillary wedge pressure [PCWP]) are used to guide therapy. Depending on the patient's serum sodium level, sufficient volumes of either lactated Ringer's or normal saline may be administered to achieve a CVP of 6 to 8 or a PCWP of 8 to 12.

If the donor continues to experience hemodynamic instability despite volume replacement and appropriate vasoactive medications, therapy with thyroid hormone (T_4), corticosteroids, and vasopressin may be instituted. Although there is inconsistent support in the literature for the use of thyroid hormone, many providers believe T_4 is essential in stabilizing the hemodynamically unstable donor and some are evaluating using it for all donors, believing it decreases the need for vasopressors and allows more organs to be transplanted (Salim, 2006).

Management of Diabetes Insipidus

One of the reasons for hypovolemia in organ donors is **diabetes insipidus (DI)**. DI develops in 40% to 70% of deceased donors due to insufficient levels of antidiuretic hormone (ADH) and results in the production of large volumes of dilute urine. Typical findings for a patient with DI include:

- Urine output greater than or equal to 300 mL/hr
- Urine specific gravity less than or equal to 1.010
- Serum sodium greater than or equal to 150
- Absent urine glucose

If the donor is producing about 200 mL/hr of urine then the nurse usually measures the hourly urine output and replaces that volume in the subsequent hour with an equivalent amount of D_5W or D5½ NS. Once the donor's urine output exceeds 300 mL/hr then either desmopressin or vasopressin is also usually administered.

COMMONLY USED MEDICATIONS

VASOPRESSIN (PITRESSIN)

INTRODUCTION

Vasopressin (Pitressin) is an antidiuretic hormone used to treat DI caused by a deficiency of endogenous vasopressin. Its effectiveness should be identifiable within minutes as shown by a decrease in urine output and an increase in urine specific gravity. Due to its vasoconstrictive effects, it may also stabilize the donor's BP and is the form of the drug of choice when the patient is hypotensive. The alternative to treatment with vasopressin is administration of desmopressin (DDAVP) 2 to 4 mcg nasally every 4 to 6 hours.

Nursing Responsibilities:
- Administering vasopressin by IV infusion, usually as a 1-Unit bolus followed by an IV infusion at a rate beginning at 0.5 to 1 Unit/hour. It may be titrated depending on urine output and systemic vascular resistance (SVR).
- Monitoring hourly urine output and urine specific gravity or osmolarity. If the donor's urine output drops below 1 mL/kg/hr, he may be given a minimal (2 mg) dose of furosemide to increase the urine flow.

Management of Ventilation

If the transplant team is considering recovering the donor's lungs then it is essential to avoid excessive fluid replacement and to prevent atelectasis. Providing sufficient fluid to maintain a CVP of 6 to 8 or PCWP of 8 to 12 while replacing fluid lost due to diuresis usually helps to prevent fluid overload and limit pulmonary edema. Aggressive pulmonary management is needed to prevent atelectasis. Many potential lung donors have a bronchoscopy to assess their lungs and aid in the prevention of atelectasis. Donors receive vigorous pulmonary hygiene and should be suctioned frequently. Ventilator settings should be reviewed carefully. The intent is to attain the highest level of oxygen concentration in the donor's blood (PaO_2) with the lowest amount of inspired oxygen (FiO_2). Usually, the plan is to maintain the PaO_2 greater than 70 and the oxygen saturation greater than 98% to 99% using tidal volumes of 8 to 12 mL/kg, FiO_2 less than 60%, and PEEP less than or equal to 5 cm H_2O (O'Connor et al., 2006; Shah & Bhosale, 2006). In addition, the use of bronchodilators and the administration of antibiotics have been shown to improve the likelihood of successful lung transplantation.

Management of Electrolyte Imbalances

The goal is to maintain the serum sodium less than 150 and the serum potassium greater than 4.0 with any acidosis corrected by mildly hyperventilating the donor to maintain a pCO_2 of 30 to 35.

Management of Hypothermia

Following brain death dysfunction of the hypothalamus often occurs. The donor becomes poikilothermic, which means that his body temperature fluctuates with the temperature of the environment. If the room is cool the donor is predisposed to hypothermia, which can be worsened by administration of cool IV fluids or ventilator air. Because hypothermia can lead to problems with coagulation and cardiac irritability and can reduce oxygen delivery to the tissues, the donor's temperature is monitored closely. The nurse might adjust the room temperature to about 90°F and administer the patient warm IV fluids or cover the patient with warming blankets to maintain a body temperature of approximately 36.5°C (98°F).

Donation After Cardiac Death

Another possibility for organ donation from deceased individuals is known as donation after cardiac death. Potential donors, known as **nonheartbeating donors**, are patients who do not meet the criteria for brain death but who are gravely ill and dying. Most have sustained a devastating nonrecoverable neurological injury that did not result in brain death. The patient, or more likely the patient's proxy, has determined in conjunction with the health care team that the patient would wish to have life-sustaining therapy withdrawn so that she could die and would want to donate her organs after death.

Evaluation of the Donor

The first step in the process is the determination that the patient would want to have life support withdrawn. After that decision has been made, the patient is evaluated first to determine if he is medically suitable as an organ donor but additionally if death will most likely occur within an hour following the withdrawal of life support. An hour is considered the maximum acceptable interval between withdrawal of support and recovery of organs for minimizing ischemic damage (Edwards et al., 2006). The University of Wisconsin has developed an evaluation tool to determine if a patient is likely to have cessation of cardiorespiratory function within an hour following withdrawal from a ventilator. The evaluation includes the following steps:

> *Step 1:* Recording the patient's type of intubation and vasopressor status
>
> *Step 2:* Recording the patient's vital signs and height and weight
>
> *Step 3:* Disconnecting the patient from the ventilator for 10 minutes then reassessing the respiratory effort (respiratory rate, tidal volume, and inspiratory force) and vital signs. The assessment is stopped if the patient's O_2 saturation drops to less than 70% or his systolic BP to less than 80.

Utilizing the scoring criteria associated with the evaluation allows prediction with more than 90% accuracy of those patients who will die within 1 to 2 hours following withdrawal of life support (Edwards et al., 2006). If cessation of cardiorespiratory effort seems likely and the patient otherwise is medically suitable as an organ donor, the family is counseled about the possibility of organ donation. Next, consents for donation and medical examiner clearance are obtained and the organ recovery team is notified. While awaiting the arrival of the organ recovery team, the patient is cared for by the hospital's normal critical care team, not the OPO. Goals of care include maintaining:

- Hemodynamic stability (which is usually not as difficult as for the brain dead donor because herniation and the disruption in autonomic response have not occurred)
- Good tissue oxygenation
- Normal electrolyte balance
- Coagulation profiles within normal limits

Collaborative Procedure

When the recovery team is in place, the patient is extubated. The team waits until the patient can be declared dead. The definition is dependent on the specific institution but is often 5 minutes of asystole on the cardiac monitor, no arterial waveform indicative of a BP or pulse, and no respiratory effort. When death occurs, the patient is pronounced dead by a physician who is not a member of the transplant team. If the patient is pronounced dead within 60 minutes of extubation, then the team begins the organ recovery process. However, if the patient continues to breathe and has a heart rhythm after 60 minutes the patient is transported to a prearranged hospital unit for palliative care.

Nursing Management

Families of patients who become nonheartbeating donors should receive support during the decision to withdraw life-sustaining technology from the patient and throughout the process of organ donation. Depending on the family, the support may be provided by the nurse, physician, social worker, or hospital chaplain. Most sources recommend that families be given the opportunity to say their farewells to the patient at a time and place of their choosing. This may take place in the ICU prior to the patient's extubation and pronouncement of death in the OR. However, some families request to stay with the patient while he is extubated and until he is pronounced dead. The Society of Critical Care Medicine (SCCM, 2001) has affirmed that families have the right to be at the patient's bedside while the patient is dying wherever that might be. Therefore, arrangements may be made for the extubation and pronouncement to occur in a room close to the OR or for the family to be present in the OR until the patient is pronounced dead. In either case it is recommended that a limited number of people be present while waiting for the pronouncement of death. Those present usually include the OPO representative responsible for caring for the donor, the physician responsible for pronouncing the patient dead, and the ICU nurse who has been providing care to the patient and who will be responsible for providing emotional support to the family. Additional emotional support will be required if the patient is one of the 5% to 10% of patients who do not have a circulatory arrest during the 60-minute time frame consistent with donation. These patients and their families will need to be provided with appropriate palliative care.

Organ Recipients

Currently there are nearly 100,000 people in the United States waiting for organ transplants. Because there are so many people waiting for only a few organs, potential organ recipients are evaluated carefully to ensure that they will benefit from the transplant. The following is a list of contraindications to most organ transplants. Some are relative and might be waived depending on the patient's circumstances.

- Age greater than 70 years
- Untreated malignancies or cancer within the last 5 years
- Active infectious process, which has not responded to prescribed therapy
- Confirmed HIV positive status
- Active hepatitis
- Active substance abuse
- Active tuberculosis
- Severe COPD when the risk of damage to the patient from anesthesia is high
- Diffuse atherosclerotic or coronary artery disease that is not repairable, ejection fraction less than 20% for patients not receiving a heart transplant
- Psychosocial or behavioral abnormalities, which would prevent adequate posttransplant treatment.
- Morbid obesity (body mass index [BMI] greater than 35).

Eligibility Criteria and Evaluation for Specific Organ Transplants

In addition to the general requirements for any organ transplantation, there are specific requirements that recipients must meet depending on the organ(s) to be transplanted.

Kidney Transplantation

There are few additional contraindications to renal transplantation, so many adults with end-stage renal disease (ESRD) are potential transplant candidates. However,

Gerontological Considerations

Eligible donors should have been in good health previously and are usually less than 70 years of age. However, age is a relative contraindication and people older than 80 have been organ donors.

Individuals considered for living donation are usually between 18 and 60 years of age.

Age greater than 70 is a contraindication to some organ transplants. However, it is relative and might be waived depending on the patient's circumstances.

Medicare covers the cost of a renal transplant and expenses during the first 3 years. However, depending on the patient's age and circumstances, after 3 years the patient may no longer qualify for Medicare and must rely on another source of funding to cover the cost of medications and other transplant-related expenses.

some people with ESRD prefer to continue dialysis and choose not to become candidates for renal transplantation. If the patient chooses to be evaluated for transplant, he should know that candidacy requirements as well as the evaluation process for kidney transplant vary according to the transplant center. Scandling (2005) describes the following criteria that are utilized by Stanford Hospitals and Clinics.

- Candidates are first cleared by their insurance. Medicare covers the cost of a renal transplant and expenses during the first 3 years. However, depending on the patient's age and circumstances, after 3 years he may no longer qualify for Medicare and must rely on another source of funding to cover the cost of medications and other transplant-related expenses. Depending on the immunosuppressants that the organ transplant recipient is receiving, the cost of medications alone may exceed $800/month.

- Next, interested candidates must attend an educational session. At Stanford, if they choose not to attend, their appointments for transplant evaluation are canceled.

- Candidates are also assessed for preexisting diseases and disorders, both those conditions listed previously that might preclude a transplant but also those, like CMV status, that would necessitate prophylaxis following transplantation.

- Finally, the candidate receives a psychosocial evaluation and the candidate's motivation and commitment to follow an intensive regimen are assessed. At Stanford, a social worker will contact the candidate's dialysis center to ensure that the candidate has demonstrated compliance with his treatment regimen and dialysis schedule.

The Candidate for Renal Transplantation

Once a person has been accepted as a candidate for renal transplantation, he is entered into the computer system maintained by UNOS. There are complex guidelines for allocation of the available kidneys to candidates on the waiting list with two overarching principles:

First, blood type O and B kidneys must be transplanted only into blood type O or B recipients except in the case of zero antigen mismatched candidates who have blood types other than O or B.

Second, it is mandatory that zero antigen mismatched kidneys be shared. A zero antigen mismatch is defined as occurring when a candidate on the waiting list has an ABO blood type that is compatible with that of the donor and the candidate and donor both have all six of the same HLA-A, B, and DR antigens. When this occurs, the kidney must be offered to that individual.

For other candidates there is a point system for kidney allocation. When information about a donor is entered into the computerized UNOS Match System, all candidates who have an ABO blood type that is compatible with the donor and who are listed as active on the waiting list are assigned points and priority based on:

- *Time of waiting:* The "time of waiting" begins when the candidate either (a) has a creatinine clearance less than or equal to 20 mL/min or (b) begins chronic maintenance dialysis.

- *Quality of antigen mismatch:* Points are assigned to a candidate based on the number of mismatches between the candidate's antigens and the donor's antigens at the HLA-DR locus.

- *Donation status:* A candidate is given additional points if she has donated an organ or an organ segment to a person within the United States.

- *Proximity:* Kidneys are allocated first locally, then regionally, and, finally, nationally.

- No points are assigned for severity of illness for allocation of kidneys on the regional or national level although physicians on the local level may take that into consideration.

Liver Transplants

In general, a donor is matched to a potential liver recipient on the basis of several factors: ABO blood type, body size, degree of medical urgency, and Model for End-Stage Liver Disease (MELD) score. The priority of any patient on the UNOS waiting list for a donor liver depends on the following factors:

- Region (donor organs are first offered locally).

- ABO type (priority is for an identical ABO blood type but compatibility is essential).

- Body size (the acceptable body range is determined by the transplant surgeon).

- Degree of medical urgency as determined by the MELD score (highest priority given to sickest patients). The MELD is a numerical scale used for adult liver transplant candidates. The individual score determines how urgently a patient needs a liver transplant within the next 3 months. The number is calculated using the most recent laboratory tests for the following lab values:
  - Bilirubin
  - INR
  - Creatinine (If the patient has been dialyzed recently, the creatinine is entered as 4 mg/dL.)

After the score is calculated, potential liver recipients are grouped at four levels on the scale (less than 10, 11 to 18, 19 to 24, and greater than or equal to 25). Patients with the highest scores are the sickest and have the most urgent need for a liver transplant. Waiting times at each MELD level are tracked. If all other factors between potential recipients are equal, waiting times at levels of illness are the determining factor in which the person receives the liver.

Heart Transplant

Hearts are allocated to candidates locally based on medical status then regionally. Every candidate older than 18 years of age awaiting heart transplantation is assigned a status code, which corresponds to how medically urgent it is that the candidate receive a heart transplant. The most severely ill candidates have at least one mechanical circulatory support device in place such as a left and/or right ventricular heart assist device, an intra-aortic balloon pump, or a total artificial heart. Candidates who are less severely ill may have implanted ventricular assist devices or continuous infusions of inotropes. In unhospitalized candidates, a reproducible VO$_2$max (the amount of oxygen required by the body as a patient exercises on a treadmill) of less than 14 mL/kg/min is an objective indication that the patient may require a transplant. ABO compatibility and body size are also factors that determine whether a candidate will receive a heart transplant from a specific donor.

In addition to the exclusion criteria mentioned previously, a heart transplant candidate might be excluded from the transplant list for:

- Age more than 65 years.
- Severe irreversible pulmonary hypertension
- Irreversible kidney or liver dysfunction not explained by underlying heart failure
- Symptomatic peripheral, renal, or cerebrovascular artery disease
- Insulin-dependent diabetes mellitus with evidence of damage to other organs
- Smoking

Likelihood of Receiving an Organ from a Deceased Donor

The number of deceased donors has remained relatively flat since 1994, whereas the number of people awaiting transplants has continued to rise. The average waiting time for various organs arranged by blood group and year as listed by UNOS (2007) is displayed in Table 15–1. According to Wolfe (2005), potential kidney transplant patients often "ask about their prospects for a transplant if they are put on the waiting list. The answer varies greatly according to where the patient lives, insurance status, age, blood type, degree of sensitization (PRA antibodies), and the HLA phenotype of the patient. However, geography plays the biggest role with more than threefold differences between regions" (p. 454).

In addition, the wait for a donated kidney for minorities may be longer than for Caucasians. This probably occurs for two reasons. First, African Americans and other minorities are three times more likely to suffer from ESRD than Caucasians. Second, transplant success rates increase when organs are matched between members of the same ethnic and racial group because they are more likely to share a common HLA phenotype. When an ethnic or racial group lacks information, has specific religious convictions, or mistrusts the medical community, they are less likely to agree to organ donation. Consequently, a lack of organs donated by minorities can contribute to longer waiting periods for transplantation.

Care of the Transplant Recipient

When delivering care to the transplant patient, the nurse should be aware of certain unique aspects of the patient's care. Those features of care include rejection and the use of immunosuppressive drugs, the increased risk for infection, specific concerns related to the organ transplanted, and psychosocial issues related to accepting an organ from another human being.

Overview of Rejection

When a patient receives an organ from a donor who is genetically different than himself, his immune system recognizes the organ as foreign and mounts an immune response to eliminate or neutralize the grafted organ. This process is known as rejection. If a solid organ transplant recipient does not receive immunosuppressant medications, then the graft will be rejected and the organ transplant will fail.

Rejection is more likely to occur when the recipient has been sensitized. Sensitization events such as previous transplants, blood transfusions, and pregnancies create antibodies that also make it harder for people to pass the crossmatch test.

TABLE 15–1

Median Waiting Time in Days for a Transplanted Organ by Organ Transplanted and Blood Group of Recipient

YEAR	ORGAN	BLOOD GROUP O	BLOOD GROUP A	BLOOD GROUP B	BLOOD GROUP AB
2001–2002	Kidney	1,840	1,135	2,093	732
2003–2004	Liver	459	350	230	75
2003–2004	Heart	241	102	98	51

Source: Based on Organ Procurement and Transplantation Network (OPTN) data as of April 1, 2007. Retrieved from http://www.optn.org.latest_Data/step2.asp

Types of Rejection

There are four types of rejection that result from different immune responses and occur at varying times post transplant. The first type of rejection, hyperacute rejection, is rare. It occurs only when the recipient has preformed antibodies to donor antigens. Thus, it develops almost immediately after the graft is transplanted into the recipient. Severe thrombosis and graft necrosis result in visible damage to the organ, the organ fails, and it must be removed.

Accelerated rejection, the second type of rejection, occurs within the first week after transplantation when the recipient has been sensitized to some of the donor antigens. Although it is usually treated aggressively with steroids and immunosuppressants, it is associated with a poor prognosis for graft survival.

Acute rejection develops in 15% to 60% of transplant recipients during the first year post transplant. Acute rejection is a cell-mediated immune response that results in T lymphocytes infiltrating the donated organ and damaging it by secreting lysosomal enzymes and lymphokines. Antirejection doses of immunosuppressants are provided; these usually reverse the process of acute rejection, and the prognosis for graft survival is good. Figure 15-2 displays the process of acute rejection with the sites of action for immunosuppressive agents.

Chronic rejection occurs months to years after organ transplantation. The process is not completely understood but probably involves a combination of humoral and cell-mediated immune responses. There is usually progressive deterioration in organ function that does not respond well to immunosuppression.

Patients who receive solid organ transplants will need to be concerned about preventing and detecting rejection for as long as they have their transplanted organ.

Donor-Recipient Compatibility Testing

Hyperacute and accelerated rejection are now rare due to requirements for ABO compatibility testing and crossmatching before all transplants. UNOS calls for retesting the ABO compatibility of the donor and recipient blood types a second time prior to transplant to prevent the tragedy of a mismatched organ. Crossmatching is also performed prior to the transplant to prevent hyperacute rejection. In a crossmatch, the blood of the donor is mixed with that of the recipient. If the blood of the recipient attacks the cells in the blood of the donor, it means that the recipient has antibodies to the tissue type of the donor. Called a "positive" crossmatch, this means that the transplant is contraindicated. If there is no reaction between the blood of the donor and the

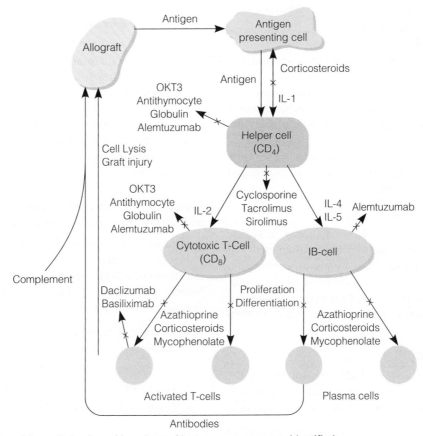

Figure 15-2 Progression of Acute Rejection with actions of immunosuppressants identified.

blood of the recipient, called a "negative" crossmatch, then the transplant may proceed.

Immunosuppression

There are three types of immunosuppressive therapy. The first two types, induction and maintenance immunosuppression, are used to prevent rejection of the transplanted organ.

Induction immunosuppression refers to the temporary use of high-dose immunosuppressants in the perioperative period when the likelihood of rejection is highest. It is used often for patients who have had kidney, intestine, and pancreas transplants, occasionally for patients with heart and/or lung transplants, and less often for patients with liver transplants (Shapiro et al., 2005). Induction most commonly involves a brief course of antibody therapy such as rabbit ATG (thymoglobulin). While the recipient is receiving induction therapy, and until the recipient's renal function stabilizes, calcineurin inhibitors may be omitted from therapy.

Maintenance therapy refers to the specific immunosuppressant medications that the organ recipient will continue to take either for as long as he lives or until the transplanted organ is removed. Most patients receive at least two different immunosuppressant medications that complement each other in an attempt to improve the effectiveness of the therapy. Current therapy often includes a corticosteroid, a calcineurin inhibitor, and, possibly, an antimetabolite.

Antirejection treatment is the use of higher doses of immunosuppressants and/or more potent IV immunosuppressants to resolve an acute episode of rejection. Treatment usually involves high-dose corticosteroid and antibody therapies.

The choice of the specific drug regimen for any type of immunosuppression depends on the transplant center but also on the organ transplanted. Medications are described by classification in the following section. All organ transplant patients receiving immunosuppressants should be assessed for signs of rejection and monitored for the development of infection.

Polyclonal Antibodies

Antibody induction is utilized for the majority of kidney transplant patients and slightly fewer than half of heart and/or lung recipients. Most commonly rabbit ATG (Thymoglobulin) is the immunosuppressant administered. However, monoclonal antibodies such as daclizumab and basiliximab are utilized in some circumstances (Shapiro et al., 2005).

Monoclonal Antibodies

Monoclonal antibodies include muromonab-CD3 (OKT3), daclizumab (Zenapex), and basiliximab. They may be used for induction or antirejection

immunosuppression but are less likely to be used than rabbit ATG. OKT3 induces a mild cytokine response syndrome (fever, headache, rigor, chills, tremor, joint pain, rash) in most patients. However, 5% to 15% of patients develop a severe response, symptoms of which include pulmonary edema, hypotension or hypertension, decreased urinary output, respiratory failure, and cardiac arrest. Other common adverse effects of monoclonal antibodies are GI distress and hypertension.

Identification and Management of Rejection

With the advent of induction protocols and the use of several new immunosuppressant agents, fewer patients are developing acute rejection. Still, it is essential that the nurse and patient know how to identify the symptoms of acute rejection and the patient know when to contact the transplant center.

- To avoid rejection, the patient should contact the transplant center if he cannot take his immunosuppressants or has missed doses.

- Because many medications interact with immunosuppressants, the patient should also contact the center when he changes any medication.

- Most transplant centers request that they be notified if one of their patients has a temperature above 37.8°C (100°F) and be called immediately if the patient's temperature exceeds 38.4°C (101.5°F).

- The recipient should notify the center promptly of the development of persistent, unusual weakness or fatigue; shortness of breath; sudden weight gain accompanied by swelling in the hands and feet; or a feeling of "not feeling right" accompanied by aches and pains, as well as any of the indications of rejection of a specific organ that are listed next.

Identification and Management of Rejection in Kidney Transplant Patients

According to Shapiro et al. (2005), only about 15% of kidney transplant patients require treatment for an acute rejection episode during their first year post transplant. Indications that a person might be experiencing an acute rejection of a transplanted kidney include:

- Increase in blood urea nitrogen (BUN) and creatinine levels with a decrease in urine output
- Weight gain, edema, and an increase in BP
- Fever, chills, and elevated white blood cells (WBCs)
- Graft swelling and tenderness

COMMONLY USED MEDICATIONS

CORTICOSTEROIDS, CALCINEURIN INHIBITORS, ANTIMETABOLITES

CORTICOSTEROIDS

Although steroids are still prescribed for the overwhelming majority of transplant recipients, there is increasing interest in developing protocols that either avoid or minimize the use of steroids (Shapiro et al., 2005). Steroids are currently used in both maintenance and antirejection immunosuppressant regimens.

Methylprednisolone/prednisone (Deltasone, Orasone) interferes with T-cell differentiation and macrophage function, impairing antigen recognition and cytotoxic response. It may be used for maintenance and antirejection therapy so the dose varies depending on the use. Oral prednisone doses may range from 2.5 to 100 mg/day in a single or divided dose, whereas IV methylprednisolone doses may vary from 250 to 1,000 mg/day.

Common Side Effects:
- The development of diabetes
- A Cushingoid appearance
- Mood swings
- Sodium and water retention

Longer term side effects include:

- The development of osteoporosis
- Aseptic necrosis of the hip
- Muscular atrophy
- Gastric ulceration
- Cataracts

Steroids are associated with more long-term adverse effects than other immunosuppressants (Lindenfeld et al., 2004).

Nursing Responsibilities:
- Administering the oral medication with food
- Monitoring baseline weight and BP
- Suggesting the patient have regular eye examinations
- Observing for signs of infection

Because steroids have been associated with bone loss, which develops rapidly beginning in the first 3 months post-transplant, the nurse should encourage the patient to be involved in weight-bearing exercise and take calcium supplementation.

CALCINEURIN INHIBITORS

Most post-transplant patients receive a calcineurin inhibitor for maintenance immunosuppression. The majority of noncardiac transplant patients receive tacrolimus (FK-506) because it is associated with fewer episodes of acute rejection 1 year after kidney transplant than cyclosporine (Shapiro et al., 2005). However, cyclosporine is often still used for patients following cardiac transplant.

Tacrolimus (Prograf) exerts its immunosuppressant effect through inhibition of cytokine production by T cells (calcineurin inhibition). It is heavily metabolized in the liver and has a narrow therapeutic window. There is wide variability between its rate of absorption and its bioavailability. Oral doses usually range between 0.075 and 0.15 mg/kg every 12 hours.

Adverse Effects: Adverse effects that occur more commonly with tacrolimus than cyclosporine include:
- Insulin-dependent diabetes mellitus.
- Diarrhea and vomiting.

- Neurological toxicity may develop and is seen as tremor, headache, numbness, and tingling.
- Nephrotoxicity is also a possibility.
- Hypertension and hyperlipidemia, although occurring with the drug, are not as common as with cyclosporine (Staatz & Tett, 2005).

Nursing Responsibilities:
- Oral therapy is preferred because of the risk of anaphylactic reactions with intravenous (IV) tacrolimus.
- The patient will need regular monitoring of BP, blood sugar, and renal function. Because many patients develop diabetes, they may need education about dietary modification, oral hypoglycemic medications, or insulin.

Cyclosporine (Neoral, Sandimmune) inhibits T-cell proliferation and differentiation without affecting other immune cells. The drug is absorbed erratically after oral administration and is metabolized in the liver. Therefore, the dose varies from patient to patient and may range from 3 to 10 mg/kg/day in divided doses.

Common Side Effects:
- The development of nephrotoxicity that can be acute and dose related.
- The majority of patients develop hypertension and hyperlipidemia.
- Neurologic toxicity is not as common as with tacrolimus.
- Hirsutism is a troublesome cosmetic side effect that has caused some patients to discontinue the drug.

Nursing Responsibilities:
- It is important that patients have their drug levels monitored as scheduled because metabolism varies among individuals and cyclosporine has a narrow therapeutic window.
- Patients also need to have their BP, weight, and kidney function monitored at regular intervals.
- If possible, nephrotoxic agents, such as contrast medium, should be avoided.

ANTIMETABOLITES

Mycophenolate mofetil (CellCept) has replaced azathioprine and is now the most widely used adjunct immunosuppressant in solid organ transplant (Shapiro et al., 2005).

Mycophenolate mofetil (CellCept) is an antiproliferative agent. It more selectively inhibits the B- and T-cell proliferation than the older agent azathioprine. Doses range between 500 and 1,500 mg twice a day.

Common Side Effects: The drug is normally well tolerated. The most common side effects, nausea, vomiting, and diarrhea, usually respond to a reduction in dose. Neutropenia and anemia are also common. Patients may be more prone to opportunistic infections than with azathioprine.

Nursing Responsibilities: The medication should be administered on an empty stomach and should be swallowed whole, never crushed or chewed.

COMMONLY USED MEDICATIONS

RABBIT ANTITHYMOCYTE GLOBULIN

INTRODUCTION
Rabbit antithymocyte globulin (Thymoglobulin) depletes lymphocytes and may work by modulating T-cell activation. The dose is 1.5 mg/kg/day IV for 3 to 14 days depending on whether it is used for induction or as an antirejection dose.

Common Side Effects:
- Fever, chills, dyspnea, joint pain, headache
- Gastrointestinal (GI) disturbances
- Hypertension
- Thrombocytopenia and neutropenia

Nursing Responsibilities: Rabbit antithymocyte globulin is administered by central line with a filter over 6 hours for the first dose and 4 hours for subsequent doses

---

Assessment of the patient should include:

- Accurate intake, output, and daily weights
- BP
- Serum levels of electrolytes, BUN, and creatinine
- Complete blood count (CBC)
- Evaluation for indications of a urinary tract infection
- Ultrasound of the bladder if postvoiding residuals are suspected
- Renal transplant ultrasound (Hoffman et al., 2006)

Corticosteroids are the mainstay of treatment for acute rejection of a transplanted kidney. They are used alone or in combination with another drug in 80% of the episodes of acute rejection. Antilymphocyte antibodies are also used in approximately 35% to 40% of patients with rabbit ATG being the drug of choice. The patient's transplant center normally directs the management of the rejection episode.

Chronic rejection of a kidney is usually first evidenced by the development of proteinuria and hypertension followed by a decline in renal function and urinary output. It develops slowly over months to years probably due to a combination of humoral and cellular immune responses. The course is not predictable and renal function fluctuates (Hoffman et al., 2006). However, the overall course is a decline in function that often results in loss of the renal graft.

Identification and Management of Rejection in Heart Transplant Patients

The percentage of patients requiring treatment for acute rejection after heart transplantation has remained consistent at approximately 40% over the past decade. Rejection is diagnosed via endomyocardial biopsies that are performed at regular intervals post transplant. Immediately post-op the biopsies are performed at least weekly with the frequency decreasing gradually to yearly postoperatively. The degree of rejection is graded depending on the amount of intercellular infiltrate and the presence of myocyte damage or necrosis (Hoffman et al., 2006). Biopsies are essential because the patient may be asymptomatic until late in the process when the ejection fraction drops and the patient develops heart failure and dysrhythmias. Acute rejection in heart transplant patients is primarily treated with corticosteroids with less than 20% of patients receiving antibodies.

Chronic rejection is the major reason for death of those heart transplant recipients who survive beyond the first year. It occurs in at least 60% of heart recipients 5 years after transplant and leads to progressive myocardial fibrosis and heart dysfunction.

Identification and Treatment of Rejection in Liver Transplant Patients

Although as many as 40% to 60% of liver transplant patients may experience an episode of rejection, usually in the first 3 months, the rate of treatment for acute rejection in the liver transplant patient has dropped over the past decade from 50% in 1993 to 24% in 2002 (Shapiro et al., 2005). The vast majority of liver transplant patients who are treated for rejection are treated with corticosteroids with less than 20% receiving antibody therapy.

Indications that a patient may be rejecting a liver and the transplant center should be notified include:

- Malaise, fatigue, and fever
- Abdominal discomfort with a swollen, tender graft
- Cessation of bile flow, change in color of bile from golden to colorless
- Dark- or tea-colored urine and clay-colored stools
- Jaundice
- Elevated bilirubin, liver enzymes, and international ratio (INR)

Assessment of the patient should include results of liver function tests, creatinine, urine output, prothrombin time (PT), INR, and bile drainage. A liver biopsy is the optimal test to distinguish between rejection of a transplanted liver, infection, or recurrent disease.

Infection

The factor most responsible for the predisposition to infection in recipients of transplanted organs is the use of immunosuppressants, which alter the body's normal protective responses. Two other major contributing factors to the patient's immediate posttransplant likelihood of infection are the preoperative condition of the patient and nosocomial factors. Nosocomial factors include surgical and/or invasive procedures, the hospital and critical care environments, the presence of multiresistant hospital organisms, and administration of antibiotics (Stitt, 2003).

Prevention of Infection

Prevention of posttransplant infection begins with pretransplant screening. As noted previously, the patient is screened for the presence of a variety of infections. Some like active tuberculosis (TB) preclude the transplant. However, if identified on screening "many common infections, such as CMV, may be prevented with the use of prophylactic regimens" (Baas, Bell, Giesting, McGuire, & Wagoner, 2003). Screening for CMV is essential because it is latent in as many as 80% of donors and recipients and remains dormant in an infected host. Although it only causes a flulike illness in immune competent individuals, it may develop into a serious illness that is difficult to treat in the immunocompromised person. Therefore, many centers treat all their transplant recipients prophylactically with either acyclovir or gancyclovir. Nearly all centers treat a recipient who has never been exposed to CMV (is seronegative) and receives an organ from a donor who has been exposed and has latent CMV (is seropositive) with gancyclovir or valganciclovir. Prophylaxis with acyclovir has also significantly decreased the incidence of reactivation of human herpes simplex virus, the most common viral infection seen in the first weeks post transplantation (Stitt, 2003).

Other preoperative strategies to prevent post-op infections may include the administration of vaccinations while the candidate is awaiting transplant. The potential recipient is usually seen by a dentist to assess oral hygiene, treat dental cavities, and extract any diseased teeth. Finally, the candidate is assessed for any other potential sources of infection and they are treated or eliminated.

Identification and Management of Infection

How frequently a recipient develops infection postoperatively depends on the type of transplant he has received and the interval post transplant. There are three time frames during which different infections occur in transplant recipients: first month, second through sixth month, and beyond the sixth month. Overall, more than 50% of allograft recipients have evidence of active infection during the first 6 months post transplantation, and infection remains the most common cause of death for all transplant recipients (Stitt, 2003).

Infections During the First Month Postoperatively. Infections that occur in the first month after transplantation are usually nosocomial infections similar to infections occurring in any surgical patient. The most common sites for infection in the first month are:

- The incision
- Lungs, especially if the person remains intubated or is mechanically ventilated
- Urinary tract via a catheter
- Biliary tree due to catheters
- Blood due to invasive IV or arterial catheters

The high level of immunosuppression during this first month exacerbates these infections in transplant recipients, but immunosuppression has not been prolonged enough for patients to be prone to opportunistic infections (Stitt, 2003).

Postoperatively, a clean, but not sterile, environment and frequent hand washing are the foundations of infection prevention for the organ transplant recipient (Stitt, 2003). Nurses should also emphasize maintaining the integrity of skin and mucous membranes, limiting the number and duration of invasive devices, and providing optimal nutritional support. Routine postoperative measures to prevent infections such as the use of incentive spirometry, deep breathing, and early ambulation are also required. In order to limit the likelihood of infection, some centers require all people entering the recipient's room to wear masks, whereas others merely exclude visitors with respiratory infections. Many centers preclude patients from having plants or flowers in their rooms because the standing water may be a source of infection.

Family and patient teaching at the time of patient discharge from the hospital should focus on self-care practices that prevent infection (Baas et al., 2003). Although Bass et al. indicate that some of these practices do not have an evidence base to support them, many transplant centers continue to instruct their patients to:

- Wash their hands before putting anything in or near their mouth and after toileting
- Wear a mask when in a crowd for the first few months post transplant
- Remove plants and flowers in vases from their homes
- Wash, peel, and/or cook all fruits and vegetables
- Avoid exposure to live vaccines
- Avoid environments contaminated by mold, fungus, or water damage
- Obtain prophylactic antibiotics prior to dental procedures

Additionally, recipients and their families are taught to report any indications of infection to the transplant center immediately. Health care providers should be suspicious anytime a recipient reports unusual symptoms because the normal signs of infection have been suppressed by the patient's required medications. Although an increase in WBC count is usually associated with infection, leukopenia may develop in response to infection of the transplant recipient. Fever and chills may not develop so the nurse may need to look at subtle changes in lab values and patient symptoms to determine the source of the infection.

Infections Occurring from the First to Sixth Month Postoperatively. Opportunistic infections are the most common cause of infections after the first month until the sixth month post transplant. Any episode of rejection that results in an increased dose of immunosuppressant medications can set the stage for the recipient to develop an opportunistic infection. The development of an opportunistic infection is due to the presence of an organism and suppression of the patient's innate immunity but also may be compounded by the presence of an immunomodulating virus. Immunomodulating viruses make the patient more susceptible to opportunistic infections. Examples of immunomodulating virus are hepatitis B and C, Epstein-Barr virus, and CMV.

CMV is the most common and most significant viral infection in solid organ transplant recipients, occurring in 20% to 60% of all such patients (Stitt, 2003). The seronegative recipient who receives an organ from a seropositive donor is most likely to develop a primary CMV infection after transplantation. However, disease may also occur with reactivation of infection in the patient who was CMV seropositive before transplantation. One of the earliest signs of active CMV infection is the nonspecific lab finding of leukopenia. However, CMV may present in a variety of ways:

- In most cases, CMV infection results in mild to moderately severe disease manifesting as episodic fevers accompanied by joint pain, fatigue, anorexia, abdominal pain, and diarrhea.

- However, CMV infection can also result in tissue invasive disease causing pneumonia, gastritis, colitis, hepatitis, retinitis, and endocarditis.

- Unfortunately, the development of CMV disease predisposes the patient to other hazards as well. CMV disease has been demonstrated to contribute to acute and/or chronic allograft injury and dysfunction as well as to an increased risk for opportunistic bacterial, viral, and fungal infections (McDevitt, 2006).

One common type of fungal infection in transplant recipients is candidiasis. Oral candidiasis, also known as thrush, can result in pronounced discomfort, preventing the patient from eating and leading to nutritional deficiencies. Therefore, frequent assessment of the patient's mouth and throat is an essential component of the nursing care of the transplant recipient. The nurse looks for white lesions scattered over the tongue and oropharyngeal mucous membranes and a red, sore throat and gums. Thrush can often be prevented by application of a topical antifungal agent.

Infections Occurring Later Than 6 Months Postoperatively.
After the first 6 months, patients are most likely to develop community-acquired infections such as influenza, staphylococcal pneumonia, and pneumococcal pneumonia. Patients who develop persistent infections in this late posttransplant period have usually required higher doses of immunosuppressive agents either because of frequent episodes of acute rejection or the development of chronic rejection (Stitt, 2003).

Care of the Patient Following Specific Organ Transplantation

Organ transplants are complex surgical procedures. Thus, the collaborative and nursing care of the patient following a transplant varies depending on the transplanted organ and the specific surgical procedure.

Kidney Transplant

The majority of patients who receive a donated organ receive a kidney. The number of people awaiting kidney transplants has increased steadily because the quality of life is usually better for patients with ESRD who receive renal transplants than those who remain on dialysis.

Surgical Procedure

Since 1954, transplanted kidneys have been placed extraperitoneally, which is in the right iliac fossa as shown in Figure 15-3. Placing a transplanted kidney in the iliac fossa is advantageous because of its close proximity to major blood vessels and the bladder. It also facilitates assessment of the transplanted kidney by palpation, auscultation, and biopsy. Finally, if removal of the graft is necessary, it can be performed with less risk to the patient. The patient's own kidneys usually remain in place following a transplant. The exceptions are for uncontrolled hypertension, tumors, recurrent infections, or stones of the kidney. In such cases, one or both of the native kidneys might be removed.

At the beginning of surgery, the donor's and recipient's renal arteries and veins are anastomosed. Once the kidney is perfused, the donor ureter is attached to the recipient's bladder. The most desirable method of attaching the ureter to the bladder involves passing the donor ureter into a tunnel carved through the posterior bladder wall and sewn to the inner bladder mucosa. This tunnel helps to prevent urinary reflux with bladder contraction and decreases the risk of bacterial infection (Winsett, Martin, Reed & Bateman, 2003). To maintain

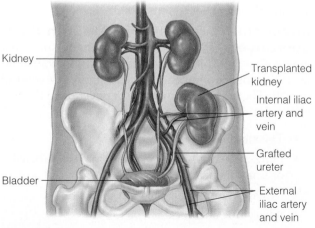

Kidney

Transplanted kidney

Internal iliac artery and vein

Grafted ureter

Bladder

External iliac artery and vein

Figure 15-3 Placement of a transplanted kidney in the iliac fossa.

the patency of the ureter, an indwelling ureteral stent is commonly placed for the first few days to weeks after surgery. The donor kidney usually begins to function immediately. The procedure typically takes about 3 hours after which the transplant recipient is transferred first to the post anesthesia care unit (PACU) then to a transplant unit.

Nursing Management

The postoperative care of the renal transplant patient includes all of the essentials of good postoperative care for any patient. However, as previously noted, strategies to prevent post-op infections are even more essential than normally. In addition, the nurse must monitor the function of the transplanted kidney and detect early signs of any complications.

The amount of urine the transplanted kidney produces immediately after it is perfused varies greatly, depending on how well the kidney was perfused prior to transplant. The nurse monitors the patient's hourly urine output and evaluates his renal function tests. On occasion, delayed graft function (DGF), defined as oliguria that necessitates dialysis during the first 7 days after kidney transplantation and that lasts a few days to weeks, may occur. Approximately 23% of patients who receive kidneys from deceased donors and 6% of patients who receive kidneys from live donors develop DGF (Winsett et al., 2003). DGF that persists for more than 1 week has an impact on long-term graft survival and is associated with an increased rate of acute rejection, decreased long-term graft survival, and decreased patient survival (Winsett et al., 2003).

Surgical complications after kidney transplant are relatively rare (Hoffman et al., 2006) and may be grouped into three different categories:

- Urological: which include urine leakage, reflux, and obstruction
- Vascular: which include renal artery or vein thrombosis
- Wound complications: which include infection and lymphocele

An obstruction from blood clots or kinking of the urinary catheter may develop early in the postoperative period. If the obstruction persists, the bladder could become overdistended, the implanted ureter might separate from the bladder, and a urine leak could develop. Therefore, the nurse maintains the urinary catheter free of clots and monitors the urine output carefully. Obstruction usually presents as a sudden decrease or cessation of urine output rather than a gradual decline. In addition, the patient may complain of cramping and clots or fibrin may be visible in the catheter. After recognizing the obstruction and determining nothing is visibly kinked, the nurse might milk the urinary catheter in an attempt to dislodge any clots. If milking is not successful and the catheter requires flushing it is done aseptically with small volumes (approximately 30 mL) and only per agency protocol.

A lymphocele is a wound complication occurring in 10% to 20% of kidney transplant recipients. Lymphatic fluid collects in either the donor or recipient lymph nodes surrounding the transplant. The fluid builds up and may obstruct the proximal ureter, resulting in decreased urine flow, or may obstruct venous drainage from the leg, resulting in edema of that leg. The patient may complain of edema of the leg on the side of the graft, tenderness over the incision, and/or mild-to-moderate abdominal discomfort. If the lymphocele has an opening to the skin surface, there is usually copious, clear drainage. An ultrasound is used to diagnose a lymphocele. Treatment, depending on the size of the lymphocele and the patient's symptoms, might include watchful waiting, aspiration, or surgical creation of a window into the peritoneal cavity (Winsett et al., 2003).

Nursing Care

Pain management is essential for all postoperative patients and there are no critical differences for pain management in the kidney transplant recipient. Pain relief must be adequate so that the patient will engage in deep breathing and coughing and be ready to get out of bed and walk the day after surgery.

Imbalanced Nutrition

The kidney transplant recipient may be malnourished postoperatively because between 40% and 70% of dialysis patients suffer from malnutrition (Tritt, 2004). Most patients begin taking sips of liquids within the first 24 hours after transplant surgery and begin eating as soon as bowel function resumes. For those patients with immediate return of renal function, there is no reason to restrict protein or potassium in the diet (Tritt, 2004). The patient's caloric needs are increased due to the stress of surgery, high-dose steroids, and possible preexisting malnutrition; therefore, the patient is usually provided a diet with 30 to 35 kcal/kg of dry weight. If the patient's oral intake is poor, then an oral nutritional supplement may be required. Although routine vitamin and mineral supplements may not be necessary, the nurse needs to review the postoperative levels of serum magnesium and phosphate because they may drop rapidly after transplant and require replacement (Tritt, 2004).

Recovery

Patients typically remain in the hospital for 3 to 5 days. Psychosocial issues are not uncommon in the first year post transplant and are discussed later in this chapter.

TABLE 15-2

Survival Following Kidney Transplant 1997–2004 Identified as Percentage of Patients or Grafts Surviving and Noted by Type of Donor (Living or Deceased)

POSTTRANSPLANT DURATION	PATIENT SURVIVIAL	GRAFT SURVIVAL	LIVING DONOR	DECEASED DONOR
1 year	96%	91.9%	95%	89%
3 years	91%	82.4%	87.9%	77.8%
5 years	85%	71.9%	79.7%	66.9%

Source: Based on Organ Procurement and Transplantation Network (OPTN) data as of April 1, 2007. Retrieved from http://www.optn.org.latest_Data/ step2.asp

Most graft failures and patient deaths are the result of chronic rejection. The survival rates for kidney transplant grafts and patients from 1997 until 2004 are displayed in Table 15–2.

Heart Transplant

Heart transplant surgery is a time-consuming intricate procedure that is performed approximately 2,300 times each year in hospitals in the United States.

Surgical Procedure

After completion of the pretransplant procedure and in synchrony with arrival of the donor heart, the heart transplant candidate is connected to a heart-lung machine. In the orthotopic technique, the recipient's heart is removed from its connections to the great arteries, leaving in place the back parts of the right and left atria. The new heart is carefully fitted and sewn to the remaining portions of the recipient atria. Anastamoses of the aorta and pulmonary artery complete the procedure. An alternative newer approach, the bicaval technique, preserves the entire donor right atrium, attaching it to the recipient's superior and inferior vena cavae. The newer technique has led to less atrial distortion, fewer conduction abnormalities, and less tricuspid and mitral valve regurgitation. It has also resulted in fewer thromboembolic events, less need for permanent postoperative pacemaker placement, and an overall improvement in heart function in the early postoperative period. Thus, the bicaval technique is now commonly used. Both techniques are displayed in Figure 15-4.

After the new heart is completely sewn in place and begins to function, the patient is removed from the heart-lung machine. With the completion of the operative procedure, one or more chest or pleural tubes are placed. Epicardial pacing wires are brought out of the chest cavity through the skin's surface, in case there is a temporary need for pacing of the heart postoperatively. The sternum is brought together with stainless steel wires, and the fatty tissues and skin are closed with absorbable sutures. Most patients are then transported to the ICU where they remain on a mechanical ventilator for 24 to 48 hours.

Postoperative Problems Related to the Surgical Procedure

Perioperative management of the heart transplant patient is in many ways similar to that of patients undergoing other major cardiovascular procedures. However,

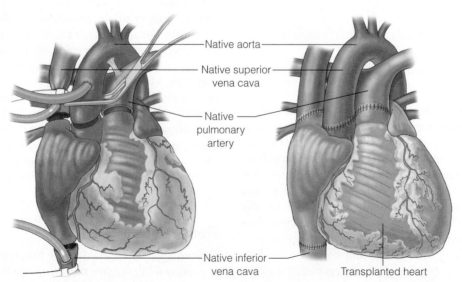

Figure 15-4 Orthotopic heart transplant bicaval technique.

there are specific problems that occur only in patients undergoing heart transplantation.

The donor heart that is placed in the recipient's chest was denervated during removal from the donor. This means that the transplanted heart will not be able to respond to autonomic stimulation. Thus the patient's resting heart rate usually ranges between 90 and 110 beats per minute (bpm). The heart can still respond to circulating catecholamines with an increase in heart rate and cardiac output. However, the heart's response to stress and exercise is delayed, as is the return to a resting heart rate after exercise. The lack of innervation also means that the heart will not respond to certain medications, such as atropine, that increase heart rate by blocking vagal stimulation of the heart. Instead, isoproterenol may be used during the postoperative period because it has a beta-adrenergic effect and can overcome sinus node dysfunction while inducing peripheral vasodilation.

Although a resting tachycardia is common post cardiac transplant, sinus bradycardia may occur if ischemia or edema of the donor sinoatrial (SA) node developed during procurement, transfer, or transplant. The bradycardia is usually temporary, resolving within 2 weeks. If necessary, the temporary pacing wires placed during surgery may be used to pace the patient. Additionally, posttransplant patients may develop dysrhythmias commonly associated with all cardiac surgeries such as atrial fibrillation.

If the older orthotopic approach was utilized to attach the atria, the patient will have two existing SA nodes. Impulses from each of the nodes (the recipient's as well as the donor's) will result in P waves on the electrocardiogram (ECG). The P waves from the recipient's native SA node are generally slower than the donor P waves and will respond to stimulation and increase or decrease in rate. However, the recipient's native P waves will be unrelated to the QRS complexes.

Other Concerns

The most common causes of death following a heart transplant are infection or rejection of the transplanted heart that were described earlier. However, cardiac allograph vasculopathy (CAV), an aggressive, diffuse form of arteriosclerosis, is common in heart transplant recipients, occurring in 40% to 50% of them 5 years after surgery. Unlike the stenoses that develop in CAD that are localized to one section of an artery, CAV can affect the entire length of an artery in the transplanted heart. The diffuse nature of the stenoses makes them less likely to be responsive to angioplasty and stenting. Therefore, heart transplanted recipients are encouraged to maintain a heart healthy lifestyle beginning as soon as possible postoperatively. The patient is usually encouraged to do the following:

- Avoid smoking
- Control his blood sugar, especially if he has diabetes
- Maintain a normal weight and BP
- Manage his cholesterol level by diet and medications (usually statins)
- Take a daily aspirin
- Engage in appropriate exercise

There is some indication that modifying the immunosuppressant medication regimen by including sirolimus or everolimus may reduce the incidence of CAV because those drugs may inhibit cellular proliferation (Hoffman et al., 2006). To determine the existence or extent of CAV in the heart transplant recipient, left heart catheterizations are done yearly.

Nursing Care

Heart transplant recipients may be debilitated and malnourished at the time of surgery. However, the focus of their nutritional support is adequate oral nutrition as soon as possible following extubation. They are started on a heart healthy diet as soon as they are able to eat after surgery.

Comfort

Management of postoperative pain is similar to pain management in any patient who has had cardiac surgery. However, unlike other cardiac surgery patients, some transplant recipients report that they can breathe easier and feel better within 24 hours of the surgery despite the sternotomy incision (Dressler, 2003).

Unfortunately, there is a more serious concern about heart transplant recipients and pain. Normally, patients with coronary artery disease experience chest pressure or pain when their hearts are not adequately perfused. However, because the hearts of transplant patients are denervated, they will not experience the warning sign of angina. There is some indication that reinnervation may occur in some patients over time (Hoffman et al., 2006). However, because the recipient may not experience angina, the nurse should emphasize the importance of maintaining a heart healthy lifestyle and having heart catheterizations as scheduled.

TABLE 15–3

Survival Following Heart Transplant 1997–2004 Identified as Percentage of Patients or Grafts Surviving

POSTTRANSPLANT DURATION	% OF PATIENTS SURVIVING	% GRAFT SURVIVING
1 year	87.7%	87.1%
3 years	79.1%	78.4%
5 years	72.5%	71.5%

Source: Based on Organ Procurement and Transplantation Network (OPTN) data as of April 1, 2007. Retrieved from http://www.optn.org.latest_Data/ step2.asp

Recovery

Most heart transplant recipients are able to resume regular activities and their normal lifestyle despite cardiac denervation, but there are cautions for patients when resuming activities. Patients are instructed on their need to have a warm-up period prior to exercising to establish circulating catecholamines. They also need to cool down slowly after exercising to allow the catecholamine levels to taper off and their heart rate to return slowly to baseline. They should also be cautioned to change their position gradually to avoid orthostatic hypotension. Most patients are encouraged to enroll in a cardiac rehabilitation program within 3 months of their transplant (Babruth, 2004) so that "they may become more comfortable with their new heart and how it deals with exercise" (Babruth, 2004, p. 35). After the initial post-op period, patients have no limits on their prescribed amount of exercise and heart transplant patients have been known to run marathons and climb mountains.

The prognosis following heart transplant depends on many factors, including age, general health, and status of the donor (Dressler, 2003). Survival rates for the first 5 years following heart transplant are displayed in Table 15–3. The 10-year survival rate after heart transplantation is approximately 45% (Dressler, 2003).

Liver Transplant

Liver transplant is a complex surgical procedure that requires a well-coordinated team for the best patient outcomes.

Surgical Procedure

The surgical procedures for liver transplantation differ depending on whether the recipient's liver is totally or partially removed, and whether a whole or partial organ is transplanted. When the entire liver is removed, all ligaments that hold it in place as well as the common bile duct, hepatic artery, and portal vein are identified and clamped. Usually a portion of the inferior vena cava is removed along with the liver. When the hepatectomy is complete, the donor liver is implanted in the recipient's abdominal cavity. After blood flow to the new liver is restored by anastamoses of the inferior vena cava, portal vein, and hepatic artery, the bile duct is anastomosed, either to the recipient's own bile duct or to the small intestine. Usually a T tube or biliary stent is placed at that time. Figure 15-5 shows the surgical technique in liver transplantation.

The surgery usually takes between 5 and 6 hours but may be longer or shorter depending on the difficulty of the operation and the experience of the surgeon. Following surgery the patient is usually transported to the ICU where he may remain for several days on a mechanical ventilator. The most common problems following liver transplant are rejection and infection (which have been discussed previously) followed by mechanical problems, recurrent hepatitis, and psychological changes (Hoffman et al., 2006).

Postoperative Problems Related to the Surgical Procedure

One of the lesser-understood problems in liver transplantation is primary nonfunction of the graft, a graft that simply fails to function. In most cases, it is clinically evident almost immediately in the OR because a functioning liver graft usually produces bile as soon as it is perfused and preexisting coagulopathies begin to improve almost immediately. The absence of bile production and the continuation of coagulation problems are early indications of graft failure.

Assessment of graft function in the postoperative period is one of the responsibilities of the nurse. The

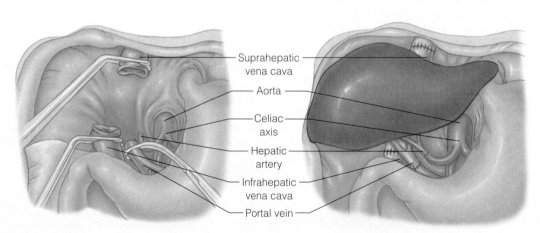

Suprahepatic vena cava
Aorta
Celiac axis
Hepatic artery
Infrahepatic vena cava
Portal vein

Figure 15-5 Surgical technique in liver transplant.

nurse carefully reviews laboratory tests and notes the appearance and amount of biliary drainage to assess graft function. The most sensitive laboratory indices of liver function are the coagulation indicators, PT (or INR), and partial thromboplastin time (PTT). A steady downward trend toward normalcy in coagulation studies as well as in following laboratory tests:

Alanine aminotransferase (ALT)

Aspartate aminotransferase (AST)

Total bilirubin

Lactic dehydrogenase

Ammonia

indicates that the transplanted liver is beginning to function (Mansarheitia & Smith, 2003). Hyperglycemia in the immediate postoperative period is an indication that the liver is responding normally by storing glycogen and converting it to glucose in response to the metabolic effects of corticosteroids.

The appearance of adequate amounts of thick dark green or gold bile in the T-tube postoperatively in conjunction with a decrease in serum bilirubin indicates that both the liver is functioning and the bile drainage system is intact. Biliary complications are relatively common, occurring in up to 15% of cases (Mansarheitia & Smith, 2003) so a T-tube is usually left open to a drainage bag for several days postoperatively. The nurse continues to observe and record the amount and color of bile drainage until the T-tube is capped. It remains clamped but in place until about 3 months after transplantation. At that time, the likelihood of biliary complications from a leak or stenosis is less, a cholangiogram is performed and if there are no leaks or stenoses, the T-tube is removed (Hoffman et al., 2006).

For a variety of reasons liver transplant recipients are at high risk for the development of pulmonary complications (Mansarheita & Smith, 2003). The reasons include:

- Atelectasis that develops from the patient spending the long surgical procedure in the supine position.
- Mechanical ventilation is necessary for a period postoperatively, predisposing the immunosuppressed patient to pulmonary infections. Efforts to wean the patient from mechanical ventilation can be thwarted by paresis or paralysis of the right hemidiaphragm if the phrenic nerve was damaged during surgery.
- The patient may be immobile for extended periods.
- Pleural effusions are common on the right side following liver transplant.

To prevent these possible pulmonary complications, nurses need to mobilize the patient as much as possible and cough or suction the patient as needed. Aseptic technique when suctioning the patient's endotracheal (ET) tube is always appropriate as is the use of a ventilator bundle to prevent complications associated with mechanical ventilation (see Chapter 3). ∞ Frequent assessment of the lungs, especially for diminished sounds at the right base caused by a pleural effusion or atelectasis, is necessary. If the effusion is large enough, it may require several thoracenteses or placement of a chest tube for drainage.

Nursing Care

Pain is common in postoperative patients and nurses must be vigilant in treating it in their patients. However, in a study of liver transplant patients by Del Barrio, Lacunza, Armendariz, Margall, and Asiain (2004) none of the participants remembered any pain. The authors believe it was because nurses utilized a pain management protocol and were very attentive to pain management postoperatively. "One patient expressed it as follows: 'The truth is that in those days I felt practically no pain, I am really quite certain about this, and I shall say again that I don't remember any pain'" (Del Barrio et al., 2004, p. 972). However, the liver transplant recipients in Del Barrio et al.'s study did recall great discomfort from thirst, heat, trouble sleeping, and restrictions to movement caused by invasive devices.

Imbalanced Nutrition

Malnutrition is a preoperative problem associated with ESLD and a postoperative complication for many liver transplant patients. However, attempts to replete the malnourished patient with liver failure often lead to hyperglycemia and an increase in the rate of complications (Pomposelli & Burns, 2002). Therefore, the goal of nutritional support is usually to provide adequate protein and energy from carbohydrates or fats equivalent to or slightly less than energy expenditure. If at all possible, nutritional requirements are provided enterally because parenteral nutrition is associated with increased risk of infection in the liver transplant recipient. Although any patient receiving immunosuppressants is at high risk for infection with parenteral nutrition, liver transplant recipients seem to be at an even higher risk due to "loss of much of their RES system" (Pomposelli & Burns, 2002, p. 345).

Conversely, as many as 40% of liver recipients are obese within 1 year of transplantation. Recipients' weights tend to increase for the first 2 years postoperatively and weight gains of 20% to 30% above pre-op weight may occur (Burke, 2003). Management is consistent with any program of weight management: careful reduction in caloric intake, accompanied by an increase in exercise.

Recovery

The first to fifth year survival rates for graft and patient postliver transplant are displayed in Table 15–4.

The causes of death in liver transplant recipients after the first year are graft failure (40%), cardiovascular

TABLE 15–4

Survival Following Liver Transplant 1997–2004 Identified as Percentage of Patients or Grafts Surviving

POSTTRANSPLANT DURATION	% OF PATIENTS SURVIVING	% GRAFT SURVIVING
1 year	87.7%	83.4%
3 years	79.9%	73.7%
5 years	74.3%	67.4%

disease (18%), infection (15%), and malignancy (8%) (Burke, 2003). The major sources of illness after the first year are clearly associated with the causes of death. Liver failure may be due to recurrence of liver diseases such as hepatitis or biliary cirrhosis. The following contributors to cardiovascular disease occur commonly:

> Hypertension occurring in between 41% and 81% of recipients
>
> Hypercholesterolemia (greater than 240 mg/dL) in 20% to 66% of recipients
>
> Diabetes occurring in 21% to 32% of recipients
>
> Obesity (body mass index [BMI] greater than 30) in 39% to 43% of recipients

Management of the precursors to cardiovascular disease in the postliver transplant patient is similar to management of any other patient with the problem. Skin cancer is the most common malignancy that develops post-transplant and is more aggressive in transplant recipients than in immunocompetent individuals. Recipients should be instructed to avoid the sun, to examine their own skin, and to have a yearly formal skin evaluation by a health care provider with referral to a dermatologist for any suspicious lesion.

Nursing Diagnoses

TRANSPLANT PATIENT

- Risk for infection related to inadequate secondary defenses (immunosuppression), malnutrition, indwelling catheters and drains or the presence of IVs and endotracheal tubes
- Risk for fluid volume excess related to renal insufficiency, steroid therapy or decreased cardiac output
- Risk for decreased cardiac output related to cardiac muscle disease
- Interrupted family processes related to illness of family member and situational crisis of transplant
- Disturbed body image related to permanent changes in body due to immunosuppressant medications and presence of donated organ

Psychosocial Issues in Transplant Recipients

During the first year following a transplant, many recipients experience some degree of psychosocial distress. The recipient's family may be overly involved in the health of the recipient with family life revolving around the recipient. If the patient received an organ from a family member, the donor and recipient may need to resolve some issues such as how much gratitude the recipient owes the donor, how close the two will remain, and the donor's fears that the recipient may not adhere to the medical regimen and adequately care for the organ. Common nursing diagnoses during this period are risk for ineffective individual coping and ineffective management of the therapeutic regimen.

Risk for Ineffective Individual Coping

According to Dew et al. (2003), numerous investigators have reported that important psychosocial issues arise during the first year following organ transplantation. Common psychosocial issues for patients and families relate to:

- Coping with the fear of rejection of the transplanted organ. Recipients and families express the most concern about this during the 6-week to 6-month period when they view their physical health as most likely to be in jeopardy (Jones, 2005).

- Accepting the changes in physical appearance that result from steroid therapy. Especially bothersome to female recipients may be the "moon face" and excessive facial hair growth that may develop from medications. Patients may feel they "no longer look like themselves" or may not be willing to socialize due to their appearance (Jones, 2005).

- Enduring the psychological highs and lows that sometimes occur as side effects of medications (Dew et al., 2003).

- Managing the complex posttransplant regimen (Dew et al., 2003). At about 6 months patients were beginning to manifest serious health-related side effects from the transplant regimen and the difficulty of continuing the treatment was becoming apparent to them.

- Integrating the transplant experience. Thirty percent of one sample of transplant recipients developed post-traumatic stress disorder (PTSD) during the first year post transplant. The symptoms ranged from having flashbacks about the transplant to inability to recall elements of the transplant to feelings of detachment from others and restricted affect. The recipients who had had an acute onset of illness and those with mild rather than severe symptoms were more likely to report PTSD (Mintzer et al., 2005). It appeared that the person's subjective appraisal of the threat was most important in the development of PTSD in this sample than the acuity of the patient's illness.

- Psychological acceptance of the transplant, for example, dealing with feelings of "split identities" or personality changes. This unsettled sense of self is most apparent at 6 months, and recipients seem to have established a new more stable sense of self by the end of the first year post transplant (Jones, 2005).
- Managing with economic and financial issues such as the high cost of medications and health care (Dew et al., 2003; Jones, 2005).

High levels of emotional distress, as well as clinically significant depression and anxiety, are more common during the first year after a transplant than during later years for all patients having organ transplants. It appears that recipients achieve relative stability after the first year (Dew et al., 2003). In heart recipients followed for 3 years following transplantation, the rate of new episodes of major depression decreased after the first year, and there were few new episodes of anxiety disorders in later years (Dew et al., 2003).

Ineffective Management of the Therapeutic Regimen

Compliance after transplantation, the degree to which patients' behaviors coincide with transplant team recommendations, is a major concern for transplant patients. Unfortunately, health care providers have not been successful at identifying ways to predict a patient's compliance with the complex posttransplant regimens (Dew et al., 2003). Therefore, it is unclear which patients are most likely to be noncompliant post transplant.

Noncompliance appears to be relatively common during the first year after transplantation and tends to worsen as time from transplantation increases. Dew et al. (2003) cite the following levels of noncompliance:

- As many as 20% of heart transplant recipients and 50% of kidney transplant recipients have been noncompliant with prescribed immunosuppressant medications during any given 12-month period.

- 5% to 26% of heart transplant recipients smoked at least once after their transplant.
- 11% to 48% of liver transplant recipients resume alcohol consumption during the first year post transplantation.

Adolescents are at particular risk to be noncompliant following transplantation. McAllister et al. (2006) found the following themes were associated with noncompliance in a qualitative study of adolescents following heart transplantation. In contrast to adolescents who adhered to medical therapy, less adherent recipients were less likely to have supportive friends and family available, more likely to have had dramatic changes in lifestyle, and more likely to have had negative cosmetic and physiological side effects from their medications. Because compliance with the medication regimen is essential for graft survival, it is important for the nurse caring for the posttransplant recipient to develop an accurate understanding of how often the recipient is complying with therapy and what factors are contributing to the recipient's difficulty in complying.

Support Groups

Many transplant patients and their families gain initial assistance and encouragement from support groups. Depending on the type of support group, patients and families may share their concerns and fears, receive educational information, share coping strategies, ask personal questions of people who have had similar problems, or receive assistance from social workers and transplant coordinators. Guest speakers may be invited to speak to the group about topics such as trends in transplantation or medications. Groups might share practical advice such as how to deal with insurance companies and where to purchase medications.

Talking with others with similar conditions can provide the new recipient with a feeling of security and comfort while assuring him that he and his family are "not alone." It is encouraging for new recipients to see how others who have had transplants for years and their families are coping. As a patient's transplant experience progresses, he may gain confidence and begin to provide assistance to others.

TRANSPLANT SUMMARY

Organ donation has been demonstrated to be an effective therapy for end-stage cardiac, liver, and renal disease. Unfortunately, due to the shortage of organs, many potential recipients spend a long time on the transplant waiting list. During their time on the waiting list, their physiological status often declines and some candidates die. The shortage of organs and resultant deaths of candidates waiting for organs has led health care providers and ethicists to consider ways to expand the

pool of potential donors. Caring for the potential donor and his family requires skill and compassion from the critical care nurse. When delivering care to the transplant recipient, the nurse recognizes there are some unique aspects to the patient's care. These include rejection, which requires the use of immunosuppressive drugs; an increased risk for infection; specific concerns related to which organ was transplanted; and psychosocial issues related to receiving an organ from another human being.

VISUAL MAP Transplant Recipient

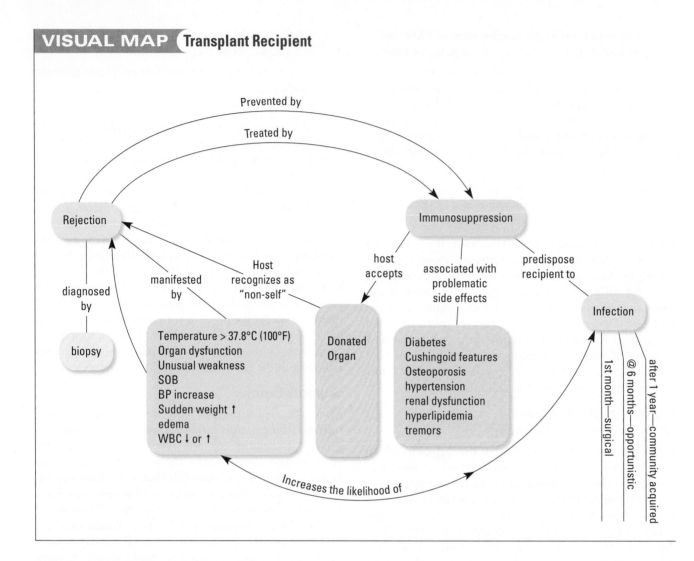

CASE STUDY

David Johnson a 22-year-old senior in college went to see his physician complaining of not feeling well. He stated that he had headaches that were increasing in frequency and that he was getting up three to four times each night to urinate. His BP was 138/96. David had been diagnosed with glomeulonephritis in high school but had avoided his health care provider since entering college.

His urinalysis revealed proteinuria and his renal ultrasound with biopsy confirmed rapid deterioration in renal function. During the next few months, his decline in renal function continued. He became depressed and stated that he was not able to attend class because he was so tired.

Some of his lab studies were: creatinine 6.1, BUN 63, potassium 5.7 (despite a low-potassium diet), Hct 26, and blood group AB positive.

David considered dialysis. However, both his sister and brother indicated that they would be willing to donate a kidney and the nephrologist concurred that if early donation was possible, David might do better. Initial testing was performed, David's sister was B positive and a 0 antigen mismatch. His brother was AB positive with no matching antigens.

1. Why is it a benefit for David to receive an organ from one of his siblings?

2. Which of David's siblings is the better choice for a donation? Why?

3. What other factors will need to be assessed about the potential donor?

David was scheduled to receive a transplant. Immediately prior to surgery, his BP was 167/92. His lab studies revealed that his creatinine was 8.1 and BUN 83. His potassium was 5.5, and Hct 26. His donated kidney began working immediately and by later that day his creatinine had decreased to 6. On day 3, he was feeling well, was up and walking, and his creatinine was 1.3, BP 132/84. He was discharged home, taking prednisone, CellCept, and tacrolimus.

4. For what symptoms should David be advised to contact his health care provider?

5. What precautions should David take to prevent infection?

About a month after discharge, David began to complain of pronounced hand tremors.

6. What is most likely to be causing the tremors?

Seven months after his transplant, David is feeling "lousy," he has gained 3 pounds in a few days, his BP is 150/90, and his creatinine is 3.4.

7. What is the most likely cause of his change in condition? What will be the probable management?

Five years following his kidney transplant, David has had three hip replacements.

8. What is the likely cause of his hip dysfunction?

See answers to Case Studies in the Answer Section at the back of the book.

CRITICAL THINKING QUESTIONS

1. What is the difference between opting in and opting out for consent for organ donation?

2. How is brain death diagnosed?

3. How can a nurse increase the likelihood that a family will donate a deceased person's organs?

4. Why is the calcineurin inhibitor, tacrolimus (FK506), preferred over cyclosporine?

5. Why are transplant recipients predisposed to develop infection?

6. Why is cytomegalovirus (CMV) a problematic infection in the transplant patient?

7. Differentiate between the four types of rejection. Which of the four types is associated with the highest morbidity and mortality for transplant recipients?

8. Why is parenteral nutrition a poor choice for provision of nutrition in the transplant recipient?

9. Why is the development of coronary artery disease of particular concern in the heart transplant recipient?

10. What factors affect patient compliance post transplantation? How can nurses improve patient compliance?

See answers to Critical Thinking Questions in the Answer Section at the back of the book.

EXPLORE MEDIALINK

http://www.prenhall.com/perrin

Additional interactive resources for this chapter can be found on the Web site at http://www.prenhall.com/perrin. Click on "Chapter 15" to select activities for this chapter.

Case Study: Transplant

Nursing Care Plan

NCLEX Review Questions

MediaLinks:
- *US Transplant—Scientific Registry of Transplant Recipients*
- The Organ Procurement and Transplant Network
- The *European International Foundation*

- *Give Life*, the transplant journey
- *Transplant Experience*
- *Transplant Living* is sponsored by Roche
- Nova: PBS
- Operation Heart Transplant or how to transplant a heart in 19 easy steps

MediaLink Applications

REFERENCES

American Academy of Neurology. (1995). Report of the Quality Standards Subcommittee of the American Academy of Neurology: Practice parameters: Determining brain death in adults. *Neurology, 45,* 1012–1014.

Baas, L. S., Bell, B., Giesting, R., McGuire, N., & Wagoner, L. E. (2003). Infections in the heart transplant recipient. *Critical Care Clinics of North America, 15,* 97–108.

Babruth, A. J. (2004). What every patient should know ... pretransplantation and posttransplantation. *Critical Care Nursing Quarterly, 27*(1), 31–60.

Burke, A. (2003). Medical management of the liver transplant patient. *Graft, 6*(2), 136–144.

Del Barrio, M., Lacunza, M., Armendariz, A. C., Margall, M., & Asiain, M. (2004). Liver transplant patients: Their experience in the intensive care unit. A phenomenological study. *Journal of Clinical Nursing, 13,* 967–976.

Dew, M. A., Manzetti, J., Goycoolea, J., Lee, R., Zomack, R., Vensak, J. L., et al. (2003). Psychologic aspects of transplantation. In *Organ transplantation: Concepts, issues, practice, and outcomes.* Retrieved March 27, 2007, from http://www.medscape.com/viewarticle/436541_3

Dosemeci, L., Cengiz, M., Yilmaz, M., & Razamoglu, A. (2004). Frequency of spinal reflexes in brain dead patients. *Transplant Proceedings, 36*(1), 17–20.

Dressler, D. (2003). Heart transplant. In *Organ transplantation: Concepts, issues, practice, and outcomes.* Retrieved March 27, 2007, from http://www.medscape.com/viewarticle/436544

Edwards, J., Mulvania, P., Robertson, V., George, G., Hasz, R., & D'Alessandro, A. (2006). Maximizing organ donation opportunities through donation after cardiac death. *Critical Care Nurse, 26*(2), 101–115.

Ehrle, R. (2006). Timely referral of potential organ donors. *Critical Care Nurse, 26*(2), 88–92.

Flowers, W., & Patel, B. R. (2000). Accuracy of clinical evaluation in the determination of brain death. *Southern Medical Journal, 93*(2), 203–207.

Henneman, E. H., & Karras, G. E. (2004). Determining brain death in adults: A guideline for use in critical care. *Critical Care Nurse, 24*(5), 50–56.

Hoffman, F. M., Nelson, B. J., Drangsbveit, M. B., Flynn, B. M., Watercott, E. A., & Zirbes, J. M. (2006). Caring for transplant recipients in a nontransplant setting. *Critical Care Nurse, 26*(2), 53–74.

Jones, J. B. (2005). Liver transplant recipients' first year of posttransplant recovery: A longitudinal study. *Progress in Transplantation, 15*(4), 345–352.

Lindenfeld, J., Miller, G. G., Shakar, S. F., Zolty, R., Lowes, B., Wolfel, E. E., et al. (2004). Drug therapy in the heart transplant recipient. Part II: Immunosuppressive drugs. *Circulation, 110,* 3858–3865.

Mansarheitia, C., & Smith, S. (2003). Liver transplantation. In *Organ transplantation: Concepts, issues, practice, and outcomes.* Retrieved March 27, 2007, from http://www.medscape.com/viewarticle/451209

McAllister, S., Buckner, E., & White-Williams, C. (2006). Medication adherence after heart transplant: Adolescents and their issues. *Progress in Transplantation, 16*(4), 317–323.

McDevitt, L. M. (2006). Etiology and impact of cytomegalovirus disease on solid organ transplant recipients. *American Journal of Health-Systems Pharmacists, 63*(Suppl.), 3–9.

Mintzer, L. L., Stuber, M. L., Deacord, D., Castaneda, M., Mesrhhani, V., & Glover, D. (2005). Traumatic stress symptoms in adolescent organ transplant recipients. *Pediatrics, 115*(6), 1640–1644.

O'Connor, K. J., Wood, K. E., & Lord, K. (2006). Intensive management of organ donors to maximize transplantation. *Critical Care Nurse, 26*(2), 94–100.

Pomposelli, J. J., & Burns, D. L. (2002). Nutrition support in the liver transplant patient. *Nutrition in Clinical Practice, 17*(6), 341–349.

Randhawa, G. (1998). Coping with grieving relatives and making a request for organs. *Medical Teacher, 20,* 247.

Rodrigue, J. R., Cornell, D. L., & Howard, R. J. (2006). Organ donation decision: Comparison of donor and nondonor families. *American Journal of Transplantation, 6,* 190–198.

Rudlow, D. L., Charlton, M., Sanchez, C., & Chang, S. (2005). Kidney and liver living donors: A comparison of experiences. *Progress in Transplantation, 15,* 185–191.

Salim, A. (2006). Organ retrieval in brain death. *The American Surgeon, 72,* 377–381.

Scandling, J. D. (2005). Kidney transplant candidate evaluation. *Seminars in Dialysis, 18*(6), 487–494.

Shah, V., & Bhosale, G. (2006). Organ donation problems and their management. *Indian Journal of Critical Care Medicine, 10*(1), 29–34.

Shapiro, R., Young, J. B., Milford, E. L., Trotter, J. F., Bustami, R. T., & Leichtman, A. B. (2005). Immunosuppression: Evolution in practice and trends, 1993–2003. *American Journal of Transplantation, 5,* 874–886.

Society of Critical Care Medicine. (2001). Recommendations for nonheartbeating organ donation. *Critical Care Medicine, 29*(9), 1826–1831.

Sommerer, C., Wiesel, M., Schweitzer-Rothers, J., Ritz, E., & Zeier, M. (2003). The living kidney donor: Giving life, avoiding harm. *Nephrology, Dialysis, Transplantation, 18,* 23–26.

Staatz, C., & Tett, S. E. (2005). Pharmacokinetic considerations relating to tacrolimus dosing in the elderly. *Drugs in Aging, 22*(7), 541–557.

Steinberg, D. (2004). An "opting in" paradigm for kidney transplant. *The American Journal of Bioethics, 4*(4), 4–14.

Stitt, N. L. (2003). Infections in the transplant recipient. In *Organ transplantation: Concepts, issues, practice, and outcomes.* Retrieved March 27, 2007, from http://www.medscape.com/viewarticle/451788

Tamburri, L. M. (2006). The role of the critical care nurse in the organ donation breakthrough collaborative. *Critical Care Nurse, 26*(2), 20–24.

Tritt, L. (2004). Nutritional assessment and support of kidney transplant recipients. *Journal of Infusion Nursing, 27*(1), 45–50.

United Network for Organ Sharing (UNOS). (2007). *U.S. transplantation data.* Retrieved March 7, 2007, from http://www.unos.org/data/default.asp?displayType=usData

Wijdicks, E. (2001). The diagnosis of brain death. *New England Journal of Medicine, 344*(16), 1215–1222.

Winsett, P., Martin, J., Reed, L., & Bateman, C. (2003). Kidney transplantation. In *Organ transplantation: Concepts, issues, practice, and outcomes.* Retrieved March 27, 2007, from http://www.medscape.com/viewarticle/443490

Wolfe, R. (2005). The state of kidney transplantation in the United States. *Seminars in Dialysis, 18*(6), 453–455.

Zink, S., & Wertlieb, S. (2006). A study of the presumptive approach to consent for organ donation: A new approach to an old problem. *Critical Care Nurse, 26,* 129–136.

Care of the Acutely Ill Burn Patient

Linda S. Edelman, RN, PhD

Learning Outcomes

Upon completion of this chapter, the learner will be able to:

1. Explain the common etiologies of burn injuries.

2. Evaluate the severity of a burn injury.

3. Describe the manifestations of an inhalation injury.

4. Explain the changes within body systems that occur following a burn injury.

5. Describe initial assessment and management of a patient with a burn injury.

6. Explain priorities in the care of the patient with major burns during the resuscitation phase.

7. Discuss wound management during the acute phase following burn injury.

8. Develop a plan to meet the needs of the burn injury patient during the rehabilitation phase.

9. Analyze the specific needs of older adult patients with a burn injury.

Abbreviations

ABLS	Advance Burn Life Support
BMR	Basal Metabolic Rate
IAP	Intra-Abdominal Pressure
TBSA	Total Body Surface Area
VAC	Vacuum-Assisted Closure

Burn injuries occur as a result of exposure to heat, chemicals, radiation, or electric current. The resulting transfer of energy from the heat source to the body initiates local changes to the integumentary system, including tissue destruction and initiation of the inflammatory cascade, which, in severe burns, can lead to a systemic response involving all body systems. Treatments range from over-the-counter topical agents for minor burns to specialized care for major burns provided in a burn intensive care unit. Specialized burn care involves skin grafting and other surgical procedures, hemodynamic monitoring, and ventilator support.

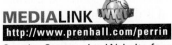

MEDIALINK
http://www.prenhall.com/perrin

See the Companion Website for chapter-specific resources at www.prenhall.com/perrin.

Over one million burn injuries occur in the United States each year, resulting in approximately 500,000 emergency department visits and 40,000 hospital admissions (American Burn Association, 2007a). Approximately 4,000 of these injuries are fatal, making burns the fourth leading cause of death from unintentional injury (American Burn Association). The majority of burn injuries and deaths occur as a result of residential fires (Runyan, Bangdiwala, Linzer, Sacks, & Butts, 1992) and 40% to 50% of these deaths could be prevented by working smoke alarms (Ahrens, 2001). Most burn injuries are unintentional, but intentional burns are forms of child and elder abuse (Pruitt, Wolf, & Mason, 2007).

Men are at increased risk for burn injury. The 2006 National Burn Repository report states that nearly 70% of burn patients admitted to U.S. burn centers are male (Kerby et al., 2006). Gender differences in rates of burn injury occur early, with males being the majority of burns occurring to individuals under the age of 16 treated in emergency departments (Rawlins, Khan, Shenton, & Sharpe, 2007). The patterns of injury are different between genders. Men are burned more often by fire/flame, whereas women experience more scald injuries (Kerby et al., 2006). Men tend to have larger cutaneous burns and are more likely to sustain inhalation injury.

Children and the elderly are at increased risk of burn injury and are more likely to die as a result of their injury. Children under 4 years of age are at particular risk for burn injury because of impulsivity and the inability to move away from a burn source. The majority of pediatric burn injuries and deaths are a result of scald injuries and residential fires. The elderly are at risk because of sensational and mobility impairments associated with aging and because of environmental risks such as living in older homes, using older appliances, and not having operational smoke alarms (Istre, McCoy, Osborn, Barnard, & Bolton, 2001). Other factors associated with increased risk of burn injury include living in rural areas, poverty, and race.

Burn rates have declined over the last several decades as have the number of hospitalizations for burn treatment. Most burns are minor and can be treated in outpatient clinics and emergency departments. More severe burns are treated in hospitals or burn centers. Burn care for these patients has also advanced dramatically during the past few decades, resulting in declining death rates. Because the majority of burns are minor, nurses in outpatient and emergency department settings must be familiar with how to assess the severity of a burn, pro- vide basic wound care, and support the unique psychosocial needs of burn patients and their caregivers. Nurses working in specialized burn centers are part of a multidisciplinary team that comprehensively treats patients through the resuscitation, acute care, and rehabilitation phases of a burn injury.

Etiology of Injury

The causes of burn injury may be thermal (heat) or non-thermal (electricity, chemical, or radiation). These etiologies all result in tissue damage; however, the causative agents and the initial treatment measures differ.

Thermal Burns

The most common burns are thermal in nature and are caused by exposure to heat. Thermal burns include fire/flame injuries, scald injuries from exposure to hot liquids or steam, and contact/friction injuries. Scald injuries are the most common form of burns, but fire/flame injuries account for the majority of deaths. The majority of thermal burns occur in the home, and the young and elderly are at particular risk.

Scald injuries may be caused by hot liquids or steam. Exposure to 120°F water for 5 minutes can cause a scald in a healthy adult (American Burn Association, 2008b). The exposure time required to sustain a scald injury is decreased to 1 second when the water temperature is 155°F (see Safety Initiatives: Burn Prevention Education). Severe burns can occur in children and the elderly at lower temperatures and exposure times. The majority of scalds occur in children less than 4 years of age. In this population, scalds are caused by pulling hot liquids onto themselves or by being placed in bath water that is too hot. The elderly and disabled individuals are at risk for scalding by hot bath water because of impaired sensation, slower reaction times, and decreased mobility. Grease and hot cooking liquid injuries are common scald injuries in adults. Kitchen-related scalds and hot tar burns are common work-related injuries.

The majority of fire/flame injuries are caused by residential fires. Many of these injuries are caused by the misuse of fuels and flammable liquids. Other fire/flame injuries are automobile related, including flash burns sustained while repairing carburetors and starting boat motors, and burns resulting from ignition of fuel following an automobile crash. Fire/flame injuries tend to be larger and more severe than other burn etiologies. These injuries account for the majority of admissions to specialized burn centers and are more likely to result in death (Pruitt et al., 2007).

Ignition of clothing is a common source of thermal injury in all age groups and is the second most common cause of fatal burns (Pruitt et al., 2007). In particular, ignition of synthetic fabrics that melt and adhere to the skin results in more severe burns.

VISUAL MAP Burns Pathophysiology

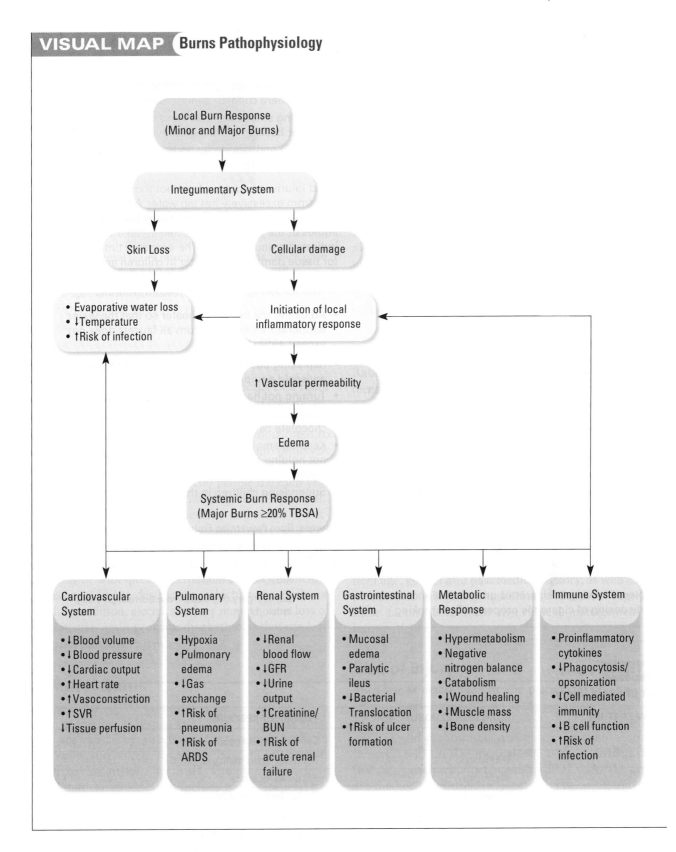

Local Burn Response
(Minor and Major Burns)

↓

Integumentary System

↓ ↓

Skin Loss   Cellular damage

↓ ↓

• Evaporative water loss   Initiation of local
• ↓Temperature   inflammatory response
• ↑Risk of infection

↑ Vascular permeability

Edema

Systemic Burn Response
(Major Burns ≥20% TBSA)

Cardiovascular System
• ↓Blood volume
• ↓Blood pressure
• ↓Cardiac output
• ↑Heart rate
• ↑Vasoconstriction
• ↑SVR
↓Tissue perfusion

Pulmonary System
• Hypoxia
• Pulmonary edema
• ↓Gas exchange
• ↑Risk of pneumonia
• ↑Risk of ARDS

Renal System
• ↓Renal blood flow
• ↓GFR
• ↓Urine output
• ↑Creatinine/BUN
• ↑Risk of acute renal failure

Gastrointestinal System
• Mucosal edema
• Paralytic ileus
• ↓Bacterial Translocation
• ↑Risk of ulcer formation

Metabolic Response
• Hypermetabolism
• Negative nitrogen balance
• Catabolism
• ↓Wound healing
• ↓Muscle mass
• ↓Bone density

Immune System
• Proinflammatory cytokines
• ↓Phagocytosis/opsonization
• ↓Cell mediated immunity
• ↓B cell function
• ↑Risk of infection

Other thermal burns include contact and friction injuries. Contact injuries occur when the body comes in contact with a hot object. Common sources of contact burns are motorcycle mufflers and campfire coals. The young, elderly, and disabled are at risk for burns caused by heating pads and blankets as well as other hot appliances. Common sources of friction burns are "road rashes" from motor vehicle accidents and, particularly in children, contact with treadmills or other fast-moving machinery.

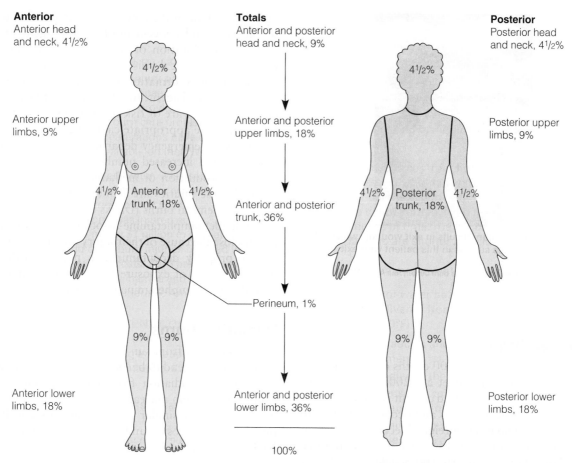

Figure 16-2 Rule of nines. The "rule of nines" is one method for quickly estimating the percentage of TBSA affected by a burn injury. Although useful in emergency care situations, the rule of nines is not accurate for estimating TBSA for adults who are short, obese, or very thin.

and Browder chart (Figure 16-3). This chart determines the percentage TBSA burned for each body part according to the age of the client. It also allows clinicians to document the percentage TBSA according to burn depth.

The calculation of burn size is very subjective. Therefore, computer programs, such as the Web-based Sage diagram, have been developed to increase the reproducibility of burn size assessments. Three-dimensional or laser imaging to calculate the surface area of wounds is a developing technology that may help increase the accuracy of burn assessments in the future (Neuwalder, Sampson, Breuing, & Orgill, 2002).

Depth of Injury

The depth of burn injury is determined by the depth of tissue destruction (Figure 16-4). A number of factors contribute to burn depth, including the etiology, temperature and duration of the burning agent, and skin thickness.

Superficial, or first-degree burns, involve only the epidermal layer of the skin, leaving the skin intact (Figure 16-5). The involved skin is pink to red in color and slightly edematous. Blisters will not form until after 24 hours if at all. The TBSA of first-degree burns is not usually included in burn size estimates because these burns will heal without scarring in 3 to 6 days. However, extensive first-degree burns may cause chills, headaches, nausea and vomiting, and considerable pain. Common etiologies of first-degree burns are sunburns and minor flash burns.

A partial-thickness, or second-degree, burn involves the epidermal and dermal layers of the skin, but the hair follicles, sebaceous glands, and epidermal sweat glands remain intact (Figure 16-6). A partial-thickness burn is further classified into either a superficial or deep second-degree burn by the amount of dermis involved. A superficial partial-thickness burn does not involve the entire depth of the dermis. The burn wound is often bright red in color and edematous.

Area	Age (years)					% 1°	% 2°	% 3°	% Total
	0–1	1–4	5–9	10–15	Adult				
Head	19	17	13	10	7				
Neck	2	2	2	2	2				
Ant. trunk	13	13	13	13	13				
Post. trunk	13	13	13	13	13				
R. buttock	$2\frac{1}{2}$	$2\frac{1}{2}$	$2\frac{1}{2}$	$2\frac{1}{2}$	$2\frac{1}{2}$				
L. buttock	$2\frac{1}{2}$	$2\frac{1}{2}$	$2\frac{1}{2}$	$2\frac{1}{2}$	$2\frac{1}{2}$				
Genitalia	1	1	1	1	1				
R.U. arm	4	4	4	4	4				
L.U. arm	4	4	4	4	4				
R.L. arm	3	3	3	3	3				
L.L. arm	3	3	3	3	3				
R. hand	$2\frac{1}{2}$	$2\frac{1}{2}$	$2\frac{1}{2}$	$2\frac{1}{2}$	$2\frac{1}{2}$				
L. hand	$2\frac{1}{2}$	$2\frac{1}{2}$	$2\frac{1}{2}$	$2\frac{1}{2}$	$2\frac{1}{2}$				
R. thigh	$5\frac{1}{2}$	$6\frac{1}{2}$	$8\frac{1}{2}$	$8\frac{1}{2}$	$9\frac{1}{2}$				
L. thigh	$5\frac{1}{2}$	$6\frac{1}{2}$	$8\frac{1}{2}$	$8\frac{1}{2}$	$9\frac{1}{2}$				
R. leg	5	5	$5\frac{1}{2}$	6	7				
L. leg	5	5	$5\frac{1}{2}$	6	7				
R. foot	$3\frac{1}{2}$	$3\frac{1}{2}$	$3\frac{1}{2}$	$3\frac{1}{2}$	$3\frac{1}{2}$				
L. foot	$3\frac{1}{2}$	$3\frac{1}{2}$	$3\frac{1}{2}$	$3\frac{1}{2}$	$3\frac{1}{2}$				
					Total				

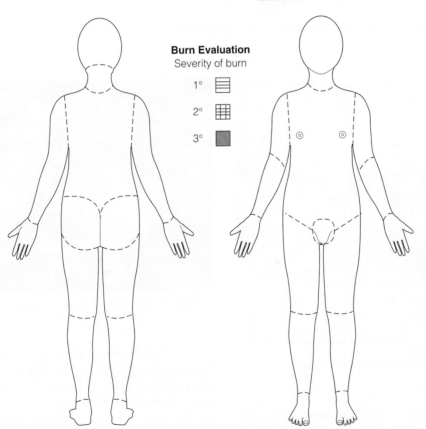

Burn Evaluation
Severity of burn

1°
2°
3°

Figure 16-3 Lund and Browder burn assessment chart. This method of estimating TBSA affected by a burn injury is more accurate than the "rule of nines" because it accounts for changes in body surface area across the life span.

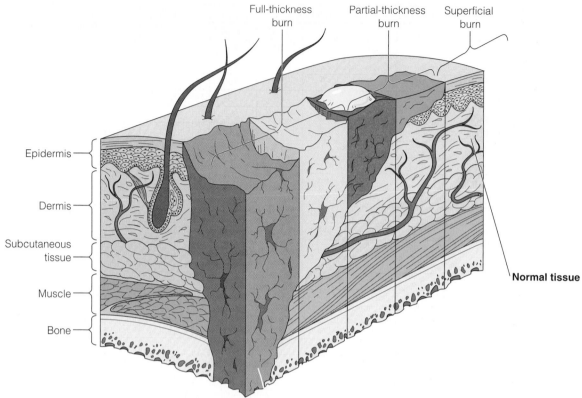

Figure 16-4 Depth of burn injury. Burn injury classification according to the depth of the burn.

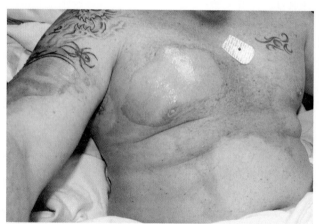

Figure 16-5 First- and second-degree burns. This patient sustained burns to the chest. The first-degree burn areas in the center of the chest and the right side of the abdomen are red but the skin is intact. The second-degree burn above the right nipple line is red and moist.
(Courtesy of University of Michigan Trauma Burn Center, Ann Arbor, MI)

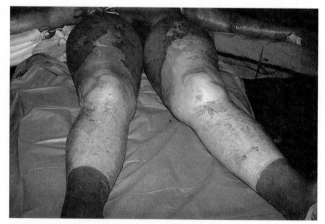

Figure 16-6 Partial-thickness burn injury.
(Courtesy of the University of Utah Burn Center)

Capillary refill is near normal. The surface is moist and thin-walled, fluid-filled blisters appear within minutes. A superficial partial-thickness burn is very painful and sensation to even very superficial pressure, such as air currents, is increased. Healing occurs within 21 days with little to no scarring. A deep partial-thickness burn involves the entire dermis. The wound appearance is white and waxy and capillary refill is decreased. The surface may be wet or dry and blisters can range from large and fluid filled to flat. When nerve fibers are destroyed, there is less pain and decreased sensation even to deep touch. A deep partial-thickness burn heals in approximately 3 weeks and scarring is likely. Initially, a deep partial-thickness burn may appear to be a full-thickness burn, but after 7 to 10 days skin buds and hair growth will be noticeable, indicating that the skin appendages are intact. However, some burns that initially appeared to be deep second-degree burns may progress to full-thickness injuries due to decreased blood supply or infection.

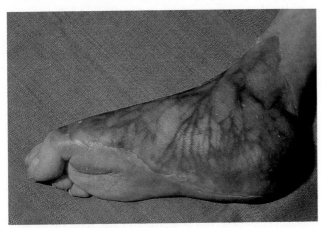

Figure 16-7 Full-thickness burn injury.
(Courtesy of University of Utah Burn Center)

A full-thickness, or third-degree, burn involves all layers of the skin, including the hair follicles, sebaceous glands, and the epidermal sweat glands (Figure 16-7). The wound color ranges from very pale to bright red; but, unlike a second-degree burn, there is little to no capillary refill and thrombosed blood vessels may be evident. The surface of the wound is dry, firm, and may have a leathery feel. A third-degree burn has no sensation to deep pressure. There is no pain because the nerve endings have been destroyed. Skin grafting is required for a third-degree burn to heal.

If the burn extends into the subcutaneous tissue, muscle, or bone, it is classified as a fourth-degree burn. The extremities may appear charred and mummified. Amputation is usually required. Fourth-degree burns are associated with high morbidity and mortality.

Other Factors Contributing to Burn Severity

Although the percentage of TBSA involved and the depth of injury are the primary classifications of burn severity, several other factors also contribute to the severity of the burn.

Location of Injury

The area of the body that is burned can contribute to severity of injury. Edema from burns to the face can cause acute airway compromise. Scarring is always a concern for individuals with burns to the face. Other body areas of concern are the genitalia, hands, and feet because of scarring and loss of function. A burn that extends over major joints also can be more serious because of the risk of developing joint contractures, resulting in loss of mobility. Injury to all of these areas can result in long-term morbidity and often require the specialized treatment provided by burn centers.

Age and Gender

Historically, mortality rates following burn injury have been the highest in the very young and the elderly. Pedi-

Gerontological Considerations

More than a thousand Americans over the age of 65 die as a result of fire each year, constituting approximately 25% of all fire-related deaths. For each decade over the age of 65, the death rate from a fire increases onefold. Because older adults are more likely to die from a major burn injury, they are best treated in a specialized burn center.

Older adults with impaired hearing often do not have fire alarms that compensate for their impairment, they may not hear an alarm, and they may not be able to evacuate a burning building promptly.

Fires caused by smoking are the leading cause of death in older adults. Fires due to smoking are especially dangerous in older adults because older adults are more likely to have concurrent respiratory problems (chronic obstructive lung disease, asthma, or lung cancer). In addition, when the older person has been smoking, his clothing or bedding is likely to be ignited early in the fire.

Approximately 3,000 older adults are injured in residential fires each year, with cooking fires being the leading cause of injuries. Because they have thinner skin, when older adults receive burn injuries they often get more severe burns at lower temperatures and in less time than younger adults. In addition, the older adult may delay seeking treatment for the burn due to a diminished sense of pain. The effect of such a delay can be devastating; when treatment is delayed from 2 to 5 hours the mortality increases fivefold.

Tap water injuries may cause fatalities in older adults if the person falls, faints, or remains in a bathtub with water that is too hot. The recommended maximum setting for home water heaters is 120°F (48.9°C). Heating pads are another common cause of minor burns that may lead to major burns in older adults with sensory or cognitive deficits.

Preexisting health conditions influence how the older adult responds to the acute injury. The patient with heart problems must be closely monitored during fluid resuscitation and a balance must be maintained between providing adequate resuscitation to the tissues and further stressing the heart. The older adult with an inhalation injury may require more ventilatory support and is at increased risk for developing pneumonia or sepsis. Wound healing is delayed in the older adult, and finding good donor sites for skin grafting can be a problem. The older adult becomes debilitated more rapidly after a burn injury and return to preburn function is more difficult.

atric patients can now survive very large and deep burns due to advances in pediatric burn care. However, mortality rates in the elderly remain high due to a number of reasons. The elderly individual with decreased mobility may have trouble extinguishing or escaping the heat source and thus may sustain a more extensive and deep burn. Elderly skin is thinner and less elastic, resulting in deeper depth of burn. Chronic health problems in the elderly decrease the ability of the body to handle the systemic stress placed on it by a burn injury.

Women are at decreased risk for burn injury but they have been reported to have increased mortality rates. Female gender has been proposed as a risk factor for mortality that is independent of age, burn size, or the presence of inhalation injury. The findings are most conclusive in women of reproductive age, suggesting that sex hormones may play a role (George et al., 2005; Kerby et al., 2006). Etiology of injury, preburn health status, and social factors may also influence the increased risk of mortality seen in women.

Concurrent Health Problems

The patient with chronic health problems has increased morbidity following a burn injury. It is important that a complete medical history is obtained from the burn patient. Particular attention should be paid to the patient with a history of cardiac, pulmonary, or renal disease because of the stress a burn injury places on these systems. Individuals with a history of diabetes, peripheral vascular disease, or impaired skin integrity may have decreased wound healing of even minor burns. Immunosuppression from disease or steroid use also increases morbidity.

Inhalation Injury

Approximately one third of patients admitted to burn centers have concomitant smoke inhalation injury (Traber, Herndon, Enkhbaatar, Maybauer, & Maybauer, 2007). The patient with an inhalation injury has a mortality rate of 5% to 8%; this risk increases to over 20% if the patient also has cutaneous burns (Sen & Gamelli, 2005). Inhalation injury results in pulmonary edema, which predisposes the burn patient to pulmonary failure, infection, and long-term pulmonary complications; these are discussed in detail later in this chapter.

Pathophysiology of Burn Injury

A burn injury rapidly invokes a multisystem physiological response (see Visual Map on page 415). The extent of this response depends on the size and depth of injury. Minor burns produce a localized response involving the integumentary system. Moderate and more severe burns result in changes that are systemic and long lasting. Major burns, those involving more than 20% TBSA, produce a pathophysiologic response involving all body systems. As a rule of thumb, therapeutic intervention is necessary in order for an individual with a major burn to survive.

Integumentary System

The skin is the largest organ in the body, accounting for 20% of the body's weight. It serves as a barrier to infection, ultraviolet radiation, and fluid loss. An important function of the skin is body temperature regulation. Touch and pressure receptors in the skin help protect the body from the environment and mechanical injury.

Anatomy of the Skin

The skin has three layers: the epidermis, the dermis, and the subcutaneous layer (refer to the layers of the skin depicted in Figure 16-1). The outermost layer, the epidermis, is a protective layer that is continually regenerating. The epidermis varies in thickness depending on location. Therefore, the sole of the foot will receive a less severe burn than the perineum when exposed to the same heat source. The epidermis is thinner in the very young and the elderly, putting them at increased risk for more serious burn injury. Keratinocytes, the primary cells of the epidermis, are produced in the basal layer and then move upward, first becoming enlarged and then flattened and stacked. At the skin surface the keratinocytes are dead and cornified, and they function as a protective barrier and in preventing evaporative water loss. The epidermis contains other cells that provide further protection. Melanocytes produce melatonin that provides skin color and shields the body from ultraviolet radiation. Langerhans cells, which migrate from the bone marrow, initiate an immune response against environmental antigens.

The second layer of the skin is the dermis, which is composed primarily of connective tissue. Also located in the dermis are fibroblasts, mast cells, and macrophages, which are important in immune regulation and the inflammatory response. The dermis provides the elasticity necessary for movement. The dermal appendages, including sweat and sebaceous glands and hair follicles, are located in the dermis. The papillary capillaries, located in the dermis, provide blood to the skin and dermal appendages. Sweat glands and arteriovenous anastomoses in the dermis are important in thermoregulation. The dermis also contains nerves and lymphatic vessels.

The third layer of the skin is the subcutaneous layer, which is composed of lobules of fat cells separated by walls of collagen and large blood vessels. The subcutaneous layer serves as a heat insulator, shock absorber, and nutritional reserve.

Burn Injury

The skin damage resulting from a burn injury depends on the amount and duration of heat as well as the body location. Because the thickness and vascularization of the skin vary, skin dissipates heat from a burn differently depending on location. If the microcirculation of the skin is not damaged by the heat source, such as in a first-degree burn, the dermis is protected. When the microcirculation is damaged, the skin cannot cool itself after the heat source is removed and the burning process continues, resulting in damage to the dermis.

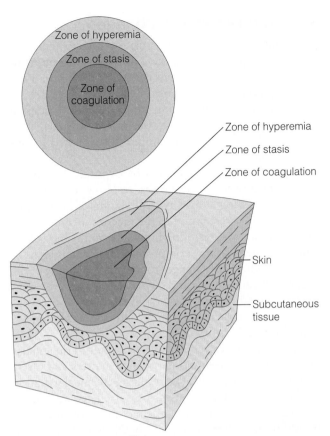

Figure 16-8 The zones of injury.

Zones of Injury. A burn injury causes a bull's-eye pattern of injury on the skin surface. The deepest part of the burn is in the center with less deep areas surrounding it to form the periphery of the injury. One to three zones of injury develop depending on the depth of injury (Figure 16-8). Third-degree burns develop all three zones, beginning with the inner **zone of coagulation**, which is the deepest part of the burn. The cells are nonviable and the microcirculation is destroyed, leaving the skin dark colored and leathery. The hard crust that forms over the nonviable necrotic tissue is called eschar. The medial **zone of stasis** is composed of viable and nonviable cells. There is damage to the microcirculation, resulting in vasoconstriction and ischemia. The skin initially appears moist or blistered and is red in color. Capillary refill is delayed. Spontaneous healing can occur, but persistent inflammation or infection can result in further loss of perfusion and subsequent conversion with the zone of coagulation. The outer **zone of hyperemia** is tissue with intact microvasculature that heals spontaneously within days. The area initially appears pink and capillary refill may be increased due to vasodilation induced by local inflammatory mediators.

Alterations in Skin Function. The skin is sterile immediately after a burn injury. Eschar develops over the burn wound and provides the perfect medium for bacterial growth. The burn wound soon becomes colonized

with bacteria and yeast, which are normal flora of the accessory glands of the skin, respiratory, and gastrointestinal tracts (Sharma, 2007). Burn patients are at risk for developing nosocomial infections. Hospital infection protocols should be followed, aseptic technique should be used when handling the burn wounds, and dressings should be changed regularly. The wound should be assessed for signs and symptoms of infection at each dressing change and appropriate treatment initiated.

Patients with large burns are more susceptible to infection and have difficulty regulating body temperature even after the burn wound is healed. Healed burned areas are more susceptible to mechanical injury as a consequence of changes in the texture of the skin and loss of sensory perception. Sun exposure should be avoided because burned areas are more susceptible to ultraviolet radiation. In addition, patients with deep partial-thickness and full-thickness burns have a decreased ability to synthesize vitamin D when exposed to sunlight.

Cardiovascular System Changes

A burn injury can cause a variety of cardiovascular system changes, particularly in individuals with preexisting cardiovascular disease. The most common cardiovascular change is hypovolemic burn shock. Other changes include alterations in cardiac rhythm and peripheral extremity vascular compromise.

Within minutes of a burn injury, increased capillary permeability in burned areas where the microcirculation is not destroyed results in edema formation. The extent of edema depends on burn severity and body parts affected. Burn edema is greatest over areas where the skin is less elastic, such as the face and genitals, and less over areas with increased elasticity, such as the extremities. Increased vascular permeability is present for approximately the first 24 hours after injury. Without intervention, burn edema decreases over the first 72 hours following injury as circulating blood volumes increase and diuresis occurs. Factors that contribute to sustained burn edema are extremes of age, burn severity, and cardiovascular compromise. In addition, fluid resuscitation can contribute to increased and sustained burn edema.

Burn Shock

Burn edema is generalized in the patient with major burns (Figure 16-9). Resulting burn shock has two components. The cellular component of burn shock is the result of damage to cells in the burn wound. Damaged cells have altered membrane potential that results in metabolic and immune changes, which are discussed in subsequent sections. The hypovolemic cardiovascular component is a result of the massive decrease in circulating blood volume as systemic edema develops. The loss of plasma blood volume results in hyperviscosity of the blood and slowed capillary circulation. Burn shock occurs when

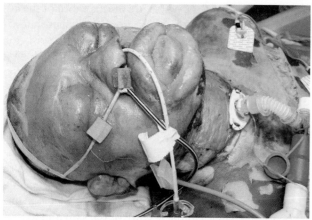

Figure 16-9 The edema associated with large burn injuries can be extensive. Patients with massive facial edema are at risk for airway obstruction.
(Courtesy of University of Michigan Trauma Burn Center, Ann Arbor, MI)

blood pressure and cardiac output decrease to compensate for blood volume losses. As a result, tachycardia and vasoconstriction occur, increasing systemic vascular resistance (SVR) and pulmonary vascular resistance (PVR). The release of inflammatory mediators suppresses myocardial contractility. Electrolyte imbalances can arise and contribute to the development of cardiac dysrhythmias.

White blood cells (WBCs) and platelets accumulate in the tissue surrounding the burn. The combination of vasoconstriction with the accumulation of WBCs and platelets contributes to decreased tissue perfusion. Decreased perfusion to the burn causes ischemia, which can progress to necrosis. Prolonged ischemia and lack of oxygen to damaged tissue can cause burn depth to increase. Large burns require fluid resuscitation to reverse burn shock and prevent further complications such as acute renal failure and cardiovascular collapse. However, despite adequate fluid resuscitation, cardiac output remains decreased in patients with large burns during the acute burn phase. Fluid status assessment and prompt alterations in resuscitation parameters is an important nursing function.

Other Cardiovascular Changes

Burns can cause myocardial changes. Electrical injuries can result in dysrhythmias or cardiac arrest by interfering with the electrical activity of the heart or by direct heat to the myocardium. Inflammatory mediators produced in response to a large thermal injury can cause myocardial ischemia, which leads to decreased contractility and cardiac output.

Peripheral vascular compromise occurs in individuals with extremity burns. Peripheral vasoconstriction from burn shock and edema contribute to decreased perfusion. Circumferential extremity burns are at risk for developing compartment syndrome in which the pressure within the muscle compartments is greater than within the microvasculature.

Respiratory System Changes

Pulmonary damage occurs either by direct inhalation injury or as part of the systemic response to burn injury. Patients exposed to smoke or heat within an enclosed place, or those near an explosion, are at increased risk for inhalation injury that can occur in the absence of cutaneous burns. Individuals with singed scalp or facial hair should be evaluated for inhalation injury.

Inhalation injury is caused by exposure of the airways to heat or toxic substances, resulting in damage to the upper and lower airways. Inhalation of heat immediately causes direct injury to the mucous membranes of the upper airways, resulting in inflammation and edema and subsequent airway compromise. Immediate signs of inhalation injury are changes to the mucosal lining of the oropharynx and larynx and include the presence of soot, hoarseness, edema, or blisters. Symptoms of direct injury occur over the first 24 hours and include stridor, hypoxia, and respiratory distress.

Injury to the lower airways is a result of the inhalation of noxious gases and particulate matters and rarely of direct thermal injury. The resulting chemical irritation of the alveolar tissue causes loss of ciliary action, increased mucus production, edema, and bronchospasm. In addition, carbon monoxide (CO), which is a compound in smoke, rapidly diffuses into the bloodstream and directly impairs oxygen utilization by displacing oxygen on hemoglobin. The patient with a lower airway injury may not initially show signs of respiratory difficulty and have normal arterial blood gases and chest x-rays for the first 24 hours, after which chest x-rays may show the development of patchy atelectasis. Inhalation injury increases the risk of developing infection, respiratory failure, and acute respiratory distress syndrome (ARDS). Morbidity and mortality are greatly increased.

Burn shock contributes to pulmonary changes following burn injury. Patients with major burns may develop pulmonary edema as a result of increased PVR. Immune system changes can increase the risk of developing pneumonia and ARDS, particularly in patients requiring mechanical ventilation for extended periods.

Gastrointestinal System Changes

The systemic vasoconstriction caused by burn shock often results in the development of paralytic ileus and mucosal edema. The patient with paralytic ileus is at risk for abdominal distention, nausea, vomiting, and hematemesis. A nasogastric tube is placed in the patient with a major burn to prevent abdominal distension and aspiration if emesis occurs. Bowel ischemia can lead to increased intestinal mucosal permeability, which allows bacterial translocation from the lumen of the gut to the mesenteric lymph nodes and systemic tissues. Bacterial translocation increases the risk of systemic infection and multiple-organ dysfunction syndrome (MODS)

(Magnotti & Deitch, 2005). Stress ulcers in the stomach or duodenum are common in burn patients. Symptoms of a stress ulcer, which can occur after the acute phase of the burn injury, include abdominal pain, hematemesis, and melenic stools. Symptoms can arise quickly, and close attention should be paid to hematocrit levels because patients often require blood transfusions.

Renal System Changes

Renal blood flow and glomerular filtration rates are greatly decreased during the hypovolemic burn shock phase of burn injury. As a result urine output is decreased and serum creatinine and blood urea nitrogen increase. Hemoglobinuria-free hemoglobin from destroyed red blood cells (RBCs) and myoglobinuria—myoglobin released from damaged muscle cells—can cause urine to be dark brown. Acute renal failure can develop if fluids are not administered and renal blood flow normalized.

Urine output is the most reliable monitor of adequate burn shock resuscitation. Every patient with a burn large enough to warrant fluid resuscitation, generally 20% TBSA or larger, should have a urinary catheter placed immediately. Urine output should be monitored hourly throughout the resuscitation phase. Fluids should be administered to maintain urine output greater than 30 mL/hr in adults or 1 mL/kg/hr in children.

Immune System Changes

The cellular component of burn shock causes immediate and severe changes to the immune system that result in prolonged immunosuppression of both the humoral and cellular immune systems. Activation of the inflammatory cascade occurs immediately after a burn injury, resulting in the systemic release of proinflammatory cytokines (Gosain & Gamelli, 2005). Products released from activated inflammatory cells increase vascular permeability and local tissue ischemia. The function of WBCs and other phagocytic cells is altered and the ability to opsonize and phagocytose bacteria is decreased. The number of circulating T cells is decreased and T helper (Th) cell production shifts to Th2 lympocytes. A decrease in Th1 cells results in decreased cell-mediated cytotoxicity. Levels of circulating antibodies are diminished. Together suppression of the humoral and cellular immune responses results in immune dysfunction that can last for over a month, putting the patient at risk for infectious complications.

Metabolic Changes

Cellular metabolism is decreased the first few days following burn injury. Oxygen consumption is decreased during hypovolemic burn shock. Cellular metabolism increases once hypovolemia has been reversed by fluid resuscitation. The basal metabolic rate (BMR) can be twice the normal rate. Even so, the body expends up to 100% more energy than it produces. Hypermetabolism results in protein catabolism, lipolysis, and gluconeogenesis. Urea and creatinine levels in the urine increase. Body weight drops quickly. Delayed wound healing, muscle wasting, and bone loss can occur. Hypermetabolism persists until wound closure. It is imperative that burn patients receive early and adequate oral or gastrointestinal nutrition to combat hypermetabolism.

Collaborative Management

Burn care is multidisciplinary. Physicians, nurses, physical and occupational therapists, pharmacists, dieticians, social workers, and case managers work together to plan and administer care. Nurses are a vital member of the burn team and often manage the continuum of care required for full recovery. Burn care is often broken down into three stages: the resuscitation, acute, and rehabilitation stages. Burn care must be as dynamic as the burn injury itself and the plan of care must be individualized and continually reevaluated.

The following section discusses the primary assessment of the burn that will determine if the burn is minor or major and where care will be delivered. Minor burns are often treated in the emergency department or outpatient clinic, and the focus of care is pain management and wound care. Large burns require hospitalization, often in specialized burn centers, for the resuscitation and acute care phases. Burn care does not end when the patient is discharged from the hospital but continues through rehabilitation and scar management.

The first step in burn care, whether at the scene or in a medical facility, is to stop the burning process. The patient should be removed from the burn source as quickly as possible while protecting the patient from further injury or endangering others. Chemical burns should be lavaged with water immediately. Any powdered chemicals should be brushed from the clothing and skin prior to lavage. Clothing and jewelry should be removed to prevent further burning; however, clothing that adheres to the skin should be left in place.

Once the burning process is stopped, the burns should be covered with dry bandages and the patient wrapped in blankets to prevent unnecessary heat loss. One exception is chemical burns that should be lavaged repeatedly with water until a determination is made how the chemical agent should be treated.

Primary Assessment

A burned patient's appearance can be startling to individuals unused to working with burn injuries. Normal skin can be covered in soot. Injured skin may range in color from white to dark brown or may be covered in large weeping blisters. The burn wound is not itself an immediately life-threatening injury; but systemic effects may be, particularly if the patient experienced inhalation or electrical burns. Therefore, the first assessment of a burn patient, whether at the scene or in the emergency department, should be a primary trauma survey beginning with the ABCs (airway, breathing, circulation).

First, the patient's airway and breathing should be assessed. If the patient is not breathing, immediate steps should be taken to establish a patent airway. The patient is evaluated for signs and symptoms of inhalation injury, including the presence of facial burns or singed facial and scalp hair, progressive stridor, and hoarseness. Humidified oxygen is administered, particularly if the patient has signs of inhalation injury. The patient may be prophylactically intubated if there are signs of progressing respiratory stress or airway edema. Procuring a secure endotracheal tube is very important because it is very difficult to reintubate a burn patient due to severe airway edema and neck swelling.

Assessment of the burn patient's circulation must be performed immediately. Heart rate and blood pressure should be reassessed frequently. At least one large-bore intravenous line should be placed and well secured. Cardiac monitoring should be initiated for all major burns. Electrical burn patients should have cardiac monitoring for 24 hours following injury to assess for dysrhythmias. Tachycardia and hypotension are expected findings immediately after a burn injury. Body temperature can decrease rapidly secondary to the loss of intact skin and the patient should be kept covered with warm blankets. Extremities should be elevated.

Once the initial ABCs have been assessed, neurological status should be examined. A burn patient should be awake and able to follow commands. Decreased neurological status or unconsciousness may indicate anoxic injury or an additional neurological injury. If the patient was involved in a fall or high-voltage electrical injury, a cervical spine collar and long board should be applied. The patient's vital information should be obtained as soon as possible, particularly if the patient has major burns and may be unable to provide information if sedation or intubation is required later.

Initial Burn Assessment

A secondary burn assessment may be started at the scene and repeated in more detail once the patient reaches the emergency department. Often the burn assessment is done in parallel with the primary assessment. A complete burn history should be obtained either from the patient or individuals present at the burn scene. Injury details such as etiology, location, and circumstances should be described in as much detail as is available. Initial vital signs and neurological status should be recorded. Part of the burn assessment is to examine the circumstances of the injury. Burns are a common form of child abuse and the patient should be evaluated for patterns of injury that are not congruent with the burn history. Adult burn patients with suspicious patterns of

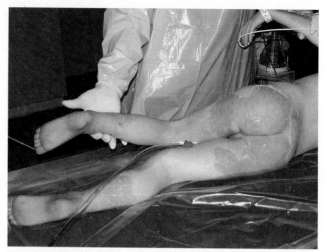

Figure 16-10 The child in this photo has a burn injury pattern that is suspicious of intentional scalding. The burns on the buttocks and feet suggest that the child was placed into hot water. (Courtesy of University of Michigan Trauma Burn Center, Ann Arbor, MI)

burns that are not in agreement with the burn history may have self-inflicted or assault-related burns or have been involved in illegal activities such as methamphetamine production. Classic patterns of burn injury that are suspicious of abuse in children include scalds with uniform depth, bilateral symmetry, and the absence of splash marks, indicating that the child was held still; multiple superficial well-defined circular burns, indicating cigarette burns; and small punctate burns indicative of electrocution with small live wires (Greenbaum, Horton, Williams, Shah, & Dunn, 2006) (Figure 16-10). Children with suspicious burn wounds often have signs of previous abuse (Greenbaum, Donne, Wilson, & Dunn, 2004). Patterns are similar for elder abuse. Hospital and state guidelines for reporting inflicted burns should be followed.

The physical assessment of the burn should be head to toe and should include examination for any signs of cotrauma. The eyes should be examined for corneal injury prior to the onset of severe edema. Signs of inhalation injury should be reassessed. Carboxyhemoglobin levels should be obtained if the patient was burned within an enclosed space or with signs indicating inhalation injury. If inhalation injury is suspected, a bronchoscopy may be performed.

The location and appearance of all burn wounds should be assessed as to size and depth of injury. The patient with deep or circumferential chest burns is at increased risk for developing respiratory problems and may require eschartomies to ensure adequate respiration. All extremities should be assessed for circumferential burns to identify areas at risk for loss of perfusion as burn edema progresses. Peripheral nerve stimulation is difficult to do on edematous areas but should be attempted if circumferential extremity burns are present.

A diagram of the burn injury should be drawn during the burn assessment using either the rule of nines or the Lund and Browder chart (see Figures 16-2 and 16-3). The percentage TBSA of second- and third-degree burns, and the total % TBSA burned, should be calculated. The % TBSA burned guides fluid resuscitation and helps in the determination of whether the patient should be transferred to a specialized burn center. The burn assessment should end with a decision as to whether the patient has a minor injury that can be treated in the outpatient setting or if the burn is severe enough to warrant hospitalization.

Transfer of the Patient to a Specialized Burn Center

The patient with a major burn injury is best treated in a specialized burn center. The American Burn Association uses the guidelines established by the American College of Surgeons Committee on Trauma (2006) to describe the burn patient who should be transported to a burn center for treatment (Table 16–2). Criteria evaluated to determine if referral is warranted include burn size, burn etiology, preexisting medical conditions, cotraumas, children first seen in hospitals without pediatric care capabilities, and individuals with specific psychosocial needs.

The closest burn center should be contacted when burn patients meet any of the referral criteria. The nurse should be prepared to provide the burn center with the following information:

- Patient demographics and past medical history, including allergies, medications, and immunization status
- Burn circumstances
- Burn size estimate and the presence or absence of inhalation injury and/or cotraumas
- Appearance of burn wound and dressings in place

- Vital signs
- Airway management
- Pain management
- Fluids and medications administered since the burn injury
- Presence of venous or arterial lines, urinary catheter, nasogastric tube
- Social history and special needs

The burn center will advise the referring emergency department or hospital on how to prepare the patient for transport, including fluid resuscitation requirements and airway management.

Burn centers are regional centers of care; therefore, patients are often transported over great distances to the nearest burn center. Air transport is the primary mode of transport for patients with major burn injuries or with cotraumas. Less severe burns may be transported by ground ambulance or private vehicle for burn center admission or evaluation in the burn outpatient clinic.

The Patient with Minor Burns

The majority of burn injuries are minor burns involving less than 20% TBSA and no full-thickness injuries. In this textbook, a minor burn is defined as any adult burn less than 20% TBSA and any pediatric burn less than 10% TBSA. However, other factors such as age, cotraumas, or preexisting medical conditions can contribute to the seriousness of a burn injury. Minor burns do not usually require hospitalization; however, some minor burns should be evaluated in a specialized burn center because of associated factors that require more intensive treatment. Therefore, a patient with a minor burn involving 10% to 20% TBSA should be considered for burn center referral. A patient with a minor burn injury who has

---

TABLE 16–2

Burn Center Referral Criteria

A burn center may treat adults or children, or both.
Burn injuries that should be referred to a burn center include the following:

1. Partial-thickness burns of greater than 10% of the total body surface area.
2. Burns that involve the face, hands, feet, genitalia, perineum, or major joints.
3. Third-degree burns in any age group.
4. Electrical burns, including lightning injury.
5. Chemical burns.
6. Inhalation injury.
7. Burn injury in patients with preexisting medical disorders that could complicate management, prolong recovery, or affect mortality.
8. Any patients with burns and concomitant trauma (such as fractures) in which the burn injury poses the greatest risk of morbidity or mortality. In such cases, if the trauma poses the greater immediate risk, the patient's condition may be stabilized initially in a trauma center before transfer to a burn center. Physician judgment will be necessary in such situations and should be in concert with the regional medical control plan and triage protocols.
9. Burned children in hospitals without qualified personnel or equipment for the care of children.
10. Burn injury in patients who will require special social, emotional, or rehabilitative intervention.

Source: Excerpted from Guidelines for the Operation of Burn Centers (pp. 79–86), Resources for Optimal Care of the Injured Patient 2006, Committee on Trauma, American College of Surgeons.

burns involving the face, hands, feet, genitalia, perineum, or major joints should be referred to a burn center. Likewise, a patient with a minor burn caused by electricity or chemicals, or with inhalation injury, is best evaluated in a burn center. The minor burn patient with preexisting medical conditions, cotraumas, or requiring special psychosocial interventions will benefit from specialized burn care.

Collaborative Management

The patient with a minor burn may present to the emergency department or outpatient clinic immediately after burn injury or days later when he or she has concerns about burn severity or infection. The patient with a minor burn that does not meet the criteria for referral to a burn center does not require formal resuscitation but should be encouraged to increase oral fluid intake for the first 24 hours post burn to replace fluids lost by localized edema. Minor burns can be very painful and anxiety invoking for the patient and family. Nursing care should encompass burn wound care and pain management. Time should be spent discussing the resources of the patient and family and concerns they have about caring for the burn. The ability of the patient to care for the wound and to be safe at home should be assessed. The patient should be given detailed instructions on wound care, pain management, and signs and symptoms of infection prior to discharge to home.

Management of Pain

The patient with a minor burn may be experiencing intense pain by the time he or she presents at a health care facility. Pain should be assessed and treated prior to beginning wound care. The patient undergoing the initial wound evaluation and debridement may require an intravenous narcotic such as morphine to achieve adequate pain control. Anxiolytics such as midazolam and lorazepam may be required if the patient is experiencing high anxiety. Nurses, working with social workers and child-life specialists, often use nonpharmaceutical methods to decrease the pain and anxiety associated with wound care. Techniques involving guided imagery, hypnosis, and relaxation can decrease the amount of pain medication needed. Oral pain medications should be prescribed for the patient to take as needed at home.

Wound Care

Wound care of minor burns involves cleaning and dressing the wound. The first step is to debride the burned area of loose tissue, wound debris, and eschar. First, the wound is gently washed with a mild antimicrobial soap or wound cleansing solution. Washing can be done with gauze pads or wet washcloths. Blistered skin should be gently removed. Eschar or loose skin that cannot be trimmed with a scissors or removed with gently washing should not be removed. Body hair in the wound and immediately around it should be shaved. The wound is rinsed with warm water or saline and patted dry with gauze or warm cloths.

Minor burn wounds that have developed thick eschar or necrotic tissue may require enzymatic debridement. A number of commercially available topical enzymes are available. The nurse should follow the directions on the product label. Generally, the enzyme is applied to the burn wound and covered with gauze followed by a wet dressing.

Dressings for Minor Burns

A wound dressing should achieve two goals: It should maintain a moist environment to facilitate wound healing and it should prevent infection. These goals are accomplished by applying a topical ointment or cream directly to the clean wound and covering the wound with a dressing. A number of topical agents are used to treat minor burn wounds. Two common topical burn wound creams are silver sulfadiazine (Silvadene) and Bacitracin ointment, which have antimicrobial properties. Ointments containing vitamins A, D, and E are commonly used to dress minor burns of the face. Once the minor wound has healed, vitamin-enhanced ointments are used to keep the skin moist.

The topical agents applied directly to the minor burn wound can be left open to air or covered with a semiopen or closed dressing (see Figure 16-11). Minor

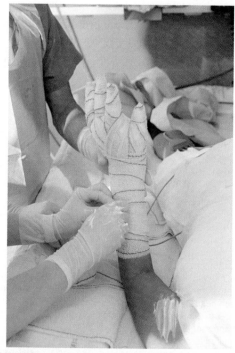

Figure 16-11 Closed method of dressing a burn.
(Courtesy of BSIP/Phototake NYC)

burns, particularly on the face and head, may be covered with a thin layer of antimicrobial cream and left open to air. The topical agent must be reapplied frequently so that the wound does not become dry. Wounds left open to air may be more painful because nerve endings are exposed to air currents. Therefore, most wound agents have nonadherent dressings placed over the topical agent. The nonadherent dressings can be covered with netting so that the wound remains semiopen to the environment. The application of gauze pads or rolls over the nonadherent dressing provides a closed dressing to the environment. Patients with closed dressings have greater mobility and are less prone to infection.

The nurse providing wound care for a minor burn should invite the patient to participate in each step. Participation can decrease pain and anxiety by allowing the patient to control the timing of each step. Participation, along with demonstration, also shows the patient how wound care should be performed. The patient and caregivers should be educated about the wound appearance and how to conduct wound care at home. It is important that the patient is informed about the signs and symptoms of infection and any other concerns specific to the wound.

Collaborative Management

Major burns differ from minor burns in that they require more intensive acute burn care, usually in the hospital setting. Burns involving greater than 20% TBSA in adults, or greater than 10% TBSA in children and adults older than 50 years, are considered major. However, third-degree burns, inhalation injury, electrical burns, or burns in individuals with preexisting health conditions may also require burn resuscitation. The patient with a major burn injury should be referred for evaluation and treatment in a specialized burn center.

Nurses are vital members of the burn team that manages and cares for major burns. An important component of nursing care for the burn patient is to discuss the care plan goals with the patient and family and to adjust goals accordingly. In many burn centers, nurses are responsible for coordinating the care provided by burn team members.

The care of a patient with major burns can be divided into three phases: the fluid resuscitation phase, the acute care phase, and the rehabilitation phase. The resuscitation phase begins with Emergency Medical Services (EMS) and continues until fluid resuscitation is complete, approximately 72 hours after injury, and the acute phase continues. The nurse is vital in administering fluids, monitoring the patient's status, and adjusting care accordingly. The acute phase lasts until the burn wound is closed, which can be weeks to months after the burn injury occurred.

Nursing Diagnoses

PATIENT WITH A BURN INJURY

- Ineffective airway clearance related to inhalation injury
- Impaired gas exchange related to inhalation injury
- Deficient fluid volume related to third spacing of fluids
- Pain related to burn injury
- Impaired skin integrity related to burn injury
- Anxiety related to sudden change in health status
- Body image disturbance related to change in physical appearance
- Risk for infection related to inadequate defense mechanisms
- Risk for imbalanced nutrition less than body requirements due to increased metabolic needs following burn injury

Nursing care focuses on promoting wound healing, preventing complications, and providing psychosocial support to the patient and family. The final rehabilitation phase focuses on restoring the burn patient's ability to function in society and can last for several years following a burn injury. Most of the rehabilitation phase occurs outside of the hospital and nursing interventions are limited.

Resuscitation Phase

The fluid resuscitation phase of burn care begins at the time of burn injury and ends with successful fluid resuscitation. Patients with major burns entering this phase should have large-bore intravenous access for fluid administration. A urinary catheter should be placed prior to administering large boluses of fluids. In men, the foreskin should be reduced to avoid paraphimosis from excess edema. A nasogastric tube should be placed and suction applied to prevent aspiration. Heart rate and blood pressure monitoring should be available.

Nursing care during the resuscitation phase is intensive. Refer to the common nursing diagnoses box for a list.

Airway Management

Laryngeal swelling and upper airway obstruction from edema can occur anytime within the first 24 hours following a major burn injury. Early intubation is encouraged because obstruction can occur rapidly, making intubation of the patient in respiratory distress difficult and risky. Intubated patients are heavily sedated and often chemically paralyzed to provide both patient comfort and decrease the risk of extubation. Management of the ventilated patient is described in Chapter 3. ∞

Airway management during the fluid resuscitation stage should begin with a thorough respiratory status assessment followed by continual monitoring. An initial chest x-ray should be taken to assess for signs of atelectasis, pneumonia, and edema. If the patient is intubated, the endotracheal tube placement should be noted. Arterial blood gases and vital signs should be obtained throughout the resuscitation phase of treatment and ventilatory adjustments made as needed. Other nursing interventions include elevating the head of the bed and turning the patient if possible, frequent suctioning, and administering humidified oxygen as ordered. Patients with burns to the neck, chest, and abdomen should be evaluated frequently for the development of compartment syndrome that can lead to ineffective breathing patterns. Compartment syndrome is discussed further in this chapter.

Inhalation Injury

The patient with head and neck burns or who was burned in an enclosed space should be further evaluated for signs and symptoms of inhalation injury. Bronchoscopy may be performed. During the resuscitation phase, manifestations of inhalation injury include high carboxyhemoglobin levels, upper airway obstruction, and pneumonitis. Nursing interventions, in addition to those described earlier, include monitoring of carboxyhemoglobin levels and observing for signs of respiratory distress associated with airway obstruction (increased respiratory rate, tachycardia, increased work of breathing, wheezing/hoarseness). If the patient was not initially intubated, the nurse should be prepared for emergent intubation. The placement and security of endotracheal tubes should be continually assessed as burn edema waxes and wanes.

Carbon Monoxide. Although all components of fire smoke are capable of damaging airway mucosa, CO can cause additional damage because it interferes with oxygen delivery. CO has a stronger affinity for hemoglobin than does oxygen and it displaces oxygen as it binds to the hemoglobin, thus impairing oxygen transport and tissue oxygenation. The primary targets of CO poisoning are the heart and brain. The level of CO bound to hemoglobin in the blood determines the symptoms. Elevated carboxyhemoglobin levels are associated with the following symptoms:

0% to 5% Normal value, no symptoms

10% to 20% Headache, nausea, dizziness, light-headedness

20% to 40% Confusion, headache, tachycardia, angina, hypertension, dysrhythmias

40% to 60% Syncope, hypotension, seizures, and coma

Greater than 60% Ventricular dysrhythmias and death

The rate at which CO is excreted by the lungs is related to the fraction of inspired oxygen in the air the person

is breathing. If a patient is breathing room air, CO will have a half-life of 3 to 4 hours. However, if the patient is breathing 100% oxygen, the half-life of CO is reduced to 30 to 40 minutes. Therefore, patients with suspected CO poisoning are provided with high-flow oxygen (90% to 100%). Many burn centers recommend the use of hyperbaric oxygen therapy (2.5 atm) if the patient has pronounced changes in his level of consciousness or if his levels of carboxyhemoglobin are high. When hyperbaric oxygen is utilized, the nurse must monitor the patient for the development of tension pneumothorax, tympanic membrane rupture, and sinus or ear pain.

Fluid Resuscitation

Burns involving greater than 20% TBSA require fluid resuscitation to counteract the intravascular fluid losses resulting from increased capillary permeability. The goal of fluid resuscitation is to perfuse the organs; however, optimal fluid resuscitation is a balance between underresuscitation, which can result in decreased perfusion, kidney failure, and organ dysfunction and overresuscitation, which can increase burn edema, elevate compartment pressures, and lead to ARDS and multiple organ dysfunction (Pham, Cancio, & Gibran, 2008).

Administration of Fluids

The American Burn Association (ABA) published the following practice guidelines for burn shock resuscitation in 2008 (Pham et al., 2008).

1) "Adults and children with burns greater than 20% TBSA should undergo formal fluid resuscitation using estimates based on body size and surface area burned."

2) "Common formulas used to initiate resuscitation estimate a crystalloid need for 2 to 4 ml/kg body weight/%TBSA during the first 24 hours."

3) "Maintenance fluids should be administered to children in addition to their calculated fluid requirements caused by injury."

4) "Increased volume requirements can be anticipated in patients with full-thickness injuries, inhalation injury, and a delay in resuscitation."

The amount of fluid administered is dependent on body and burn size. Several formulas are used to fluid resuscitate burn patients (Warden, 2007). The most commonly used formula is the Parkland Formula that recommends 4 mL per kg body weight per % TBSA administered during the first 24 hours following a burn injury. Half of the total resuscitation volume is given in the first 8 hours. An example of how to calculate the Parkland Formula for an adult burn patient is shown in Table 16–3. Pediatric patients require more fluids per body weight. Pediatric formulas often follow the Parkland Formula but add basal fluid requirements, which

TABLE 16–3

Calculating Fluid Needs for an Adult Patient

Formulas: Parkland Formula (for resuscitation)	2–4 mL × kg body weight × % TBSA
Maintenance Formula: (Basal fluid requirement + Evaporative water loss)	$(1{,}500 \text{ mL} \times m^2) + [(25 + \% \text{ TBSA burn}) \times m^2 \times 24 \text{ hr}]$

EXAMPLE OF HOW TO CALCULATE FLUID RATES FOR AN ADULT BURN PATIENT

Patient: 71-year-old male burned in a house explosion	Weight: 86 kg Height: 188 cm TBSA: 26% BSA[a]: 2.1 m^2

RESUSCITATION FLUIDS (FIRST 24 HOURS)

PARKLAND FORMULA + BASAL REQUIREMENTS[b]	CALCULATION
Parkland Formula (24-hour total)	4 mL × 86 kg × 26% TBSA = 8,944 mL
Basal Requirements (24-hour total)	1,500 × 2.1 m^2 = 3,150 mL
24-hour fluid total	8,944 + 3,300 = 12,094 Ml
Fluid administration rate 1st 8 hours ($^1/_2$ of 24-hour total) 2nd and 3rd 8 hours ($^1/_2$ of 24-hour total)	6,047 mL/8 hr = 756 mL per hour 6,047 mL/16 hr = 378 mL per hour

MAINTENANCE FLUIDS

Maintenance Formula (24-hour total)	$(1{,}500 \times 2.1 \ m^2) + [(25 + 26\% \text{ TBSA}) \times 2.1 \ m^2 \times 24 \text{ hr}]$ = 5,720 Ml
Fluid administration rate	5,720 mL/24 hr = 240 mL per hour

Source: From Mosteller, R. D. [1987 October 22]. Simplified calculation of body surface area [Letter]. *New England Journal of Medicine, 317* [17], 1098.

[a] BSA can be calculated with a BSA calculator (many are available on the Internet) or by using a formula. One common formula is the Mosteller formula: BSA (m^2) = ([Height(cm) × Weight(kg)]/ 3,600)$^{1/2}$.

[b] Not all burn centers add basal requirements to the Parkland Formula when resuscitating burn patients. The nurse should be familiar with the practice of the burn center treating the patient.

are an additional 1,500 cc for each m^2 of body surface area (BSA). Some burn centers also add basal fluid requirements to the Parkland Formula when resuscitating adult burn patients. Recent studies have found that most current burn patients receive fluid volumes exceeding 5 to 7 mL per kg of body weight per % TBSA (Pham, Schrag, Hargraves, & Bach, 2005). Because fluid resuscitation volumes are calculated for the first 24 hours post burn, patients transferred from great distances to a burn center must have resuscitation fluid rates adjusted to account for the total amount of fluids administered prior to admission.

The goal of resuscitation is for the patient to maintain adequate urine output on a maintenance rate of fluids. The fluid maintenance volume is determined by the patient's recommended fluid intake (basal fluid requirement) plus evaporative water loss. Maintenance fluid calculations take into account the patient's BSA and the % TBSA burned. The following formula is used to calculate the daily maintenance fluid rates following successful resuscitation for adult burn patients: $(1{,}500 \text{ mL/}m^2) + [(25 + \% \text{ TBSA burn}) \times m^2 \times 24] =$ total maintenance fluid (mL) to be given over 24 hours (Warden, 2007). An example of how to calculate main-

tenance fluids for an adult burn patient is shown in Table 16–3.

Crystalloid fluids are most commonly used for burn resuscitation. Crystalloid fluids are electrolyte-based fluids that diffuse easily from the bloodstream. Lactated Ringer's solution is the fluid of choice for burn resuscitation because it is slightly hypotonic, treating both intravascular volume losses and extracellular sodium losses. Hypertonic saline is occasionally used for burn resuscitation because it draws water back into the intravascular space by osmosis. Several studies have suggested that hypertonic saline results in hypernatremia and subsequent acute renal failure.

Colloids, such as albumin, plasma, or dextran, have been used to replenish the plasma proteins lost by the administration of high volumes of crystalloids during burn resuscitation (Pham et al., 2008). Colloids given after the first 12 to 24 hours post burn may decrease overall fluid requirements and edema formation (Pham et al., 2008). Nonetheless, the use of colloids remains controversial; a recent Cochrane review of the literature states that there is no evidence that resuscitation with colloids reduces the risk of death in burn, trauma, or surgical patients (Perel & Roberts, 2007). Antioxidant therapy, such as administration of ascorbic acid (vitamin C), may decrease overall fluid requirements following burn injury (Pham et al., 2008).

Monitoring of Resuscitation

Nursing roles during resuscitation include administering fluids and continually monitoring and assessing the patient's status. Hourly urine output measurement is the gold standard by which burn resuscitation is monitored. The ABA practice guidelines state that "Fluid resuscitation, regardless of solution type or estimated need, should be titrated to maintain a urine output of approximately 0.5–1.0 ml/kg/hr in adults and 1.0–1.5 ml/kg/hr in children" (Pham et al., 2008). Fluid type and rates are adjusted hourly based on urine output. Depending on the protocol used, fluid rates are gradually decreased as urine output is maintained. Burn resuscitation is considered successful when the patient has adequate urine output after 2 hours of fluids administered at maintenance rate.

Vital signs are also monitored. Acceptable parameters include a heart rate less than 120 beats per minute; a blood pressure that is normal to slightly hypertensive; and clear lung sounds. Arterial blood gases are useful indicators of the patient's status during resuscitation. Elevated base deficit and increased lactate levels occur when systemic perfusion is compromised (Ahrns, 2004). Base deficit and lactate levels can remain elevated in burn patients considered adequately resuscitated based on urine output measurements, and mortality is increased in patients whose levels do not correct over time (Ahrns, 2004; Pham et al., 2008). Whether base excess and lactate levels should be used to determine resuscitation endpoints remains controversial.

Invasive cardiac output monitoring is sometimes used in elderly patients or patients who are not responding to standard treatment. A pulmonary artery wedge pressure less than 18 mm Hg is an indicator that resuscitation is adequate, but this measurement should always be used in adjunct to urine output and other parameters.

Electrolyte status should be monitored during burn resuscitation. Burn shock can result in hyper- or hypokalemia. Hyperkalemia, accompanied by hyponatremia, can occur during the initial fluid shift from potassium leaking out of damaged cells and is treated by correcting metabolic acidosis. Hypokalemia can result from fluid loss at the burn wound or hemodilution from fluid resuscitation. Hyponatremia can occur in conjunction with hypokalemia. Fluid rates should be adjusted if fluid excess occurs, and potassium should be replaced with careful monitoring. Crystalloid fluids and restriction of free water will usually correct sodium deficits.

Fluid resuscitation is considered complete when the patient's fluid rates are at maintenance levels for 2 hours with adequate urine output. At that time dextrose containing crystalloid solutions may be used.

Abdominal Compartment Syndrome

A complication of excess fluid resuscitation is an accumulation of abdominal fluid, resulting in high intra-abdominal pressure. Subcutaneous edema and eschar in patients with abdominal burns contribute to further increase intra-abdominal pressures (IAPs). Intra-abdominal hypertension places the burn patient at risk for developing secondary abdominal compartment syndrome. If abdominal compartment syndrome remains untreated, the risk of organ failure and death is high. The patient undergoing fluid resuscitation for major burns should be monitored for development of intra-abdominal hypertension. Bladder pressure, measured via the patient's urinary catheter, is the most common measurement of IAP. Intra-abdominal hypertension occurs when bladder pressures exceed 30 mm Hg, but patients with bladder pressures as low as 15 mm Hg may have intra-abdominal hypertension and be at risk for abdominal compartment syndrome (Hershberger, Hunt, Arnoldo, & Purdue, 2007; Kramer, Lund, & Beckum, 2007). The treatment for intra-abdominal hypertension includes decreasing crystalloid fluid rates and administering colloid fluids such as albumin (Hershberger et al., 2007). The patients with circumferential abdominal burns may require abdominal escharatomies to decrease IAP and prevent abdominal compartment syndrome.

Abdominal compartment syndrome is diagnosed by sustained intra-abdominal hypertension along with abdominal tightness, difficulty in providing adequate ventilation due to increased inspiratory pressures, and increasing oliguria in spite of fluid therapy. Abdominal compartment syndrome often requires abdominal decompression either by the insertion of a percutaneous catheter to drain the excess fluid or by laparotomy to relieve abdominal pressure. Decompression laparotomy results in an open abdomen that is covered by a dressing until the wound can be surgically closed.

Collaborative Management

Initial management of large burn wounds involves debridement, assessment, and wound coverage. The goals of wound management at this stage are to decrease fluid and electrolyte losses, prevent infection, and decrease the risk of developing compartment syndrome.

The initial wound management usually occurs in the patient's room. The nurse should have multiple towels, drapes, wound care solutions, and wound dressings available. Wound care can result in the patient becoming chilled so precautions, such as warm blankets and increasing the room temperature, should be taken to maintain the patient's body temperature. The patient should be premedicated for pain. Wound care involves moving the patient; therefore, all lines and the endotracheal tube should be secured. Members of the burn team performing wound care wear protective gowns, masks, and gloves to decrease the risk of nosocomial infections. Dressings applied at the scene or emergency department should be gently removed.

Debridement of the major burn wound involves cleaning the burn wound with warm water or sterile saline and antimicrobial soaps or wound cleansers. Loose skin and debris is removed using wet washcloths or gauze. Fluid-filled blisters and skin tags are trimmed with a scissors. Hair in or around the wound should be shaved. The debrided wound is washed with warm water or saline.

Assessment of the major burn wound includes description of the body location, size, and depth of injury. Circumferential burns of the neck, chest, abdomen, and extremities should be assessed further for the development of compartment syndrome. The patient with facial burns should be assessed for corneal injuries, and ocular lubrication should be applied to prevent corneal ulceration.

The major burn wound is dressed similarly to a minor burn. Silver sulfadiazine is the most common topical agent used. Bacitracin is commonly used on facial burns. Large gauze pads or gauze wrap are used to cover the wounds and secured in place with netting. Extremity burns are wrapped circumferentially starting at the distal end of the extremity and moving proximally. Individual fingers and toes are wrapped separately. Gauze dressings on the extremities can be secured with elastic bandages. Bandages must be loose enough to allow for edema formation. Windows into the bandages are often made to give nurses access to extremity pulse points. Depending on the products used, wound care is performed once or twice daily. After the patient's wounds are dressed, the patient should be placed under warm blankets and the temperature closely monitored.

Compartment Syndrome

Circumferential burn wounds to the neck, chest, abdomen, and extremities are at risk for developing compartment syndrome. The burn eschar constricts the burned area at the same time that edema is causing subcutaneous fluid expansion. The net result is impaired circulation to the involved area. Compartment syndrome can arise rapidly at any time during the resuscitation phase. The nurse continuously assesses areas with circumferential burns for tautness, lack of color or capillary refill, coolness, and numbness and tingling. Pulses peripheral to burned extremities are assessed. Doppler ultrasound is used to assess for blood flow in the extremities. The nurse should assess the patient with circumferential burns to the neck and torso for signs indicative of compartment syndrome including decreased lung sounds, respiratory distress, and increased ventilatory needs.

Compartment syndrome is prevented by performing an escharotomy (Figure 16-12). The physician uses a

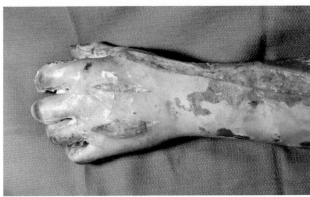

Figure 16-12 Escharotomy. The surgical procedure consists of removing the eschar formed on the skin and underlying tissue following severe burns. The procedure is particularly helpful in restoring circulation to the extremities of clients when scar tissue forms a tight, constrictive band around the circumference of a limb.
(Courtesy of Michael English, M.D./Custom Medical Stock Photo, Inc.)

scalpel or electrocautery to cut through the eschar, which releases tension and permits blood flow to the area. Escharotomies are usually performed at the bedside. The nurse should be prepared to assist in draping and monitoring the patient during the procedure. The escharotomy incisions are packed with gauze for at least 24 hours after which the incisions can be treated similarly to the burn wound. Nursing interventions following an escharotomy include monitoring the patient for blood loss and assessing for further signs of compartment syndrome. The original escharotomy incisions may need to be extended if edema progresses and pressures continue to rise. Occasionally, pressure below the fascia develops and fasciotomies are performed.

Pain Management

The patient with a large burn injury experiences excruciating pain, particularly in areas where the burn is not full thickness. During the resuscitation phase, the burn patient is treated with intravenously administered narcotics. Continuous infusions of morphine or fentanyl are common. Narcotics are titrated according to the patient's pain responses, and boluses are given for anticipated procedures such as wound care. Anxiolytics are often prescribed prior to procedures. It is important that the nurse continually assesses the patient for pain. Ventilated patients who are chemically paralyzed also require medication for pain. Hospital protocols for assessing pain in these patients should be followed.

Acute Phase

The resuscitation phase ends within 24 to 72 hours postburn injury. Intravenous fluid requirements decrease as the extravasation of intravascular fluids ends. Clinically, the acute phase of burn care begins when the burn patient can maintain adequate urine output while receiving only maintenance rates of intravenous fluids. Following burn resuscitation, the patient enters into a hypermetabolic state that lasts until after the wound is healed. Characteristics of hypermetabolism are increased body temperature, tachycardia, increased caloric needs, and weight loss.

Burn care during the acute phase focuses on supporting the patient as the burn wounds heal. Support includes maintenance of respiratory and circulatory status, wound care, pain management, infection control, nutritional support, physical therapy, and psychosocial support. Every member of the burn team is actively enrolled in this phase of burn care. Nursing coordinates patient care throughout this phase, maintaining constant communication with other members of the burn team, the patient, and the patient's family.

The burn patient requires ongoing assessment of circulatory and respiratory status during the acute burn phase. Fluid and electrolyte requirements can be variable during this stage depending on surgical procedures, infections, and nutritional status. Transfusions may be required to correct for blood loss. Tachycardia and fever are common throughout this stage because of the hypermetabolic response. Ventilatory requirements gradually decrease as burn edema subsides. Frequent suctioning is required to clear the lungs. The patient with inhalation injury may require prolonged ventilation and is at increased risk for pneumonia and other pulmonary complications. The patient is extubated after gradual periods of weaning. Tracheostomies are often performed if the patient fails ventilator weaning or requires prolonged ventilatory support for other reasons.

Wound Management in the Acute Phase

Once burn resuscitation is complete, the burn team can begin aggressive wound care management. Areas of first- and second-degree burns can be managed with wound care. Deep second-degree burns can heal without surgical intervention unless the wound becomes necrotic due to impaired circulation or infection. Third-degree, or full-thickness, burns require surgical intervention to heal.

Surgical Management in the Acute Phase

Perhaps the most important progress in modern burn care is early excision and coverage of full-thickness burn injuries (Muller, Gahankari, & Herndon, 2007). The purpose of excision and coverage is to remove the eschar and other debris of a full-thickness burn, leaving viable tissue exposed. Morbidity is decreased if the patient with major burns undergoes excision and closure within the first week of injury. Early surgical intervention slows the inflammatory response, decreases wound colonization, and attenuates the hypermetabolic response (Muller et al., 2007; Sheridan, 2002).

The patient with major burns may require multiple excisional procedures staged over several days. Excision is performed using electrocautery or a dermatome. Burned tissue is removed in thin slices until bleeding occurs and viable dermis or subcutaneous tissue is visible. Excision can result in considerable blood loss and blood transfusions may be necessary.

Once the burn wound is excised, it is covered with either a skin graft (autograft) or other biological or biosynthetic coverings (Table 16–4). Coverage decreases insensible water loss and allows healing to begin. The type of coverage is dependent on the amount of unburned skin the patient has to donate for skin grafting, patient status, and the preferences of the burn surgeon.

Autografting

Autografting is a procedure that involves removing thin slices of unburned skin from an unburned "donor" site and placing it on top of the excised burn wound (Figure 16-13). Autografts are intended to be permanent. Donor sites may be "harvested" more than once if the patient requires multiple skin grafting procedures. Donor skin can be placed directly onto the burn (sheet graft) or meshed to increase the burn surface area covered. Meshed autografts result in more scarring and are placed, when possible, on the back, buttocks, and thighs. The patient with large areas to be grafted and limited donor sites may have meshed autografts placed on more visible body areas such as the trunk, arms, and lower extremities. Sheet grafts are applied to the hands and face to decrease the risk of scarring and loss of function.

Biological and Biosynthetic Dressings

Biological skin coverings can be used to cover excised burn wounds when the patient does not have enough donor sites to provide autograft coverage. Cadaver skin (allograft) is often used to cover excised skin or widely meshed autograft. Tissue typing is not performed; therefore, allograft results in a temporary coverage until it sloughs from the wound bed. An allograft provides a barrier against mechanical trauma, bacterial infection, and water loss (Sheridan, 2002).

Cultured autologous epithelial cells manufactured by Genzyme are the only commercially available permanent skin covering available in the United States. The cost of autologous epithelial autograft is considerable and use is reserved for patients with very large burns and few donor sites. Specific wound care protocols are implemented when cultured epithelial autografts are used and only experienced wound care nurses should care for these wounds.

A number of commercial biosynthetic and synthetic skin substitutes are available (see Table 16–4). Permanent biosynthetic products, such as Integra and Alloderm, are composed of biological and synthetic materials and serve as a dermal replacement over which autograft is placed. Other products, such as Biobrane, Aquacel, and Acticoat, serve as temporary protective coverings over wide-meshed autografts, donor sites, and partial-thickness burns.

TABLE 16-4
Wound Dressings

BIOLOGIC WOUND DRESSINGS

NAME	DESCRIPTION	TYPE	MANUFACTURER
Autograft	Graft of patient's own skin. Can be full or partial thickness. Can be "reharvested" multiple times from the same donor site.	Permanent	
Allograft	Graft from human cadaver. Can be fresh or cryopreserved. Often placed over autograft. Covers large wound areas and aids in revascularization of the wound. Eventually rejected.	Temporary	
Cultured epithelial autograft (CEA)	Composed of patient's own keratinocytes cultured with mouse fibroblasts to form an epidermal autograft, and then attached to a petrolatum gauze backing. Used as a permanent skin replacement in patients with large burns. Requires a small biopsy of healthy skin.	Permanent	Genzyme Corporation

BIOSYNTHETIC WOUND DRESSINGS

Integra	Bilayer skin replacement system comprised of dermal and epidermal layers. Collagen-based dermal layer serves as matrix for revascularization. The silicone-based epidermal layer controls moisture loss. When revascularization is adequate, the silicone layer is removed and covered with a thin layer of autograft.	Permanent	Integra LifeSciences Corporation
Alloderm	Acellular dermal matrix made from donated human skin that is placed directly on the wound bed and covered with a thin layer of allograft. Provides matrix for revascularization of the allograft.	Permanent	LifeCell Corporation
Biobrane	Biosynthetic dressing applied to second-degree burns or other partial-thickness wounds. Collagen bound dressing that adheres firmly to the wound until epithelialization occurs.	Temporary	Smith & Nephew

SYNTHETIC WOUND DRESSINGS

NAME	DESCRIPTION	TYPE	MANUFACTURER
Aquacel	Silver-impregnated dressing used on partial-thickness burns, skin grafts, and donor sites. Can be left in place for up to 14 days, reducing the need for painful dressing changes.	Temporary	Convatec
Acticoat	Antimicrobial barrier dressing consisting of three layers: absorbent core sandwiched between silver-coated adherent polyethylene net layers. Antimicrobial properties effective for 3 days. Low wound adherence decreases pain of dressing changes. Used on partial-thickness burns, skin grafts, and dermal substitutes.	Temporary	Smith & Nephew
DuoDerm	Hydrocolloid dressing that adheres to moist wounds.		Convatec
Kaltostat	Calcium alginate dressing that absorbs exudate from moderate to heavily draining wounds. Used on donor sites.		Convatec

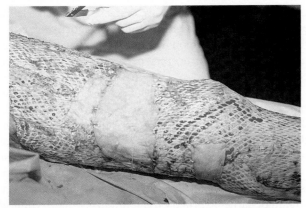

Figure 16-13 A meshed autograft applied to third-degree burn areas.
(Courtesy of University of Utah Burn Center)

Major Burn Dressings

The patient with large burns requires extensive wound care. Wound care is often conducted in a hydrotherapy room where the patient is placed on a shower table or in a hydrotherapy tank for cleansing using antimicrobial soap or wound cleansing agents. Nursing interventions include premedicating the patient for pain and anxiety, monitoring the patient's pain, vital signs, and temperature during the dressing change. The burn wounds can be in varying stages of healing and include wounds that have not been excised, grafted wounds, and donor sites, all of which require specific care. Each dressing change should include a visual assessment of the wounds for signs of infection, wound healing, or graft loss.

Burn wounds that have not been excised or that will heal without surgical intervention are usually treated with silver sulfadiazine or other silver-coated dressings. Facial burns are treated with antimicrobial ointments such as Bacitracin or vitamin A, D, and E cream. Burns to the ear can result in chondritis and loss of the ear cartilage. The burned ear should be treated with antimicrobial agents and protected from mechanical pressure caused by wound dressings, pillows, or endotracheal tube ties.

Vacuum-assisted closure (VAC) is frequently being used on partial-thickness wounds. A sponge connected to a tube is placed over the wound and covered with an adhesive occlusive dressing. When the tube is attached to the VAC pump, a negative pressure is created over the wound.

Skin grafts require meticulous wound care and each burn center has developed protocols for graft care. In the operating room, the fresh skin graft is covered with a moist dressing such as impregnated mesh gauze or silver-impregnated dressings. The dressing is covered with bulky gauze and wrapped securely. The initial dressing may remain in place for up to 3 days if no complications such as bleeding or signs of infection are noted. Initially the grafted skin is very fragile so mechanical forces should be avoided when cleaning and dressing the wound.

Donor sites can be very painful. Wound care and dressings are similar to minor burns. Dressings that can remain in place for several days are commonly used to decrease the pain associated with dressing changes. Donor sites heal within 10 to 14 days, at which time they can be reharvested.

Nursing Care

During the acute phase of burn care the nurse is a vital member of the burn team and continuously interacts with team members and the patient to ensure appropriate patient care. The nurse is involved with wound management as discussed earlier. Other nursing concerns during this phase include pain management, prevention of infection, nutritional support, involvement of physical therapy, and psychosocial support. Find these and other common nursing diagnoses in the Nursing Diagnoses box.

Pain Management

Pain is a constant for the patient with large burns. In fact, pain control becomes a more significant issue as the acute phase of burn care progresses and the wounds include donor sites. Background pain is a result of exposed nerve endings within the burn injury and donor sites, as well as pain associated with straightening and flexing burned areas during routine movements. Background pain can be interrupted with periods of increased breakthrough pain that is difficult to relieve with pain medications. The patient experiences additional procedural pain related to surgeries, dressing changes, and physical therapy sessions. As the patient becomes more alert, an-

ticipatory pain and anxiety can become overwhelming to the point where patient progress is limited.

Narcotics are the most common medications used to treat burn pain. Continuous infusion of intravenous morphine is standard of care for ventilated patients. Once a patient is extubated and able to swallow, intravenous narcotics are transitioned to oral forms. Nonsteroidal anti-inflammatory drugs are often used in conjunction with narcotics. Pain is often decreased if patients are allowed to control some aspects of their pain management. Anxiety resulting from fear and loss of control can increase pain levels if not treated. Anxiolytics are commonly administered in conjunction with pain medications. Donor site itching contributes to patient discomfort and should be treated with oral medications and topical emollients.

Pain should be continually monitored during the acute burn phase. Treatment should be individualized and take into account patient history, burn size, anticipated procedures, and patient coping strategies. Nursing interventions include providing adequate background and procedural pain and anxiety control and assisting the patient with nonpharmacologic pain-reducing therapies such as distraction or guided imagery. Nurses can help alleviate anxiety by providing the patient with information about procedures and encouraging participation in wound care and physical therapy.

Prevention and Management of Infection

Infections are responsible for approximately 75% of deaths following burn injury (Sharma, 2007). Burn patients are at risk for developing infections secondary to altered skin integrity, respiratory endothelium damage from inhalation injury, and alterations in the immune response. The presence of blood and urinary catheters and prolonged intubation contributes further to the risk of infection.

Staphylococcus aureus and *Pseudomonas aeruginosa* are the most frequently isolated organisms from patients in burn units (Sharma, 2007). Fungal and antibiotic resistant organisms can result in life-threatening infections. Infections arise from endogenous sources, including normal flora of the skin, upper respiratory tract, and gastrointestinal tract. Exogenous sources from the hospital environment are responsible for the majority of infections. The most common mode of transmission of exogenous organisms is via hospital personnel or contaminated equipment.

The ABA has published guidelines to define infections and sepsis in burn patients (Greenhalgh et al., 2007). Sepsis is defined as "a change in the burn patient that triggers the concern for infection" and is the point at which antibiotics are started and the search for the cause of infection initiated. Causes of infection include organisms from the respiratory tract (pneumonia), bloodstream or catheter, urinary tract, or burn wound. Clinical signs of a burn wound infection include changes in wound appearance such as erythema, early separation of

---

COMMONLY USED MEDICATIONS

TOPICAL BURN MEDICATIONS

SILVER SULFADIAZENE (SILVADENE, SSD, THERMAZENE)

Desired Effect: Used for both partial- and full-thickness burns, it has broad-spectrum bactericidal action against many gram-negative and gram-positive bacteria. Application is painless but the drug does not penetrate eschar.

Nursing Responsibilities:
- Monitoring the patient's white blood count
- Identifying any signs of infection
- Monitoring for the development of a rash and discontinuing the medication if one develops

Side and/or Toxic Effects: Some patients develop transient leucopenia, which usually improves over the course of therapy. A few patients develop hypersensitivity.

MAFENIDE ACETATE (SULFAMYELON)

Desired Effect: Used for partial- and full-thickness burns, it is an antimicrobial cream or solution containing mafenide (which is related to the sulfonamides). It has broad-spectrum bacteriostatic action against many gram-positive and gram-negative bacteria. It does penetrate eschar, it is absorbed systemically, and application can be painful.

Nursing Responsibilities:
- Monitoring for signs of fungal infection because no fungal coverage is provided
- Assessing and treating pain associated with dressing changes
- Monitoring for acid-base imbalances—especially metabolic acidosis
- Assessing the patient's respiratory function
- Discontinuing use if a rash develops

Side and/or Toxic Effects: Patients may develop metabolic acidosis if they are unable to hyperventilate to compensate for the metabolic acidosis that the drug induces. Patients may develop a hypersensitivity reaction manifested by a rash on their unburned skin.

BACITRACIN

Desired Effect: Applied to superficial and facial burns that are left open to the environment, it is effective against gram-negative organisms and application is painless.

Nursing Responsibilities:
- Monitoring for signs and symptoms of hypersensitivity and discontinuing use if a rash develops
- Monitoring for signs of infection
- Reapplying frequently to prevent the wound from becoming dry

---

burn eschar, or progression of the wound depth. Wound infections are diagnosed by objective findings from wound biopsies or swabs and tissue histology. Antibiotic sensitivities are performed to guide the pharmacological treatment. Infected wounds are sometimes treated with surgical excision to remove the infected tissue.

Controlling the risk of infection in patients with large burns is an important part of nursing care and should include the following goals:

- Prevention of transmission of organisms to patients or personnel. Strict hand-washing protocols should be implicated for personnel and visitors en-

tering patient rooms. Some burn centers require that anyone coming in contact with patients with large burns must wear gloves and protective gowns. All equipment should be cleaned prior to patient contact.

- Aggressive management of the burn wound. Aseptic technique should be followed. Wound care should progress from sites at most risk of infection to sites at least risk, and care should be taken to not contaminate the burn wound with normal flora from the bowel. The wound should be monitored for signs and symptoms of infections and treated appropriately. The nurse should be familiar with the actions of topical and systemic antibiotics.

- Close monitoring of signs and symptoms of infection. Bacterial cultures should be ordered per hospital protocol and systemic antibiotics prescribed appropriately. Infected lines should be removed or replaced.

Nutritional Support

During the acute phase of burn care, the patient is in a hypermetabolic state and total energy needs can be 100 times normal. Early and aggressive nutritional support within 24 to 48 hours of burn injury is required to promote wound healing and decrease the risk of sepsis. The goal of nutritional support is to meet the patient's caloric needs and maintain a positive nitrogen balance.

Nutritional support can be provided orally if the burn patient is able to eat. However, the patient with a large burn usually requires enteral nutritional support in order to meet caloric requirements. Enteral feeds can be delivered to the stomach or the small intestine. Postpyloric feeding decreases the risk of aspiration. The burn patient receiving enteral feeds should have a nasogastric tube placed and feeding should begin slowly to assess the patient's tolerance.

Nutrition requirements are based on the patient's age and burn size. A number of formulas are used to estimate daily caloric needs, including the Curreri and Harris-Benedict formulas (Saffle & Graves, 2007). Formulas vary widely and no one formula has been shown to correlate well with actual energy expenditure. In addition, burn patients' caloric needs fluctuate widely during the acute burn phase. Formulas are used as a guide to estimate caloric needs but must be adjusted according to measurements of the patient's nutritional and clinical status.

Enteral nutrition must contain complete nutrition for the burn patient. A variety of commercially available nutritional products are available. The main source of calories is from carbohydrates. The increased caloric needs put the burn patient at risk for hyperglycemia. Tight glucose monitoring and control is important, even in patients with no history of glucose intolerance. Protein catabolism is a result of burn hypermetabolism. Enteral nutrition must be high protein to prevent catabolism. The current protein recommendation is 1.5 to 2.0 grams protein per kilogram body weight per day (Saffle & Graves, 2007). Enteral nutrition contains a small quantity of fat to prevent essential fatty acid deficiencies. Micronutrients are often included in enteral nutrition. Vitamins A, C, D, iron, zinc, and selenium are considered beneficial to the burn patient. The amino acids glutamine and arginine are commonly added supplements because of their positive roles in immune function and wound healing (Saffle & Graves, 2007).

A patient with a large burn injury often experiences dysphagia as a result of prolonged intubation. Speech therapists assess the patient's ability to swallow without aspiration before the patient is allowed to take liquids or food by mouth. As the patient is able to tolerate oral feeding, enteral feeds are gradually decreased until oral intake matches caloric needs. Daily calorie counts help determine when the patient no longer requires enteral nutritional support. Because hypermetabolism lasts well past healing of the burn injury, the burn patient must be encouraged to eat high-caloric high-protein diets supplemented with vitamins and minerals in order to meet their nutritional needs.

Nutritional status is assessed in several ways (Saffle & Graves, 2007). Body weight changes over time can indicate whether a patient is receiving enough calories to maintain body weight. Body weight is not an accurate day-to-day predictor of nutritional status because of edema. Indirect calorimetry, which measures resting energy expenditures, is the gold standard for measuring nutritional status (Prelack, Dylewski, & Sheridan, 2007). When done weekly, indirect calorimetry shows changes in clinical status over time and allows for caloric intake to be adjusted accordingly. Indirect calorimetry is not available in many hospitals. Therefore, nitrogen balance is widely used to assess nutritional status. Twenty-four-hour urine samples are collected at least weekly to determine urea nitrogen levels and calculate nitrogen balance. A positive nitrogen balance indicates that the patient is taking in more protein than he is using.

Enteral feeding is not tolerated in patients with a number of conditions, including ileus, duodenal ulcers, or pancreatitis. Total parenteral nutrition (TPN) is administered to patients who cannot tolerate enteral feeds. TPN should be used judiciously in burn patients because it has been associated with increased infection rates in trauma patients and increased mortality in burn patients (Saffle & Graves, 2007).

Physical Therapy

Physical therapy is an important part of the acute phase of burn care. The nurse works closely with physical therapists to prevent pressure wounds, promote wound healing, and prevent the formation of scars and joint contractures. The patient with a major burn injury is immobile for periods secondary to chemical paralysis or sedation. The immobilized patient is at risk for developing pressure wounds. The nurse continually assesses and repositions the patient. In the immobilized patient, physical therapy is limited to range of motion.

The burn patient with burns over joints can develop contractures as the burn wound heals that impede mobility. The nurse works with physical therapy to properly position the patient and apply splints that prevent the formation of joint contractures. As the burn wounds heal, the physical therapist assesses the need for pressure garments, custom-made elastic garments that apply uniform pressure over the wound. Pressure garments, if worn correctly, reduce scarring and prevent the formation of hypertrophic scars. The patient may wear pressure garments for up to 2 years after sustaining a major burn injury.

The physical therapist ambulates the burn patient as soon as the patient is stable. As the patient becomes stronger, physical therapy exercises to increase strength and improve function are implemented. Physical therapy sessions can be very painful for the patient, and the burn nurse works with the therapist to ensure that the patient is properly medicated for pain and anxiety prior to each session.

Psychosocial Support

A major burn injury can result in a psychological crisis for the patient and family. Fear, loss of control, and disruption of the family structure contribute to the psychological devastation. Often the burn patient or family members have mental health histories or addiction problems that are exacerbated by the trauma of burn injury. The nurse works with members of the burn team, including social workers, psychologists, and child-life specialists, to provide psychological support to the patient and family.

— • • • —

Supporting the Patient

A burn injury is a frightening and traumatic event for the patient regardless of severity. The patient's preinjury cognitive status, psychological health, coping skills, and social support networks all contribute to the way the patient responds psychologically to the burn injury (Blakeney, Rosenberg, Rosenberg, & Faber, 2008). The nurse assesses preinjury psychological status upon admission, obtaining information from the patient and the family. Information about how the patient has handled stressful events in the past is helpful in planning care. The patient with a large burn initially may not be aware of the extent of injury. As the patient becomes more alert, the patient becomes cognizant of the fact that a life-changing, if not life-threatening, event has occurred. This realization can bring feelings of fear that contribute to the pain and anxiety. The nurse works to alleviate these feelings by providing the patient information about the plan of care and allowing the patient and family some control in care decisions. The patient's room should be made as comfortable as possible. Placing favorite objects in the room and playing the patient's favorite music can help orient the patient and decrease anxiety.

The patient with a large burn injury may use strategies such as dissociation, disintegration, and depersonalization to cope with the burn injury (Blakeney et al., 2008). The nurse must be aware of the coping strategies the patient is using and work with the patient to adopt strategies that are conducive to healing. It is not uncommon for the burn patient to experience feelings of hopelessness, despair, and depression as body image changes and functional limitations become apparent. Antidepressants are often prescribed to treat depression. The nurse helps the patient and family adapt and set realistic goals toward which to work.

The psychosocial aspects of burn care are often physically and emotionally difficult for the nurse. As the patient recovers, dependence on nursing staff can increase. Hopelessness and despair can cause the patient to act out in anger or to withdraw in tears. The nurse must be compassionate yet firm in setting boundaries with the patient. Most importantly, the nurse should encourage the patient to verbalize feelings followed by reassurance that the patient's feelings are normal after a burn injury. The nurse should avoid personal judgment of the patient's actions. The burn team supports the patient, family, and each other as the patient adapts psychologically.

Most patients do recover from the emotional trauma of a burn injury and return to productive fulfilling lives. The nurse provides the patient with resources to help complete this recovery, including further psychological evaluation and therapy and burn survivor networks. Burn survivor groups include support groups led by psychosocial burn team members at most burn centers and burn survivor networks. Often the first burn survivor a burn patient meets is him- or herself. Networking with other burn survivors can alleviate feelings of isolation. Numerous online and national burn survivor networks exist. The Phoenix Society is one such network that provides many psychosocial resources for burn survivors and their family.

Supporting the Family

Following a major burn, the nurse provides immediate comfort and support to the patient's family as they see their loved one for the first time. The first visit is frightening for family members, as the patient may be heavily sedated, on a ventilator, and so edematous as to be unrecognizable. The nurse should work with other members of the burn team to educate the family to the burn unit layout, the sounds and smells, and the need for infection control practices. A child-life specialist, if available, can prepare small children to see their family member, using dolls and role-playing. Once the family is at the patient's bedside, the nurse educates the family to the lines and machines attached to the patient. The family is encouraged to talk to and touch the patient. The

nurse must be prepared to answer the family's questions about the patient's status and prognosis in a way that instills hope without being misleading. The nurse is often responsible for introducing family members to other members of the burn team and ensuring that the family comprehends the plan of care for the patient.

Once the burn patient enters the acute phase of burn care, the nurse works with the family to provide emotional support to the patient. It is natural for family members to go through periods of hopelessness even as the patient improves. The nurse helps the family develop coping strategies and connects the family with support services as needed. The nurse should be aware of issues specific to the family such as financial concerns, family dynamics, and the ability to cope. Discord among family members is not uncommon. Hospital security policies are put in place if the nurse perceives that the safety of hospital staff or the patient is threatened by family members or visitors.

Many burn centers have support groups for family members. Families should be encouraged to attend sessions even if the patient is not stable enough to attend. Communication with other family members helps validate feelings. Burn unit social workers, or trained volunteers, facilitate support group dialogue and answer questions about the burn healing process.

Rehabilitation Phase

The rehabilitation phase of burn care begins when the patient is no longer acutely ill and most of the burn wounds are covered. The rehabilitation phase begins in the hospital and continues post discharge as the patient regains function and recovers emotionally. For the patient with large burns, the rehabilitation phase may continue for several years during which the patient wears pressure garments, continues physical therapy, and has reconstructive surgeries.

Nursing Management

Burn patients with very large burns are now surviving. Restoring quality of life and appearance have become important measures of successful burn care. Nursing care during the resuscitation phase can help the burn patient achieve optimal recovery. The primary nursing intervention during this phase is to support the patient's physical and emotional healing. This includes preparing the patient and family for discharge and ensuring that the patient is connected to resources in his or her home community to facilitate continued healing.

During the rehabilitation phase, physical healing focuses primarily on wound healing. There are additional factors that the nurse should address with the patient and family during this phase. Because altered immune function is sustained throughout the healing phase, the burn patients may be susceptible to infections and colds. Appropriate precautions should be taken, including avoiding unnecessary exposure to people with colds or infections and maintaining up-to-date immunizations. The recovering burn patient should be educated about signs and symptoms of infection and should seek prompt medical treatment. Hypermetabolism is sustained for 9 to 12 months following burn injury (Hart et al., 2000). The patient's weight should be monitored closely throughout the rehabilitation phase. The patient may still require supplemental enteral nutrition or high-caloric nutritional supplements to maintain a positive energy balance. Large burn injuries have been associated with bone density losses, and the patient may be at increased risk for osteoporosis and pathologic fractures (Evans, 2007). Thermoregulation disturbances continue throughout the rehabilitation phase and the patient may experience heat intolerance.

Wound and Scar Management

The rehabilitation phase of burn care begins when the patient's wounds are primarily covered. Wound management consists of final closure of the burn wound, assessing for signs of infection, and scar management. The patient and family are taught wound care prior to discharge from the hospital. Post discharge the patient is followed as an outpatient regularly for the duration of the rehabilitation phase.

During the rehabilitation phase, the burn wound becomes a scar. The burn scar continues to develop for up to 2 years post injury. Proper wound and scar management helps the burn scar become lighter in color and more pliable. The patient with large burns is at risk for developing a number of scar-related complications during this time. The nurse works with physical and occupational therapists to assess scar development and develop appropriate treatment modalities to prevent complications. The patient's tolerance for exercise is measured over time. Active exercise is encouraged to maintain or rebuild muscle mass, decrease edema, and reduce the risk of deep vein thrombosis.

Hypertrophic Scarring

Second-degree burn wounds extend into the dermis, synthesizing collagen to form a scar. In areas of the wound with granulation tissue, collagen deposition can be disorganized, resulting in the development of a hypertrophic scar that is erythematous and raised. Hypertrophic scarring occurs most often in nongrafted burns that took longer than 2 weeks to heal or along the edges of skin grafts. Children and individuals with darker skin pigments are more susceptible. Hypertrophic scarring can be prevented or greatly reduced by the application of pressure garments. Pressure over time helps the collagen bundles align in a more parallel fashion and reduces hypervascularity and cellularity. Keeping the skin soft and pliable with ointments and massage also helps reduce the hypertrophic scar.

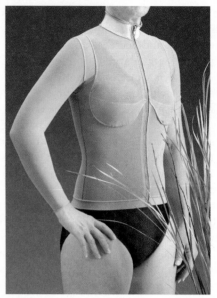

Figure 16-14 The patient may wear custom-made elastic pressure garments for 6 months to 2 years post injury. (Photo © Gottfried Medical, Inc., used with permission)

The burn patient may be required to continuously wear pressure garments for up to 2 years following injury (Figure 16-14). Physical or occupational therapists measure the patient at different times to ensure that the garments fit correctly and provide continuous pressure. The patient is educated about the importance of wearing the garments continuously during this time and how to protect fragile skin under the garments with lubrication. Pressure garments can be uncomfortable to wear, causing itching and heat intolerance. Therefore, patient compliance can be an issue. The nurse works with the burn team to encourage compliance. Over-the-counter or prescription medications to decrease itching are often prescribed.

Wound Contractures

Wound contractures occur as a result of scar formation over joints, which limit joint movement. Contractures are prevented by exercise, body positioning, joint splinting, and pressure dressings. Prevention begins during the acute phase of burn care and continues through the rehabilitation phase. During the rehabilitation phase, the nurse works with physical and occupational therapy to ensure that the patient is exercising and that appropriate body positioning is maintained using splints and other devices (Figure 16-15).

Contractures are treated by applying splints to the affected area and by specific range-of-motion exercises. The splints are worn for prescribed times. An important nursing intervention is to assess the patient's compliance. Contractures that are not responding to exercise and positioning may require surgical incision of the scar tissue to "release" the contracture of a joint. The excised scar is closed by primary closure, z-plasty, or skin grafting (Huang, 2007).

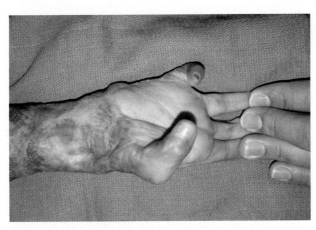

Figure 16-15 Burn contracture.
(Courtesy of JPD/Custom Medical Stock Photo, Inc.)

Other Wound Complications

The maturing burn scar is fragile and susceptible to wound breakdown from shearing and pressure. The burn nurse assesses the patient for signs of wound breakdown and makes sure that wound dressings and pressure garments are fitted properly. Wound breakdown can occur after the patient is discharged from the hospital. The patient and family are provided education about protecting the wound from breakdown and how to care for open wounds that develop.

Neuropathies can develop as a result of scar formation, edema, or improper positioning of splints or dressings. The nurse assesses peripheral pulses and sensation throughout the rehabilitation phase. Symptoms of neuropathies include severe burning pain, increased or decreased sensation, abnormal sensation, and cold intolerance (Warden & Warner, 2007). The nurse works with physical and occupational therapists to position splints and dressings appropriately. Edema can be prevented by elevating edematous limbs.

Heterotopic bone ossification, the abnormal formation of bone, is a rare complication of burn injury. Heterotopic formation is more likely to occur in a joint that had an overlying deep burn and which was immobilized for a long period. Early joint mobility in the acute burn phase is important in preventing this complication. During the rehabilitation phase, the patient is assessed for range of motion. A symptom of heterotopic bone formation is the patient's reluctance to move a joint that previously had good range of motion. The patient is taught the importance of continuing range-of-motion exercises for joints near the burn injury.

Pain During the Rehabilitation Phase

Pain during the rehabilitation phase of burn care is characterized as an aching pain (Meyer, Patterson, Jaco, Woodson, & Thomas, 2007). As in the acute phase, the burn patient experiences procedural pain and background pain. Oral opioids, acetaminophen, or nonsteroidal anti-inflammatory medications provide adequate pain relief for most patients. Once the patient's pain is treated, itching and anxiety should be addressed as separate issues. Pain and anxiety medications should be tapered during the rehabilitation phase. The nurse, working with psychosocial burn team members, can use nonpharmacological therapies to decrease pain and anxiety.

Psychosocial Support

During the rehabilitation phase, the burn patient becomes aware of the extent of the burn injury and the effect of appearance, function, and activities of daily living. The patient experiences feelings of grief and loss for the "preburn self." Feelings of hopelessness and loss of autonomy often result in the patient becoming angry with the burn team and family members (Blakeney, Rosenberg, Rosenberg, & Faber, 2008). The burn team works with the patient to combat these feelings by setting limits, defining achievable goals, and providing as much autonomy as possible. The patient and family are provided with information about the psychological recovery from a burn injury and future disfigurement and functional abilities. The patient and family may benefit from attending a burn support group where they meet other burn survivors who validate their own experiences and instill hope for the future.

Reintegration into Society

The burn team begins to prepare the patient for reintegration into society prior to discharge. For the patient with a large disfiguring burn, reintegration is a daunting anxiety-provoking step. The patient fears rejection and ridicule from acquaintances and strangers seeing the burn scars for the first time. Both the patient and family worry that they will not be able to manage activities of daily living and burn-specific care at home. The burn team works to alleviate these concerns by encouraging the patient and family to be independent prior to discharge. The patient and family are encouraged to practice interacting with others by taking short trips outside the hospital prior to discharge. The burn team may also work with the patient's community to ease social reintegration. Groups important to the patient can be provided with education about burns and be given the opportunity to ask questions about how to best assist and encourage the patient.

After discharge the burn patient faces many physical and psychosocial challenges. The nurse assesses the patient's coping abilities during outpatient clinic visits. During this time the patient may begin experiencing heightened levels of depression, anxiety, or signs of posttraumatic stress disorder. The patient who has altered behavior may benefit from consultation with a psychiatric or mental health care provider.

The patient's family members must also learn to cope with the long-term consequences of the burn injury. A major burn injury often results in loss of income and changed family roles. The family may feel ill equipped to care for the patient's physical and psychosocial needs. Prior to discharge, the burn team assesses the family's ability to care for the patient at home and provides the family with references for local services that can ease the transition.

Recent studies have shown that individuals who sustained a major burn injury as a child or adult report that their quality of life is high. Quality of life in young adults who sustained a 30% or larger TBSA burn as children was comparable to age-matched population controls 2 years following injuries (Baker, Russell, Meyer, & Blakeney, 2007). Many years after injury, quality of life in patients who sustained very large burns (70% to 98% TBSA) as children remained comparable to that of nonburned individuals, even with lingering physical limitations (Sheridan et al., 2000). Other studies have shown that adult patients also report good quality of life after a large burn injury. Size of injury, age of the individual when burned, nonburn physical illness, psychological disorders, and social connectedness have been shown to contribute to quality of life post burn (Anzarut, Chen, Shankowsky, & Tredget, 2005; Moi, Wentzel-Larsen, Salemark, Wahl, & Hanestad, 2006). Therefore, patients with a major burn injury can go on to lead full and rewarding lives. The nurse can help patients and families recognize that quality of life can be good and to provide them with support services to help them achieve this goal.

BURN SUMMARY

Burns are painful injuries that involve every major body system. Even a minor burn can be a very stressful event for a patient. A major burn is an often life-threatening injury. The patient endures countless medical procedures, intense physical therapy, and much pain. In addition, the physical scarring and loss of function associated with a large burn contribute to psychological stresses. The nurse caring for the burn patient must be aware of both the physical and psychological issues associated with burn care. Most burn injuries are minor and treated in emergency departments or clinics, where the nurse assesses

Nursing Care

Nursing care of the burn patient is challenging yet rewarding. Even minor burns can require complex care in the emergency department or clinic setting. Nursing interventions for the minor burn injury include wound care, assessing for signs and symptoms of infection, pain management, and psychosocial evaluation.

Care of the patient with serious burns is often delivered in specialized burn centers by a dedicated multidisciplinary burn team. The burn team is comprised of the following members: physicians, nurses, physical and occupational therapists, dieticians, pharmacists, psychologists, and social and child-life workers. Other disciplines, such as recreational therapists, speech therapists, and other medical specialists, are consulted as needed. Nursing members of the burn team include advance practice nurses, burn nurses, and case-managers to name a few. Most nurses working with burn patients are Advance Burn Life Support (ABLS) certified and many are certified in intensive care or pediatric specialties. The nurse caring for the burn patient is a vital member of the burn team. The nurse provides bedside care and communicates the patient status to other members of the burn team and the family. The nurse provides continuity of care throughout the three phases of burn care. See the Nursing Diagnoses box for a specific list.

and cares for the wound while monitoring and treating pain and anxiety. The nurse working in a specialized burn center is part of a multidisciplinary team providing intensive care to patients with burn injuries. In this setting, the nurse cares for the burn patient through the continuum of burn care: from resuscitation to rehabilitation. Because of the broad depth of knowledge a nurse must have to care for a major burn, burn nursing is challenging. However, the rewards of following a patient with severe burns from intensive care to the time when the patient is functioning fully in society are many and great.

CASE STUDY

Jon Lewis, a 21-year-old student at a university, was trapped in his room during a house fire. In an attempt to escape the fire, he opened the door from his room, burning his forearms, face, and chest, then turned and jumped arms first through his second-floor window. On the ground he was met by firemen who rushed him to the burn trauma center at the university hospital 5 minutes away.

Jon arrived in the emergency department (ED) of the burn trauma center 10 minutes post burn.

1. Should the burning process have stopped? If not, what care is indicated to stop the process?

2. What findings would lead the burn team to suspect an inhalation injury?

3. What should the ED team do immediately if they suspect an inhalation injury?

4. How should the extent and depth of his burns on his chest, forearms, and face be assessed?

5. Why is lactated Ringer's the preferred fluid for fluid resuscitation? How is the amount of fluid required calculated? How will the nurse know if fluid resuscitation is adequate?

On further evaluation, Jon was found to have compression injuries of his T5-7 vertebrae and a severed muscle and tendons in his right arm.

6. How did he probably sustain these injuries?

Following initial management in the ED, Jon was transported to the burn trauma unit of the hospital.

On admission to the burn trauma ICU, he was ventilated, had dressings applied to his chest, arms, and face, and was receiving 800 mL/hr of lactated Ringer's. His vital signs were: BP 184/92, heart rate 110 bpm, respirations 12, oxygen saturation 94%.

7. What additional information should the nurse obtain from the ED team?

8. What complications might the nurse anticipate?

9. What preventive strategies should the nurse initiate immediately?

See answers to Case Studies in the Answer Section at the back of the book.

CRITICAL THINKING QUESTIONS

1. What are the most common etiologies of burn injury for each of the following age groups?
   a. Children
   b. Adults
   c. Older adults

2. What are the differences in manifestations between a partial- and a full-thickness burn?

3. What findings would indicate a possible inhalation injury?

4. What changes occur within the vasculature following a burn injury? What implications do these changes have for patient management?

5. What are the priorities of care immediately after a patient with a severe burn injury arrives at a hospital?

6. How are full-thickness burn wounds managed?

7. What are some of the psychological issues that confront burn victims?

8. Why are very young and very old people likely to have more severe burn injuries?

See answers to Critical Thinking Questions in the Answer Section at the back of the book.

EXPLORE MEDIALINK

http://www.prenhall.com/perrin

Additional interactive resources for this chapter can be found on the Web site at http://www.prenhall.com/perrin. Click on "Chapter 16" to select activities for this chapter.

Case Study: Burn Trauma

Nursing Care Plan

NCLEX Review Questions

MediaLinks:
- University Hospital's Burn Center, University of Utah
- Burnsurgery.Org

- Clinical Review: ABC of Burns
- Center for Disease Control and Prevention
- Fire Deaths and Injuries Fact Sheet
- American Burn Association
- Phoenix Society for Burn Survivors

MediaLink Applications

REFERENCES

Ahrens, M. (2001). *The U.S. fire problem overview report: Leading causes and other patterns and trends*. Quincy, MA: NFPA Fire Prevention and Analysis.

Ahrns, K. S. (2004). Trends in burn resuscitation: Shifting the focus from fluids to adequate endpoint monitoring, edema control, and adjuvant therapies. *Critical Care Nursing Clinics of North America, 16*(1), 75–98.

American Burn Association (2008a). Burn incidence and treatment in the US: 2007 fact sheet. Retrieved April 15, 2008, from: http://www.ameriburn.org/resources_factsheet.php

American Burn Association. (2008b). *Scald injury prevention: Educator's guide*. Chicago: Author.

American College of Surgeons. (2006). Guidelines for the operation of burn centers. In Committee on Trauma & American College of Surgeons (Eds.), *Resources for optimal care of the injured patient* (pp. 79–86). Chicago: Author.

Anzarut, A., Chen, M., Shankowsky, H., & Tredget, E. E. (2005). Quality-of-life and outcome predictors following massive burn injury. *Plastic and Reconstructive Surgery, 116*(3), 791–797.

Baker, C., Russell, W., Meyer, W., & Blakeney, P. (2007). Physical and Psychologic rehabilitation outcomes for young adults burned as children. *Archives of Physical Medicine Rehabilitation, 88,* S57–64.

Baker, S. P., O'Neill, B., Ginsburg, M. J., & Li, G. (1992). *The injury fact book* (2nd ed.). New York: Oxford University Press.

Blakeney, P. E., Rosenberg, L., Rosenberg, M., & Faber, A. W. (2008). Psychosocial care of persons with severe burns. *Burns, 34,* 433–440.

Danks, R. R., Wibbenmeyer, L. A., Faucher, L. D., Sihler, K. C., Kealey, G. P., Chang, P., et al. (2004). Methamphetamine-associated burn injuries: A retrospective analysis. *Journal of Burn Care and Rehabilitation, 25*(5), 425–429.

Evans, E. B. (2007). Musculoskeletal changes secondary to thermal burns. In D. N. Herndon (Ed.), *Total burn care* (3rd ed., pp. 652–666). Philadelphia: Saunders Elsevier.

George, R. L., McGwin, G., Jr., Schwacha, M. G., Metzger, J., Cross, J. M., Chaudry, I. H., et al. (2005). The association between sex and mortality among burn patients as modified by age. *Journal of Burn Care and Rehabilitation, 26*(5), 416–421.

Gosain, A., & Gamelli, R. L. (2005). A primer in cytokines. *Journal of Burn Care and Rehabilitation, 26*(1), 7–12.

Greenbaum, A. R., Donne, J., Wilson, D., & Dunn, K. W. (2004). Intentional burn injury: An evidence-based, clinical and forensic review. *Burns, 30*(7), 628–642.

Greenbaum, A. R., Horton, J. B., Williams, C. J., Shah, M., & Dunn, K. W. (2006). Burn injuries inflicted on children or the elderly: A framework for clinical and forensic assessment. *Plastic and Reconstructive Surgery, 118*(2), 46e–58e.

Greenhalgh, D. G., Saffle, J. R., Holmes, J. H. T., Gamelli, R. L., Palmieri, T. L., Horton, J. W., et al. (2007). American Burn Association consensus conference to define sepsis and infection in burns. *Journal of Burn Care and Research, 28*(6), 776–790.

Hart, D. W., Wolf, S. E., Mlcak, R., Chinkes, D. L., Ramzy, P. I., Obeng, M. K., et al. (2000). Persistence of muscle catabolism after severe burn. *Surgery, 128*(2), 312–319.

Hershberger, R. C., Hunt, J. L., Arnoldo, B. D., & Purdue, G. F. (2007). Abdominal compartment syndrome in the severely burned patient. *Journal of Burn Care and Research, 28*(5), 708–714.

Huang, T. (2007). Management of contractural deformities involving the axilla (shoulder), elbow, hip, knee, and ankle joints in burn patients. In D. N. Herndon (Ed.), *Total burn care* (3rd ed., pp. 727–740). Philadelphia: Saunders Elsevier.

Istre, G. R., McCoy, M. A., Osborn, L., Barnard, J. J., & Bolton, A. (2001). Deaths and injuries from house fires. *New England Journal of Medicine, 344*(25), 1911–1916.

Kerby, J. D., McGwin, G., Jr., George, R. L., Cross, J. A., Chaudry, I. H., & Rue, L. W., 3rd. (2006). Sex differences in mortality after burn injury: Results of analysis of the National Burn Repository of the American Burn Association. *Journal of Burn Care and Research, 27*(4), 452–456.

Kramer, G. C., Lund, T., & Beckum, O. K. (2007). Pathophysiology of burn shock and burn edema. In D. N. Herndon (Ed.), *Total burn care* (3rd ed., pp. 93–106). Philadelphia: Saunders Elsevier.

Magnotti, L. J., & Deitch, E. A. (2005). Burns, bacterial translocation, gut barrier function, and failure. *Journal of Burn Care and Rehabilitation, 26*(5), 383–391.

Meyer, W. J. I., Patterson, D. R., Jaco, M., Woodson, L., & Thomas, C. (2007). Management of pain and other discomforts in burned patients. In D. N. Herndon (Ed.), *Total burn care* (3rd ed., pp. 797–818). Philadelphia: Saunders Elsevier.

Moi, A. L., Wentzel-Larsen, T., Salemark, L., Wahl, A. K., & Hanestad, B. R. (2006). Impaired generic health status but perception of good quality of life in survivors of burn injury. *Journal of Trauma, 61*(4), 961–968; discussion 968–969.

Muller, M., Gahankari, D., & Herndon, D. N. (2007). Operative wound management. In D. N. Herndon (Ed.), *Total burn care* (3rd ed., pp. 177–195). Philadelphia: Saunders Elsevier.

Neuwalder, J. M., Sampson, C., Breuing, K. H., & Orgill, D. P. (2002). A review of computer-aided body surface area determination: SAGE II and EPRI's 3D Burn Vision. *Journal of Burn Care and Rehabilitation, 23*(1), 55–59; discussion 54.

Perel, P., & Roberts, I. (2007). Colloids versus crystalloids for fluid resuscitation in critically ill patients. *Cochrane Database System Review* (4), CD000567.

Pham, H. H., Schrag, D., Hargraves, J. L., & Bach, P. B. (2005). Delivery of preventive services to older adults by primary care physicians. *Journal of the American Medical Association, 294*(4), 473–481.

Pham, T. A., Cancio, L. C., & Gibran, N. S. (2008). American Burn Association practice guidelines: Burn shock resuscitation. *Journal of Burn Care and Research, 29*(1), 257–266.

Prelack, K., Dylewski, M., & Sheridan, R. L. (2007). Practical guidelines for nutritional management of burn injury and recovery. *Burns, 33*(1), 14–24.

Pruitt, B. A., Wolf, S. W., & Mason, A. D. J. (2007). Epidemiological, demographic, and outcome characteristics of burn injury. In D. N. Herndon (Ed.), *Total burn care* (3rd ed., pp. 14–32). Philadelphia: Saunders Elsevier.

Rawlins, J. M., Khan, A. A., Shenton, A. F., & Sharpe, D. T. (2007). Epidemiology and outcome analysis of 208 children with burns attending an emergency department. *Pediatric Emergency Care, 23*(5), 289–293.

Runyan, C. W., Bangdiwala, S. I., Linzer, M. A., Sacks, J. J., & Butts, J. (1992). Risk factors for fatal residential fires. *New England Journal of Medicine, 327*(12), 859–863.

Saffle, J. R., & Graves, C. (2007). Nutritional support of the burned patient. In D. N. Herndon (Ed.), *Total burn care* (3rd ed., pp. 398–419). Philadelphia: Saunders Elsevier.

Sen, S., & Gamelli, R. L. (2005). Burns and inhalation injury. In M. P. Fink, E. Abraham, J.-L. Vincent, & P. M. Kochanek (Eds.), *Textbook of critical care* (5th ed., pp. 691–697). Philadelphia: Saunders Elsevier.

Sharma, B. R. (2007). Infection in patients with severe burns: Causes and prevention thereof. *Infectious Disease Clinics of North America, 21*(3), 745–759, ix.

Sheridan, R. L. (2002). Burns. *Critical Care Medicine, 30*(Suppl. 11), S500–514.

Sheridan, R. L., Hinson, M. I., Liang, M. H., Nackel, A. F., Schoenfeld, D. A., Ryan, C. M., et al. (2000). Long-term outcome of children surviving massive burns. *Journal of the American Medical Association, 283*(1), 69–73.

Traber, D. L., Herndon, D. N., Enkhbaatar, P., Maybauer, M. O., & Maybauer, D. M. (2007). The pathophysiology of inhalation injury. In D. N. Herndon (Ed.), *Total burn care* (3rd ed., pp. 248–261). Philadelphia: Saunders Elsevier.

Warden, G. D. (2007). Fluid resuscitation and early management. In D. N. Herndon (Ed.), *Total burn care* (3rd ed., pp. 107–118). Philadelphia: Saunders Elsevier.

Warden, G. D., & Warner, P. M. (2007). Functional sequelae and disability assessment. In D. N. Herndon (Ed.), *Total burn care* (3rd ed., pp. 781–787). Philadelphia: Saunders Elsevier.

Care of the Patient with Sepsis

Kathleen Perrin, PhD, RN, CCRN

Learning Outcomes

Upon completion of this chapter, the learner will be able to:

1. Differentiate between systemic inflammatory response syndrome (SIRS), sepsis, severe sepsis, and septic shock.

2. Describe evidence-based prevention strategies for ventilator-associated pneumonia (VAP), central venous catheter site infections, and surgical site infections.

3. Perform a nursing assessment of the patient with SIRS and severe sepsis.

4. Discuss the elements of the sepsis resuscitation bundle.

5. Compare and contrast the use of three vasoactive medications in the management of septic shock.

6. Describe the elements in the sepsis management bundle.

7. Evaluate methods used to reduce fever in a febrile patient.

8. Explain the process of disseminated intravascular coagulation.

Abbreviations

APC	Activated Protein C
FDPs	Fibrin Degradation Products
IL	Interleukin
MRSA	Methicillin-Resistant *Staphylococcus Aureus*
TNF	Tumor Necrosis Factor

Severe sepsis, the presence of infection, inflammation, and organ dysfunction, is a complex, costly, and frequently lethal syndrome with a hospital mortality rate that approached 29% worldwide in 2001. It is such a disturbing health problem that an international task force was mobilized to study and recommend evidence-based solutions to the problem. Infection prevention strategies and evidence-based interventions advocated by the Surviving Sepsis Campaign (2004) are beginning to improve outcomes for septic patients.

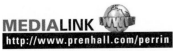

MEDIALINK
http://www.prenhall.com/perrin

See the Companion Website for chapter-specific resources at www.prenhall.com/perrin.

Inflammatory Immune Response in Septic Shock

Severe sepsis is a complex process that is not completely understood. However, it seems the body responds to sepsis in three general ways: inflammation, thrombosis, and fibrinolysis. This process is displayed in Figure 17-1.

Pathophysiology Review

The inflammatory phase of sepsis begins in response to an infectious organism as white blood cells release proinflammatory cytokines such as tumor necrosis factor (TNF) and interleukins (IL). Normally, anti-inflammatory cytokines are also produced so inflammation is limited. The endothelium is affected at the same time and the coagulation cascade and complement system are activated. In most circumstances, these mechanisms isolate the **infection**. In severe sepsis, bacteria and neutrophils continue to stimulate the proinflammatory cytokines, overwhelming the anti-inflammatory cytokines and resulting in a systemic inflammatory response. The abundance of proinflammatory cytokines causes additional damage

to the endothelium, a fluid shift from capillaries into the damaged tissues, and further activation of the coagulation cascade.

With activation of the coagulation cascade, thrombin is produced. The presence of thrombin causes additional inflammation and results in new endothelial damage and a procoagulant state. Normally, this procoagulant state is balanced by the presence of anticoagulation mediators such as activated protein C (APC). However, APC is deficient in sepsis and the procoagulant state can result in the formation of miniscule clots that obstruct the microvasculature and limit tissue perfusion.

In the final stage, fibrinolysis is delayed (possibly because of endothelial damage) and the balance between clot formation and breakdown is disrupted. In severe sepsis what began as a local response to infection escalates to a systemic disease due to imbalances in the compensatory mechanisms. The imbalances that occur in the normal processes of inflammation, coagulation, and fibrinolysis result in systemic inflammation, with the potential for impaired perfusion of multiple organs, and coagulation disturbances.

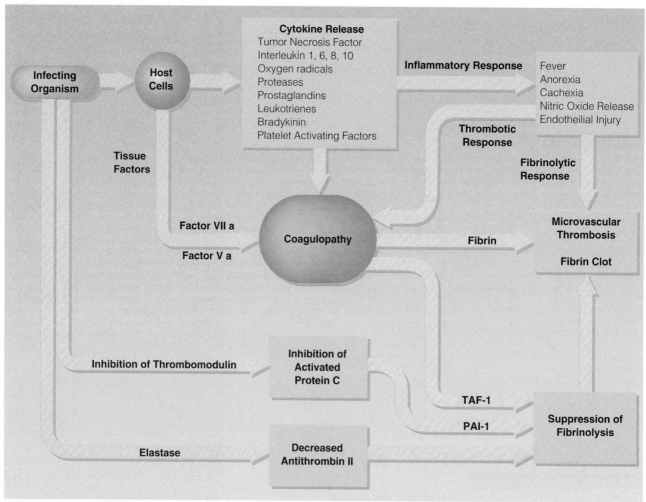

Figure 17-1 Inflammatory immune response in septic shock.

VISUAL MAP Infection, Sepsis, and Disseminated Intravascular Coagulation

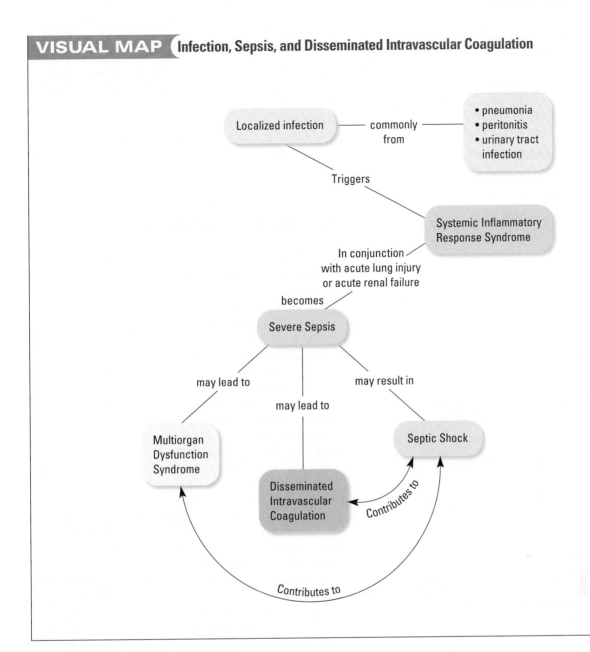

Incidence and Prevalence

Severe sepsis is a costly illness that is likely to increase in incidence. According to Angus et al. (2001), severe sepsis had an annual incidence of nearly three quarters of a million cases in the United States with a hospital mortality rate approaching 29% in 2001. Because sepsis rates rise sharply with age, Angus et al. predict that as the nation ages the incidence of sepsis will increase and there will be almost a million cases of sepsis in the United States by the year 2010.

Sepsis is more likely to be lethal in the older adult. In Angus et al.'s study, the overall hospital mortality rate was 28.6%, but it approached 38% in those 85 years or older. The impact of age on outcome was most important for previously healthy older adults.

The majority of septic patients, approximately 70% of them, receive care in an intensive care, coronary care, or intermediate care unit. In fact, sepsis is the leading problem in European intensive care units (Kortgen, Hofmann, & Bauer, 2006). The care of a septic patient in a critical care unit is expensive; Kortgen et al. calculated the cost of care as 20,000 to 30,000 euros per patient. Per-patient costs for the condition were highest in infants, nonsurvivors, intensive care unit (ICU) or surgical patients, and patients with dysfunctions of four or more organ systems. However, because sepsis affects the elderly disproportionately, more than half of all annual costs—$8.7 billion—were spent on care of septic patients 65 years or older.

The Surviving Sepsis Campaign (2004) is a joint effort of the European Society of Intensive Care Medicine, the International Sepsis Forum, and the Society of Critical Care Medicine. The focus of the campaign is improving the diagnosis, survival, and management of patients with sepsis by addressing the challenges associated with it.

"The Surviving Sepsis program aims to: increase awareness, understanding and knowledge, change perceptions and behavior; increase the pace of change in patterns of care, influence public policy, define standards of care in severe sepsis and reduce the mortality associated with sepsis by 25% over the next 5 years."

Predisposing Factors

There are a variety of factors that increase an individual's risk for developing sepsis. These factors include:

- Advanced age (older than 85 years)
- Compromised immune status such as
  - Alcohol misuse
  - Cancer
  - Immunosuppressant therapy
  - Positive human immunodeficiency virus (HIV) status
- Chronic illness such as:
  - Diabetes mellitus
  - Chronic renal failure
  - Hepatitis
- Invasive interventions such as central line catheters and endotracheal intubation
- Malnutrition
- Surgical/invasive procedures, especially intra-abdominal surgery
- Sequential infections treated with broad-spectrum antibiotics

Causes

Nguyen, Rivers, and Abrahamlan (2006) analyzed multiple studies of both community- and hospital-acquired severe sepsis and **septic shock**. They determined that the most common sources of infection were the following:

Lungs (35%)

Abdomen (21%)

Urinary tract (13%)

Skin and soft tissues (7%)

Other sources (8%)

Unknown source (16%)

This was true as long as the patient was less than 65 years of age; among older patients the urinary tract source was the most common source of infection.

Prevention of Hospital-Acquired Infections

Hospital-acquired infections are associated with increased lengths of hospital stay as well as increased costs. At the very least the development of an infection can be uncomfortable for the patient and worrisome for the patient and family. Catheter-related bloodborne infections and surgical site infections increase the likelihood that the patient will develop severe sepsis or multisystem organ dysfunction and spend time in intensive care. Other hospital-acquired infections such as ventilator-associated pneumonia are linked to an increased risk of patient death. Therefore, nurses and other health care providers need to be vigilant about utilizing evidence-based practices to prevent nosocomial infections.

Ventilator-Associated Pneumonia Protocols

Ventilator-associated pneumonia (VAP) is an airway infection that develops at least 48 hours after a patient is intubated, most commonly a week later. Preventing pneumonia associated with ventilator use is of special importance because VAP is the leading cause of death from hospital-acquired infections (Institute for Healthcare Improvement [IHI]). Death from VAP exceeds the rate of death from central line infections, severe sepsis, or respiratory tract infections in the nonintubated patient. In addition to making it more likely that the patient will die, VAP also prolongs the patient's illness and hospitalization. It results in more time spent on the ventilator, more days in the ICU, and more time in the hospital after discharge from the ICU. Due to the increased amount of care required, the development of VAP adds an estimated $40,000 to a typical hospital admission.

According to Seckel (2007), VAP develops in between 9% and 27% of intubated patients. Bacteria usually enter the respiratory tract after colonizing the oral cavity, sinuses, trachea, or stomach. The normal flora of the oral cavity changes within 48 hours of hospital admission to more virulent flora, whereas stomach contents become colonized with bacteria when the pH of the stomach is altered for stress ulcer prophylaxis. VAP may develop when there is aspiration of these contents or when bacterial colonies develop on the endotracheal tube (Seckel).

Two crucial steps in reducing the morbidity and mortality due to ventilator-associated pneumonia are application of evidence-based practices to reduce the occurrence of pneumonia and early recognition and treatment of VAP should it develop. The IHI recommends that every health care institution implement the "Ventilator Bundle, a series of interventions related to ventilator care that, when implemented together, will achieve significantly better outcomes than when implemented individually."

The key components of the IHI ventilator bundle are:

- Elevation of the head of the bed
- Daily "sedation vacations" and assessment of readiness to extubate
- Peptic ulcer disease prophylaxis
- Deep venous thrombosis prophylaxis

PURPOSE: To significantly reduce methicillin-resistant *Staphylococcus aureus* (MRSA) infection by reliably implementing five components of care recommended in the IHI guidelines

RATIONALE: Health care-associated infections remain a major cause of disability, death, and increased cost of health care. Treatment of infections has become more complex because of the alarming rise in antibiotic resistance. Infections caused by MRSA are particularly problematic because their incidence has increased in the past decade and they are often lethal. Moreover, MRSA accounted for 63% of *S. aureus* infections acquired in ICUs in the United States in 2004.

HIGHLIGHTS OF RECOMMENDATIONS:
In order to reduce MRSA infections, the IHI recommends that organizations start with these five components of care:

1. Hand hygiene. Adequate hand hygiene involves wearing gloves during patient care and properly washing hands after the gloves are removed.

2. Decontamination of the environment and equipment. Because MRSA can survive on table tops, bed rails, and computers, these surfaces must be adequately decontaminated.

3. Active surveillance cultures. These cultures identify colonized patients and allow for implementation of isolation and adequate decontamination of surfaces to prevent transmission. Although the nares are the most common site for colonization, 15% to 25% of patients harbor MRSA in their axillae, 30% to 40% in their perineum, and 40% on their hands and arms.

4. Contact precautions for infected and colonized patients. Contact precautions interrupt the important modes of MRSA transmission. If nurses wear gloves during contact with patients with MRSA or while in the immediate environment of patients with MRSA, the likelihood that the nurses will contaminate their hands is decreased. Wearing a gown can protect nurses from contaminating their clothing when caring for colonized or infected patients.

5. Device bundles: See ventilator and central line bundles in Chapter 3 and Chapter 5, respectively.

Source: Reduce Methicillin-Resistant *Staphylococcus aureus* (MRSA) Infections

Available: http://www.ihi.org/IHI/Programs/Campaign/MRSAInfection.htm

---

Additional interventions recommended to prevent VAP include:

- Washing hands before and after contact with each patient (Tolentino-DelosReyes, Ruppert, & Shyang-Yun, 2007)

- Use of a continuous-suctioning endotracheal tube (Seckel, 2007)

- Change of ventilator circuit no more often than every 48 hours (Tolentino-DelosReyes et al., 2007) or no longer routinely changing the patient's ventilator circuit (Seckel, 2007)

- Preventing oral-tracheal contamination (Aragon & Sole, 2006)

Elevation of the Head of the Bed

Elevation of the head of the bed (HOB) to at least 30 degrees is recommended because it reduces the risk of aspiration of oropharyngeal contents. IHI guidelines advocate that it be standard procedure for all patients (especially for those receiving gastric feedings) to have their HOB elevated to 30 degrees unless there is a compelling reason, such as hemodynamic instability or the presence of an intra-aortic balloon pump, for them to have their HOB lower. Because the constant elevation of the HOB may result in increased lumbosacral pressure,

nurses need to be vigilant about assessing skin breakdown and providing pressure relief for patients.

Daily Sedation Vacations

Daily "sedation vacations" and assessment of readiness to extubate are recommended because reducing the amount of time on a ventilator decreases the patient's potential for exposure to VAP. There is concern among some nurses about the safety of interrupting sedation; therefore, most institutions have specific policies outlining for whom and when sedation interruption should be attempted. The evidence demonstrates that appropriate use of daily interruption of sedation to determine readiness to wean decreases patients' time on a ventilator, length of stay in ICU, and length of hospital stay without increasing unplanned extubations (Aragon & Sole, 2006). For additional information about sedation vacations, see Chapter 3.

Peptic Ulcer Prophylaxis

Peptic ulcer prophylaxis is recommended for ventilated patients for two reasons. First, there is a higher incidence of stress ulceration in critically ill patients. Next, critically ill intubated patients lack the ability to protect their airway, and the effects of aspirating acidic contents may be worse than aspirating material with a higher pH. Increasing the pH of gastric contents with H_2-receptor inhibitors may protect against a greater pulmonary inflammatory response if gastrointestinal contents are aspirated. The Surviving Sepsis Campaign Guidelines concluded that histamine receptor inhibitors are the preferred agents because they are more effective than sucralfate. Proton pump inhibitors have not been fully evaluated but they do not increase gastric pH as much as H_2-receptor inhibitors.

Deep Vein Thrombosis Prophylaxis

The IHI recommends deep venous thrombosis (DVT) prophylaxis because when it is applied as part of "a package of interventions for ventilator care, the rate of pneumonia decreases precipitously." The IHI believes that interventions to decrease DVTs remain excellent practice in the general care of ventilated patients. When determining which type of prophylaxis is appropriate, the IHI recommends balancing the increase in the risk of bleeding that may occur if anticoagulants are used with the fact that sequential compression devices are often not consistently applied to patients. For example, the devices may be removed for extensive periods when patients are away from the ICU for procedures. For additional information about DVT prophylaxis, see the safety initiative in Chapter 9 ∞ titled "Reducing Surgical Complications: Venous Thromboembolism (VTE) Prophylaxis."

Additional Evidence-Based Approaches to Prevention of Ventilator-Associated Pneumonia

Hand washing before and after patient contact has been demonstrated to be the single most important means of preventing infection (Aragon & Sole, 2006). The Center for Disease Control and Prevention (CDC) recommends alcohol-based products for hand hygiene. The CDC advises that hand hygiene should also include avoiding artificial nails and keeping natural nails short.

Seckel (2007) recommends use of a continuous subglottal suctioning tube to reduce the incidence of VAP (Figure 17-2).

In 2004, the American Association of Critical-Care Nurses (AACN) issued guidelines advising the use of an endotracheal tube (ET) with a dorsal lumen above the cuff (CASS tube). Such a tube permits continuous suction and prevents accumulation of tracheal secretions in the subglottic area. If a CASS tube is not inserted when the patient is initially intubated, the tube should not be changed to a CASS tube due to the increased likelihood of infection from reintubation. Aragon and Sole (2006) recommend maintaining cuff pressures in a traditional ET tube above 20 mm Hg to prevent VAP but indicate that further studies are needed to confirm this practice.

In the past ventilator circuits were changed at regular intervals, ranging from every 8 hours to every 2 days. Current recommendations are to change ventilator cir-

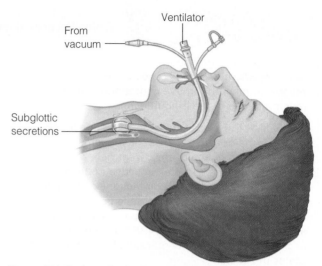

Figure 17-2 Endotracheal tube with evacuation lumen.

cuits no more often than every 48 hours (Tolentino-Delos-Reyes et al., 2007) or not to routinely change the patient's ventilator circuit (Seckel, 2007). Some sources now recommend that ventilator circuits be changed only when they are visibly soiled or are not functioning properly.

There is insufficient evidence about whether the provision of routine oral care with specific products decreases the incidence of VAP. The AACN (2006) noted in a practice alert that although several studies that included oral care as part of a VAP prevention bundle showed a decrease in the incidence of VAP, the specific contribution of oral care to the reduction in VAP was unknown. Most ICUs have specific policies for the delivery of oral care, usually requiring toothbrushing at least twice a day with a chlorhexidine product and differentiating comprehensive oral care (including toothbrushing) from oral cavity moisturizing.

The American Dental Society recommends tooth brushing at least twice a day to limit dental plaque, a source of bacteria, whereas chlorhexidine appears to prevent the overgrowth of more virulent bacteria in the mouth. However, the most appropriate technique for oral care and whether rinse, gel, or paste is the most effective way to apply the chlorhexidine are still being researched. The AACN recommends that nurses ensure their ICU has a written oral care policy and that they adhere to that policy. See Figure 17-3 for an example of an oral care cleansing system.

Preventing Venous Catheter-Related Bloodstream Infections

Central venous catheters (CVCs) are being used more frequently in patient care. The IHI estimates that 48% of ICU patients have CVCs, accounting for 15 million central venous catheter-days every year. Compared to peripherally inserted catheters, CVCs carry a significantly greater risk

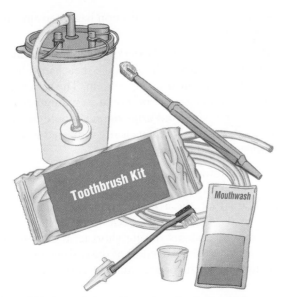

Figure 17-3 An oral cleansing and suctioning system.

of infection, accounting for nearly 90% of catheter-related bloodstream infections. Todd (2006) notes that approximately 80,000 such infections occur annually in ICUs. Mortality attributable to these infections is between 4% and 20% so between 500 and 4,000 patients in the United States die annually due to CVC-related bloodstream infections. In addition, nosocomial bloodstream infections prolong hospitalization by a mean of 7 days and increase the cost of a patient's care during a hospitalization by $3,700 to $29,000.

The IHI advocates use of the central line bundle, a group of evidence-based interventions for patients with intravascular catheters that, when implemented together, result in better outcomes than when implemented individually. The key components of the central line bundle are:

- Hand hygiene: Hands should be cleansed prior to contact with patients with waterless cleaning solution or if visibly soiled with soap and water. Alcohol-based products are recommended because they require less time, they act faster, they are less likely to irritate the skin, and they are more likely to be used.

- Maximal barrier precautions upon insertion: Full barrier precautions means that cap, mask, sterile gown, sterile gloves, and full body drapes are required during insertion of CVCs.

- Chlorhexidine skin antisepsis: Chlorhexidine 2% in alcohol 70% has been demonstrated to be the most effective agent for cleansing the skin. Cleansing should include a friction scrub for 30 seconds followed by 2 minutes of drying the site (Aragon & Sole, 2006).

- Optimal catheter site selection, with subclavian vein as the preferred site for non-tunneled catheters site: Selection is determined based on

individual patient issues. However, when possible, use of the subclavian vein has been associated with fewer bloodstream infections.

- Daily review of line necessity with prompt removal of unnecessary lines.

Once the CVC has been established, hand hygiene and sterile gloves are required for dressing changes. There is insufficient evidence to support the recommendation for a specific type of dressing. However, frequency of dressing change is dependent on dressing type. It is recommended that gauze dressings be changed every 2 days or as needed, whereas transparent dressings may be left in place for up to 7 days. There is evidence to suggest that IV tubings should be changed no more frequently than every 72 hours but should be replaced by at least 96 hours. However, tubings should be changed more frequently when blood products, propofol, or lipids are administered (AACN, 2005).

Surgical Site Care

Surgical site infections are common in hospitalized patients, occurring in 2% to 5% of clean extra-abdominal surgeries and up to 20% of intra-abdominal surgeries. Patients who develop surgical site infections are 60% more likely to spend time in ICU, average 7 days more in the hospital, and have twice the mortality of patients who do not develop infections. Two methods that have been advocated for prevention of surgical site infections are the administration of an appropriate antibiotic and the avoidance of shaving of the surgical site. Clear evidence exists that providing an appropriate antibiotic no more than 1 hour prior to the surgical incision and discontinuing the antibiotic 24 hours after surgery (48 hours after cardiac surgery) results in fewer surgical site infections. There is no convincing evidence to recommend in favor of hair removal from the surgical site prior to surgery. However, strong evidence exists that if hair removal is considered necessary, shaving should not be performed. Instead hair removal with a depilatory or an electric clipper is recommended immediately before surgery (Bolton, 2006).

Preventing Urinary Tract Infections

Indwelling urinary catheters are inserted in approximately four million Americans each year and are used in the majority of critical care patients. Not surprisingly, because they are used so frequently, catheter-associated urinary tract infection (CAUTI) is one of the most common nosocomial infections in ICUs worldwide. Nosocomial bacteriuria develops in 25% to 40% of patients requiring a urinary catheter for more than 7 days. Although CAUTI may result in a moderate increase in cost and length of stay, it is not usually associated with an increase in mortality.

Risks for Development of Catheter-Associated Urinary Tract Infections

Laupland et al. (2005) identified the following factors and noted the associated relative risks for development of a CAUTI:

Prolonged catheterization (longer than 6 days)	5.1–6.8
Female gender	2.5–3.7
Catheter insertion outside operating room	2.0–5.3
Other active sites of infection	2.3–2.4
Diabetes	2.2–2.3
Malnutrition	2.4
Azotemia (creatinine greater than 2.0 mg/dL)	2.1–2.6
Monitoring of urine output	2.0
Drainage tube below level of bladder and above collection bag	1.9
Antimicrobial drug therapy	0.1–0.4

Guidelines for Prevention of Catheter-Associated Urinary Tract Infections

Aragon and Sole (2006) emphasize that data on preventing UTIs stem from guidelines that were developed by the CDC in 1981. Laupland et al. (2005) note that there have been no randomized controlled clinical trials demonstrating the effectiveness of the practices usually recommended to prevent, or at least delay, the onset of CAUTI. Nevertheless there are recommendations for preventing CAUTIs. The guidelines include:

- *Avoiding Unnecessary Catheterizations:* The use of indwelling urinary catheters should be limited to circumstances when they are absolutely necessary (such as for monitoring urine output accurately in a critically ill patient), and catheters should be removed as soon as they are no longer needed. Studies have indicated that as many as 40% of catheters are inserted unnecessarily or left in place too long.

- *Insertion Using Aseptic Technique:* Catheters should be inserted by trained health care professionals using aseptic technique, including sterile gloves, a fenestrated sterile drape, and an antiseptic, such as 10% povidone-iodine or 2% aqueous chlorhexidine.

- *Maintaining a Closed Drainage System:* After a catheter is inserted, strict maintenance of a closed drainage system can limit the overall risk of CAUTI to less than 25% for up to 2 weeks.

- *Ensuring Dependent Drainage and an Unobstructed Urine Flow:* The collection tubing and bag should always remain below the level of the patient's bladder with the drainage tubing always above the level of the collection bag to ensure constant drainage.

- *Minimizing Manipulation of Urine Collection System:* Caregivers should wash their hands before touching the drainage system. The catheter and the drainage system should be manipulated as little as possible, and urine output should be monitored hourly only when clearly indicated by the patient's condition.

Potential future solutions include the use of antimicrobial urinary catheters. Johnson, Kuslowski, and Wilt (2006) state that there is fair quality evidence that antimicrobial urinary catheters can prevent bacteriuria in hospitalized patients during short-term catheterization. However, the effectiveness of the catheters depends on the antimicrobial coating, and the cost implications remain undefined.

Assessment of the Septic Patient

Early recognition of the septic patient is key to the initiation of early goal-directed therapy and better patient outcomes. Therefore, it is essential that critical care nurses recognize the manifestations of SIRS, sepsis, and septic shock and assess their patients for them.

Recognition of the Patient with Systemic Inflammatory Response Syndrome

The first phase of the septic process, the **systemic inflammatory response syndrome** (SIRS), has been described as the presence of two or more of the following:

- Temperature greater than 38°C (100.4°F) or less than 36°C (96.8°F)
- Pulse greater than 90 beats per minute
- Respiratory rate greater than 20 breaths/minute or $PaCO_2$ less than 32 torr
- White blood cells (WBCs) greater than 12,000/mm³ or less than 4,000/mm³

Although an international consensus panel convened in 2001 reaffirmed this definition of SIRS there has been some dissatisfaction with the criteria because they are both sensitive and nonspecific. Giuliano (2007) attempted to identify which of the parameters in the syndrome were most predictive of sepsis. She determined that 80% of septic patients could be identified on the basis of a temperature greater than 38°C and a mean arterial pressure (MAP) less than 70 mm Hg. Her findings also suggested that hypothermia might not be a valid indication of early sepsis; instead it might occur late in the septic process when the body is unable to mount an appropriate thermal response to infection. She noted that other physiological parameters and laboratory tests might be helpful in the early identification of sepsis.

Recognition of the Patient with Sepsis

Sepsis is defined as the development of SIRS accompanied by the presence or presumed presence of infection. In addition to meeting the criteria for SIRS, patients who have developed sepsis usually have at least two of the following clinical signs:

- Chills
- Hypotension
- Decreased skin perfusion
- Decreased capillary refill or mottling
- Decreased urine output
- Significant edema or positive fluid balance (more than 20 mL/kg over 24 hours)
- Hyperglycemia (plasma glucose greater than 120)

The patient with sepsis should be assessed to identify localizing signs of infection. Some of the common origins of infection for hospitalized patients are displayed in Figure 17-4.

In order to assist in identifying the source of infection the nurse should consider the following:

- Does the patient have a cough or a change in the character of his sputum that might indicate a pulmonary source of infection?
- Is the patient experiencing nausea, vomiting, or diarrhea? Does he have abdominal pain or rebound tenderness that might indicate an abdominal source of infection?
- Has the patient been experiencing dysuria, frequency of urination, or pain at the costovertebral angle that could be indicative of a renal source of infection?
- Does the patient have a new murmur or a change in a murmur, possibly indicating endocarditis?
- Does the patient have a headache or a change in mental status or neurological findings that might indicate a neurological focus of infection?
- Does the patient have redness, tenderness, or drainage at the sites of any implants, catheters, or medical devices (Henker & Carlson, 2007)?

Recognition of the Patient with Severe Sepsis and Septic Shock

Severe sepsis occurs when dysfunction of two or more organ systems develops in response to hypoperfusion. It can develop either slowly or suddenly but once it has developed, patient outcomes are not as likely to be positive. Therefore, the nurse caring for a septic patient needs to be vigilant about monitoring the patient for the development of any of the following signs of organ dysfunction:

- Acute lung injury indicated by tachypnea and/or hypoxemia
- Coagulation abnormalities or thrombocytopenia
- Neurological dysfunction indicated by a sudden change in mental status with possible confusion or psychosis
- Renal dysfunction evidenced by a decreased urine output for at least 2 hours and an increase in serum creatinine greater than 0.5 mg/dL
- Liver dysfunction indicated by jaundice, coagulopathy, decreased protein C levels, and increased D-dimer levels
- Gastrointestinal injury indicated by stress ulceration, ileus (absent bowel sounds), and malabsorption
- Cardiac dysfunction indicated by tachycardia, dysrhythmias, hypotension with decreased CVP or PA pressures, and either high or low cardiac outputs
- Hypotension with lactic acidosis

Septic shock, the most severe form of sepsis, is defined as the presence of sepsis and refractory hypotension. Refractory hypotension is a systolic blood pressure (BP) less than 90 mm Hg, an MAP less than 65 mm Hg, or a decrease of 40 mm Hg in systolic BP that is unresponsive to a crystalloid fluid challenge of 20 to 40 mL/kg.

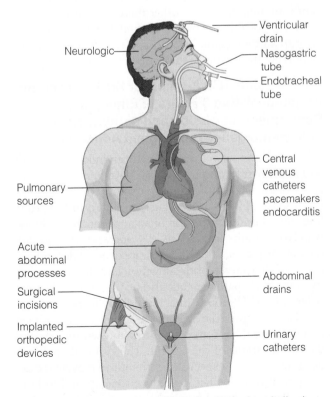

Figure 17-4 Possible sources of infection in the hospitalized patient with sepsis.

Diagnostic Criteria

A number of laboratory abnormalities are also correlated with the presence of sepsis. These include:

- Leukocytosis (white count greater than 12,000/mm^3) and a shift to the left of neutrophils. However, a peaking fever appears to be more sensitive than leukocytosis to predict bacteremia.

- Thrombocytopenia (platelet count less than 100,000)

- Hyperglycemia (plasma glucose greater than 120 mg/dL)

- Plasma C reactive protein level greater than 2 SD above normal

- Coagulation abnormalities (international ratio [INR] greater than 1.5 or an activated partial thromboplastin time (aPTT) greater than 60s)

- Hyperbilirubinemia (plasma bilirubin greater than 4 mg/dL)

- Increased lactate (greater than 1 mmol/L)

In addition, computerized tomography (CT) scans may be used to identify possible abscesses, and chest or abdominal x-rays may reveal infectious processes.

Collaborative Management

Collaborative management of sepsis is based on the understanding that interventions to optimize the patients' hemodynamic status instituted early in the septic process reduce mortality. It appears that accurate diagnosis and definitive management of severe sepsis and septic shock must occur within the first 6 hours of the onset of symptoms for the best outcomes (Otero et al., 2006). This makes sense because the purpose of the interventions is to prevent further organ dysfunction. If interventions are delayed until after organ and cellular dysfunction develop, then the strategies designed to provide the cells with more oxygen are unlikely to be helpful. Therefore, many health care institutions have developed guidelines based on the Surviving Sepsis Guidelines to ensure that patients with severe sepsis are identified early and are managed appropriately.

Sepsis Resuscitation Bundle

When a patient is identified with severe sepsis, septic shock, and/or lactate greater than 4 mmol/L (36 mg/dL), there are seven evidence-based goals known as the sepsis resuscitation bundle that the Surviving Sepsis Campaign states should be completed within the first 6 hours. For the best outcomes, the appropriate bundles should be instituted in the emergency department (ED) even before the patient is transferred to an ICU (Dellinger et al., 2008). Management of sepsis in the ED

and the first few hours in the ICU may also be referred to as early goal-directed therapy. As with the sepsis bundles, specific physiological parameters are assessed and interventions are instituted to aid in the resuscitation of the patient. The goals for care and the therapies utilized in both approaches are comparable. See Figure 17-5 for the Emergency Department Guidelines for Severe Sepsis form.

Bundle Element 1: Measure Serum Lactate

A serum lactate greater than 4 mmol/L is often present in patients with severe sepsis or septic shock and may develop in response to anaerobic metabolism due to hypoperfusion. Although elevated lactate levels may result from other causes such as decreased clearance by the liver, obtaining a serum lactate is essential to identifying inadequate tissue perfusion in patients who are not yet hypotensive but who are at risk for septic shock. Identification of septic patients prior to the deterioration of their vital signs allows for early goal-directed therapy and decreases both morbidity and mortality.

Bundle Element 2: Obtain Blood Cultures Prior to Antibiotic Administration

Of patients presenting with a clinical syndrome of severe sepsis or shock, 30% to 50% have positive blood cultures. Therefore, blood should be obtained for culture in any critically ill septic patient. The Surviving Sepsis Campaign (2004) recommends that blood cultures be obtained as soon as possible after the onset of fever and chills. Russell (2006) recommends also culturing the patient's sputum, urine, and other fluids such as a draining wound or possibly cerebrospinal fluid. Obtaining cultures prior to antibiotic administration offers the best hope of identifying the organism that caused the patient's sepsis.

Bundle Element 3: Administer Broad-Spectrum Antibiotic Within 3 Hours of Emergency Department Admission and Within 1 Hour of Nonemergency Department Admission

Administration of an appropriate antimicrobial agent within the first few hours after the development of sepsis is one of the few interventions that clearly reduce mortality in sepsis (Liberman & Whelan, 2006). In fact, each hour that the administration of an appropriate antibiotic is delayed results in a nearly 8% increase in mortality (Powers & Jacobi, 2006). The choice of agent depends on the suspected source of the infection and the susceptibility of the likely pathogen but also on the patient's history. After 48 to 72 hours, the multidisciplinary team reassesses the appropriateness of the antimicrobial regimen by reviewing the results of cultures and sensitivities and the clinical status of the patient. The eventual goal is to use a single narrow-spectrum antibiotic to prevent the development of resistance, to reduce toxicity, and to limit costs. Patients should begin therapy with a full loading dose of each antimicrobial. However, because patients

EMERGENCY DEPARTMENT GUIDELINES FOR SEVERE SEPSIS

Note: *Not Part of Medical Record*

Return to EMERGENCY DEPARTMENT

Patient Information

- Screening for "SEVERE" Sepsis Completed:

  - 2 of 4 SIRS criteria positive, infection, "and"
  - Hypotensive *after* fluid challenge (1,000 mL crystalloid) "or"
  - Lactate *over* 4

- 1. Document Time protocol initiated : ____:____
  - (Notify Intensive Care MD and ICU charge nurse)

- 2. Confirm appropriate Antibiotics are ordered (1 hour goal)
  - Cultures drawn

- 3. Central Line Placement:
  - Central Line Checklist completed
  - Procedure Verification completed

- 4. Level CVP monitor and document initial reading
  - Initial CVP: _____ mm Hg
  - Time of CVP:____:____

- 5. **Administer fluids** for **goal CVP** (500 mL Q 30 minutes)
  - CVP *over* 12 mm Hg if intubated
  - CVP *over* 8 mm Hg if not intubated

  - 500 mL Normal Saline/LR given, time: ____/____ CVP _____ mm Hg
  - 500 mL Normal Saline/LR given, time: ____/____ CVP _____ mm Hg
  - 500 mL Normal Saline/LR given, time: ____/____ CVP _____ mm Hg

- 6. Start **Pressors** for MAP *under* 65 mm Hg at anytime during resuscitation

  - Intial MAP: _____ mm Hg
  - Time: _____

  Document Initial Pressor used:

  - Levophed   (0–25 mcg/min)   rate: _____ mcg/min
  - Dopamine   (0–20 mcg/kg/min)   rate: _____ mcg/kg/min
  - Neosynephrine   (0–180 mcg/min)   rate: _____ mcg/min

- 7. For Hypotension (MAP under 65 mm HG) refractory to initial pressor start:

  - Vasopressin   0.04 units/min   rate: _____ units/min

- 8. Draw **Mixed Venous Gas,** time ____:____

- 9. Transfer to ICU, time: ____:____

- 10. Document Goals obtained:

Activate SEPSIS PATHWAY

ABX In 1Hr

Fluids for CVP

Pressors for MAP

Mixed Venous Gas

SEPSIS TREATMENT GOALS:

- CVP on transfer = _____ mm Hg
- MAP on transfer = _____ mm Hg
- Mixed Venous = _____ %
- Antibiotics administered: Time ____:____

Figure 17-5 Emergency department guidelines for severe sepsis.
(Courtesy of the Elliot Hospital, Manchester, NH)

with sepsis often have abnormal renal or hepatic function, the pharmacist should be consulted to ensure that the prescribed dose results in serum concentrations that are both clinically effective and minimally toxic.

Bundle Element 4: In the Event of Hypotension and/or Serum Lactate Greater Than 4 mmol/L

Step 1: Deliver an initial minimum of 20 mL/kg of crystalloid or a colloid equivalent.

The severe sepsis resuscitation bundle calls for an initial fluid challenge of a minimum of 20 mL/kg of crystalloid in cases of suspected hypovolemia or actual cases of serum lactate greater than 4 mmol/L (36 g/dL).

- To deliver a fluid challenge, the nurse infuses the prescribed fluid volume (usually 500 to 1,000 mL) over approximately 30 minutes.
- The nurse anticipates that the patient's BP and heart rate will begin to normalize quickly if the challenge has been successful. An adequate response to a fluid challenge for the patient with sepsis is defined as a MAP greater than 70 with a heart rate less than 110 bpm.
- Fluid volume requirements vary greatly among septic patients and may be difficult to predict. Therefore, the fluid challenge may be repeated if the patient does not respond adequately. The 20 mL/kg of crystalloid merely represents the minimally acceptable initial fluid volume. If repeated fluid boluses are required, a central venous pressure (CVP) line may be inserted to guide fluid administration (see Bundle Element 5).
- Nearly all septic patients will require appreciably more intake than output so the nurse recognizes that I&O alone cannot guide fluid replacement.
- The nurse is responsible for monitoring the patient closely during the fluid challenge for evidence of pulmonary and systemic edema. If pulmonary edema develops, the fluid challenge is ended.

A colloid equivalent is an acceptable alternative to crystalloid, and an equivalent dose generally ranges from 0.2 g/kg to 0.3 g/kg depending on the colloid. To this point there have been no studies that show a clear benefit to either fluid. However, because the volume of distribution is greater for crystalloids than for colloids, resuscitation with crystalloids requires more fluid to achieve the same goals and results in more edema.

Step 2: Apply vasopressors for hypotension not responding to initial fluid resuscitation to maintain a MAP greater than 80 mm Hg.

It is important to follow the MAP rather than the systolic BP because it is more likely to reflect actual tissue perfusion. Because the vasopressor will be titrated to the MAP, a reliable BP should be continuously available. Therefore, direct monitoring of the BP through the radial artery is usually indicated. The insertion of the arterial line may be delayed until the patient has been transported to the ICU, whereas the delivery of vasopressors should be through a CVC as soon as one is available. (See Chapter 5 ∞ for information on arterial lines.)

Although vasopressor agents are recommended, there remain concerns about their potential for inappropriate or detrimental use (Dellinger et al., 2008). When vasopressors are used in patients who have not received adequate fluid resuscitation, they produce additional vasoconstriction that may worsen organ perfusion. Even if the patient has received adequate fluid volume, there is concern that vasopressors may increase BP and perfusion to some organs at the expense of perfusion to the intestine and kidneys. Finally, too high a BP has the potential to increase left ventricular workload to an unsustainable level and worsen heart failure in the patient with preexisting heart disease. Therefore, the nurse needs to continually and carefully assess renal and cardiac functioning when vasopressors are added to the treatment regimen.

Choice of Vasopressors. The choice of vasopressor varies with the institutional protocol or the specific physician. Norepinephrine or dopamine is the first-choice for a vasopressor agent to correct hypotension in septic shock (Dellinger et al., 2008). Vasopressin use might be considered in patients with refractory shock despite adequate volume replacement and high-dose conventional vasopressors.

Bundle Element 5: In the Event of Persistent Hypotension Despite Fluid Resuscitation (Septic Shock) and/or Lactate Greater Than 4 mmol/L

Step 1: Achieve a CVP of greater than or equal to 8 mm Hg unless the patient is mechanically ventilated (then maintain a CVP of 12 to 15).

Patients should receive the initial minimum 20 mL/kg fluid challenge prior to placement of a CVC. If the patient does not respond adequately to the initial fluid challenges then the physician may insert a CVP line so that repeated fluid challenges may be delivered until the target value is achieved. According to the guidelines, while focusing on the goal of attaining a CVP greater than 8, it is also necessary to achieve central or mixed venous oxygen saturation targets. If a patient is hypovolemic and has a hematocrit less than 30%, it is appropriate for the patient to receive packed red blood cells.

COMMONLY USED MEDICATIONS

DOPAMINE, NOREPINEPHRINE, AND VASOPRESSIN

DOPAMINE: A VASOPRESSOR, INOTROPIC AGENT, AND CARDIAC STIMULANT

Desired Effect: Dopamine increases MAP primarily by increasing stroke volume and increasing heart rate. It has a minimal effect on systemic vascular resistance. When administered by continuous infusion, dopamine should begin to have an effect within 2 to 5 minutes.

Nursing Responsibilities: Dopamine is administered by continuous IV infusion. Initial range of the infusion may be 2 to 5 mcg/kg of body weight per minute. If doses higher than 15 and 20 mcg/kg/min are required, adding another vasopressor should be considered.

The nurse should monitor BP every 2 to 5 minutes after beginning a continuous infusion of dopamine. Dopamine may be titrated up or down every 10 to 30 minutes to obtain a MAP of 80. The lowest dose possible to attain the MAP should be utilized.

In addition to monitoring the MAP, the nurse should assess the heart rate and monitor pattern, CVP, and urine output.

If dopamine is administered through a peripheral IV line, extravasation may cause severe irritation, necrosis, or sloughing of tissue. Therefore, if at all possible, dopamine should be administered through a CVC. Should that not be possible, a large vein should be utilized and the IV infusion site should be observed frequently.

Potential Side and/or Toxic Effects: With moderate to high doses, an increase in heart rate may occur. Therefore, the nurse monitors the patient for the development of symptomatic tachycardia.

With doses approximating the maximal dose, pronounced vasoconstriction may occur. Therefore, the nurse should assess the patient for a decrease in urine output and decreased peripheral pulses with cool or mottled extremities.

NOREPINEPHRINE: A POTENT ALPHA-ADRENERGIC AGONIST WITH SOME BETA-ADRENERGIC EFFECTS

Desired Effects: Due to its vasoconstrictive effects, norepinephrine usually results in a significant increase in MAP with little change in heart rate or cardiac output. It seems to be more effective than dopamine at reversing hypotension in septic shock patients resistant to fluid resuscitation. Initial response should begin in 1 to 2 minutes of IV administration.

Nursing Responsibilities: Norepinephrine is administered by continuous IV infusion. Usual maintenance range of the infusion is 2 to 12 mcg/min. The usual maximum dose is 25 mcg/min.

The nurse should monitor BP every 2 to 5 minutes after beginning a continuous infusion. Norepinephrine may be titrated up or down cautiously to obtain a MAP of 80. The lowest dose possible to attain the MAP should be utilized.

In addition to monitoring the MAP, the nurse will assess the heart rate and monitor pattern, CVP, and urine output continuously during administration.

If at all possible norepinephrine should be administered through a CVC. If norepinephrine is administered through a peripheral IV line, severe vasoconstriction may result. Veins in the hands, ankles, and legs should be avoided but a large antecubital vein can be acceptable if necessary. Blanching along the vein is an indication of extravasation that can lead to severe tissue necrosis, sloughing, and gangrene.

If extravasation does occur, phentolamine (Regitine) 5 to 10 mg diluted in 10 to 15 mL of normal saline is injected liberally throughout the tissue to prevent necrosis.

Potential Side and/or Toxic Effects: Side effects are rare when used as directed. However, previously there was concern that the vasoconstriction occurring with norepinephrine could result in deterioration of renal functioning. This does not appear to be the case. Instead, by increasing the MAP norepinephrine appears to increase glomerular filtration and renal function. However, the nurse should be certain to monitor the urine output and serum creatinine of the patient receiving norepinephrine.

Septic shock may be accompanied by a reduced vascular response to catecholamines. Thus a patient may have had adequate volume replacement and be receiving high doses of vasopressors but still remain hypotensive. In such circumstances, a continuous infusion of low-dose arginine vasopressin might be utilized.

VASOPRESSIN: A SYNTHETIC HORMONE, AN ANTIDIURETIC, A POTENT VASOCONSTRICTOR

Desired Effects: An increase in MAP without an increase in cardiac index or heart rate should be detectable within 1 hour of the institution of a continuous infusion of vasopressin 0.04 units/min. At this dose, there should not be a decrease in urine output.

Nursing Responsibilities: Vasopressin has been associated with a decrease in cardiac output in some studies of patients with septic shock. Therefore, the nurse should continue to observe the patient for adequate tissue perfusion and cardiac output.

End-organ perfusion, specifically gastrointestinal (GI) and liver perfusion, has been reduced in some patients in septic shock receiving vasopressin. Therefore, the nurse should routinely assess liver and GI function.

Potential Side and/or Toxic Effects: In higher doses, vasopressin has been associated with arrhythmias, bradycardia, hypertension, myocardial infarction (MI), and abdominal cramping.

Overdose can result in water intoxication.

Administering blood increases the oxygen delivery to the ischemic tissue while increasing the CVP.

Step 2: Achieve a central venous oxygen saturation ($ScvO_2$) greater than or equal to 70% or mixed venous oxygen saturation (SvO_2) greater than or equal to 65%.

Measurement of central or mixed venous saturation is an estimate of the oxygen saturation of the blood returning to the right side of the heart. Both values correlate with measurement of extraction of oxygen from the blood by body tissues and therefore are indications of the balance between oxygen supply and demand. A decline indicates that the demand of the tissues is exceeding the oxygen delivery. The presence of low values in patients with early sepsis is associated with higher morbidity and mortality (Otero et al., 2006).

An increase in the $ScvO_2$ or SvO_2 may be accomplished in either of two ways. The first is through blood transfusions as was described previously. The second strategy involves attempting to improve the patient's hemodynamic profile with inotropes. Provided that the patient has received adequate amounts of fluid and the CVP is 8 mm Hg, it may be that cardiac output remains insufficient to meet the metabolic demands of the body. A dobutamine infusion (up to a maximum of 20 μg/kg/min) may be employed to increase oxygen delivery to the periphery and prevent further organ dysfunction due to hypoperfusion and ischemia.

Sepsis Management Bundle

The sepsis management bundle reflects what evidence suggested were the interventions to be instituted within the first 24 hours for patients with severe sepsis, septic shock, and/or lactate greater than 4 mmol/L (36 mg/dL). Unlike the elements of the sepsis resuscitation bundle, individual elements of the sepsis management bundle have not received uniform support because they have not consistently been shown to prolong survival or decrease mortality in the patient with septic shock. In addition, some of the elements have been associated with significant side effects. However, the Surviving Sepsis Campaign (2004) has recommended that each of the elements be assessed and, if appropriate, that the interventions be instituted.

Bundle Element 1: Administer Low-Dose Steroids by a Standard Policy

The nurse should administer low-dose steroids for septic shock in accordance with a standardized ICU policy. If not administered, the nurse documents why the patient

---

COMMONLY USED MEDICATIONS

DOBUTAMINE: AN INOTROPE, PRIMARILY A BETA-ADRENERGIC AGENT

Desired Effect: Dobutamine increases the contractility of cardiac muscle and enhances microcirculation blood flow and organ perfusion. A dose of 5 mcg/kg/min can improve capillary perfusion in patients with septic shock (Powers & Jacobi, 2006). It may take up to 10 minutes to see the peak effects of a specific dose.

Nursing Responsibilities: Adequate preload is essential for optimal benefit from dobutamine therapy so the nurse ensures that the appropriate fluid resuscitation has taken place.

Dobutamine is administered as a continuous IV infusion. Administration may begin at 2.5 mcg/kg/min and be titrated up by increments of 2.5 mcg/kg/min every 15 to 20 minutes to prevent sudden drops in BP (Otero et al., 2006).

Potential Side and/or Toxic Effects: If the dobutamine infusion causes hypotension, a norepinephrine infusion may be started to counteract the vasodilatory effects of dobutamine and maintain the desired MAP.

Heart rate should be monitored continuously during the administration of dobutamine. If the patient develops sinus tachycardia, the dose of dobutamine might be decreased, dobutamine therapy discontinued, or the type of vasopressor might be changed.

Because dobutamine increases the force of contraction of the heart, the patient should be assessed for the development of chest discomfort, an increase in the number of premature ventricular complexes (PVCs), and ST segment and T-wave changes, and the physician should be notified. The development of myocardial ischemia is more likely in the event of an increase in heart rate and is an indication to decrease or stop the infusion.

---

did not qualify for low-dose steroids based on the standardized protocol.

Low-dose steroids have been indicated for the patient in septic shock because they limit the duration of the shock and in some studies have decreased mortality. These results may be due to the effect of corticosteroids on vascular tone or to the ability of corticosteroids to attenuate the inflammatory response without causing immunosuppression. Current recommendations are for IV corticosteroids (usually hydrocortisone 200 to 300 mg/day for 7 days in three or four divided doses or by continuous infusion) to be administered to patients with septic shock who, despite adequate fluid replacement, require vasopressor therapy to maintain adequate BP. One advantage of administration of hydrocortisone by continuous infusion as opposed to bolus is that continuous infusion appears to promote normoglycemia in septic patients. The nurse needs to observe the patient for the development of hyperglycemia, nosocomial sepsis, and recurrent septic shock because they are more common when corticosteroids are administered.

Bundle Element 2: Administer Drotrecogin Alfa (Activated) by a Standard Policy

In a large double-blind study, human recombinant activated protein C (drotrecogin alfa activated) decreased mortality by 6% in patients with severe sepsis and decreased mortality by 13% in patients at high risk for death (Rivers et al., 2001). Although use of Drotrecogin Alfa (also called recombinant human activated protein C) is included in the sepsis management bundle, it is not consistently advocated or utilized. According to Liberman and Whelan (2006), some of the reasons why it is not consistently used are:

- Irregularities in the original study could have affected interpretation of the data.
- It is only recommended for patients with severe sepsis and the highest risk of death.
- It is associated with a significantly increased risk of bleeding.
- When utilized in clinical practice, the mortality rates have been higher than those reported in clinical trials.
- The average cost per patient is $6,800.

Although some sources recommend evaluating the patient and administering Drotrecogin Alfa as soon as possible, Nguyen et al. (2006) recommend delaying consideration and use of the drug until after identification of the source of the infection and any surgical procedure required to control it.

Recombinant human protein C is indicated only for patients with severe sepsis at the highest risk for death. Checklists to determine if a patient is a candidate are available. A simple summary is that the patient must meet the criteria for SIRS, have two or more organs that

COMMONLY USED MEDICATIONS

DROTRECOGIN ALFA (ACTIVATED), RECOMBINANT HUMAN PROTEIN C, OR XIGRIS— AN ANTITHROMBOTIC

Desired Effect: The mechanism for the drug's ability to enhance survival in patients with severe sepsis is not completely understood. However, effects may be due to the drug's ability to provide endothelial protection as well as anti-inflammatory, antithrombotic, and profibrinolytic actions. The dose, 24 mcg/kg/hr, is infused through a dedicated IV line over 96 hours.

Nursing Responsibilities: Because of the drug's antithrombotic and profibrinolytic effects, the drug should be stopped 2 hours before any invasive procedure and not restarted until an hour after a minor procedure or 12 hours after hemostasis following surgery.

The patient should be continuously observed for signs of bleeding. If clinically important bleeding develops, the physician should be notified and the infusion should be stopped.

Potential Side and/or Toxic Effects: Bleeding is the most common side effect; usually patients develop ecchymoses or GI bleeding. The risk of bleeding is increased in patients who are receiving other agents that affect coagulation.

are dysfunctional, and have an APACHE score greater than 25. It is contraindicated in patients who have had active internal bleeding, a variety of intracranial or intraspinal lesions, and recent surgery or trauma.

Bundle Element 3: Maintain Glucose Control of Greater Than 80, but Less Than or Equal to 150 mg/dL

Following initial stabilization of patients with severe sepsis, blood glucose should be maintained at less than 150 mg/dL. The rationale and a protocol for instituting glycemic control utilizing a continuous infusion of insulin are available in Chapter 13. ∞ Recently, concerns have arisen about the cost-effectiveness of tight glycemic control as well as the potential for adverse effects, especially hypoglycemia, when it is utilized for septic patients (Martin, 2007).

Bundle Element 4: Maintain a Median Inspiratory Plateau Pressure (IPP) Less Than 30 cm H₂O for Mechanically Ventilated Patients

Patients with sepsis are at an increased risk for developing acute respiratory failure, and nearly 50% of patients with severe sepsis develop acute respiratory distress syndrome (ARDS). For a detailed description of ARDS, see Chapter 3. ∞ High tidal volumes should be avoided in patients prone to the development of ARDS. Current recommendations are for "low" tidal volume (6 mL/kg/lean body weight) as a goal in conjunction with the goal of maintaining end-inspiratory plateau pressures of less than 30 cm H₂O to prevent further lung injury.

Collaborative Management

In addition to the bundle elements, an essential collaborative intervention for management of the septic patient is source control and identification and eradication of the source of infection. As previously described, patients with sepsis should be evaluated to determine the source of the infection. In addition to identifying localizing signs of infections, reviewing the exposure history with the patient or family, and performing diagnostic tests such as CT or magnetic resonance imaging (MRI) may be useful. When the source of infection is identified, it should be eliminated if possible. Source control might involve the drainage of an abscess, the debridement of infected necrotic tissue, the removal of a potentially infected device, or the definitive control of a source of ongoing microbial contamination. The nursing management of the patient is dependent on the specific site of the infection and the type of surgery performed for source control.

Nursing Care

The patient with sepsis may experience a variety of sources of discomfort, including discomfort from medical devices and pain at the site of the infection. Management of a septic patient's pain will vary depending on the specific source of the pain. See Chapter 1 ∞ for a general discussion of pain management in the critically ill patient. In addition, most septic patients are febrile and may experience discomfort from their fever or the efforts of health care providers to reduce their fever.

Comfort

Uncomplicated fever is an important immunologic defense mechanism. Therefore, unless a fever is severely elevated, the patient is very uncomfortable, or the patient is at risk for compromise from the fever, there may be no

Gerontological Considerations

Rates for severe sepsis rise sharply with age. There are 0.2 case per 1,000 population among children but 26.2 cases per 1,000 adults over the age of 85.

Mortality is also greater in older individuals. The mortality rate is 10% in children and 38% for adults over the age of 85.

Among adults over the age of 65, the most common source of infection is the urinary tract.

Multiple organ dysfunction syndrome is more likely to occur following severe sepsis in older patients when they have preexisting organ dysfunctions.

More than half of the $8.7 billion in annual cost for severe sepsis is spent on care of septic patients 65 years or older.

VISUAL MAP Fever

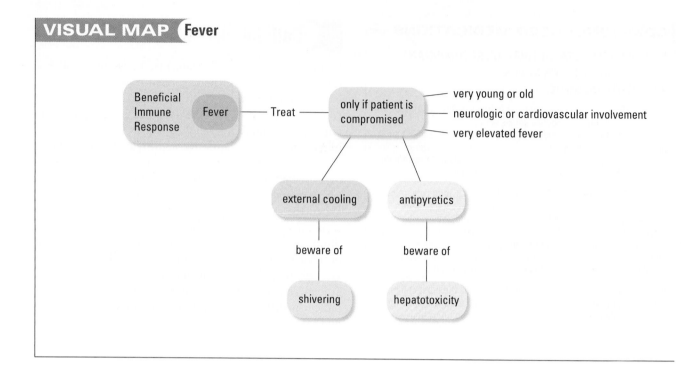

attempt to actively reduce the fever. According to the Joanna Briggs Institute (2001), there is no consistent definition of what constitutes too high a fever. However, patients are usually defined as febrile when their fevers reach 38.3°C (101°F), and interventions are often instituted for fevers higher than 39°C (approximately 102°F). Critical care nurses need to observe their patients with fever to determine if the fever is resulting in cardiovascular compromise or excessive metabolic demands. Fevers are more likely to result in compromise in very old patients, neonates, neurological patients with increased intracranial pressure or seizures, and patients with cardiovascular disease. See Visual Map.

Commonly used interventions to reduce fever such as the use of antipyretic drugs and external cooling should be evaluated in terms of potential risks. Although antipyretics are usually instituted for fevers higher than 39°C (102°F), reducing such fevers does not necessarily improve patient outcomes (Henker & Carlson, 2007). Acetaminophen, one of the most commonly used antipyretics, is erratically absorbed when administered via nasogastric tube, often resulting in elevated drug levels in critically ill patients. Repeated therapy at recommended doses can result in drug accumulation, and hepatotoxicity has developed in some patients. Thus, some health care providers recommend alternating doses of acetaminophen with ibuprofen. However, according to the Joanna Briggs Institute (2001), such a scheme can result in the potential for excessive doses. When acetaminophen is administered every 4 hours with ibuprofen every 6 hours, not only is it possible for the recommended daily dose to be exceeded but it is unclear which antipyretic should be administered at the twelfth hour (acetaminophen or ibuprofen, or both). If acetaminophen and ibuprofen are

alternated every 2 hours the recommended number of total daily doses is exceeded. When administering antipyretics, the critical care nurse needs to be attentive to the total daily dose of acetaminophen that the patient is receiving as well as to the patient's liver function.

Henker and Carlson (2007) note that exogenous cooling should be considered when a critically ill patient's fever exceeds 39.5°C (103°F). ICU nurses rarely use tepid sponges to cool patients because tepid sponges are unlikely to be successful and most patients find them very uncomfortable.

- More commonly an external cooling (hypothermia) blanket is utilized to cool the patient.
- Of particular concern when instituting exogenous cooling is the potential for the patient to shiver. Shivering causes an increase in the metabolic rate of 100% to 200% and increases body temperature. Thus, it should be prevented.
- In order to prevent shivering, the nurse might:
  - Use higher temperatures on the cooling blanket
  - Keep the patient's hands and feet off the blanket
  - Sedate and paralyze the patient. Sedating or paralyzing a patient with drugs that suppress shivering during external cooling results in a more rapid reduction of fever and reduced energy expenditure than if the patient were treated with antipyretic drugs alone (Axelrod, 2000).
- The utilization of an external cooling blanket requires continuous, accurate assessment of the patient's core temperature.
- Usually the blanket is turned off when the patient's temperature is about 1°C above the desired temperature.

Nutrition

The Surviving Sepsis Campaign (2004) states that it is important to provide nutritional support for the septic patient both to meet nutritional requirements and to limit the likelihood of hypoglycemia. The metabolic needs of patients in sepsis change as their temperatures fluctuate. For example, for every 1°C increase in a patient's temperature, the patient's metabolic requirements increase by approximately 10%. Whenever possible, nutritional requirements are met by enteral nutrition because it prevents translocation of bacteria from the GI tract as well as limits sources of bloodstream infections. Currently, supplementation of enteral feedings with glutamine to enhance the immune system is being evaluated. Enteral feedings supplemented with extracts of fish and borage oils as well as the antioxidant vitamins C and E are also being investigated to see if they can improve outcomes in septic patients.

Unfortunately, it is not always possible to meet the nutritional needs of septic patients with enteral feedings, in which case parenteral feedings are indicated. Standard total parenteral nutrition (TPN) solutions may not be metabolized well in septic patients so specialized solutions may be used. Because the nutritional requirements of septic patients are complex and undergoing revision, a nutritionist or a nutrition protocol should be consulted to determine each patient's specific requirements for calories and nutrients. See Chapter 1 ∞ for more information about nursing responsibilities in administration of enteral and parenteral nutrition.

Prevention and Detection of Complications

The most common complications of sepsis are **multiple organ dysfunction syndrome (MODS)** and **disseminated intravascular coagulation (DIC)**. MODS is defined as altered organ function in an acutely ill patient such that homeostasis cannot be maintained without intervention. DIC is defined as systemic intravascular activation of the coagulation cascade with fibrin formation and deposition in the microvasculature, resulting in simultaneous thrombic and hemorrhagic complications. The most effective way to prevent both of these complications is to identify the septic patient early and initiate definitive management of severe sepsis within the first 6 hours of the onset of symptoms.

Multiple Organ Dysfunction Syndrome

MODS develops in severe sepsis in response to a series of factors. First, older patients may have preexisting organ dysfunctions that make organ failure more likely to develop. Initially in all patients, tissue damage develops at the site of an infection, resulting in damage to the endothelial layer of blood vessels with release of vasoactive and procoagulant mediators. This results in localized increased vascular permeability and shunting. When SIRS develops the response to the circulating mediators becomes systemic. A major contributor to the development of tissue ischemia may be that in response to the circulating procoagulants, platelets, red cells, and thrombin form microaggregates in blood vessels and impede blood flow to vital organs. Additionally, proinflammatory cytokines and other mediators may cause generalized endothelial dysfunction, resulting in extensive capillary leakage in organs such as the lungs, liver, heart, and kidney. As more organs fail, the mortality rate from MODS increases. When one organ fails the mortality rate is about 7%, whereas when four organs fail the mortality rate approaches 70%. Therefore, the nurse caring for a septic patient needs to be vigilant about monitoring the patient for the development of any of the following signs of organ dysfunction:

- Acute lung injury (ALI) indicated by tachypnea, hyperventilation (arterial pH less than 7.35, and pCO_2 less than 32), and/or hypoxemia.
  - Assessment and management of the patient with ALI/ARDS is discussed in Chapter 3. ∞ However, as noted in the sepsis management bundle, high tidal volumes should be avoided in septic patients. Current recommendations are for "low" tidal volume (6 mL/kg/lean body weight) as a goal in conjunction with the goal of maintaining end-inspiratory plateau pressures of less than 30 cm H_2O to prevent further lung injury.
- Coagulation abnormalities or thrombocytopenia.
  - Assessment and management of the patient with DIC is discussed later in this chapter.
- Neurological dysfunction indicated by a sudden change in mental status with possible confusion or psychosis progressing to coma.
- Renal dysfunction evidenced by a decreased urine output (less than 0.5 mL/kg/hr) and elevated serum creatinine.
  - Assessment and management of the patient with acute renal failure is discussed in Chapter 14. ∞ However, evidence suggests that consultation with a nephrologist as soon as renal dysfunction is suspected results in better patient outcomes.
- Liver dysfunction indicated by jaundice, coagulopathy, decreased protein C levels, and increased D-dimer levels.
  - Assessment and management of the patient with liver failure is discussed in Chapter 14. ∞
- Gastrointestinal injury indicted by stress ulceration, ileus, and malabsorption.
- Cardiac dysfunction indicated by tachycardia, dysrhythmias, hypotension with decreased CVP or PA pressures, and either high or low cardiac outputs.

If the nurse recognizes that the patient is developing organ failure, she should notify the physician and prepare to institute the appropriate interventions. There is no specific care for the patient with MODS other than the supportive care indicated for the dysfunctional organ(s) and management of the underlying condition. However, the earlier that interventions are instituted, the more likely the outcome is to be positive.

Disseminated Intravascular Coagulation

Although sepsis is the most common cause of DIC, it may also develop following a variety of other conditions. Common other precursors of DIC (often called triggers) include:

- Traumatic injuries, especially multiple trauma, burns, and crush injuries
- Obstetrical complications such as abruptio placenta, placenta previa, retained dead fetus, and eclampsia
- Embolisms, whether fat, amniotic fluid, or pulmonary
- Immunological disorders such as transfusion reactions and transplant rejection
- Malignancies
- Shock accompanied by acidosis

Figure 17-6 displays how DIC progresses once it has been triggered. In DIC, the trigger causes excessive activation of the normal coagulation cascade. Either the extrinsic coagulation pathway is activated by mas-sive tissue destruction (e.g., crush injury) or the intrinsic pathway is activated through endothelial cell injury (e.g., shock with acidosis). Next, thrombin production, which should be balanced by chemical mediators such as proteins S and C, is not and continues unrestrained. The excessive thrombin production activates fibrinogen, resulting in the formation of fibrin. Fibrin is deposited throughout the microcirculation, leading to obstruction of blood vessels and ischemic tissue damage. As the fibrin deposits are formed, platelets and coagulation factors are consumed, leading to a deficiency of clotting factors, and the patient begins to bleed. The bleeding may be intensified as the clots are lysed, resulting in fibrin degradation products (FDPs) because the FDPs are anticoagulants. Thus, the patient develops simultaneous thrombic and hemorrhagic complications.

Patient Assessment. Patient assessment is geared at identifying the manifestations that result from the excessive thrombosis formation and bleeding. These signs may appear acutely as a profound clotting/bleeding disorder or may develop slowly as a chronic, partially compensated process. How rapidly DIC develops is partially dependent on the intensity of the trigger but is also related to the condition of the patient's liver, bone marrow, and endothelium. Some patients present primarily with bleeding abnormalities; others present with manifestations from microemboli. The critical care nurse must be aware of the various possible manifestations of DIC and must be prepared to notify the physician if DIC is suspected.

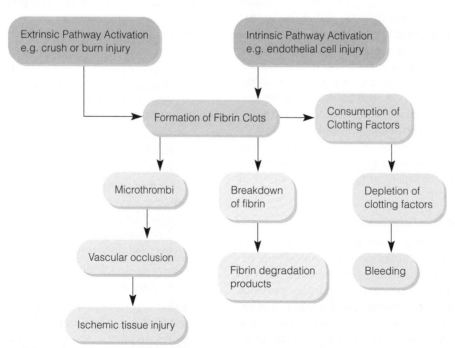

Figure 17-6 Overview of disseminated intravascular coagulation.

Initially, the patient may show manifestations of thrombosis and microemboli:

- Occlusion of blood vessels may be seen as cyanosis and/or gangrene, especially of the digits. There may actually be a demarcation line between the viable and necrotic tissue visible on the fingers or toes, and the patient may complain of pain in the digits.

- Pulses may be diminished.

- Inadequate perfusion of the brain may result in a CVA or present as an altered level of consciousness.

- Inadequate renal perfusion may be identified by a decrease in urine output, an increase in serum creatinine, or pain at the costovertebral angle.

- The patient may complain of abdominal tenderness and have diminished or absent bowel sounds that may indicate an ileus or a bowel infarction.

As clotting factors are depleted, the patient begins to ooze or bleed from multiple sites:

- In chronic DIC, there may be only a slight oozing of blood.

- In acute DIC the patient may bleed heavily from IV sites, arterial lines, urinary catheters, surgical sites, the GI tract, and mucous membranes.

- The patient may also have ecchymoses on the palate, gums, and skin.

- Bleeding in the pulmonary tree may be evidenced as hemoptysis.

- If the patient begins to hemorrhage from any of these sites then the signs of symptoms of hemorrhagic shock may become evident.

Diagnosis of Disseminated Intravascular Coagulation.
The diagnosis of DIC is made based on the presence of an underlying disorder that is likely to lead to DIC, the clinical presentation of the patient, and laboratory values.

No single definitive test for DIC exists, so the nurse examines a series of lab tests to determine the likelihood of DIC. The tests include:

- Platelet count (normally 150,000 to 400,000). A value of less than 50,000 is suggestive of DIC. However, a drop of 50% from baseline may also be indicative.

- FDPs (normally less than 10 mcg/mL). A value greater than 40 mcg/mL or rising values are suggestive of DIC.

- D-dimer (normally less than 250 ng/mL). Higher values may be indicative of DIC but the test is less sensitive than FDPs because a positive D-dimer may result whenever a large clot is being dissolved.

- Fibrinogen (normally 200 to 400 mg/dL). Levels may be normal very early in the disorder or in mild DIC. A value of less than 100 or falling values are suggestive.

- Prothrombin time ([PT], normally 11 to 12.5 seconds). Any elevation is suggestive of DIC.

- Activated partial thromboplastin time (normally 30 to 40 seconds). Prolongation is suggestive of DIC; critical values are greater than 70 seconds.

Collaborative Management

The most important intervention for DIC is identification and treatment of the underlying disorder.

Identifying and Treating the Trigger

When the trigger is an easily identifiable and treatable cause, such as an abruptio placenta, the outcome is likely to be better than if the trigger cannot be identified or is difficult to treat. Aggressive treatment of the underlying disorder is always indicated because if treatment fails, the mortality rate for DIC is high.

Restoring the Balance of Clot Formation, Dissolution, and Inhibition

Geiger (2003) notes that maintaining hemostasis is not an easy task requiring delicate balancing of clot formation, dissolution, and inhibition. To this end, clotting factors that have been consumed in the process of DIC may be replaced. Replacement of these factors is more likely to aid in rebalancing the coagulation disorder if the trigger has been identified and removed.

Platelet replacement may be provided if the patient is actively bleeding and the platelet count is dangerously low. There is no uniform agreement about an appropriate level for platelet transfusions in DIC, with recommendations ranging between 20,000 and 40,000. As with all blood transfusions, consent is required prior to platelet transfusions. Platelets are administered using filter tubing at an infusion rate of 4 to 8 mL/kg/hr.

Depending on laboratory findings, and if the patient continues to bleed, other clotting factors may also be replaced. The PT/INR may be used to guide administration of fresh frozen plasma. If the fibrinogen level is less than 100 mg/dL, cryoprecipitate may also be given because it contains 5 to 10 times more fibrinogen than plasma. Baird, Keen, and Swearingen (2005) recommend that 10 units of fibrinogen be given for every 2 to 3 units of fresh frozen plasma.

Theoretically, administering heparin should decrease the consumption of clotting factors and slow the process of DIC. Although heparin has been used for many years, it has not been shown to be consistently effective in practice. Baird et al. (2005) state that heparin may be useful when the trigger for DIC is a carcinoma or if the trigger for DIC is not reversible. Geiger (2003) notes that it may be a therapeutic indication for heparin when the patient demonstrates severe organ dysfunction from microemboli. If heparin is used, the patient should have an obvious thrombosis and it should be administered in low doses such as 5 to 10 units/kg/hr. During administration, the nurse observes the patient closely to detect any increase in the amount or rate of bleeding.

Supporting Organ Perfusion and Function.

Supporting and maintaining adequate organ and tissue perfusion are crucial to patient survival. Specific interventions depend on the patient's underlying condition and the degree of hemorrhage:

- IV fluids may be sufficient to maintain adequate perfusion in some patients. However, if blood loss is pronounced, then packed red blood cells may be administered. (See Chapter 8 ∞ for guidelines on administration.)
- The nurse monitors the patient's BP, heart rate, CVP or PAWP, and oxygen saturation at least every 2 hours and more often if necessary.
- The physician should be notified if the heart rate changes more than 10% from baseline or if the MAP drops below a specified level (often 65 to 70 mm Hg).

The nurse also closely monitors the function of the patient's various organ systems, especially neurological and renal functioning:

- Neurological screening, such as the Glasgow Coma Scale, should be performed at least every 2 hours.
- Urine output should be measured every hour to 2 hours, and creatinine should be reviewed on a daily basis.
- The nurse checks the adequacy of peripheral perfusion by assessing and documenting the pulses, sensations, movement, capillary refill, and warmth of each of the extremities at least every 2 hours.
- The nurse closely observes the patient for any increased bleeding, noting the presence of ecchymoses, documenting the presence of obvious bleeding, and testing any suspicious secretions for the presence of blood.

The patient should also be protected from further tissue injury:

- The nurse avoids inserting any invasive devices (including rectal thermometers) unless absolutely necessary.

- After an IV is removed, the nurse holds pressure for 3 to 5 minutes to ensure hemostasis.
- Mouth care is provided gently with soft massage of the gums to remove debris.
- Soft clots should not be removed but should be allowed to fall away on their own.

Providing Pain Relief. It is essential to assess the patient at regular intervals for pain because pain is one of the hallmarks of tissue ischemia. The nurse questions the patient hourly, when possible, concerning the presence, location, intensity, and duration of any pain. The development of pain in a new location may be an indication of new microemboli. Pain may also be the result of bleeding into confined spaces, especially joints. After carefully evaluating the pain and notifying the physician, if necessary, the nurse provides the appropriate medication.

▌ Nursing Care

Patients who develop DIC and their families are often highly anxious. Some patients were already critically ill and DIC represents a serious, potentially lethal complication. Other patients, especially pregnant women with abruptio placenta, were anticipating a joyous event and have encountered a crisis. Pronounced bleeding from multiple sites can be very frightening for both the patient and the family. The nurse needs to be willing to explain repeatedly to the patient and family what is occurring, what the likely cause is, and how the health care team is attempting to intervene. Additional guidelines about how to communicate with critically ill patients and their families are provided in Chapter 2. ∞

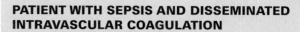

Nursing Diagnoses

PATIENT WITH SEPSIS AND DISSEMINATED INTRAVASCULAR COAGULATION

- Infection related to inadequate primary defenses
- Decreased cardiac output related to decreased ventricular filling (decreased preload)
- Deficient fluid volume related to failure of regulatory mechanisms and increased metabolic rate
- Interrupted family processes related to serious injury of family member
- Risk for ineffective tissue perfusion: peripheral, renal, GI, cardiovascular, cardiopulmonary, and cerebral related to hypotension and hypovolemia

VISUAL MAP Septic Shock and Disseminated Intravascular Coagulation

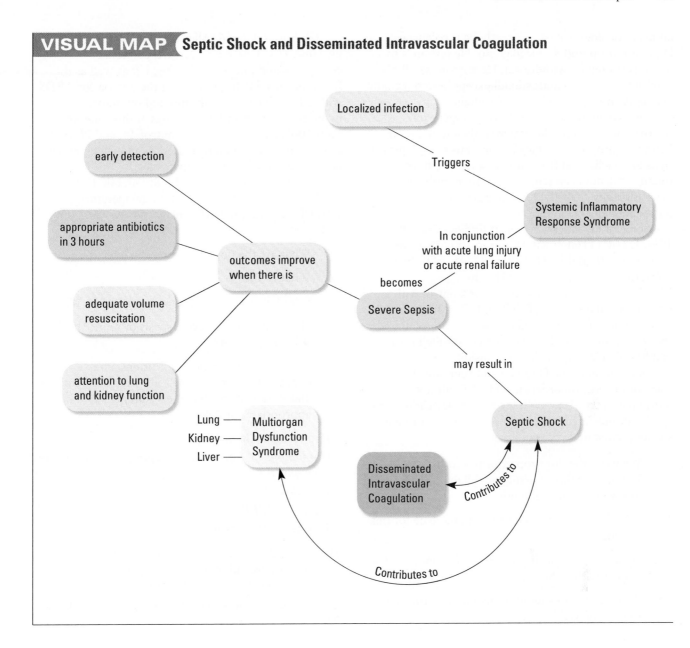

SEPSIS SUMMARY

Severe sepsis is a complex illness that develops after a localized infection triggers the inflammatory response syndrome, resulting in the failure of one or more organ systems. In the past it was associated with high morbidity and mortality. Recently, early goal-directed therapy has led to improved outcomes for septic patients. However, treatment of severe sepsis remains complicated, especially if patients are not diagnosed promptly, do not receive adequate volume resuscitation, or are not treated with appropriate antibiotics within the first 3 hours.

CASE STUDY

Allen Hale, 27 years old, was admitted to the eight-bed ICU of a community hospital after running a red light in his car and colliding with another car. He is being transferred to the operating room (OR) to evacuate a left parietal subdural hematoma. His concomitant injuries include a flail chest with pulmonary contusions, for which he is being mechanically ventilated, and a fractured left femur. His blood alcohol level on admission was 200 mg/dL (0.2% weight/volume) and there was indication of marijuana on his toxicology screen. Currently he is receiving Diprivan (propofol) 45 mcg/kg/min. He responds to noxious stimuli by withdrawal. He withdraws all his extremities from noxious stimuli except his left leg, and his pupils are equal and reactive to light.

On arrival in the ICU following surgery for removal of a subdural hematoma, Allen remains on Diprivan (propofol) 45 mcg/kg/min. His neurological signs are unchanged from pre-op, and his left leg fracture has not been repaired but an immobilizer is in place (dorsalis pedis (DP) and posterior tibial (PT) pulses are palpable in the left foot).

Some of his other assessment findings are: BP 109/71, HR 111/min, RR 18, Temp 100.6°F, urine output 20–30 mL/hr, pH 7.28, pCO_2 46, pO_2 99, O_2 saturation 97%, Hgb 10, and Hct 30.

His ventilator settings are: Assist Control with a rate of 18, tidal volume (TV) 800, FiO_2 50%, PEEP 5. Lung sounds are diminished on the left with scattered rhonchi on the right. He has a left chest tube in place and has bilateral equal chest expansion.

In addition to the Diprivan and ventilator settings some of his post-op orders include: IV antibiotics, morphine sulfate 2 mg q 4h for pain, Foley catheter to gravity drainage, nasogastric tube to low continuous suction, maintain left leg in immobilizer.

1. What are the three top priorities for nursing care? List at least three nursing or collaborative interventions for each priority.

2. What additional concerns would there be for this patient?

3. What are the priority concerns when managing a patient with a chest tube?

4. What measures should be instituted at this time to prevent VAP?

On hospital day 6, Allen became increasingly unstable. His chest x-ray revealed pulmonary contusions and pneumonia on the left as well as the fractured ribs. He began to meet the criteria for ARDS with diffuse bilateral infiltrates and refractory hypoxemia. His ventilator settings at this time were: FiO_2 100%, TV 800, Assist Control 24, and PEEP 7. His Diprivan had been increased to 55 mcg/kg/min but he was becoming increasingly restless.

Other findings included: BP 80/50, HR 120 bpm, RR 28, urine output 18–20 mL/hr, temperature 101.4°F, pH 7.22, pO_2 109, pCO_2 54, WBC 32,000, Hgb 8, Hct 28.

5. What are the possible sources of infection?

6. What is SIRS?

7. Is it likely that Allen is developing SIRS? Why?

8. Has he developed severe sepsis or septic shock? Why or why not?

9. Explain the rationales, indications, and contraindications for the following interventions and state whether the interventions would be appropriate for Allen:

Drotrecogin Alpha (Xigris)

Continuous IV infusion of norepinephrine bitartrate (Levophed)

Low-dose dopamine

Increase in PEEP

Increase in the amount of sedation

10. Are there indications that Allen is in danger of developing failure of other organs? If yes, what are the indications?

See answers to Case Studies in the Answer Section at the back of the book.

CRITICAL THINKING QUESTIONS

1. Why is severe sepsis a costly illness? Why is it likely to become more costly?

2. How does elevating the head of the bed for a ventilated patient decrease the incidence of ventilator-associated pneumonia?

3. What interventions are included in evidence-based management of a central venous catheter?

4. Why is shaving a surgical site preoperatively no longer indicated?

5. What assessment findings would indicate to the nurse that the patient had developed systemic inflammatory response syndrome (SIRS)?

6. What questions should the nurse consider when attempting to localize the source of a patient's infection?

7. What are the elements of the sepsis resuscitation bundle?

8. Which of the elements of the sepsis management bundle are controversial? Why?

9. When should a patient's fever be treated?

10. Why does disseminated intravascular coagulation result in both thrombosis and bleeding?

See answers to Critical Thinking Questions in the Answer Section at the back of the book.

EXPLORE MEDIALINK

http://www.prenhall.com/perrin

Additional interactive resources for this chapter can be found on the Web site at http://www.prenhall.com/perrin. Click on "Chapter 17" to select activities for this chapter.

Case Study: Sepsis

Nursing Care Plan

NCLEX Review Questions

MediaLinks:
- AACN Practice Alerts
- Institute for Healthcare Improvement

- Ventilator Bundle
- Central Line Bundle
- Surviving Sepsis Campaign
- Sepsis Resuscitation and Management Bundles

MediaLink Applications

REFERENCES

American Association of Critical-Care Nurses (AACN) Practice Alert. (2005). *Practice alert: Preventing catheter-related bloodstream infections*. Retrieved April 9, 2008, from http://www.aacn.org/AACN/practiceAlert.nsf/vwdoc/pa2

American Association of Critical-Care Nurses (AACN) Practice Alert. (2006). Practice alert: Oral care in the critically ill. *AACN News, 23*(8), 4. Retrieved April 9, 2008, from http://www.aacn.org/AACN/practiceAlert.nsf/vwdoc/pa2

Angus, D. C., Linde-Zwirble, W. T., Lidicker, J., Clermont, G., Carcillo, J., Pinsky, M., et al. (2001). Epidemiology of severe sepsis in the United States: Analysis of incidence, outcome, and associated costs of care. *Critical Care Medicine, 29*, 1303–1310.

Aragon, D., & Sole, M. L. (2006). Implementing best practice strategies to prevent infection in the ICU. *Critical Care Clinics of North America, 18*, 441–452.

Axelrod, P. (2000). External cooling in the management of fever. *Clinical Infectious Diseases, 31*, S224–S229.

Baird, M. S., Keen, J. H., & Swearingen, P. L. (2005). Manual of critical care nursing: Nursing interventions and collaborative management (5th ed.). St. Louis, MO: Elsevier Mosby.

Bolton, L. L. (2006). Evidence corner: Preventing surgical site infection. *Wounds, 18*(7), A20–A22.

Dellinger R. P., Levy, M., Carlet J. M., Bion, J., Parker, M., Jaeschke, R., et al. (2008). Surviving Sepsis Campaign guidelines for management of severe sepsis and septic shock. *Critical Care Medicine, 36*, 296–327.

Geiger, H. (2003). Disseminated intravascular coagulopathy. *Dimensions of Critical Care Nursing, 22*(3), 108–116.

Giuliano, K. K. (2007). Physiologic monitoring for critically ill patients: Testing a predictive model for early

detection of sepsis. *American Journal of Critical Care, 16*(2), 122–131.

Henker, R., & Carlson, K. K. (2007). Fever: Applying research to bedside practice. *AACN: Advanced Clinical Care, 18*(1), 73–87.

Institute for Healthcare Improvement. Ventilator bundle. Retrieved May 17, 2007, from http://www.ihi.org/IHI/Topics/CriticalCare/IntensiveCare/Changes/ImplementtheVentilatorBundle.htm

Institute for Healthcare Improvement. *Central line bundle*. Retrieved May 17, 2007, from http://www.ihi.org/IHI/Topics/CriticalCare/IntensiveCare/Changes/ImplementtheCentralLineBundle.htm

Joanna Briggs Institute. (2001). Management of the child with fever: Evidence-based practice information sheets for health professionals. *Best Practice, 5*(5), 1–6.

Johnson, J. R., Kuslowski, M. A., & Wilt, T. J. (2006). Systematic review: Antimicrobial catheters to prevent urinary tract infections in hospitalized patients. *Annals of Internal Medicine, 144*, 116–126.

Kortgen, A., Hofmann, G., & Bauer, M. (2006). Sepsis—Current aspects of pathophysiology and implications for diagnosis and management. *European Journal of Trauma, 1*, 3–9.

Laupland, K. B., Bagshaw, S. M., Gregson, D. B., Kirkpatrick, A. W., Ross, T., & Church, D. L. (2005). Intensive care unit–acquired urinary tract infections in a regional critical care system. *Critical Care, 9*(2), R60–R65.

Liberman, J. D., & Whelan, C. T. (2006). The evolving treatment of sepsis. *Journal of Clinical Outcomes Management, 13*(4), 227–234.

Martin, G. S. (2007). SAFE, VASST, LIPOS, CORTICUS and more: Implications for the surviving sepsis campaign guidelines. *Medscape.* Retrieved April 8, 2008, from http://medscape.com/viewprogram/6954_pnt

Nguyen, H. B., Rivers, E. P., & Abrahamlan, F. M. (2006). Severe sepsis and septic shock: Review of the literature and emergency department guidelines. *Annals of Emergency Medicine, 48*(1), 28–54.

Otero, R. M., Nguyen, H. B., Huang, D. T., Gaieski, D. F., Goyal, M., Gunnerson, K. J., et al. (2006). Early goal directed therapy in severe sepsis and septic shock revisited: Concepts, controversies, and contemporary findings. *Chest, 130*(5), 1579–1595.

Powers, J., & Jacobi, J. (2006). Pharmacologic treatment related to severe sepsis. *AACN Advanced Critical Care, 17*(4), 423–432.

Rivers, E., Bryant, N., Haustad, S., Ressler, J., Muzzin, A., & Knoblich, B. (2001). Early goal-directed therapy in the treatment of severe sepsis and septic shock. *New England Journal of Medicine, 345*, 1368–1377.

Russell, J. A. (2006). Management of sepsis. *New England Journal of Medicine, 355*, 1699–1713.

Seckel, M. (2007). Implementing evidence-based practice guidelines to minimize ventilator-associated pneumonia. *AACN News, 24*(1), 8–9.

Sepsis resuscitation and management bundles. Retrieved April 7, 2008, from http://www.survivingsepsis.org/node/156

Surviving Sepsis Campaign. (2004). Retrieved April 8, 2008, from http://www.survivingsepsis.org/aboutcampaign

Todd, B. (2006). Emerging infections: Preventing bloodstream infections. *American Journal of Nursing, 106*(1), 29–30.

Tolentino-DelosReyes, A. F., Ruppert, S. D., & Shyang-Yun. (2007). Evidence-based practice: Use of the ventilator bundle to prevent ventilator acquired pneumonia. *American Journal of Critical Care, 16*(1), 20–27.

Caring for the ICU Patient at the End of Life

Kathleen Perrin, PhD, RN, CCRN
Marianne Matzo, PhD, APRN, BC, FAAN

Learning Outcomes

Upon completion of this chapter, the learner will be able to:

1. Describe the four categories defined by Copnell by which death occurs in the ICU.

2. Evaluate the advantages and disadvantages of family presence during CPR.

3. Discuss best practices for nurses when speaking with a bereaved family.

4. List the criteria for death by neurological criteria (brain death).

5. Explain possible ways to discuss limiting of further therapy such as instituting a Do Not Resuscitate (DNR) order with a patient and/or patient's family.

6. Compare and contrast substituted judgment and the best interests standard for decision making for an incapacitated patient.

7. Discuss the needs of families of dying patients.

8. Describe collaborative management of patients' symptoms at the end of life.

9. Explain sources of conflict at the end of life.

Abbreviations

DNR   Do Not Resuscitate
ENA   Emergency Nurses' Association

When critically ill patients die, it may be unexpected. However, it is more likely to be following discussion with the patient and family and withdrawal or withholding of life-sustaining technology. Care of the dying patient in the intensive care unit (ICU) focuses on meeting the needs of the dying patient and his family.

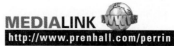

MEDIALINK
http://www.prenhall.com/perrin

See the Companion Website for chapter-specific resources at www.prenhall.com/perrin.

VISUAL MAP **End of Life Overview**

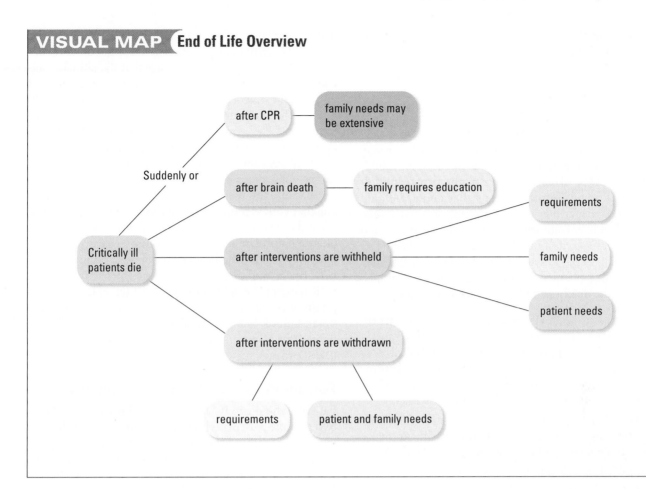

Review of Some Ethical End Legal Concepts

For the past 20 years in the United States, an emphasis has been placed in medical ethics on the principle of respect for persons. A derivation of this principle is that the patient should be the primary decision maker about his health care as long as he is competent. **Advance directives** were developed to allow competent patients to indicate in advance the kind of health care treatment they would desire should they become incapacitated at the end of their lives. Patients may use an advance directive to indicate a preference for specific treatments to be provided or withheld (medical directive) and/or to designate an individual (health care proxy) to make treatment decisions for them. Once signed the directives are legally enforceable. However, patients or their proxies may change their minds about the treatments described in the directive at any time, even during a patient's final illness. Recently, there has been a movement away from a reliance on patient autonomy toward a "shared decision" paradigm stimulated in part by studies showing that patients want their families involved in their health care decision making and that many favor joint decision making with their health care providers (Carlet et al., 2004).

When considering what care should be provided to a patient, many health care providers and patients weigh the benefits and burdens of the treatment. Some ethicists refer to this balancing of effects as proportionalism, derived from the medieval principle of double effect. The principle of double effect acknowledges that many treatments not only have benefits (good effects) but also impose substantial burdens (bad effects). In proportionalism, not only must the benefits outweigh the burdens but the person choosing the treatment also must intend the good effect rather than the bad one. When using this methodology, a person weighs the circumstances, his intentions, and the consequences to determine the least harmful result (McGhee, 2007). For example, when a nurse is providing morphine for dyspnea to a dying patient, he intends the medication to decrease the patient's anxiety and dyspnea, thus improving the patient's comfort, and the nurse accepts the possibility that it may decrease the patient's respiratory rate.

Many ethicists and health care providers believe not just that curative treatment should be forgone when a patient is clearly dying but that palliative care is ethically and legally appropriate and even necessary. In **palliative care** the emphasis of care shifts from the pursuit of a cure to the provision of comfort. The goal of palliative care is the achievement of the best quality of life for dying patients and their families.

Extent of the Problem

Although families and patients usually associate critical care with the promise of modern medicine and the expectation of a cure for the patient, the limits of medicine may be reached and the patient may die. Angus et al. (2004) found that 22% of deaths of hospitalized patients followed ICU admission; that means that about 540,000 American patients die after ICU admission each year. Thus, ICU nurses routinely encounter dying patients and need to be prepared to provide expert care to them.

Copnell (2005) noted that although ICU deaths may be classified as planned or unplanned, a better approach is to view the deaths as falling into four categories:

- Death that occurs despite all efforts on the part of clinicians. (This may be called "failed CPR" and accounts for approximately 10% of ICU deaths. It includes patients who die suddenly following traumatic injuries and patients who have been receiving maximal support for days or even weeks.)
- Death that occurs following demonstration of lack of brainstem functioning. (This is usually known as **brain death** and represented 8% of deaths in one study in a tertiary care center.)
- Death that occurs following a decision not to initiate one or more interventions such as ventilation, intubation, dialysis, enteral feeding, or vasopressors. (This may be known as "limitation" because a decision is made not to institute a medical therapy because the therapy is unlikely to benefit the patient.)
- Death that occurs after a decision to withdraw one or more therapies that have already been initiated but are not benefiting the patient. (This is often termed "withdrawal.")

The vast majority of ICU deaths in the United States, approximately 70% to 90%, follow either limitation or withdrawal of medical interventions. Limitation and withdrawal usually have two phases: the first is the "process of shared decision making that leads from the pursuit of cure or recovery to the pursuit of comfort and freedom from pain," whereas the second "focuses on the humanistic and technical skills that must be enlisted to ensure the needs of the patient and family are met" (Truog et al., 2001).

Death That Occurs Despite All Efforts on the Part of Clinicians

Approximately 10% of the time, patients receive aggressive interventions, including **cardiopulmonary resuscitation**

(CPR), until the end of life. Weil and Fries (2005) in a review of current management and outcomes of CPR concluded, "there is no secure evidence that the ultimate outcomes after cardiopulmonary resuscitation in settings of in-hospital cardiac arrest have improved in more than 40 years." They indicate that the current survival rate may be as high as 17%, a modest increase from 14% documented in the past. Some groups of patients, such as patients with renal failure, cancer, and multisystem organ failure, rarely survive following a cardiac arrest.

Because the survival rate is so low, some ethicists argue that CPR is a futile intervention and ought not to be offered to every patient. Moreover, resuscitation is most likely a painful or at least an uncomfortable process. The patient's ribs may be broken, endotracheal intubation is performed, and electric shocks may be delivered. Yet CPR remains the default option for intervention for hospitalized patients, even those patients with multisystem organ failure. It is provided unless the patient or the patient's proxy agrees to a written **Do Not Resuscitate (DNR)** order.

Family Presence During Resuscitation

Patients who die in ICUs following CPR usually fall into two groups: patients who were admitted within the previous 2 days with devastating but potentially survivable injuries such as severe traumatic injuries, and patients who refuse or for whom their families refuse to have a DNR order written. In both of these circumstances the family may not have had the opportunity to come to terms with the devastating nature of the injury and the realization that modern health care is unable to cure the patient. This is one of the reasons why many health care practitioners are advocating that family members be present during CPR. There are a number of benefits to family presence during resuscitation such as:

- Family members may be able to ask questions and gain a sense of reality about the critical illness.
- Family members may be able to provide comfort and support to the patient.
- Family members usually realize that the health care team has tried heroically to keep the patient alive.
- After seeing the patient's last moments, family members are less likely to be haunted by what they imagine might have occurred during that time.
- If the patient dies, family members usually cope better with their loss.
- Staff are reminded of the patient's personhood (Halm, 2005).

Few patients survive and communicate following resuscitation, so it is difficult to determine the patient's perspective on having the family present during CPR. In one study (Eichorn, Meyers, & Guzzetta, 2001) that examined a few patients who survived resuscitation attempts, patients reported feeling "comforted, supported, and less afraid" when family members were in the room during resuscitation.

Opponents of family presence usually are concerned that the health care team will not be able to function optimally if family members are present. They worry that family members may not be aware of all of the patient's medical conditions and there may be a breach of confidentiality. Opponents of family presence are often worried about the effects of the family on the hospital staff. They fear that more staff will be needed during CPR because someone will need to meet the needs of the family. They believe that the staff will experience more stress, resulting in performance anxiety (Halm, 2005). Opponents also believe that family members may misunderstand what they see and hear during the code, possibly resulting in lawsuits. Research has not supported these concerns. Thus, there has been steadily growing interest in allowing family members to be present during resuscitation of their loved one under certain circumstances.

Helping the Family to Decide

When the nurse is helping family members to decide whether or not they should stay with their loved one during resuscitation, seven steps should be followed (using the mnemonic device "in-or-out") (Riwitis & Twibell, 2006, p. 14).

1) **I**: Introduce yourself to the family.
2) **N**: Now: Explain the patient's current status.
3) **O**: Outcome: Explain the possible results.
4) **R**: Relationships: Learn who makes the decisions.
5) **O**: Option: Provide the choices.
6) **U**: Understanding: Assess comprehension.
7) **T**: Time: Take action.

Guidelines for Family Presence

If a family member decides that she would like to be present, Mason (2004) recommends the following guidelines be followed:

- The nurse should initially find out the family member's relationship to the patient and ask for identification.
- The nurse should determine if the family member is able to follow instructions about being in the room, such as stepping away from the bed during defibrillation. If family members want to go in but are very emotional, it may be possible to get them to cooperate by looking them in the eye and saying, "You'll need to pull yourself together if you want to go into the room and be of help to your loved one." Emergency Nurses' Association

(ENA) guidelines recommend that people who appear to be under the influence of drugs or alcohol or who are abusive should not be permitted in the room.

- If the patient is conscious, the nurse should ask the patient's permission. If not, and if the hospital does not have a written policy on family presence, the nurse should get the permission of the person responsible for the care, such as the physician in charge of the code.
- A trained facilitator such as a nurse, social worker, or chaplain should prepare the family for how their loved one will appear, what they will see in the room, and what they can do. The facilitator should stay with the family while they are in the room to provide them with explanations and instructions (such as to stay away from the bed during defibrillation).
- Even if the family stays in the room for only 5 or 10 minutes, they need to be debriefed afterward. The facilitator should ask them how they are feeling and encourage them to describe their experience or to ask any questions they may have about what they witnessed.

Working with the Bereaved Family

After a patient has died, the ICU nurse often is involved in comforting the bereaved family. According to Truog et al. (2001) best practices when speaking with bereaved families and loved ones include:

- If the family has not been at the hospital and the death is unexpected, contacting them and explaining they should come to the hospital rather than saying outright over the phone that the patient has died
- Providing privacy for the family and loved ones during the discussion
- Beginning conversations with words of condolence such as "I'm so sorry for your loss" unless such words are not appropriate in the family's religious tradition (e.g., Judaism)
- Maintaining eye contact and touching the family member if appropriate
- Avoiding the use of jargon such as "CPR" or "vent"—instead the nurse should use words like "heart stopped" and "we tried to restart it" or "the breathing machine"
- Listening to the family rather than rushing to speak, and particularly avoiding the use of clichés such as "She lived a long (or good) life" because they may not be well received by the family
- Offering private time for the family to be with the patient after death and before the body is removed from the unit

Brain Death

Brain death is defined as the irreversible loss of brain function including the function of the brainstem. The frequency with which a nurse encounters a patient declared dead by neurological criteria will depend on the type of institution where the nurse is employed, with nurses employed in tertiary medical centers encountering more patients. However, the total number of brain-dead potential donors in the United States is estimated to be between 10,500 and 13,800 annually (Ehrle, 2006).

Meeting the Criteria

The Quality Standards Sub-Committee of the American Academy of Neurology (1995) has established guidelines for the determination of brain death. These guidelines are only appropriate for use with adults over the age of 18 who do not have severe electrolyte, metabolic, or acid-base imbalances; have not ingested drug overdoses or poisons; and have a core body temperature greater than 32°C (90°F). There are three cardinal findings that are necessary for the determination of brain death. These are coma, absence of brainstem reflexes, and apnea:

- Coma is determined by the lack of motor responses or grimacing to noxious stimuli.
- Absence of brainstem reflexes is determined by pupils 4 mm or larger that do not respond to light, and the absence of all of the following reflexes: oculocephalic, oculovestibular, corneal, gag, and cough.
- Apnea is identified by removing the patient from the ventilator for approximately 8 minutes and placing him on 100% oxygen by T piece. The patient is observed to determine that there are no respiratory movements.

The determination of brain death may be confirmed by using additional criteria. The tests for brain death are described in detail in Chapter 15. ∞ Once these tests have been completed and confirmed, the patient may be declared dead using brain death criteria.

Communicating with Families About Brain Death

When the patient has been declared dead by neurological (brain death) criteria, health care providers must be very careful about their choice of words (Truog et al., 2001). One common mistake for a health care provider to make is to say something such as, "Your (family member) has been diagnosed with brain death. He will die shortly after we take him off the ventilator." This may confuse the family, who may not understand that the patient has been pronounced dead and removing the ventilator is essentially removing a useless mechanical device from a person who has already died. Instead a nurse might confirm, "Your family member has been pronounced dead be-cause he has no functional brain activity. We will be removing the ventilator shortly but would like to answer any of your questions before we proceed."

Donation Request

The United States has a system of required request, which means that all institutions receiving Medicare or Medicaid funds must notify the organ donor bank of impending deaths and ask the families of potential donors for permission to procure organs and tissues. The request for organs and tissues should be done separately from the notification to the family that the patient has died and is most effective when done by a specially trained individual from the Organ Procurement Organization (OPO). Thus both members of the OPO and hospital staff will be communicating with the patient's family.

To ensure that the entire health care team communicates the same message to the family, the OPO recommends "huddles." Huddles are short coordinated, frequent discussions between health care providers and OPO personnel whose goal is to meet the unique needs of the potential donor's family. Huddles have been identified as one of the key evidence-based practices to improve donation rates (Ehrle, 2006).

Whether or not the family agrees to donation, it is important that the nurse spend time with the family, preparing them for the patient's imminent death and explaining to them what will occur (Matzo, 2006). Families need to believe that the potential donor is valued as a person. Therefore, patients who are considered to be brain dead should be treated in such a way as to maximize integrity and minimize discomfort, even though by definition they do not feel pain (Evans, 2004). Evaluation and care of the prospective deceased donor is described in Chapter 15. ∞

Death That Occurs Following a Decision to Limit Therapy

Most patients who die in critical care units in the United States have had some potential therapies withheld prior to their death. Therapies that may be limited prior to a patient dying include among others: CPR, dialysis, ventilation, intubation, and vasopressors. Many Americans prefer to have aggressive medical care delivered and resources expended until the patient's prognosis becomes apparent, and physicians, nurses, patients, and families are certain that it is appropriate to limit interventions.

One of the most difficult issues in critical care is to determine when a patient is actually dying. The Support Principal Investigators reported in a landmark study (1995) that it was not apparent that the patient was dying until about 2 days before the patient died. Patients and families may consider DNR orders before limitation of other medical interventions because resuscitation is only instituted when the patient's heart or respiration has already stopped, and what is being considered is an attempt, probably futile, to revive the patient, not a limitation of care.

Do Not Resuscitate

In 1995, the Support Principal Investigators found that, "nearly half of the patients who had a desire for CPR to be withheld did not have a DNR order written during their hospitalization. Nearly one-third of those patients died before discharge." The 10 years since the study has not shown any significant improvement, with CPR still being infrequently addressed in the hospital orders or medical records of patients who undergo CPR during their hospital stay (Mirza, Kad, R. & Ellison, N , 2005). Because CPR has a small chance (17%) of being successful, it is not clearly futile. Thus, the decision about resuscitation is value laden, is not purely medically determined, and is one in which patients and families should participate. Resuscitation is clearly an intrusive, expensive, and, possibly, painful medical intervention, so health care providers, ethicists, and lawyers are in agreement that patients and families may decline the intervention if they believe it will offer minimal benefit or be too burdensome. Therefore, if a patient is in the hospital, either the patient or the patient's family ought to be asked if CPR should be performed or withheld should the patient have a cardiac or respiratory arrest.

Unfortunately, many health care providers are uncomfortable about initiating a discussion about DNR orders with patients and families. Often, it is the nurses who have been listening to the patients' and families' concerns about prognoses and treatment choices who alert the physicians to the patients' and families' willingness to discuss resuscitation. Nurses can begin such discussions by interjecting questions about prognosis and DNR beliefs into the casual conversation of daily care, thus developing trust before attempting to identify the patient's wishes (Matzo & Ramsey, 2006). Nurses may start by providing some patient education, saying, "This is what is happening now and we're going to try this treatment." Then they might ask the patient, "Have you thought about what you would want if this didn't work or if you didn't get better? What would you want to happen?"

Many ICU patients are incapable of making a decision for themselves, causing nurses and other health care providers to turn to advance directives or families and loved ones to learn the patient's preferences. Applicable advance directives are uncommon; so the nurse may need to carefully query the family to help them articulate the patient's desires. A nurse might approach family members as she had the patient, educating the families about the treatments and asking similar questions. If the nurse believes that death could be imminent, she might directly and immediately ask about the patient's wishes for resuscitation. Asking specific questions about CPR is essential. When patients or family members are asked if they want "everything done," they will often say "Yes" only to declare later, "I didn't mean that."

Saying they do not want everything done for a dying family member or loved one often makes people feel as if they are abandoning the dying patient. There are other ways to tactfully ask if a patient should be resuscitated. A nurse could say something like: "We are doing all that we can to try to cure your family member, however she is not improving. We would like to keep her comfortable rather than try to restart her heart if it stops, do you agree?" The response may be very different than if the nurse asked, "Do you want everything done?" Nurses may need to spend a significant amount of time explaining the concept of DNR in understandable terms to patients and families so that they can give informed consent (Perrin, 2006).

Nurses should emphasize to patients and families that consent to a DNR order does not imply consent to limit other medical interventions or a decision to switch to a goal of comfort rather than cure. These are separate issues that may be discussed simultaneously or at a later time. Consenting to a DNR does not imply that the patient will receive less care. Patients with DNR orders in ICUs frequently receive more nursing time and nursing care.

Although the decision to withhold CPR is often the first limitation of treatment, it is common for other therapies to be withheld as well. These therapies are usually withheld under the understanding that although it is possible to provide them and they might offer some marginal benefit to the patient, instituting them is more likely to result in prolonging the patient's dying than survival with meaningful quality of life. In other words, when weighing the benefits and burdens of treatment, the burdens clearly outweigh the benefits and treatment can be declined.

Limitation of therapy usually follows a discussion among members of the health care team, the patient, and family. In the best situation, patients can state their desires for limitation of therapy or, if they are incapacitated, they have advance directives that are clearly pertinent to the situation so that family and health care providers are able to follow the patient's wishes. However, it is uncommon for patients to have made their wishes for therapy known and legally enforceable prior to hospitalization.

Advance Directives

Advance directives, although originally regarded as the solution for dealing with incapacitated patients, are now recognized as having had "little demonstrated impact" (Tulsky, 2005) for several reasons:

- First, despite considerable publicity since the advent of the Patient Self Determination Act in 1991, the majority of Americans have failed to complete advance directives; in fact 90% of the patients an ICU nurse encounters will never have made one (Boyle, Miller, & Forbes-Thompson, 2005).

- Second, if the patient has completed a directive the responsible person may be unable to locate it, it may be out of date, or it may not provide adequate guidance in the clinical situation.

- Third, if the directive appoints a health care proxy who is empowered to make decisions for the patient, the health care proxy may or may not have a clear understanding of the patient's preferences (Engelberg, Patrick, & Curtis, 2005). If the health care proxy has not discussed the specific circumstances with the patient prior to the hospitalization, the most commonly recommended means for the health care proxy to make a decision are by the substituted judgment or best interests standards:
  - In the substituted judgment standard, the health care proxy imagines himself as the patient in the particular situation and determines what the patient would want. This can be difficult depending on the ability of the health care proxy to see the situation from the point of view of the patient.
  - In the best interests standard, the health care proxy makes a decision based on what he believes is in the best interests of the patient. Bailey (2006) argues that when using the best interests standard, the decision maker is essentially making the determination that the quality of life the patient would experience is, or would be, so poor that it is worse than no life at all. It can be extremely difficult for a health care proxy or family member to objectively determine when the anticipated degree of the patient's body integrity and function will have deteriorated to such a point.
- Finally and perhaps most importantly, a completed directive is no substitute for a person who has had a conversation with the patient who understands the patient's goals and values. When patients have had discussions with their prospective health care proxy, the potential health care proxy displays a better understanding of what is important to the patient at end of life and may be more likely to accurately follow patient preferences. There are a few questions that are useful for the nurse to ask that might help to clarify the wishes of the patient. The nurse might wish to know:
  - Has the patient spoken to anyone about the terms of the advance directive?
  - With whom did the patient speak?
  - What was discussed?
  - What are the patient's wishes in her or his own words?

Patients generally want their health care proxies to be family members and although they want the family member to voice their perspective about what type of care should be provided, most want the decision making to be shared between their loved ones and their physician (Nolan et al., 2005).

Thus the nurse may be responsible for coordinating a discussion between members of the health care team, the family, and the patient about goals of patient care. Conflict may develop when families, patients, or health care team members have differing views about what is in the patient's best interests or what ought to be the goals for patient care. For example, is the patient dying and should care be limited? The nurse has an important role in promoting effective communication and preventing conflict between health care providers, patients, and families. Tulsky (2005) states that developing trust is an essential first step in developing a relationship with a potentially dying patient and her family and an important factor in avoiding conflict and coming to a realistic decision about end-of-life care. Tulsky recommends these steps that the nurse can follow for establishing trust:

- Encourage patients and families to talk and identify and acknowledge the family's feelings as well as the difficulty of the situation by asking something such as: "I'm sure this illness has been a lot for you to absorb quickly. How are you coping with it?"
- Maintain a higher ratio of family member-to-health care provider speaking time; therefore, listening, asking clarifying questions, and tolerating silence are important skills for nurses.
- Do not contradict or put down other health care providers yet recognize patient concerns by saying something such as: "I hear you saying that you don't feel you are being heard by the physicians. I'd like to make certain you have a chance to voice all your concerns."
- Acknowledge errors.
- Be humble by setting a nonthreatening tone.
- Demonstrate respect for family members by saying something such as: "I'm so impressed by how involved you have been with your father throughout his illness." Also by assuming that the family members are operating in what they believe to be the patient's best interests unless there is proof to the contrary.

Gerontological Considerations

There are significant demographic and clinical variations in the rates of ICU use at the end of life. Older patients and those with more chronic illnesses have the highest rate of end-of-life ICU use, consuming a significant proportion of its resources.

However, the proportion of patients who die in the ICU and the proportion of patients who receive mechanical ventilation decline after patients reach age 85 (Seferian & Afessa, 2006).

Conveying Bad News

Once trust has been established, the nurse and other members of the health care team must assist the family to understand what is happening to their family member so that they can plan for the future. When dealing with potentially dying, critically ill patients this often involves conveying or helping the family to accept "bad news." Peel (2003) notes that patients and families expect to hear "bad news" initially from the physician either in an individual meeting or during a family or multidisciplinary team meeting. However, people in crisis, as these families and patients are, usually need repeated explanations of the same information (Perrin, 2006). Thus, the nurse will need to continue to convey and reaffirm the bad news. The challenge is to deliver the news consistently in a sensitive manner at an appropriate time. Best practices for discussing bad news according to Buckman (1992) include:

- Finding out what is already known
- Finding out how much information the patient and/or family want to know
- Sharing information, starting from their viewpoint and step by step bringing them closer to medical facts
- Responding to their reactions, using an empathic approach
- Explaining the treatment plan and prognosis, summarizing, and making a contact

Truog et al. (2001) add the following recommendation:

- Not forcing decisions, that is, allowing the patient and family time to absorb information and discuss their concerns

In addition, Downey, Engelberg, Shannon, and Curtis (2006) recommend that the nurse talk with the patient and family about their cultural needs and attempt to meet them. Truthfulness and how to deliver bad news are often culturally derived values so the Society for Critical Care Medicine (SCCM) recommends that when there is a choice of providers, the provider's culture should be matched to the patient's (Davidson et al., 2007). In some cultures, it may be traditional for the patient's family to be the sole recipients of information. If the patient refuses to hear information and defers to his family, the SCCM states that the "informed refusal" should be respected. Information about the patient's illness and its prognosis should then be delivered in a culturally relevant and appropriate manner to his family and the outcome of such discussions documented in his medical record.

Evidence is beginning to accumulate that frequent multidisciplinary team and family meetings to set goals for patient care during an ICU stay are most likely to result in an appropriate and coordinated plan of care and to reduce conflict. Boyle et al. (2005) recommend an initial meeting of the multidisciplinary team, patient (if possible), and family within 72 hours of the patient's ICU admission if the patient is at risk for death. During this meeting, medical facts and treatment options should be reviewed, a plan of care devised, and criteria to judge whether the plan is succeeding or not developed. Additional meetings may then be held to judge the success or failure of the plan and to determine the goals of patient care. To avoid potential conflict, Boyle et al. (2005) also recommend using a screening tool to identify patients and families who are at high risk for conflict. These families are further evaluated by a social worker and recommended for additional interventions, such as regular family meetings or an ethics consult, if appropriate.

Limitation of Care

Once the family, patient, and health care team acknowledge that the patient may be dying, there are a number of interventions that may be withheld so that the dying process is not prolonged. However, this does not mean that the patient does not receive nursing care. The goal of the nursing care will usually change from cure to comfort but most studies demonstrate that ICU nurses spend more time with their dying patients, not less. There may be no more that medicine can do to cure but there is a great deal that nursing can do to comfort and care.

Common interventions that may be withheld include ventilation, dialysis, and enteral feeding. There is little controversy surrounding limiting the first two of these because they are both aggressive and intrusive. However, there has been a resurgence of controversy surrounding the limitation of food and fluid to the terminally ill. Because food is associated with nurturance and care in many cultures and religions, withholding food and fluid may seem unacceptable and unethical to some families and health care providers. Many people believe that food and fluids should always be provided to patients because they represent simple, ordinary means of care. However, at some point in the dying process, additional food and fluid appear to offer little benefit and may be very burdensome to a patient. Studies of aggressive nutritional support, including tube feeding, of patients with cancer have demonstrated no benefits in length of survival. In fact, qualitative studies and practitioner experiences suggest that such aggressive feeding may harm the patient.

According to Zerwekh (1987), providing artificial fluid replacement once the patient's organs have begun to fail may be a contributing factor in the development of peripheral edema; ascites; increased respiratory secretions, which may result in dyspnea; and increased gastrointestinal secretions, which may result in nausea and vomiting. Nurses in one hospice service noted that their patients who did not receive IV fluid replacement did not have difficulty with respiratory secretions and did not require suctioning. The comfort experienced by these patients who were allowed to take only the food and fluid they desired was in stark contrast to the suctioning required by patients who had IV fluids administered (Dolan, 1983).

During terminal dehydration, patients do not appear to be experiencing pain. There is some indication that the increase in circulating endorphins resulting from ketosis may provide a natural analgesic effect at the end of life (Meares, 1994). Thus, providing food and fluids by artificial means, such as IVs or nasogastric tubes, appears to offer more burdens than benefits for the dying patient. When the burdens so clearly outweigh the benefits of treatment, there is no ethical imperative to offer the treatment. Consensus supports the practice that patients be offered only the oral food and fluid they desire at the end of life, even if they desire very little (Brody, Campbell, Faber-Langedoen, & Ogle, 1997).

Family Needs

While the patient is probably dying, the nurse should attend to the needs of both the family and the patient. Truog et al. (2001) reviewed research studies and summarized the needs of families of patients dying in ICUs.

Families Need to Be with the Dying Patient.

Evidence suggests providing a private room with unlimited visiting hours if possible. Restrictions on the number of people visiting and children and pets visiting should be lifted if at all possible. If, however, the family is unable to be with the patient, they should be reassured that it is acceptable for them to remain at home and that a nurse will stay with the patient until the end (if this is likely to be true).

There is ongoing discussion about whether palliative care should be provided in the environment of the ICU. Some argue that the high-tech environment is not appropriate for dying patients and that they would be better served on a palliative care or medical surgical unit. Nurses often argue that if the patient and family have formed a bond with the nursing staff, death is likely to occur soon, and the bed is not urgently needed, that allowing the patient to die in the ICU promotes continuity of care and comfort for patient and family. Some ICUs have established "palliative care packages" to convert the high-tech environment into a more comfortable space for the dying patient and family.

Families Want to Be Helpful to the Dying Patient.

The nurse can show the family how to provide care to the patient. It will depend on the family what care they will want to provide. A few families may want to bathe the patient. However, for most patients, the nurse can show the family how to moisten the patient's lips, reposition the patient, or soothe the patient. The nurse might encourage the family to bring in music or read to the patient so that they feel they have been able to provide some comfort.

Families Need to Be Assured of the Patient's Comfort.

Some health care providers and ethicists argue that if the patient is showing agonal respirations or having a "death rattle" even if the patient does not appear to be uncomfortable, it may be appropriate to medicate her for the benefit of the family (Truog et al., 2001). Otherwise, all appropriate medications for pain, nausea, and dyspnea should be administered aggressively. Evidence-based strategies for management of symptoms in a dying patient are discussed in detail later in the chapter.

Families Need to Be Informed About the Patient's Condition.

There are many different ways to keep the family informed about what is happening:

- Family members can be provided with an electronic pager when they leave the unit so they can be notified of any significant event or need for them in the unit.

- A family member should be provided with the telephone number of the unit and told that one member of the family is welcome to call if the family is anxious and needs an update.

- Families should be able to identify the physician and nurse who have primary responsibility for caring for the patient. A family member should feel free to ask the physician and nurse to explain the patient's treatment at any time.

It is not just the ability to receive information that is important to the family; the family must believe that the information is accurate and trustworthy. To ensure this members of the health care team should offer a consistent message to the family. Nurses and all health care providers should be careful of the way they use language; families will often interpret the phrase "He had a good day" as the patient is getting better. The team should discuss the likely prognosis and agree about what they will say to the family. However, they will have to acknowledge that medical prognoses are not always certain and help the family to understand that it is not possible to know exactly how things will progress or when. Tolerating such ambiguity can be difficult for families, and the support of clergy and social workers is often essential.

Families Need to Be Comforted and Allowed to Express Their Emotions.

According to Morse (2001), people who are suffering have two distinct patterns of behavior requiring different types of nursing interventions. The first behavior pattern is enduring. In this phase the family member has not acknowledged the full impact of the situation and is attempting to control her emotions and the situation. She may appear rigid, does not display any emotion, and interacts minimally with people around her. The second phase is emotional suffering. During that phase, the person acknowledges what is occurring and starts to respond emotionally. In order to move forward, the person must enter the phase of emotional suffering. However, any person may move between the phases depending on the situation. For example, a family member may display emotional suffering in the waiting room but enduring when in the room with the patient. The nurse should comfort people differently depending on which behaviors they are displaying.

Morse's research (2001) has indicated that while people are enduring, the nurse should comfort them by:

- Respecting the person's need for physical space and not touching or hugging him or her. Morse calls touching or being empathetic to the person at this stage "side swiping" because it will undermine the person's enduring.
- Reinforcing enduring strategies by saying: "You are doing such a good job"—talking to the patient, sitting by the bedside—or "You're holding up well."
- Explaining what is happening, offering anticipatory guidance, and providing potential time frames for what is occurring.
- Being with the person in silence.

When the person is displaying emotional suffering, Morse's evidence suggests that the nurse may comfort her by becoming engaged with the sufferer's emotion (2001). The nurse might utilize the following:

- Positioning (The nurse places herself directly in line with the person's vision so that eye contact must be made between the two.)
- Touching (The nurse might hug, stroke, or pat the person to create a physical connection with her.)
- Appropriate use of verbal responses (The nurse might use therapeutic empathy, informing reassurance, humor/distraction, or confrontation.)
- Sharing in the experience (The nurse might convey sympathy, commiseration, compassion, consolation, or reflexive reassurance to the patient.)

Death That Occurs Following Withdrawal of Life-Sustaining Technology

The withdrawal of medical interventions already in progress has been practiced in critical care units in the United States for the past 20 years. To understand why such a position is ethically justifiable, one must acknowledge that modern medicine is not capable of curing all conditions and that it is capable of imposing inordinate suffering on patients in attempts to prolong their lives. If an ongoing medical treatment is not capable of benefiting the patient, most ethicists do not view withdrawing the treatment as the direct cause of the patient's death. The cause of death in such a circumstance would be the relentless progression of the patient's disease. Thus, when an intervention is neither enhancing the care of the patient nor promoting the patient's recovery, the intervention may be withdrawn. Therapies that support a variety of physiological functions may be withdrawn. The following is an abbreviated list:

Cardiovascular:	Vasopressors
	Pacemakers and implantable cardioverter/defibrillators
	Intra-aortic balloon pumps
	Ventricular assist devices
Respiratory	Mechanical ventilation
	Supplemental oxygen
	Artificial airways
Renal	Dialysis
	Hemofiltration
Neurological	Cerebral spinal fluid drainage
Immunologic	Treatment of infection with anti-infectives

The guideline suggested by Truog et al. (2001) to determine if it is appropriate to continue an intervention at the end of life is whether the intervention will provide symptom relief; enhance functional status; or lessen emotional, psychological, or spiritual distress. Thus, simple laboratory tests or chest x-rays that might cause discomfort and would only provide unneeded information might be discontinued. However, a more sophisticated intervention such as cerebral spinal fluid drainage might be continued even when it is not curing the patient but it is providing symptom relief. The decision to continue each intervention is based on the specific patient's comfort, so an intervention that might be used for one patient might be withdrawn from another. For example, a patient might have an antibiotic continued if it decreases the pain and fever from otitis media, whereas a different patient might have an antibiotic withheld if there is no available access and the patient is not experiencing discomfort or fever from the infection.

One of the most common modalities withdrawn at the end of life is ventilator therapy. There has been a continuing debate about the best method for withdrawing mechanical ventilation (Truog et al., 2001). One approach, terminal weaning, which is favored by Campbell, Bizek, and Thill (1999), involves the gradual reduction in settings on the ventilator: a change to synchronized intermittent mechanical ventilation with pressure support, a decrease in the respiratory rate, a reduction in the FIO_2, and finally discontinuation of the ventilator and provision of humidified room air by T piece. The other common approach, terminal extubation, involves removal of the endotracheal tube (ET) and discontinuation of the ventilator. Campbell et al. (1999) recommend rapid terminal weaning, believing that it is a humane process in the unconscious patient and the patient is usually comfortable. Other authorities suggest that the family may find a terminal wean less morally troublesome than terminal extubation and that it may be a better choice if the patient has large quantities of oral or respiratory secretions. Advocates of terminal extubation state that it does not prolong the dying process, that it cannot be mistaken for a therapeutic wean when the patient may be improving, and that when the patient has had the ET tube removed, he or she appears more "normal" to the family. There is not sufficient data to determine which method is preferable. Approximately 54% of physicians practice both methods of withdrawal, 33% prefer terminal weaning, and 13% prefer terminal extubation (Truog et al., 2001).

Dialysis is another therapy that may be withdrawn either following a patient's request or when death appears imminent in a critically ill patient. Unlike terminal extubation, where the median length of patient survival is hours following withdrawal of therapy, the mean length of survival following discontinuation of dialysis is 8 to 9 days (Brody et al., 1997) although some patients may survive for weeks. Most patients, nearly 65%, appear to die comfortable deaths, providing excessive IV fluid administration is avoided and the patient is permitted oral fluids as desired for comfort. If the patient does receive excessive fluid administration, he or she may develop dyspnea.

Nursing Care

Once the decision is made that therapy will be limited or withdrawn and there will be no attempt to stop the dying process, the goal of patient care is comfort. The nurse needs to recognize that each time he cares for an actively dying patient, it will be a unique event. The symptoms will vary and the nurse needs to adapt institutional guidelines and the recommendations described next to the needs of the specific patient.

Nursing Diagnoses

INTENSIVE CARE UNIT PATIENT AT THE END OF LIFE

- Anticipatory grieving related to perceived impending death
- Ineffective breathing related to the dying process
- Interrupted family processes related to illness of family member and possible conflict among family members
- Impaired verbal communication related to endotracheal intubation, dyspnea, and fatigue
- Risk for ineffective coping related to diagnosis of serious illness and personal vulnerability
- Risk for spiritual distress related to challenged beliefs and value systems

Dyspnea

"Dyspnea is a form of suffering and is probably the most important symptom that must be relieved for patients dying in the ICU" (Truog et al., 2001, p. 2339).

Collaborative Management

When a ventilator is withdrawn, regardless of whether terminal wean or terminal extubation is utilized, most patients receive anticipatory dosing of sedatives or pain medication to prevent them from experiencing a sudden increase in dyspnea. "As a general rule, the doses of medications that the patient has been receiving hourly should be increased by two or threefold and administered acutely before withdrawing mechanical ventilation" (Truog et al., 2001, p. 2339). With appropriate dosing, patients should appear comfortable, and research indicates that administration of high doses of medication to relieve symptoms does not hasten patients' deaths (Campbell et al., 1999; Vitella, Kenner, & Sali, 2005). Campbell et al. (1999) have validated that a simple subjective comfort scale correlates well with objective measures and can be used to assess comfort and to identify the need for medication in the patient being terminally weaned. They recommend rating alertness, calmness/agitation, physical movement, muscle tone, heart rate, respiratory response, and facial tension using a modified version of the COMFORT scale that does not include the blood pressure. (See Table 18–1.) Higher scores on the scale indicate greater patient distress and the need for more medication. The optimal dose of medication is "determined by increasing the dose until the patient responds" (Brody et al., 1997, p. 653).

The following are recommendations for the use of medication to relieve dyspnea during terminal weaning or extubation. However, as noted previously, it is essential that medication and dose be individualized to relieve the symptoms of the specific patient.

The nurse may utilize nonpharmacological means in conjunction with medication to relieve dyspnea. Positioning the patient to encourage chest expansion may offer the patient some sense of relief. The most comfortable position for the patient will depend on her underlying condition, which might be sitting up, leaning over a bedside table, or lying on a side. The administration of oxygen enhances the comfort of some patients. However, there is some evidence that patients who have been terminally extubated may be less responsive and appear more comfortable if they become hypoxic before becoming hypercarbic. Thus, some clinicians prefer not to provide oxygen to dying patients who are being weaned or extubated. If an electric fan is allowed in the unit, the sensation of coolness and air blowing on the patient's face may produce some relief of breathlessness. The goal of collaborative management is to have a patient who appears to both health care providers and family to be dying peacefully without untoward respiratory difficulty.

TABLE 18-1

The COMFORT Scale

ALERTNESS	CALMNESS/ AGITATION	RESPIRATORY RESPONSE	PHYSICAL MOVEMENT	BLOOD PRESSURE (MAP)	HEART RATE	MUSCLE TONE	FACIAL EXPRESSION	POINTS
Deeply asleep	Calm	No coughing and no spontaneous respiration	No movement	Below baseline	Below baseline	Totally relaxed; no tone	Totally relaxed	1
Lightly asleep	Slightly anxious	Spontaneous respiration with little or no response to ventilation	Occasional, slight movement	Consistently at baseline	Consistently at baseline	Reduced	Normal; no facial tension evident	2
Drowsy	Anxious	Occasional cough or resistance to ventilator	Frequent, slight movement	Infrequent elevations of 15% or more (1–3/observ.)	Infrequent elevations of 15% or more (1–3)	Normal	Tension evident in some facial muscles	3
Fully awake and alert	Very anxious	Actively breathes against respirator or coughs regularly	Vigorous movement limited to extremities	Frequent elevations of 15% or more (>3/observ.)	Frequent elevations of 15% or more (>3)	Increase tone and flexion of fingers and toes	Tension evidence throughout facial muscles	4
Hyper alert	Panicky	Fights ventilator, coughing or choking	Vigorous movement, including torso and head	Sustained elevation ≥15%	Sustained elevation ≥15%	Extreme muscle rigidity and flexion of fingers and toes	Facial muscles contorting and grimacing	5

Source: Used by permission of Oxford University Press, *Journal of Pediatric Psychology.*
MAP, mean arterial pressure.

COMMONLY USED MEDICATIONS

MORPHINE SULFATE—AN OPIOID

INTRODUCTION

Morphine is the preferred analgesic for use with a dying patient in ICU because it is potent, has a wide therapeutic range, acts rapidly when given intravenously, and is relatively inexpensive. An alternative, if needed, would be fentanyl, but much lower doses would be utilized because of its high potency.

Desired Effects: Desired effects that should become apparent 5 minutes after IV administration and last for 1½ to 2 hours (longer in patients with renal or hepatic impairment) include: analgesia, sedation, respiratory depression, vasodilation, and relief of air hunger.

Nursing Responsibilities:
- Anticipatory dosing prior to weaning or extubation. The usual dose is 5 to 10 mg IV or if the patient has been receiving morphine, two to three times the patient's usual bolus dose.
- Initiation of an ongoing morphine infusion, usually at a rate of 50% of the bolus dose/hour, immediately following the anticipatory bolus dose.

- Assessment of the patient's level of calmness/agitation, physical movement, muscle tone, heart rate, respiratory effort, and facial tension. If the patient is displaying symptoms indicative of discomfort then the morphine dose should be titrated up slowly every 5 to 15 minutes with the goal of eliminating tachypnea, coughing or choking, agitation, excessive movement of the head and torso, diaphoresis, and grimacing.
- Consistent documentation of the patient's symptoms as an indication for additional morphine administration as well as a description of the patient's response to the initial dose and any necessary increases in dose.
- Reliance on patient symptoms for medication administration rather than preestablished guidelines.

Side and/or Toxic Effects:
- Hypotension and decreased level of consciousness are anticipated side effects and should not result in a reduction in the dose of morphine. In fact, Campbell et al. (1999) removed the blood pressure parameter from the COMFORT scale because it did not supply necessary information and resulted in patient discomfort.

Anxiety

There are multiple causes of anxiety at the end of life, including poorly controlled pain, hypoxia, dyspnea, metabolic imbalances, medication side effects, and psychological distress. When the patient appears anxious or morphine alone does not adequately control a patient's dyspnea, a benzodiazepine may be used for its effect on anxiety, fear, and the autonomic responses that accompany dyspnea.

▌ Collaborative Management

The nurse may utilize nonpharmacological means in conjunction with medication to relieve anxiety. It may help to dim the lights and silence the alarms in the patient's room, thus limiting stimulation around the patient. The family may be allowed to visit without restrictions and clergy or social services may be contacted to provide support and alleviate psychological distress. In a dying patient who is less responsive, anxiety may be caused by urinary retention or constipation. Urinary retention might be treated with a Foley catheter but constipation in the immediate period near death is only treated if the patient is experiencing pronounced discomfort. It is not appropriate to search for metabolic causes for anxiety by performing laboratory tests at this time because the procedures may inflict pain and they are not usually successful in establishing the cause (Kazanowski, 2006). The goal of collaborative management is to utilize pharmacological and nonpharmacological interventions so that the patient appears to both health care providers and family to be dying peacefully without undue restlessness, anxiety, or fear.

COMMONLY USED MEDICATIONS

LORAZEPAM—A BENZODIAZEPINE

INTRODUCTION
Lorazepam is more rapidly acting, less expensive, and may have fewer respiratory and cardiovascular depressive effects than other benzodiazepines such as diazepam or midazolam.

Desired Effects: Desired effects that should peak about 30 minutes after IV administration include sedation and decreases in anxiety and restlessness. Benzodiazepines have a synergistic sedative effect with morphine and 75% of patients undergoing withdrawal of life support receive a combination of the two drugs. According to Brody et al. (1997), benzodiazepines should be first-line pharmacological therapy for anxiety in the dying patient.

Nursing Responsibilities:
- Administration of an anticipatory bolus dose (often two times the patient's normal bolus dose given IV) prior to terminal weaning or extubation
- Documentation of the patient's level of anxiety and response to medication
- Titration of the dose dependent on the benzodiazepine utilized and the patient's symptoms

Family

It is often difficult for the family to wait with the patient after life-sustaining technology has been withdrawn. Family members often anticipate that the patient will die immediately after the removal of the technology. However, this is frequently not the case. In one study the median patient survival was 2.3 hours and in another 3.5 hours following terminal weaning from a ventilator. The family usually needs assistance coping while the patient is actively dying. The needs of families of dying ICU patients are described earlier in this chapter. In addition to meeting those needs, the ICU nurse may offer assistance to the family of a patient who has had life-sustaining technology withdrawn by:

- Creating a quiet environment with soft lighting and turning off or dimming all monitors and alarms in the patient's room
- Assuring the family that the patient is being provided with all possible pharmacological and physical means to promote comfort
- Assessing the patient and family frequently and responding to needs as soon as possible, thus reassuring the patient and family that the patient will not be abandoned
- Explaining the signs of the dying process that the patient is exhibiting and providing some anticipatory guidance about when death might occur
- Acknowledging how difficult it may be for the family to tolerate the uncertainty and to wait while the dying process progresses
- Allowing the family to choose the option not to remain with the patient
- Offering to help arrange for religious or cultural observances that might comfort the patient and family

The family also needs to be aware that a small subset of patients, between 6% and 11%, do not die for a significant period following extubation and a few patients may even survive for weeks following hospital discharge.

Meeting the Spiritual Needs of the Dying Patient and Her Family

The SCCM recommends that the spiritual needs of patients be assessed by the health care team and findings that affect health and healing be incorporated into the plan of care (Davidson et al., 2007). However, when Nelson, Mulkerin, Adams, and Pronovost (2006) assessed 16 ICUs for best practices in care and communication, they found that spiritual support was addressed only 38% of the time, which was less than any of the other items. The SCCM defines *spiritual support* as encouraging and respecting prayer and adherence to cultural traditions so that patients and families may cope with illness, death, and dying (Davidson et al., 2007). Hospitals may have formal spiritual counseling by a chaplaincy service or more informal efforts by staff to accommodate the spiritual traditions and cultural needs of patients and families.

In either case, at the end of life, it is important to offer the patient and family an opportunity to consider the spiritual dimension of life. Some of the spiritual issues that a patient or family may want to explore are:

- The role of suffering in life
- Questions about meaning, purpose, and hope
- Ethical considerations
- Grief and loss issues

Patients and families may also need someone to assist them with either religious or nonreligious rituals of healing and closure. A hospital chaplain can assist with the appropriate rituals or may find a suitable religious adviser. However, if the nurse is comfortable and the patient and/or family requests it, the nurse might pray with the patient or assist with the religious ritual, especially if she is from the patient's cultural and religious tradition.

Conflict at the End of Life

There are times when the health care team, patient, and family are not able to come to agreement about how best to care for the dying patient. The patient, a member of the patient's family, or a member of the health care team may want to continue lifesaving treatment even though the others involved in treatment decision making believe the patient is dying. Occasionally, conflict may arise when either the patient or a family member asks that the patient be assisted to die.

Continuation of Life-Sustaining Treatment

Most of the time, when death is imminent, consensus can be reached among the health care providers, the patient, and the family so that life-sustaining interventions are not provided and the patient is able to die peacefully. However, sometimes consensus cannot be reached and conflict develops about what life-sustaining technology to provide. One reason why conflict may develop is that trust was not established early in the hospitalization. If a nurse suspects that lack of trust is the reason for conflict, he might validate his suspicion by saying, "From the experiences you describe, I imagine it may be difficult for you to trust us." If lack of trust is the primary reason the patient and family want to continue life-sustaining care, the nurse should act to reestablish trust; the nurse might emphasize what is being done for the patient, and the nurse can offer to fa-

cilitate getting another opinion from a health care provider who is trusted.

Disagreement about treatment may also result when decision makers do not share a common understanding of the patient's prognosis and therefore a common goal for the patient's care. Nurses suggest "presenting a realistic picture" and clarifying what the "silent patient" is experiencing (Robichaux & Clark, 2006) to the family and members of the health care team to help them recognize that the patient is dying. To help clarify the goal of therapy, a nurse might ask, "What do you think is going on?" or "What do you think will likely happen if we continue this therapy or if we do CPR?"

Sometimes the issues underlying the conflict about continuation of life-sustaining therapy are difficult to uncover or resolve. The conflict may result from a family member or a health care provider experiencing guilt about the care of the patient. For example, the spouse or physician may have ignored a symptom, which treated earlier could have resulted in a better outcome for the patient. There may be secondary gains for a family member from the patient remaining alive. The patient and family may come from a religious tradition that does not permit the withdrawal of life-sustaining therapy. For example, many observant Orthodox Jews believe that everything possible must be done to prolong a patient's life and termination of a life-sustaining treatment such as mechanical ventilation is prohibited (Carlet et al., 2004). In such situations, it may not be possible to reach a consensus about limiting care.

The situation becomes even more complex when a family member demands an intervention that the health care team considers to be futile. Medical **futility** may be defined as any treatment that is without benefit (that does not provide palliation, restoration, or cure) to the patient. The problem with such a definition is that most life-sustaining interventions can be shown to have some small possibility of benefit and the futility of their use is not always obvious to family members (Pfeifer & Kennedy, 2006). However, the health care providers, especially the nurses, who are continuing the treatment, realize how extremely slim the possibility of benefit is and how substantially the patient is suffering while enduring it. Therefore, they may object to continuing to provide it. In fact, the continuation of life-sustaining therapies in patients who are dying is one of the major sources of moral distress for critical care nurses (see Chapter 1). ∞

When the health care team, patient, and family cannot reach a consensus about the continuation of life-sustaining treatment, the issue should be referred to the hospital's ethics committee. The Joint Commission requires hospitals to have an ethics committee to aid in the resolution of such difficult issues. Some states, such as Texas, have laws that delineate procedures that must be followed prior to, during, and after ethics committee deliberations about futile treatment. After reviewing the case, the ethics committee might recommend either supporting the continuation of life-sustaining therapy or limiting treatment. In Texas, if the ethics committee recommends discontinuation of life-sustaining treatment, the patient and proxy must receive written notification of a 10-day treatment limit with an option to request transfer to another facility. If they cannot find another facility to accept the patient, then the life-sustaining treatment is discontinued after the 10th day (Pfeifer & Kennedy, 2006).

Assisted Death

When death is assisted, the health care provider purposely takes an action that directly results in the patient's death. If it is **voluntary euthanasia**, the patient requests the action be taken to end his life; in **involuntary euthanasia**, the action to end the patient's life is taken without the patient's consent. A study by Emanual, Fairclough, Daniels, and Clarridge (1996) suggests that approximately 12% of oncologists have assisted a patient to die but the study does not distinguish between voluntary and involuntary euthanasia. In one of the first published studies of nurse's practices of assisted death, Matzo and Emanual (1997) compared oncology nurses' and oncology physicians' practices. More physicians than nurses assisted their patients in dying (11% versus 1%). However, nurses were more likely than physicians to have performed patient-requested euthanasia (4% versus 1%). In a controversial study by Asch (1996) regarding assisted death in the ICU, nurses were asked about their practices regarding the use of large doses of narcotics. By the way the question was worded it may have been difficult for respondents to determine if they were being asked about pain management or about assisting a patient to die. However, Asch reported that 16% of critical care nurses had assisted their patients to die.

Most health care providers who assist a patient's death state that they are acting out of compassion. They argue that they assisted a patient's death because the patient's life was no longer worth living and that the burdens of the life far outweighed the benefits. They cite such reasons as the patient was suffering unbearably or the family and health care team were unable to reach a decision to withdraw futile, life-sustaining treatment so the patient was forced to suffer needlessly. They may also declare that the patient would never have wanted to

live in her or his current condition and would have requested interventions be halted if she or he had a voice.

Although the public supports the general concept of assisted death by physicians, oncology patients in pain usually do not (Emanual et al., 1996). Perhaps the reason is that people who are dying, whose quality of life may appear limited to others, do not want to have health care providers empowered to determine if their lives are worth living or not. In fact, only 3% of Americans would want their health care providers to make a decision and commit involuntary euthanasia on their behalf if they were not conscious and could not express their wishes (Blendon, Szalay, & Knox, 1992). Thus, there is little support for those health care providers who contend that in assisting their patients to die they are acting in accordance with their patients' wishes.

There are numerous other arguments against the use of assisted death. First, most medical and nursing professional organizations, including the American Nurses Association and the American Association of Critical-Care Nurses, state that their members have a primary duty not to harm, which prohibits them from intentionally causing a patient's death. Most religious groups profess that human life should be respected and health care providers should never intentionally cause their patients' death. Advocates for the poor and homeless wonder how long it would take before sick, vulnerable, poor people would begin to be euthanized if euthanasia were allowed in this society, where 42 million Americans lack health insurance and cost containment is becoming one of the most important medical values. Hospice nurses question whether palliative care would continue to receive adequate funding and referrals, or whether patients would experience pressures to die quickly and stop being a burden. Caring for a deteriorating or dying person takes time, a scarce commodity in our society. Finally, assisting a patient to die is illegal in most of the United States.

It is not clear how often ICU nurses are asked by patients or their families to end a patient's life. Studies of Japanese and Australian nurses (Tanida et al., 2002) indicate that 50% of nurses have been asked at least once to end a patient's suffering by ending his life. Thus, it is appropriate for a nurse to think about how she would respond to the request by either the patient or a family member to end the life of a suffering patient. One possible response is: "I cannot help you to end your suffering by ending your life but I will help you to live the rest of your life with dignity."

END OF LIFE SUMMARY

Although some critically ill patients die unexpectedly or following CPR, the majority of ICU patients die following withdrawal or withholding of life-sustaining technology. Caring for a grieving family and a dying patient

takes excellent communication skills. The nurse must be able to help the patient and his family understand that the patient is probably dying and make decisions about the type of care the patient desires.

VISUAL MAP (**End of Life Summary**)

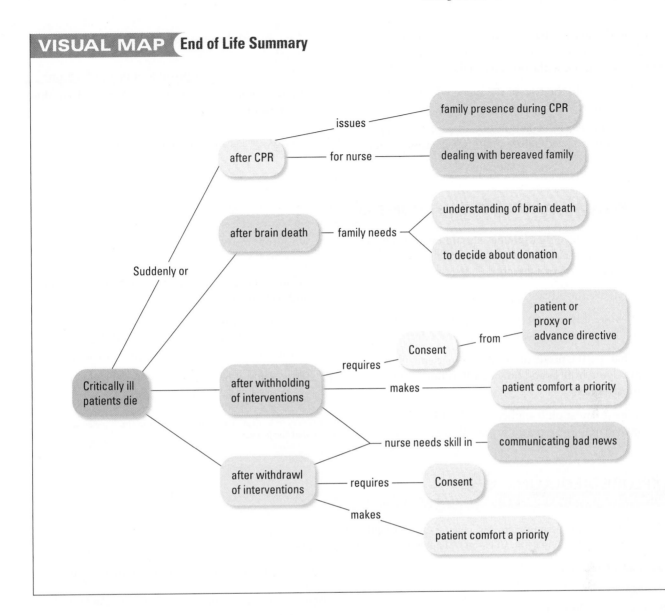

Armand Gregoire is a 78-year-old widower whose only significant medical history was a permanent pacemaker placed 4 years previously for a sinus bradycardia of 38–42 beats per minute. The pacemaker had been placed so that he could continue to scuba dive. His only over-the-counter (OTC) medication was an occasional Tylenol for joint pain and he was taking no prescribed medications.

At 6 A.M. on a Friday morning Armand experienced severe left arm pain. He drove himself to the emergency department of the nearest hospital, but by the time he arrived the pain was crushing and he was showing signs of heart failure. He was prepared immediately for cardiac catheterization then transferred to the operating room (OR) for a quadruple bypass. After transfer to the cardiac surgical ICU, he did not regain consciousness. Over the next 2 days, he

developed worsening heart failure as well as acute renal failure and could not be weaned from the ventilator.

Armand had never completed an advance directive. So the cardiac surgeon approached Armand's next of kin, his stepson, for permission to begin dialysis. The stepson's response was immediate, "My Dad would not want to be dialyzed. He wouldn't even want that breathing machine. He's been depressed, saying he wants to die and waiting for my Mom to come and get him for the past 4 years. No, I won't consent to it."

The cardiac surgeon believes that Armand has cardiogenic shock from which he can recover. The surgeon wants to start dialysis without the stepson's approval because Armand never completed an advance directive. The surgeon says that if he doesn't provide dialysis, he would not be giving Armand every chance to live and would feel as if he were killing Armand.

However, the stepson has now decided that not only does he not want his father to be dialyzed but he wants the ventilator to be withdrawn as well.

1. What should the role of the nurse who is caring for Armand be?

2. What further information does the nurse caring for Armand need before making a decision about what to do?

3. How should the nurse decide what ought to be done?

4. What are the nurse's possible courses of action?

5. What do you believe the nurse ought to do in this circumstance?

See answers to Case Studies in the Answer Section at the back of the book.

CRITICAL THINKING QUESTIONS

1. Do you believe that families should be allowed to witness resuscitation attempts on their family member? Why or why not?

2. What are the advantages of advance directives?

3. Why are advance directives currently of limited use for patients in critical care?

4. What are the needs of families of patients who are dying in ICU and how can ICU nurses meet those needs?

5. Why do most philosophers and health care providers believe that it is ethical to limit and/or withdraw medical interventions from critically ill patients?

6. What is the difference between terminal weaning and terminal extubation?

7. How do most philosophers and health care providers differentiate between withdrawing of medical interventions and assisted death?

8. How might a nurse act to resolve conflict about goals of care at the end of life?

See answers to Critical Thinking Questions in the Answer Section at the back of the book.

EXPLORE MEDIALINK
http://www.prenhall.com/perrin

Additional interactive resources for this chapter can be found on the Web site at http://www.prenhall.com/perrin. Click on "Chapter 18" to select activities for this chapter.

Case Study: End of Life

Nursing Care Plan

NCLEX Review Questions

MediaLinks:
- University of Washington, Topics in Medical Ethics: Futility
- Recommendations for End-of-Life Care in the Intensive Care Unit: The Ethics Committee of the Society of Critical Care Medicine

- Papers by the ACP-ASIM End-of-Life Care Consensus Panel
- University of Minnesota, End-of-Life Care: An Ethical Overview
- Current Projects of the End-of-Life Research Program
- Promoting Excellence in End-of-Life Care
- American Association of Critical Care Nurses
- End Link: Resources for End-of-Life Care

MediaLink Applications

REFERENCES

Angus, D. C., Barnato, A. E., Linde-Zwirble, W. T., Weissfeld, L. A., Watson, R. S., Rickert, T., et al. (2004). Use of intensive care at the end of life in the United States: An epidemiologic model. *Critical Care Medicine, 32*(3), 638–643.

Asch, D. A. (1996). The role of critical care nurses in euthanasia and assisted suicide. *New England Journal of Medicine, 334*(21), 1374–1379.

Bailey, S. (2006). Decision making in acute care: A practical framework supporting the best interests principle. *Nursing Ethics, 13*(3), 284–291.

Blendon, R. J., Szalay, U. S., & Knox, R. A. (1992). Should physicians aid their patients in dying? The public perspective. *Journal of the American Medical Association, 267*(19), 2658–2662.

Boyle, D. K., Miller, P. A., & Forbes-Thompson, S. A. (2005). Communication and end-of-life care in the intensive care unit: Patient, family, and clinician outcomes. *Critical Care Nursing Quarterly, 28*(4), 302–316.

Brody, H., Campbell, M. L., Faber-Langedoen, K., & Ogle, K. S. (1997). Withdrawing intensive life sustaining treatment—recommendations for compassionate clinical management. *The New England Journal of Medicine, 336*(9), 652–656.

Buckman, R. (1992). *How to break bad news: A guide for health care providers.* Baltimore: Johns Hopkins University Press.

Campbell, M., Bizek, K. S., & Thill, M. (1999). Patient responses during rapid terminal weaning from mechanical ventilation: A prospective study. *Critical Care Medicine, 27*(1), 73–77.

Carlet, J., Lambertus, G. T., Antonelli, M., Cassell, J., Cox, P., Hill, N., et al. (2004) Challenges in end-of-life care in the ICU: Statement of the 5th International Consensus Conference. *Intensive Care Medicine, 30*, 770–784.

Copnell, B. (2005). Death in the pediatric ICU: Caring for children and families at the end of life. *Critical Care Nursing Clinics of North America, 17*, 349–360.

Davidson, J. E., Powers, K., Hedayat, K. M., Tieszen, M., Kon, A. A., Shepard, E., et al. (2007). Clinical practice guidelines for support of the family in the patient-centered intensive care unit. *Critical Care Medicine, 35*(2), 605–622.

Dolan, M. B. (1983, January). Another hospice nurse says. *Nursing 83*, 51.

Downey, L., Engelberg, R. A., Shannon, S. E., & Curtis, R. (2006). Measuring intensive care nurses' perspectives on family-centered end-of-life care: Evaluation of 3 questionnaires. *American Journal of Critical Care, 15*(6), 568–579.

Ehrle, R. (2006). Timely referral of potential organ donors. *Critical Care Nurse, 26*(2), 88–93.

Eichorn, D. J., Meyers, T., & Guzzetta, C. (2001). Family presence during invasive procedures and resuscitation: Hearing the voice of the patient. *American Journal of Nursing, 101*, 48.

Emanual, E., Fairclough, D. L., Daniels, E. R., & Clarridge, B. R. (1996). Euthanasia and physician assisted suicide: Attitudes and experiences of oncology patients, oncologists, and the public. *Lancet, 347*, 1805–1810.

Engelberg, R. A., Patrick, D. L., & Curtis, R. J. (2005). Correspondence between patients' preferences and surrogates' understandings for dying and death. *Journal of Pain and Symptom Management, 30*(6), 498–509.

Evans, B. (2004). Stroke, coma, and brain death. In M. Matzo & D. Sherman (Eds.), *Gerontological palliative care nursing* (pp. 212–230). St. Louis, MO: Mosby.

Halm, M. A. (2005). Family presence during resuscitation: A critical review of the literature. *American Journal of Critical Care, 14*(6), 494–511.

Kazanowski, M. (2006). Symptom management in palliative care. In M. Matzo & D. Sherman (Eds.), *Palliative care nursing: Quality care to the end of life* (2nd ed.). New York: Springer.

Mason. D. (2004). *Family presence*. NSO: Nurses' Service Organization. Retrieved September 2006, from http://www.nso.com/newsletters/advisor/2004_fall/family.php?phppse-ssid=4278eeff71b994b707a01ef4fe7a2c

Matzo, M. (2006). Peri-death nursing care. In M. Matzo & D. Sherman (Eds.), *Palliative care nursing education: Toward quality care at the end of life* (2nd ed., pp. 443–467). New York: Springer.

Matzo, M., & Emanual, E. J. (1997). Oncology nurses' practices of assisted suicide and patient-requested euthanasia. *Oncology Nursing Forum, 24*(10), 1725–1732.

Matzo, M., & Ramsey, G. C. (2006). Legal aspects of end-of-life care. In M. Matzo & D. Sherman (Eds.), *Palliative care nursing education: Toward quality care at the end of life* (2nd ed., pp. 187–220). New York: Springer.

McGhee, J. (2007). Health care ethics. In K. Perrin & J. McGhee (Eds.), *Ethics and conflict* (2nd ed., pp. 1–12). Sudbury, MA: Jones and Bartlett.

Meares, C. J. (1994, May/June). Terminal dehydration: Review. *American Journal of Hospice and Palliative Care*, 10–14.

Mirza, A., Kad, R., & Ellision, N. (2005). Cardiopulmonary resuscitation is not addressed in the admitting records of the majority of patients who undergo CPR in the hospital. *American Journal of Hospice and Palliative Care, 22*(1), 20–25.

Morse, J. (2001). Toward a praxis of suffering. *Advances in Nursing Science, 24*(1), 47–59.

Nelson, J. E., Mulkerin, C. M., Adams, L. L., & Pronovost, P. J. (2006). Improving comfort and communication in the ICU: A practical new tool for palliative care performance measurement and feedback. *Quality Safe Health Care, 15*, 264–271.

Nolan, M. T., Hughes, M., Narendra, D. P., Sood, J. R., Terry, P. B., Astrow, A. B., et al. (2005). When patients lack capacity: The roles patients with terminal illnesses would choose for their physicians and loved ones in making medical decisions. *Journal of Pain and Symptom Management, 30*(4), 342–353.

Peel, N. (2003). The role of the critical care nurse in the delivery of bad news. *British Journal of Nursing, 12*(16), 966–971.

Perrin, K. O. (2006). Communicating with seriously ill and dying patients, their families, and their health care providers. In M. Matzo & D. Sherman (Eds.), *Palliative care nursing education: Toward quality care at the end of life* (2nd ed., pp. 221–245). New York: Springer.

Pfeifer, G. M., & Kennedy, M. S. (2006). Understanding medical futility. *American Journal of Nursing, 106*(5), 25–26.

Quality Standards Sub-Committee of the American Academy of Neurology. (1995). Practice parameters: Determining brain death in adults (summary statement). *Neurology, 45*, 1012–1014.

Riwitis, C., & Twibell, R. S. (2006). Family presence during resuscitation: The in's and out's. *American Nurse Today, 1*(2), 12–15.

Robichaux, C., & Clark, A. P. (2006). Practice of expert critical care nurses in situations of prognostic conflict at the end of life. *American Journal of Critical Care, 15*(5), 480–489.

Seferian, E. G., & Afessa, B. (2006). Adult intensive care use at the end of life: A population-based study. *Mayo Clinic Proceedings, 81*(17), 896–901.

Support Principal Investigators. (1995). A controlled study to improve care for seriously ill hospitalized patients. *Journal of the American Medical Association, 274*(20), 1591–1598.

Tanida, N., Asai, A., Ohnishi, M., Naguta, S. K., Fukui, T., Yamazaki, Y., et al. (2002). Voluntary active euthanasia and the nurse: A comparison of Japanese and Australian nurses. *Nursing Ethics, 9*(3), 313–322.

Truog, R. D., Cist, A. F., Brackett, S. E., Burns, J. P., Curley, M. A., Danis, M., et al. (2001). Recommendations for end-of-life care in the intensive care unit: The Ethics Committee of the Society of Critical Care Medicine. *Critical Care Medicine, 29*(12), 2332–2346. Retrieved September, 2006, from http://www.sccm.org/pdf/EndofLife.pdf

Tulsky, J. (2005). Beyond advance directives: The importance of communication skills at the end of life. *Journal of the American Medical Association, 294*(3), 359–364.

Vitella, L., Kenner, D., & Sali, A. (2005). Sedation and analgesia-prescribing patterns in terminally ill patients at the end of life. *American Journal of Hospice & Palliative Care, 22*(6), 465.

Weil, M. H., & Fries, M. (2005). In-hospital cardiac arrest. *Critical Care Medicine, 33*(2), 2825–2830.

Zerwekh, J. V. (1987, July/August). Should fluid and nutritional support be withheld from terminally ill patients? *American Journal of Hospice Care*, 37–38.

Appendix A: Normal Laboratory Values

According to the National Council of State Boards of Nursing, nurses should know the normal values and recognize deviations from normal for the following laboratory tests.

LABORATORY TEST		NORMAL VALUE
Arterial Blood Gases		
pH		7.35 to 7.45
PaO_2		80 to 100 mm Hg
SaO_2		93% to 96%
$PaCO_2$		35 to 45 mm Hg
HCO_3		22 to 26
Mixed Venous Gases		
SvO_2		60% to 75%
Serum Levels		
Glucose (fasting)		70 to 110 mg/dL
Blood urea nitrogen (BUN)		5 to 25 mg/dL
Creatinine		0.5 to 1.5 mg/dL
Sodium		135 to 145 mEq/L
Potassium		3.5 to 5.3 mEq/L
Magnesium		1.5 to 2.5 mEq/L
	or	1.8 to 3.0 mg/dL
Total calcium		9 to 11 mg/dL
Phosphorus/phosphate		1.7 to 2.6 mEq/L
	or	2.5 to 4.5 mg/dL
Lactate		
Arterial blood		0.5 to 2.0 mmol/L
Venous blood		0.5 to 1.5 mmol/L
Cholesterol		
Total		desired less than 200 mg/dL
LDL		60 to 160 mg/dL
HDL		29 to 77 mg/dL
Albumin		3.5 to 5.0 g/dL
Total protein		6.0 to 8.0 g/dL
ALT (SGPT)		10 to 35 units/L
AST (SGOT)		8 to 38 units/L
Ammonia		5 to 45 mcg/dL
Bilirubin		
Indirect		0.1 to 1.0 mg/dL
Direct		0.1 to 1.2 mg/dL

LABORATORY TEST (continued)	**NORMAL VALUE** (continued)
PT	10 to 13 seconds
INR	for anticoagulant therapy utilized after the person has been stabilized on anticoagulant therapy—depending on the reason for anticoagulation
	2.0 to 3.5 × the control
PTT	60 to 70 seconds
APTT	20 to 35 seconds
Bleeding time (Ivy method)	3 to 7 minutes
Hemoglobin A$_1$C (nondiabetic)	2% to 5%
Hematocrit	
Male	40% to 54%
Female	36% to 46%
Hemoglobin	
Male	13.5 to 17 g/dL
Female	12 to 15 g/dL
Erythrocyte sedimentation rate (ESR)	
Wintrobe method	
Male	0 to 9 mm/hr
Female	0 to 15 mm/hr
Platelet count	150,000 to 400,000 μl
White blood cell count	4,500 to 10,000 μl (mm^3)
Differential	
Neutrophils (total)	50% to 70% or 2,500 to 7,000/μl (mm^3)
Segmented	50% to 65% or 2,500 to 6,500/μl (mm^3)
Bands	0% to 5% or 0 to 500/μl (mm^3)
Eosinophils	1% to 3% or 100 to 300/μl (mm^3)
Basophils	0.4% to 1% or 40 to 100/μl (mm^3)
Monocytes	4% to 6% or 200 to 600/μl (mm^3)
Lymphocytes	25% to 35% or 1,700 to 3,500/μl (mm^3)

Urine

pH	4.5 to 8 (average 6)
Specific gravity	1.005 to 1.030
	1.015 to 1.024 with normal fluid intake
White blood cell count	3 to 4
Protein	2 to 8 mg/dL

Appendix B: Hemodynamic Formulas and Normal Values

Blood pressure preferably 120/80 mm Hg

$$\text{Mean arterial pressure (MAP)} = \frac{\text{systolic pressure} + (\text{diastolic pressure} \times 2)}{3}$$

MAP should be greater than 60 mm Hg for adequate perfusion

Normal range for MAP is 70 to 90 mm Hg

$$\text{cardiac output} = \text{heart rate} \times \text{stroke volume}$$

Cardiac output is normally 4 to 8 L/min

The cardiac output may be adjusted for the size of the patient by calculating the cardiac index.

$$\text{Cardiac index} = \frac{CO}{BSA}$$

Cardiac index is normally 2.8 to 4.2 L/m^2

$$\text{Systemic vascular resistance (SVR)} = \frac{(MAP - RAP + 80)}{CO}$$

SVR is normally 800 to 1,300 dyne/sec/cm^5

PVR (pulmonary vascular resistance) is normally 37 to 250 dyne/sec/cm^5

Normal values for pressures from a pulmonary artery line:

CVP/RA pressure	2 to 6 mm Hg
RV pressure	15–25/0–8 mm Hg
PA pressure	15–25/8–15 mm Hg
PAWP	8 to 12 mm Hg

Normal value for a mixed venous oxygen saturation:

SvO$_2$	60% to 75%

Appendix C: Medication Infusion Calculations

It is important to recalculate all IV infusions to be certain they are infusing at the appropriate rate even though many IV pumps now perform the calculations. The pump may be in error or the person who programmed the pump may have made an error.

To calculate medication infusion rates, the following formula can be utilized:

$$Dose = Rate \times Concentration$$

With two of the factors, the third can always be calculated. It is rarely necessary to calculate concentration because that is nearly always given. Dose is often prescribed so a common way this formula may be adapted is to determine a rate. To calculate the rate, the formula becomes:

$$\frac{Dose}{Concentration} = Rate$$

In addition, sometimes it is necessary to add conversion factors for minutes/hour, micrograms/milligrams, and/or kilograms.

Dose

The drug to be administered determines the dose. It may be prescribed in mg/hr, mg/min, or mcg/kg/min. It is necessary to review the physician's order and normal dosing for the medication to determine the dose.

Rate

Because IV pumps are utilized to administer these medications, the rate will always be in mL/hr. When the dose and concentration are known, then it is the rate that is being calculated (which is most often the case). If the rate is known and it is the dose that is uncertain, the rate may be identified by checking the IV pump. Depending on the medication and the specific pump, pump rates may be set at 0.1-mL intervals.

Concentration

The pharmacy will always provide the drug in a known concentration, and the concentration should be clearly visible on the label of the IV bag or bottle. The concentration may be in mg/mL, units/mL, or mcg/mL. It is particularly important to verify the concentration of the drug at the beginning of a shift or whenever a new bag or bottle is hung.

Units/hour

Example: Heparin

The prescribed dose is 1,200 U/hr of heparin. The label states that there are 20,000 U/500 mL of fluid. To calculate the rate to set the IV pump, complete the following steps:

The first step is optional: Many people prefer to simplify the concentration before they begin calculations. Often the simplified concentration will be available on the IV label.

$$\frac{20,000 \text{ U}}{500 \text{ mL}} = \frac{40 \text{ U}}{1 \text{ mL}}$$

When the formula Dose = Rate × Concentration (D = R × C) is used, to calculate rate, the formula must be converted to:

$$\frac{Dose}{Concentration} = Rate/hour \quad or \quad \frac{1,200 \text{ U}}{40 \text{ U/mL}} = Rate/hour$$

By canceling out one of the zeros in the units in the top and bottom of the fraction, the fraction can be simplified to

$$\frac{120}{4 \text{ mL}} = Rate/hour$$

After dividing, the rate is determined to be 30 mL/hr

Milligrams/hour (mg/hr)

Example: Midazolam

Calculating milligrams per hour is similar to calculating units per hour. An example would be a midazolam infusion. If a midazolam infusion was running at 5 mL/hr (5 mg/hr) and the dose was to be decreased by 20% to determine the minimum effective infusion rate, how should the dose and rate be adjusted?

To determine 20% of 5, multiply 5 by 0.2 (5 × 0.2 = 1)
To reduce the rate by 20%, subtract 1 from 5 (5 − 1 = 4)
The new dose for the infusion is 4 mg/hr

The concentration of the midazolam infusion is 100 mg/100 mL
This can be simplified to 1 mg/1 mL
The formula needed is:

$$\frac{Dose}{Concentration} = Rate/hour$$

$$or \quad \frac{4 \text{ mg}}{1 \text{ mg/mL}} = Rate \ hour \quad Therefore, the rate is 4 mL/hr$$

Milligrams/minute (mg/min)

Example: Lidocaine

To calculate the rate for medications delivered in milligrams per minute, it is necessary to add an additional step and a conversion factor for minutes to hours because the medication is prescribed in mg/min and IV pumps are set to infuse in mL/hr.

A lidocaine infusion is prescribed to run at 3 mg/min. The available concentration is 1 g in 250 mL. This is equivalent to 1,000 mg/250 mL and can be simplified to 4 mg/mL.

$$Rate \text{ (mL/hr)} = \frac{Dose \times conversion \ factor \ (60 \ minutes/hour)}{Concentration}$$

$$Rate \text{ (mL/hr)} = \frac{3 \text{ mg/min}}{4 \text{ mg/1 mL}} \times 60 \text{ minutes/hour}$$

After division and canceling of minutes and milligrams,
Rate = 45 mL/hr

Micrograms/minute (mcg/min)

Example: Norepinephrine (Levophed)

This calculation is similar to milligrams per minute except it is necessary to perform an additional step and convert from milligrams to micrograms. This time, instead of calculating for rate, the example will demonstrate how and why one might calculate for dose.

A nurse has been titrating a Levophed drip upward to maintain a MAP greater than 60 for a patient in septic shock. The concentration of the Levophed is 4 mg in 500 mL and the medication is currently infusing at 30 mL/hr. How many mcg/min of Levophed is the patient receiving?

The concentration can be simplified by converting milligrams to micrograms and reducing the fraction. It is 4,000 mcg/500 mL or 8 mcg/mL.

The appropriate formula because it is the dose that is desired is:

$$\text{Dose} = \frac{\text{rate} \times \text{concentration}}{\text{conversion factor (60 minutes/hour)}}$$

$$\text{Dose (mcg/min)} = \frac{30 \text{ mL/hr} \times 8 \text{ mcg/mL}}{60 \text{ minutes/hour}}$$

After division and canceling of units,

$$\text{Dose} = 4 \text{ mcg/min}$$

Micrograms/kilogram/minute (mcg/kg/min)

Example: Dopamine

A physician has prescribed a dopamine infusion to increase a patient's blood pressure. The infusion is prescribed to begin at 5 mcg/kg/min. The patient weighs 70 kg and the dopamine is available 400 mg/250 mL. What rate should the nurse begin the infusion?

There are numerous additional steps needed for this calculation, including converting milligrams to micrograms, adjusting for the patient's weight, and converting minutes to hours (to set the IV pump).

To simplify the concentration 400,000 mcg/250 mL = 1,600 mcg/mL

$$\text{Rate (mL/hr)} = \frac{\text{dose (5 mcg/kg/min)} \times \text{pts weight (70 kg)} \times 60 \text{ min/hr (conversion)}}{\text{concentration (1,600 mcg/mL)}}$$

$$\text{Rate} = 13.125 \text{ mL/hr}$$

Answers to Case Study and Critical Thinking Questions

Chapter 1: Answers to Case Study Questions

1. In situations where emergent care is required, if the team is unable to obtain informed consent, then consent is presumed due to the urgency of the situation and the health care team should provide treatment.

2. The nurse might explain to the sister that there are two common ethically accepted modes for making surrogate decisions. The first is the best interests standard in which the sister would decide what she believes is in the best interests of Allen. For example, she might decide that because Allen needed an adequate airway and nutrition to stay alive, it would be in his best interests to have the procedures. The second method is substituted judgment in which the surrogate (in this case the sister) decides what she thinks Allen would have decided had he been able to make the decision. For example, she might say, "Allen never wanted to live with a tracheostomy, ventilator, or tube feeding. He would never have consented to these interventions so I will not either."

3. Although nurses are often told that they should be able to provide care without discrimination to all patients, sometimes this is very difficult to do. In Angela's case, she is most likely a conscientious nurse who recognizes biases toward Allen that she might not be able to hide completely while providing care. Asking for another assignment in this situation would seem to be a legitimate request. However, the nurse leader would want to suggest that Angela take an opportunity to discuss her unresolved feelings about caring for Allen.

Chapter 1: Answers to Critical Thinking Questions

1. In a "closed ICU," a dedicated ICU team that includes a critical care physician provides patient care. Because the critical care team knows one another and has common expectations and an established communication pattern, patient outcomes appear to be better when patients are cared for in a closed system.

2. In part, because of the complexity and high degree of coupling of care, health care errors are most common in critical care areas. Complex care is usually also highly technological care, and technology also contributes to the error rate.

3. An underlying assumption of the synergy model is that optimal patient outcomes occur when the needs of the patient and family are aligned with the competencies of the nurse.

4. Many critically ill patients are intubated and unable to communicate even their most basic needs clearly. Thus, even though they may have a clear preference, they may be unable to communicate it. Other patients may be incapacitated temporarily due to pain, depression, or unconsciousness.

5. a. Could treatment of another problem obviate the need for a restraint?
   b. Is the restraint the least restrictive and invasive alternative possible?
   c. Will the use of the restraint outweigh the risks (physical, emotional, and ethical) associated with its use?
   d. Are the restraints absolutely necessary for patient safety?

6. The AACN believes there is evidence that the moral distress experienced by critical care nurses has a substantial impact on health care. According to its evidence, as many as half of critical care nurses may have left a unit due to moral distress. In addition, nurses who experience moral distress may lose the capacity to care for their patients and experience psychological and physiological problems.

7. There are a variety of self-care practices that nurses can employ for their own health and well-being but also because they may aid in the prevention of compassion fatigue. These include:
   - Make a commitment to self-care.
   - Develop strategies for letting go of work.
   - Develop strategies for acquiring adequate rest and relaxation.
   - Plan strategies for practicing effective daily stress reduction.

Chapter 2: Answers to Case Study Questions

1. 4.5 mg

2. 9.1 mg/hour

3. These doses are at the high end of therapeutic doses. They usually are reduced by 30% to 50% if the patient is also receiving an opioid (and Harold is). Thus, these doses might be too high.

4. a. Notify the physician.
   b. Adjust the rate of midazolam infusion based on the appropriate concentration and physician's recommendation.
   c. Continue to monitor the patient and titrate the rate to the desired response level of the patient.
   d. Report the occurrence in the appropriate manner and complete the appropriate forms.

5. The standard concentration used for calculation of the drip rate on the pump was 0.5 mg/mL, whereas the dose of midazolam prepared by the pharmacy was 1 mg/mL. Thus, the patient received twice the intended dose of midazolam per hour.

6. Reporting errors can allow for systemwide changes that improve patient care. Things that might have helped in this situation include:
   Automatic notification by the pharmacy or pump when a drug is to be given at a high dose
   Use of only one concentration of each medication by the hospital with the pumps programmed for that concentration
   Checking the concentration of medication in the bag and on the pump each time a medication is hung
   Having two nurses check sedative and narcotic doses
   Thorough education concerning new products, particularly IV pumps
   Appropriate use of pain and sedation assessments

7. The initial high level of pain coupled with the provision and subsequent infusion of a dose of midazolam at the high end of the therapeutic spectrum and lack of ongoing sedation assessment initiated the problem. The nurse's unfamiliarity with a new pump compounded the problem.

Chapter 2: Answers to Critical Thinking Questions

1. The AACN states that the characteristics of critically ill patients are resiliency, vulnerability, stability, complexity, predictability, resource availability, participation in care, and participation in decision making.

2. Patients describe their needs as:
   - Being thirsty
   - Having tubes in their mouth and nose
   - Not being able to communicate
   - Being restricted by tubes/lines
   - Being unable to sleep
   - Not being able to control themselves

3. Responsive patients indicate that they need their nurses to be kind, patient, and attentive to their needs, offering frequent verbal reassurances, knowing what information is important, and providing it. Nurses should recognize how frustrating communication can be for ventilated patients. When communicating with ventilated patients, nurses should do the following:
   - Routinely ask patients about their feelings and their state of mind.
   - Ask permission before beginning nursing care and procedures.
   - Evaluate patients' understanding of the information conveyed to them by asking simple yes/no questions.

4. By using a valid reliable pain assessment tool such as the CPOT displayed in Table 2-1.

5. By using a valid reliable tool such as the AACN Sedation Assessment Scale displayed in Table 2-2 or the VAMASS displayed in Table 2-3 and titrating the sedative to a predetermined level on the chosen sedation scale.

6. Nutritional support should be administered enterally if at all possible because it is associated with a much lower risk of infection and better outcomes than parenteral nutrition. In part this lower infection rate may occur because enteral feeding prevents translocation of bacteria from the GI tract, which can occur when the GI tract is inactive.

7. The advantages of open visiting hours include family satisfaction; improved communication between family, patient, and staff; more emotional support for the patient as well as physiologic benefits for the patient; and opportunities for enhanced family and patient education. Disadvantages include: discomfort of staff and the staff's unfounded concerns that the patient will be stressed or unable to receive needed care.

8. Information should be provided in a timely manner to families in an appropriate setting and delivered by a caring individual, preferably a physician, at least initially. The health care team should deliver a consistent message. In addition, regular family conferences, written instructional guides, a consistent family contact member, and a consistent nurse providing care may also help to meet the communication needs of families.

Chapter 3: Answers to Case Study Questions

1. The medication that he received for the seizures or for his intubation might have caused his blood pressure to drop. It is also possible that it interacted with the Toprol he was taking on a routine basis.

2. Elevate the HOB to at least 30 degrees.
   Monitor for gastric distention.
   Maintain a proper cull pressure in the ET tube (greater than 20 cm H_2O).
   Change the ventilator circuit only when it is soiled.
   Limit secretions in the oropharynx; use chlorhexidine for oral care.
   Use narcotics and sedatives carefully; provide daily sedation vacation.
   Wash hands.
   Provide stress ulcer prophylaxis.
   Turn the patient at least every 2 hours.
   Institute DVT prevention strategies.

3. Most institutions would recommend supporting his blood pressure with volume and/or vasopressors so that his HOB could be maintained at 30 degrees of elevation or higher.

4. He would not be a candidate for attempting a sedation vacation or withdrawing sedation at this time.

5. His ET tube will need to be repositioned (it should be 2 to 3 cm above the carina), so the nurse will need to notify the appropriate people in the agency and anticipate that the tube will be repositioned.
   The nurse has indications that the patient has infiltrates and a consolidation, so aggressive pulmonary hygiene with frequent repositioning is warranted. The nurse should check the patient's WBC (it was 21,000), determine

if a sputum culture had been sent, and notify the appropriate people.

6. Mr. Donnelly's misuse of alcohol and cigarette smoking could predispose him to the development of ARDs.

7. He is just mildly hypercapneic (norm $PaCO_2$ 35 to 45) but he has been able to compensate with a slightly elevated bicarbonate (norm 22 to 26), thus maintaining his pH in the normal range. His oxygen saturation and PaO_2 are acceptable, maintained by an FiO_2 that is within the recommended range.

8. As noted in #7, the FiO_2 is within the recommended range, as are the PEEP and tidal volume for a man of his weight.

9. In this mode, the client sets the rate independently; however, when breathing in excess of the set rate patients receive the tidal volume they can pull using their own strength. They are controlling the rate as well as volume with the ventilator serving as a "backup." The client is not allowed to breathe at less than the set rate, ensuring an adequate minute volume, but can breathe additional breaths if he has a drive to breathe.

10. The mode is called synchronized because if the client initiates a breath when it is almost time for a set volume breath, the ventilator will synchronize with the patient's respiratory effort. This prevents the machine from trying to deliver a breath at the same time a client is trying to exhale.

Chapter 3: Answers to Critical Thinking Questions

1. ALI may be caused by such direct insults to the lungs as chest trauma with pulmonary contusion, pneumonia, aspiration, near drowning, pulmonary edema, inhalation injury, pulmonary embolus, radiation, or eclampsia. It may also be caused indirectly by insults occurring from sepsis, burns, multiple transfusions, drug overdose, acute pancreatitis, and intracranial hypertension.

   Although all of these have a different initial mechanism, they result in a common pathway of inflammation with damage to the capillary and alveolar membranes and ARDS.

2. The progression of ALI is frequently divided into three stages: exudative, proliferative, and fibrotic. Disruption of alveolar capillary membrane permeability is at the crux of ALI pathophysiology. During the first phase, known as the exudative phase, the capillary membrane begins to leak, and protein-rich fluid fills the alveoli, profoundly disrupting gas exchange.

   The proliferative phase begins 7 to 10 days after onset. Type II alveolar cells sustain damage, limiting the production of surfactant, resulting in further loss of alveolar function. This decrease in available alveolar surface area results in VQ mismatch and hypoxemia.

   The final phase is called the fibrotic phase because the altered healing process results in development of fibrotic tissue in the alveolar capillary membrane. The resulting alveolar disfigurement contributes to decreased lung compliance and worsening pulmonary hypertension.

3. The early manifestations of ARDS are tachycardia and tachypnea that seem incongruent with the rest of the patient findings. The hallmark is hypoxemia that is unresponsive to oxygen administration.

4. Historically mortality rates for older adults with ARDS (69% to 80%) were higher than for younger adults. More recently, older adults have not been shown to have significantly higher mortality rates from ARDS unless they have underlying renal, cardiac, and/or neurological disease.

5. Tidal volumes of 4 to 6 mL/kg of body weight reduced mortality as well as decreasing days on the ventilator. The lower tidal volumes result in alveolar hypoventilation, resulting in a rise in serum CO_2 levels. PEEP provides additional surface area in the alveoli to enhance gas exchange; setting PEEP at levels between 14 and 16 cm H_2O can return collapsed alveoli to a functional status. In addition, FiO_2 is set at less than 60%, if possible, to minimize the potential for oxygen toxicity, and plateau pressures are maintained below 30 cm H_2O, if possible.

6. Three nursing priorities when caring for the patient with ARDS are:
   Provision of effective ventilation
   Maintenance of tissue oxygenation
   Prevention of sepsis and potential MSOF

7. a. Oxygen concentration (FiO_2): Amount of oxygen in gaseous admixture delivered to the client
   b. Tidal volume: Volume of gas delivered in one cycle
   c. Rate: Minimal number of breaths per minute
   d. Inspiratory:expiratory ratio: Ratio of time of inspiration to time of expiration; may be reversed in conditions where lungs are noncompliant
   e. High-pressure limit: Ventilator will not exceed this pressure in delivering volume; pop-off mechanism prevents excessive pressure
   f. Pressure support: Positive pressure used to decrease the client's work of breathing
   g. Positive End Expiratory Pressure (PEEP): Positive pressure left in the lungs at the end of expiration; prevents atelectasis and may enhance oxygenation at higher levels

Chapter 4: Answers to Case Study Questions

1. Epinephrine 1 mg IV, repeated every 3 to 5 minutes. The first or second dose of epinephrine may be replaced by one dose of vasopressin 40 units IV.

2. Epinephrine and vasopressin are both potent peripheral vasoconstrictors; therefore, the implication is that they may increase coronary and cerebral perfusion pressure during CPR.

   After the second shock, continued CPR, and the administration of epinephrine and vasopressin, the team prepares for another shock. The "all clear" sign is given and you watch the monitor as the shock is delivered. The following is the rhythm that you see:

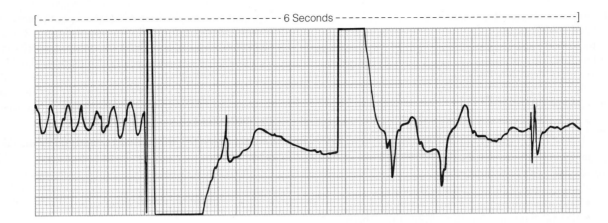

3. Assess the patient for a pulse, as it appears his dysrhythmia may have converted to a sinus rhythm.

4. An antidysrhythmic will be important to prevent a return of the ventricular dysrhythmia; amiodarone 150 mg IV bolus followed by a 1 mg/min infusion for 6 hours and then a 0.5 mg/min maintenance infusion over 18 hours.

5. Possible causes include hypovolemia, hypoxia, acidosis, hyper- or hypokalemia, hypomagnesemia, hypoglycemia, cardiac tamponade, tension pneumothorax, or thrombosis.

   Labs should include arterial blood gases to check for hypoxia and acidosis, potassium, magnesium, and glucose. The patient should also have a chest x-ray to rule out a pneumothorax and should be assessed for cardiac tamponade and thrombosis.

Chapter 4: Answers to Critical Thinking Questions

1. a. Automaticity
   b. Excitability
   c. Conductivity
   d. Contractility

2. Most patients have an underlying cardiac problem such as a valvular disease or electrolyte imbalance. Also, they may be unable to tolerate the rapid rhythm that occurs at the onset of AF.

3. Patients with AF are at high risk for embolic strokes.

4. a. Rate control with chronic anticoagulation is recommended for most AF patients.
   b. Coumadin (warfarin) is used unless the patients are in a low-risk group or have contraindications to its use.
   c. Beta blockers (atenolol, metroprolol) and calcium channel blockers (diltiazem, verapamil) are recommended for rate control as an outpatient; digoxin should be considered as second-line therapy for patients who do not respond to these medications.
   d. For patients requesting cardioversion, either synchronized cardioversion or pharmacological conversion is appropriate.

   e. To minimize the risk of embolic stroke in patients electing cardioversion, either transesophageal echocardiogram (TEE) or 3 weeks of anticoagulation prior to cardioversion is acceptable. Both strategies are followed by 3 to 4 weeks of anticoagulation.

5. Third-degree heart block, also known as complete heart block, occurs when the impulses from the atria are not conducted through the AV junction. Therefore, there is no relationship between the atria (P waves) and the ventricles (QRS waves). The PR interval varies and the QRS is usually wide and the heart rate slow (less than 40 to 60).

6. Pacemakers can fail by failing to pace or capture as well as by oversensing and undersensing.

Chapter 5: Answers to Critical Thinking Questions

1. Factors affecting oxygen supply are oxygen saturation (SaO_2) of the hemoglobin, the oxygen dissolved in the blood (pO_2), hemoglobin level, and cardiac output. Factors affecting oxygen demand are metabolic rate and stressful states.

2. The four determinants of cardiac output are heart rate, preload, afterload, and contractility. Myocardial fiber stretch from an adequate end diastolic volume or preload is required to optimize contractility. If the volume becomes too large, the myocardial fibers are overstretched, leading to failure.

3. a. Nursing actions are to ensure that the pressure bag is inflated to 300 mm Hg. Ensure there is adequate saline solution in the flush bag. Use the fast flush device on the pressure monitoring system to clear the tubing of blood.
   b. This will cause the arterial line to be overdamped.

4. Patients who would be candidates for a pulmonary artery catheter are those needing:
   • Assessment of oxygen supply and demand
   • Monitoring during high-risk cardiovascular procedures
   • A diagnosis such as HF
   • Guidance during fluid or medication therapy

5. Factors elevating the RA pressures are:
   - Fluid volume excess
   - Right ventricular failure
   - Pulmonary hypertension
   - Tricuspid stenosis or insufficiency
   - Pulmonic stenosis or insufficiency
   - Pulmonary embolism

6. a. The complication of a catheter stuck in wedge is that blood flow distal to the catheter has stopped, thus risking pulmonary tissue ischemia.
   b. Nursing actions include:
      - Ensure that all the air is out of the syringe.
      - Try repositioning the patient.
      - NEVER flush the PA catheter when the catheter is stuck in wedge as this can lead to PA rupture.
      - Notify the physician or advanced practice nurse to reposition the catheter.
      - If the nurse's institution allows, withdraw the PA catheter until the PA waveform appears.

Chapter 6: Answers to Case Study Questions

1. Signs and symptoms indicating hypovolemia in this patient include:
   - Hypotension
   - Tachycardia
   - Pale skin color
   - Delayed capillary refill
   - Absent distal pulses
   - Change in mental status

2. Lab tests indicating hypovolemia include:
   - Elevated BUN
   - Elevated sodium
   - Decreased hemoglobin
   - Decreased Hct

3. As the patient's circulating volume and blood pressure decrease, the baroreceptors in the carotid arteries and aortic arch send signals to the medulla in the brainstem. The cardiac accelerator center and the vasoconstrictor center are stimulated. The cardiac accelerator center causes an increase in heart rate and stroke volume. The vasoconstrictor center causes arterioles and veins to constrict, delaying capillary refill and reducing the quality of the peripheral pulses.

4. At face value the saturation of 96% appears within normal limits. However, in this patient the amount of hemoglobin available for saturation is reduced. Therefore, the saturation level is 96% of the available hemoglobin of 5.6. The supply side of the tissue oxygenation is reduced in this patient.

5. Factors contributing to this massive GI bleed are:
   - Esophageal varices
   - Cirrhosis likely leading to abnormal coagulation studies
   - Abnormal coagulation studies prolonging clotting time
   - Remote excessive drinking history

6. Immediate collaborative management in this patient includes rapid fluid resuscitation first with isotonic crystalloids such as 0.9% normal saline then blood products. The nurse must ensure that the large-bore intravenous catheters placed by EMS are patent and functional. The nurse should anticipate that the physician or advanced practice nurse will place a central line for additional vascular access. Use of a rapid fluid delivery device should be anticipated. Delivery of high-flow oxygen should continue and the nurse should anticipate the possibility of intubation and mechanical ventilation. Placement of a large-bore nasogastric tube is indicated to decompress the stomach, preventing aspiration as well as quantifying the amount of GI bleeding.

7. Initially, isotonic crystalloid intravenous fluids should be given followed by blood products. Isotonic crystalloid intravenous fluids include 0.9% normal saline and lactated Ringer's solution. Crystalloid administration only will not correct the patient's limited oxygen-carrying capacity.

Chapter 6: Answers to Critical Thinking Questions

1. Signs and symptoms indicating hypovolemia in this patient include:
   - Hypotension
   - Tachycardia
   - Pale skin color
   - Delayed capillary refill
   - Absent distal pulses
   - Change in mental status

2. In hypovolemic shock the heart rate is increased and the MAP, CVP/RA, and PAWP are decreased, reflecting a reduced preload. A reduction in circulating volume may also lead to a reduction in SV and CO/CI.

3. A positive response to fluid therapy would be indicated by an increasing CVP to a normal range, MAP of at least 60 mm Hg, and urine output greater than 0.5 to 1 mL/kg/hr.

4. The primary neurohormonal mechanisms involved in response to heart failure are the sympathetic nervous system and the renin-angiotensin-aldosterone system. In response to a decreased cardiac output, activation of the sympathetic nervous system releases norepinephrine, causing increases in vasoconstriction, heart rate, and contractility. Activation of the renin-angiotensin-aldosterone system further increases vasoconstriction through the activation of angiotensin II, a potent vasoconstrictor. Activation of the renin-angiotensin-aldosterone system also stimulates aldosterone, expanding fluid volume through sodium reabsorption.

5. Systolic dysfunction is impaired left ventricular contractility with a reduced ejection fraction. The ejection fraction is the percentage of blood ejected from the left ventricle with each contraction—normal is 55% to 75%. This impaired contractility leads to a reduction in cardiac output. Diastolic dysfunction appears when the ventricle is normal size but hypertrophied, leading to loss of left ventricular diastolic relaxation and distensibility. This preserves the normal ejection fraction but impairs filling, leading to elevated filling pressures and pulmonary artery wedge pressures.

6. The acutely ill patient with heart failure will exhibit signs and symptoms and laboratory alterations from the effects of basically two major dysfunctions: decreased cardiac output leading to volume overload and end-organ hypoperfusion.

   Volume overload leads to dyspnea on exertion, orthopnea, paroxysmal nocturnal dyspnea (PND), peripheral edema, abdominal pain and distention, weight gain, crackles on pulmonary auscultation, elevation of venous pressures (CVP, PAWP), and presence of S_3 or S_4 upon cardiac auscultation.

End-organ hypoperfusion is manifested by decreased exercise tolerance, fatigue, dizziness, syncope or near syncope, palpitations, hypotension, tachycardia, cool extremities, delayed capillary refill, and decreased urinary output. Older adults are much more likely to display end organ hypoperfusion by confusion than younger adults.

7. BP, PA pressure, and CVP are all usually elevated in the presence of heart failure.

8. The management of the patient involves both pharmacologic and nonpharmacologic measures. Lifestyle modifications are important in all patients with heart failure. These include smoking cessation, restriction of alcohol consumption, salt restriction, weight reduction in obese patients, and cardiac rehabilitation in stable patients. One of the mainstays of treatment for the heart failure patient is medications directed at the neurohormonal activation of the sympathetic nervous system and the renin-angiotensin-aldosterone system. By blocking the neurohormonal activation, symptoms of heart failure are reduced and progression of the disease is slowed. Leading drug categories in this process are beta blockade, ACE inhibitors, and angiotensin II receptor blockers (ARBs). In some patients the use of aldosterone antagonists will also be beneficial.

9. The signs of deterioration include dyspnea at rest, tachycardia, reduced oxygen saturation, crackles on lung auscultation, hypotension, worsening cough, new dysrhythmias, elevation of PAWP, and reduction in CO/CI.

10. Aggressive oxygen administration, administration of venodilators, and possible administration of positive inotropic therapy.

11. Maintenance of adequate ventilation and tissue oxygenation.

12. Isotonic solutions are infused into the vascular space and stay there long enough to expand the intravascular space. Hypotonic solutions, like 0.45% NS, do not stay in the intravascular space long enough to expand the circulating volume.

Chapter 7: Answers to Case Study Questions

1. Common causes of chest discomfort are acute myocardial infarction, peptic ulcer disease, acute coronary syndrome, pericarditis, and aortic dissection. A nurse in the emergency department needs to assist in a quick assessment to assist with the differential diagnosis.

2. These leads point to damage in the anterior wall of the left ventricle. This is usually due to an occlusion of the left main or the left anterior descending coronary artery. Infarctions in this area of the myocardium carry the highest mortality rate.

3. STEMI is an infarction of the full thickness of a region of the myocardium. It is caused by thrombosis over an atherosclerotic plaque occluding a coronary artery and starving the supplied area of the myocardium of oxygen. Acute coronary syndromes are a spectrum of conditions of myocardial is-

chemia in which there are possibly no ST elevations on the ECG and can include unstable angina and an NSTEMI.

4. This patient has multiple risk factors for the development and progression of acute coronary syndrome. They include hypertension, obesity, stressful work environment, stressful family life, increased caloric intake, no exercise, high blood cholesterol, and borderline diabetic.

5. The patient will need to have a CK-MB to assess for specific myocardial muscle damage. A hemoglobin A_1C is needed to assess for glycemic control. Troponin T is needed for a measurement of the muscle damage, myoglobin, especially if it is elevated with the first 2 hours of chest pain. C-reactive protein will be used to assess inflammation of the coronary system. Chest x-ray is needed to rule out pulmonary causes of chest pain.

6. Upon arrival to the emergency department the patient is placed in a semi-Fowler's position to allow for comfort and proper cardiovascular functioning. An intravenous line should be started to keep the vein open for immediate access for the administration of emergency drugs. Medications and treatments are then started in a standard progression.
   - Aspirin—Aspirin is given first and consists of four "baby strength" aspirin or the equivalent of 325 milligrams. It is used to prevent platelet aggregation and the formation of blood clots in the coronary vasculature.
   - Nitroglycerin—This is given if the patient's systolic blood pressure is above 90 mm Hg. It can be given in either the sublingual form, which will reduce the pain that is currently present, or the intravenous form to prevent future episodes.
   - Supplemental oxygen—Oxygen is administered at 2 to 4 liters per nasal cannula to increase myocardial oxygenation. The oxygen saturation level of 92% is used as a guideline for the proper amount of oxygen to be administered.
   - Morphine—Morphine sulfate is given in a dose of 2 to 5 mg intravenous every 5 to 30 minutes as needed. Morphine is used for both pain management and as an antianxiety medication. If this medication is given first it can mask the patient's perception of pain and mask the underlying cause of ischemia.
   - Vital signs should be taken at frequent intervals.
   - Electrocardiogram—This should be obtained within the first 10 minutes of arrival.

   The patient will also be evaluated with a series of blood tests and cardiac markers.

Chapter 7: Answers to Critical Thinking Questions

1. The most common cause of STEMI is reduced myocardial perfusion from an occlusive thrombus that developed on a ruptured portion of atherosclerotic plaque. This can cause damage to various areas of the myocardium, but depriving the heart muscle of oxygen.

   Unstable angina is pain that occurs more often and in unpredictable patterns. It can occur while the patient is at rest as well as with minimal exertion and causes the patient limited activity. Unstable angina is actually the beginning of a process that can lead to an NSTEMI.

The differentiation is based on clinical presentation, laboratory data, and patient history.

2. An STEMI is caused by occlusive thrombus composed of platelets and thrombin. Aspirin is an antiplatelet agent that stops platelet aggregation.

3. Troponins are molecules that regulate the interaction of actin and myosin in muscle. Troponins are released into the blood from damaged muscle. Cardiac troponins I and T are specific to cardiac muscle, are highly sensitive to ischemia and necrosis, and correlate with the amount of myocardial damage. The main drawback to the use of troponins is that the level may not rise until after 12 hours of myocardial damage.

4. The main electrolyte disturbances are hypercalcemia, hypocalcemia, hypokalemia, and hyponatremia. Calcium, sodium, and potassium are all needed for proper function of the heart. The most important level for the nurse to monitor during hospitalization and treatment of ACS is the potassium level. Many of the cardiac drugs can interfere with the body's absorption of potassium. If the level of potassium falls below 3.5, the patient is at risk for developing lethal cardiac rhythm disturbances, such as ventricular tachycardia.

5. The pain of ACS is treated with aspirin for its antiplatelet effects; nitroglycerin as a vasodilator; and morphine sulfate, an opioid, to control pain and anxiety.

6. The most common complications of a myocardial infarction are:
Heart failure due to left ventricular dysfunction from decreased myocardial blood supply and decreased ventricular wall motion.
Dysrhythmias, especially atrial and ventricular, are very common post myocardial infarction. These are caused by the release of catecholamines, hypokalemia, and the parasympathetic response.
Pericarditis, which is the inflammation of the pericardial sac, can also occur. This happens frequently after invasive cardiac surgery and is self-limiting.

7. Fibrinolytic agents such as eptifibatide (Integrelin), tirofiban (Aggrastat), and abciximab (ReoPro) are agents that break down fibrin. When used in conjunction with early aspirin therapy, these agents will dissolve the thrombus blocking the coronary artery and restore blood flow to the vessel, and thus oxygen to the heart muscle.

8. A coronary artery bypass graft is indicated for the patient who has failed medical management, has more than two diseased coronary vessels with significant blockage, may not be a candidate for PCI, or has failed a PCI attempt with ongoing chest discomfort.

Chapter 8: Answers to Case Study Questions

1. His ABCs have been quickly reviewed. It is now time for a full set of vital signs and further assessment (and reevaluation) of his breathing, circulation, and neuro status to account for the increased confusion and belligerence.

2. The indications of a flail chest are dyspnea, pain in the chest wall, and paradoxical movement of the chest wall. The size and severity of the pulmonary contusion often determine the treatment that a person with a flail chest will require.

3. A flail chest may be splinted initially. The patient may need intubation and mechanical ventilation to stabilize the ribs and to prevent pneumonia. Allen's level of consciousness is deteriorating and he may need emergent intubation.

4. He most likely has extensive blood loss. Allen may have lost large amounts of blood into both his left leg fracture and the pulmonary contusion under his left chest wall injury. He will need volume and possibly blood replacement.

5. Allen's confusion will need additional assessment. It could be due to hypoxia, hypotension and poor cerebral perfusion, head injury, intoxication, or other possibilities.

6. Initially, pulses will need to be checked below the level of the fracture. It will be x-rayed and splinted. When and how it will be treated will depend on the severity of his other injuries and the nature of the fracture.

7. Allen's increasing confusion and belligerence will complicate his abdominal assessment. His abdomen will be observed for any indication of injury and his bowel sounds will be auscultated before his abdomen is palpated.

Chapter 8: Answers to Critical Thinking Questions

1. Methylprednisolone 2,250 mg IV over 15 minutes.

2. The patient needs to be assessed for blood at the urinary meatus and any indication of pelvic trauma before the catheter is inserted. The physician should perform a digital rectal exam before the catheter is inserted.

3. The primary assessment includes: Airway, Breathing, Circulation, and Disability.
   The secondary assessment includes: Exposing the patient to check for other injuries, getting a Full set of vital signs, Giving comfort, doing a Head-to-toe assessment, obtaining an accurate History, and Inspecting the patient's posterior.

4. A variety of factors might contribute to the trauma score dropping. The drop could be due to the patient receiving pain medication with a subsequent drop in BP and respiratory rates coupled with a change in neuro status. With initial catecholamine release following trauma, some patients sustain their vital signs and do not deteriorate until they are medicated and their pain is relieved. This is not uncommon in patients with chest wall injuries. It could also be due to inadequate volume repletion and the beginnings of shock, which can become more apparent after pain medication.

5. Chest tubes may be inserted to allow air or blood to drain from the pleural space.

6. The patient and family would need to understand the reason for the fasciotomy, that sensation and circulation should have returned to the affected limb so that any recurrence of symptoms should be reported, that there will be daily moist sterile dressings, and that additional surgery and possibly skin grafting will be needed to close the wound.

Chapter 9: Answers to Case Study Questions

1. These findings most likely indicate a lesion on the left side of his brain and an increase in intracranial pressure. An increase in the systolic blood pressure occurs with increased intracranial pressure and increases cerebral perfusion. This

compensatory mechanism can occur as long as the brain's ability to autoregulate is intact.

2. Mannitol decreases intracranial pressure while reducing cerebrovascular resistance and increasing cerebral blood flow.

    Nursing responsibilities are: If the 15%, 20%, or 25% solutions are utilized, the nurse administers mannitol through an in-line filter. Mannitol may cause hypotension after rapid administration, especially in volume-depleted patients. Therefore, it is important that the patient be euvolemic and the nurse administer a bolus dose no more rapidly than over 15 to 30 minutes. Mannitol increases the osmolality of the blood, with optimal osmolality between 300 and 320 mOsm. If repeated doses of mannitol are given, the nurse monitors the serum osmolality every 4 to 6 hours and ensures that it remains less than 320 mOsm. The nurse also monitors the urine output to ensure that it is at least 30 to 50 mL/hr and reviews the lab results, looking specifically for hyponatremia and hypokalemia.

3. Because the origin of the bleeding is arterial, the hematoma accumulates rapidly and must be evacuated immediately. Patient outcomes are often good if the condition is identified promptly and the patient is taken to the OR for immediate surgical evacuation of the hematoma.

4. Sedation is often used to control agitation associated with ventilation in head-injured patients although it has not been shown to affect patient outcomes. Propofol is a sedative-hypnotic anesthetic, which decreases ICP but does not improve mortality. One advantage of propofol is that in most patients, the dose may be lowered or discontinued and within about 10 minutes an accurate neurological assessment can be obtained. Long-term and high-dose uses are associated with significant morbidity, specifically the propofol infusion syndrome.

5. The nurse has specific responsibilities when caring for a patient whose CSF is being drained through an external ventricular drain, including:
    • First the transducer and stopcock must be leveled at the tragus of the ear or higher as determined by the neurosurgeon.
    • If continuous drainage is being utilized, it is essential that the level is maintained as the patient moves or is repositioned.
    • The amount of drainage as well as the color, clarity, and presence of sediment are noted at least hourly.
    • Also hourly, the nurse accurately determines the ICP by temporarily turning off continuous drainage.

6. Depending on the institution, the nurse might have standing orders to provide additional stat mannitol or to acutely hyperventilate Adam while notifying the physician.

Chapter 9: Answers to Critical Thinking Questions

1. Normally, the intracranial pressure is kept in a range between 5 and 15 mm Hg by a mechanism known as compliance. When the volume of one of the components increases, the body may respond by:
    • Displacing CSF into the lumbar cistern
    • Reabsorbing more CSF
    • Compressing veins and shunting of blood out of the venous sinuses

These compensatory mechanisms allow for small increases in the volumes of components in the skull to occur without a significant increase in intracranial pressure.

2. Secondary injury produces ongoing increases in intracranial pressure and additional damage to the patient who has sustained a brain injury. These secondary insults are remediable—thus, preventing or limiting them is one of the major ways that the long-term outcomes from cerebral injury can be improved.

3. Admission motor score on the Glasgow Coma Scale.

4. An intracranial pressure of 34 is significantly elevated and a cerebral perfusion pressure of 50 is low. The nurse will need to check standing orders and to notify the physician. Actions that might be indicated include draining CSF, providing mannitol, changing the patient's position, changing the amount or type of IV fluid, or providing sedation carefully.

5. In the United States an average of 1.4 million traumatic brain injuries (TBIs) occur each year, resulting in 235,000 hospitalizations and 50,000 deaths. Head injuries represent 2% to 3% of all causes of deaths and 26% to 68% of trauma deaths. These large numbers of injuries are especially problematic because TBI is one of the most disabling of injuries. Approximately 5.3 Americans are living with long-term or lifelong disability following hospitalization for a TBI. In addition, in the first 3 years postinjury, patients recovering from a TBI are more likely to report binge drinking, develop epilepsy, and die.

6. Epidural hematomas usually occur in conjunction with a skull fracture and result from a laceration of the middle meningeal artery causing bleeding between the dura mater and the skull. Approximately half of the patients who suffer this injury demonstrate the classic presentation of an initial loss of consciousness followed by a lucid interval then a sudden reloss of consciousness with rapid deterioration in neurological status. Because the origin of the bleeding is arterial, the hematoma accumulates rapidly and must be evacuated immediately. Patient outcomes are often good if the condition is identified promptly and the patient is taken to the OR for immediate surgical evacuation of the hematoma. Subdural hematomas usually are the result of countercoup injuries, occurring on the opposite side of the skull from the injury just below the dura. In contrast to an epidural hematoma, this hematoma is usually the result of venous bleeding, often originating with the stretching of bridging veins. Subdural hematomas are classified as acute, subacute, and chronic. The presentation and management depend on the specific type.

7. The initial priorities in the management of any trauma patient are the same—the ABCs with assessment and treatment of any injury upon discovery. When these are completed then D (Disability), the neuro assessment, begins.

8. In order to prevent shivering, the nurse might:
    • Use higher temperatures on the cooling blanket (as high as 23.9°C) (75°F) so that the patient's temperature does not drop as rapidly.
    • Wrap the patient's arms and legs in cloth towels and position them so they are off the blanket.

- Place a bath blanket between the patient and the hypothermia blanket to prevent burning the patient's skin.
- Sedate or even paralyze the patient.

9. The classic presentation of meningitis includes fever; headache; neck stiffness; photophobia; nausea; vomiting; and changes in mental status such as irritability, lethargy, confusion, and coma. When a patient complains of the symptoms and displays the classic signs of meningitis on focused neurological assessment, the patient should bypass the usual history taking and proceed immediately to definitive diagnosis and emergent management.

10. Between 10% and 25% of patients experiencing a severe TBI develop seizures during the first week after a traumatic injury. Seizure activity in the first week may cause secondary brain damage as a result of increased metabolic demands, raised intracranial pressure, and excess neurotransmitter release. Therefore, the nurse needs to be vigilant in observing for the development of such seizures, notify the physician immediately should a patient experience a seizure, and anticipate that anticonvulsant therapy may be indicated.

Chapter 10: Answers to Case Study Questions

1. • Monitor respiratory status. (The patient is at risk for impaired breathing due to possible damage of cerebral tissues.)
   - Monitor cardiac status. (The patient's BP is already elevated and further increase may cause complications. Cardiac monitor will reveal if arrhythmia is present.)
   - Monitor neurological status. (Frequent monitoring of neurological status is needed to detect changes and impending complications.)
   - Monitor temperature. (The patient's temperature is already elevated. Hyperthermia develops when the hypothalamus is affected.)
   - Initiate NPO status. (The patient may be at risk of a swallowing deficit and further assessment will be needed when stable.)

2. • Accurate time of symptom onset
   - Any recent medical, surgical, or trauma events
   - Risk factors (Note any of the following as risk factors: male gender, over 55 years of age, prior stroke, TIAs or MI, carotid or other artery disease, hypertension, atrial fibrillation, hyperlipidemia, diabetes mellitus, tobacco use, excessive alcohol use, obesity, inactivity, and sickle cell anemia.)
   - Medications (particularly antihypertensive, antiplatelet, and anticoagulant agents and over-the-counter medications such as aspirin)

3. The admission assessment revealed a history of hypertension, carotid stenosis, and TIAs.

4. • Neuroimaging (ideally, a CT or MRI should be ordered within 45 minutes and read within 20 minutes of patient arrival to the ED).
   - Lab services: Blood tests that should be obtained immediately are CBC, chemistry, and coagulation profiles. A chest x-ray and ECG should be performed within 45 minutes of arrival to ED.

5. His treatment options depend on the time since his arrival in the ED and the capabilities of the hospital to which he has been transported. If his arrival is timely and the hospital has immediate radiological and neurological consultation, an IV thrombolytic might be provided. In a tertiary center, the thrombolytic might be provided to the appropriate cerebral artery, or another invasive method of ensuring arterial patency might be attempted. If he arrived outside the safe time frame for thrombolysis, treatment would involve watchful waiting with management of increased intracranial pressure and prevention of complications.

6. • Risk for falls
   - Dysphagia
   - Dysphasia
   - Immobility
   - Incontinence
   - Constipation
   - Skin breakdown

Chapter 10: Answers to Critical Thinking Questions

1. The most common generalized symptoms of a brain tumor are headache, nausea, vomiting, drowsiness, visual problems, and changes in personality.

   Focal symptoms are more specific symptoms that result from tumor irritation of brain tissue. Focal symptoms include hearing problems such as ringing or buzzing sounds or hearing loss, decreased muscle control, lack of coordination, decreased sensation, weakness or paralysis, difficulty with walking or speech, balance problems, or double vision.

2. The decrease in cerebral edema may occur because glucocorticoids directly affect vascular endothelial cell function and restore normal capillary permeability. In addition, dexamethasone may cause cerebral vasoconstriction.

   Nursing responsibilities are: Side effects from glucocorticoid therapy are common, so it is important to determine that the patient is among the 70% to 80% of patients who benefit from the therapy if it is to be continued. To avoid adverse effects, the dose is adjusted to the minimum that will control the patient's symptoms. Even at the lowest appropriate dose, typical doses given to patients with brain tumors have the potential to suppress the hypothalamic-pituitary-adrenocortical (HPA) axis. If the dose is to be discontinued, it should be tapered to allow the HPA axis time to recover. In addition, if the steroids are abruptly discontinued, rebound edema may occur and the patient may have an abrupt return of neurological symptoms. Tapering schedules for dexamethasone vary depending on the length of time the patient has been on the steroid and the patient's symptoms.

   Potential Side/Toxic Effects: Adverse effects are dose and time dependent, with as many as 50% of patients experiencing at least one toxic symptom. Common effects include euphoria, with excessive feeling of well-being and insomnia; increased appetite, especially for sweets; weight gain; hyperglycemia, particularly in diabetics; hypertension; muscle weakness in the legs (the patient may complain of inability to climb stairs or arise from chairs); stomach ulcer; and increased risk of infection.

   The nurse may need to educate the patient and family concerning muscle weakness because they may fear it is an indication of worsening neurological function. Dietary counseling is important to prevent excessive weight gain and high blood sugars. Nurses should encourage the patient to take steroids with food and avoid aspirin and nonsteroidal anti-inflammatory agents to prevent gastric ulceration and bleeding. When patients with brain tumors receive steroids for a prolonged period, their CD4 count may drop sufficiently to predispose them to opportunistic infections. Nurses should inspect the mouths of these patients to detect the presence of oral and esophageal candidiasis. To prevent the development of pneumocystis pneumonia, Bactrim might be administered.

3. The nursing responsibilities include:
   Maintaining head of the bed elevated 30 to 45 degrees
   Providing a moustache dressing
   Assessing for CSF leakage on the dressing
   Discouraging the patient from sneezing and blowing the nose
   Assessing the patient for a visual field defect
   Assessing pituitary function and identifying the presence of diabetes insipidus

4. Pneumatic compression boots and graduated compression stockings have been shown to decrease the occurrence of VTEs without increasing ICP. An alternative is the use of compression boots prior to, during, and for 24 hours after the surgery followed by low-dose heparin 5,000 units twice a day or enoxaparin 40 mg/day.

5. The two major categories of CVA, hemorrhage and ischemia, are totally opposite conditions. Whereas hemorrhage is defined as rupture of a blood vessel and too much blood within the closed cranial cavity, ischemia is defined as too little blood supply with inadequate oxygen and nutrients to part of the brain.

6. The four major neuroanatomic stroke syndromes are middle cerebral artery occlusions, anterior cerebral artery occlusions, posterior cerebral artery occlusions, and vertebrobasilar artery occlusions.

7. A deterioration in mental status, such as restlessness or lethargy, and the development of focal neurological deficits, most likely hemiparesis or dysphasia, suggest that the patient might be developing vasospasm. Symptoms may wax and wane, changing from minute to minute. They tend to become more apparent when the patient's blood pressure drops and less obvious when the blood pressure increases.

8. Screening for dysphagia is essential in a stroke survivor because it is a very common complication and is associated with the development of aspiration pneumonia. To determine if a patient has a swallowing deficit, the nurse might use the following swallow screening criteria. Prior to swallow screening, the nurse should:
   • Evaluate lung sounds and obtain the most recent vital signs, including temperature.
   • Evaluate the ability of the patient to follow directions.
        If the patient demonstrates any of the following problems at any time during the assessment, the nurse should cease the evaluation, keep the patient NPO, and ask the MD for a speech therapy order for a swallowing evaluation: coughing before, during, or after a swallow.
   • Gurgly/wet vocal quality or any voice changes
   • Need to swallow two or more times to clear

   • Excessive length of time to move food to the back of the throat to swallow
   • Pocketing of food
   • Excessive secretions
        The nurse should consider each of the following when doing a swallow screening:
   a. Does the patient have facial weakness or a droop?
   b. Does the patient have difficulty with arousal?
   c. Does the patient have an absent gag reflex?
   d. Given one bite of applesauce, does the patient cough or clear her throat?
   e. Given one sip of water, does the patient cough or clear her throat?
   f. Given consecutive sips of water, does the patient cough or clear her throat?
   g. Given a graham cracker or saltine, does the patient have difficulty chewing, any oral residue, and can the patient cough/clear the throat?
   h. Does the patient need to swallow more than one time per bite/sip?

Chapter 11: Answers to Case Study Questions

1. The first priority in Barbara's care should be the maintenance of her airway while she is vomiting. If her airway has been ensured then the nurse must attend to her hemorrhagic shock.

2. The nurse will need additional assessment information, especially a rapid full physical assessment, including: what is her respiratory status, how well is she perfusing (manifestations of shock) her MAP, and is she still oriented? The nurse will also want to review some lab data such as how many units of blood have been typed and crossed for her and how many are available, what are the rest of her lab studies—specifically her clotting studies? What is the current plan? Will Barbara be undergoing endoscopy? If so, when? If not, what measures will be attempted to decrease the bleeding?

3. Barbara has longstanding liver disease and it is likely that her clotting studies will reveal an abnormality. She is currently retching and vomiting and that will make bleeding from varices more severe.

4. She has severe liver disease, including a previous bleed, and she is continuing to drink alcohol. All of these factors contribute to the likelihood that she would rebleed.

5. Gastric lavage might be performed prior to endoscopy or erythromycin might be administered in an attempt to clear the stomach of blood and clots, thus making it easier to locate the source of the bleeding. Additionally, the critical care nurse should:
   • Maintain NPO status ideally.
   • Ensure informed consent.
   • Remove dentures.
   • Monitor baseline vital signs, including temperature and oxygen saturation.
   • Provide patient/family education.
   • If the patient is being mechanically ventilated, consult the endoscopist and respiratory therapy related to temporarily adjusting ventilator setting to maximize oxygenation during sedation.

6. Endoscopic sclerotherapy involves injecting a sclerosing (hardening) solution into the varix to stop the bleeding by causing a thrombosis and obliteration of the vein. The nurse should monitor for complications, including chest discomfort, sclerosant-induced esophageal ulcers, strictures, and perforations. Esophageal variceal ligation (EVL) involves suctioning the varix into the scope cylinder and deploying a band around the varix. The band strangulates the varix, causing thrombosis and obliteration. Both are effective therapeutic modalities in stopping the bleeding in the majority of the patients. Esophageal band ligation is considered the primary endoscopic therapy. It has fewer complications than sclerotherapy. However, in situations where there is severe active bleeding and poor visibility, banding may be more difficult. The use of endoscopic therapy in combination with a vasoactive agent (octreotide) is more successful than either therapy alone.

7. Barbara has only been home for about a week. It is unclear how much she was able to drink during that week and she may not undergo alcohol withdrawal during this hospitalization.

8. The nurse completes an assessment of Barbara, reviews her lab findings, and notifies the physician.

9. Barbara has most likely developed hepatic encephalopathy. The collaborative management involves identifying and treating precipitating factors (in this case the upper GI bleed and hypokalemia), determining Barbara's serum ammonia level, and using lactulose or oral antibiotics to lower the level.

10. Barbara is at high risk for either an invasive or surgical procedure to lower portal pressure. However, once she is no longer actively bleeding and has stabilized, only reduction in portal pressure will be likely to prevent her from recurrent bleeding.

Chapter 11: Answers to Critical Thinking Questions

1. When exposed to repeated doses of alcohol, the central nervous system (CNS) becomes accustomed to the depressant effects of the alcohol and produces adaptive changes in an attempt to function normally. In the absence of or with a significant decrease in the amount of alcohol, chaos erupts within the CNS. When alcohol is no longer acting as a depressant, the compensatory actions cause excessive CNS excitability. It is analogous to having an accelerator without a brake. The time course of withdrawal is determined by the time it takes to restore balance.

2. The nurse should obtain a complete history in a nonthreatening manner from the patient and/or family. It is important to consider a patient's nonverbal responses, anxiety, and presence or absence of eye contact for clues. The nurse questions the patient/family related to:
   • Current and past alcohol use and family history of alcohol problems
     —Abuse and dependence are more prevalent in families where first-degree relatives have been afflicted
   • Quantity and frequency/pattern of alcohol use
     —Severity can depend on duration and quantity of consumption.
     —Patients/families may underreport consumption and abuse or deny it.

   • History of liver disease or other alcohol-related illnesses and previous withdrawals

   Additionally, a standardized questionnaire should be utilized to detect dependency. There are several reliable and valid questionnaires available. One such questionnaire is the CAGE. It is a simple, fast, short, reliable, and valid questionnaire. The acronym helps the clinician to recall the following questions:
   • Have you ever felt the need to **CUT** down on drinking?
   • Have you ever felt **ANNOYED** by criticism of your drinking?
   • Have you ever had **GUILTY** feelings about your drinking?
   • Have you ever had an **EYE** opener first thing in the morning to steady your nerves or get rid of a hangover?

3. The CIWA-AR is the scale most commonly used to assess the intensity of withdrawal and to provide appropriate medical therapy.

4. DTs are the most severe complication of alcohol withdrawal and patients who develop DTs may die.

5. Alcoholic hallucinosis can manifest 12 to 24 hours after the last alcohol ingestion. With alcohol hallucinosis the patient experiences perceptual disturbances—usually visual, auditory, or tactile phenomena—without sensorial alterations. Patients are fully conscious and aware of their environments, acknowledging that the hallucinations are related to the substance dependence and withdrawal. The distinction from DTs is that in DTs the patient experiences disorientation and global confusion.

6. The following are all safety concerns for a patient with AWS who may be confused, disoriented, and hallucinating: Accurate assessment and appropriate medication administration per protocols (vital signs and LOC) Implementation of one-to-one continuous observation and monitoring Institution of fall protocols relative to disorientation and sedation Seizure precautions Aspiration precautions Physical restraints to prevent injury to patient and staff

7. Benzodiazepines are the foundation of pharmacological therapy for AWS. These agents serve as a substitute for alcohol by acting on inhibitory GABA mediators replacing the depressant effects on the CNS. As a substitute for alcohol, they counteract hyperactivity, thus known to have "cross tolerance." In addition to their sedative-hypnotic effect, they also have anticonvulsant properties and less adverse effects than other drugs in this classification. Benzodiazepines have been proven to be safe and effective in preventing and reducing withdrawal severity, including seizures and delirium.

   The nurse anticipates that the route of administration and dosing will be guided by the clinical picture and the kinetic properties of the benzodiazepine chosen. The therapeutic goal is to achieve light somnolence. Evidence of light somnolence is that the patient sleeps when not stimulated, yet is easily arousable when sleeping. Intravenous administration has the quickest onset. For severe withdrawal, the nurse can expect to be administering larger doses of intravenous benzodiazepines.

8. When AWS develops in critically ill patients, it may compound and confuse an already difficult situation.

9. In acute liver failure, there is sudden dramatic loss of liver function. It is a medical emergency with a high mortality rate. Treatment is dependent on the specific cause. Chronic liver failure is usually the result of excessive alcohol misuse, viral hepatitis, or nonalcoholic fatty liver disease. It may eventually result in cirrhosis.

10. Acetaminophen overdose is dangerous because untreated it has the potential to result in acute liver failure and/or death.

11. N-acetylcysteine (NAC) (Mucomyst) is an antidote that counteracts the effects of acetaminophen toxicity. When administered within 12 hours of ingestion of a single dose it can eliminate significant hepatic injury. Oral dosing is initiated on nonpregnant patients with a functioning GI system and no indications of hepatotoxicity. The loading dose is 140 mg/kg followed by 17 doses of 70 mg/kg every 4 hours. It is typically available in a 20% solution (200 mg/mL) and is diluted to a 5% solution with fruit juice, a carbonated beverage, or water.

12. Portal hypertension develops over time, is asymptomatic, and is responsible for an array of complications that can markedly reduce patients' life expectancy. The following complications are directly attributable to portal hypertension: ascites, variceal hemorrhage, hepatic encephalopathy (HE) (portosystemic encephalopathy [PSE]), and hepatorenal syndrome.

13. The nurse will need to assess the patient's hemodynamic status and neurological functioning and complete an abdominal assessment, specifically noting any indications of liver disease. The nurse will also want to review liver enzymes, serum albumin, clotting studies, serum electrolytes, and CBC.

14. The nursing responsibilities for a patient with ascites include:
Assisting with paracentesis as appropriate
Maintaining sodium and fluid restriction
Providing diuretic therapy
Evaluating the effectiveness of the therapy
Educating the patient and family about therapy
    The nursing responsibilities for a patient with hepatic encephalopathy include:
Assessing the patient's respiratory, safety, and neurological status
Reviewing the patient's blood ammonia
Identifying and correcting precipitating factors
Providing medical therapy (lactulose or oral antibiotics as indicated)

Chapter 12: Answers to Case Study Questions

1. He is dehydrated and requires immediate fluid resuscitation.

2. It is confirmed by his vital signs; his blood pressure is low and his heart rate is high despite volume replacement. His cvp is equivocal.

3. His recent heavy alcohol intake is likely the precipitating factor.

4. His pancreatitis is likely severe based on his age, his pain, his hypoxia, volume status, and WBC. His Hct at 45 would

seem to indicate hemoconcentration and the potential for pancreatic necrosis. His serum amylase indicates that he most likely has pancreatitis but the amylase level is not a reliable predictor of the severity of pancreatitis.

5. Sudden, severe epigastrum pain often peaking within 30 to 60 minutes and lasting hours to days is the hallmark of pancreatitis. It results from irritation and edema of the inflamed pancreas and, in severe cases, the release of pancreatic enzymes into the surrounding tissues.

6. The two essential collaborative interventions are fluid resuscitation and pain relief.

7. Deficient fluid volume related to severe fluid shift.

Chapter 12: Answers to Critical Thinking Questions

1. The most frequent cause of GI bleeding in older adults is the development of GI ulcers in people who are taking NSAIDs for arthritis. NSAIDs can cause local and systemic effects that promote mucosal damage.

2. Older adults are more likely to present with nonspecific signs such as dehydration and abdominal cramping. The most common manifestations of GI bleeding in other age groups are hematemesis, hematochezia, and melena.

3. Typically, the patient with a UGI bleed presents with hematemesis and/or melena, whereas an LGI bleed is suspected in patients with hematochezia. Though helpful in evaluating the source, stool color is not absolute. Both UGI and LGI bleeders can have melena and a patient with a massive UGI bleed can have hematochezia.

4. Total fluid deficit cannot be accurately predicted and fluid resuscitation should remain rapid rate as long as blood pressure remains low. Other clinical parameters guiding resuscitation are vital signs, urine output, mental status, and peripheral perfusion. The nurse anticipates that the patient's vital signs shall begin to normalize and the urine output will increase within 15 to 20 minutes of the challenge.

5. Postprocedural nursing responsibilities of the critical care nurse include:
   • If not intubated, maintain recovery position (left lateral decubitus) to protect the airway until the patient is fully awake:
     —EGD patients may have a topical anesthetic sprayed to the throat area, which may impair swallowing.
   • Monitor vital signs, including temperature and oxygen saturation, level of pain, and consciousness until the patient returns to baseline (typically every 10 to 15 minutes for 30 minutes to an hour, then per ICU protocol, more frequently depending on acuity).
   • Monitor for potential complications:
     —Gastrointestinal blood loss (rebleeding)
     —Perforation
     —Aspiration
     —Adverse reaction to procedural sedation medications

6. The exact mechanism as to how the different predisposing factors induce pancreatitis is uncertain. General consensus regarding pathogenesis is autodigestion. The acinar cells are damaged, causing inappropriate activation of trypsinogen to trypsin. Trypsin activates a cascade of other enzymes

that begin digestive functions in the pancreas, resulting in inflammation and tissue damage. The normal defense and inhibitory mechanisms are overwhelmed by the large amounts of activated enzymes.

The release of inflammatory mediators causes increased vascular permeability with varying degrees of edema, hemorrhage, and necrosis.

7. The acute physiology and chronic health evaluation (APACHE II) and Ranson's early prognostic signs are two commonly used systems to determine the severity of pancreatitis. In addition, there is a CT scan severity grading system. The most critical markers of severity are organ failure (especially MSOF) and pancreatic necrosis. Most recently the hematocrit is being investigated as a possible prognostic marker for the presence of necrotizing pancreatitis.

8. The two priorities of care are providing fluid resuscitation and pain relief.

Chapter 13: Answers to Case Study Questions

Chapter 13 has two cases indicated as Case 1 and Case 2.

Case 1

1. Initial, concurrent interventions may include the following:
   * Perform a more in-depth assessment, including all body systems.
   * Initiate ECG monitoring.
   * Obtain blood glucose (at bedside).
   * Obtain laboratory studies:
     —Blood for CBC, chemistry panel (electrolytes, glucose, creatinine, BUN), glomerular filtration rate, liver function studies, clotting studies, arterial blood gases
     —Urine for glucose, ketones, and culture
     —Possible cultures: wound, sputum, blood
   * Start intravenous fluids for hydration. Normal saline would be anticipated based on the low blood pressure and high pulse rate.
   * Insert urinary catheter for strict assessment of output.
   * Reassure the patient.
   * Call next of kin or significant other.

2. The following laboratory results are needed to calculate serum osmolarity:
   * Na+ 132, Glucose 644, BUN 31
   * Serum osmolarity calculation: $(2 \times \text{sodium}) + (\text{serum glucose}/18) + (\text{BUN}/2.8)$.
     —$(2 \times 132) + (644/18) + (31/2.8) =$
     —$(264) + (35.7) + (11.07) = 310.77$
     —Serum osmolarity = 311 mmol/liter

3. The serum osmolarity of 311 is elevated. Normal serum osmolarity is 280 to 300 mmol/liter. This elevated serum osmolarity is a result of elevated glucose. Fluid will shift from interstitial and cellular tissues to the vascular space in an attempt to dilute the serum. Osmotic diuresis will result in dumping of glucose and electrolytes, causing electrolyte depletion.

4. The following laboratory results are needed to calculate the anion gap:
   * Na+ 132, K+ 6.2, Chloride 105, Bicarbonate 17

* Anion gap calculation: (Sodium + potassium) − (chloride + bicarbonate)
  —$(132 + 6.2) - (102 + 17) =$
  —$138.2 - 119 = 19.2$
  —Anion gap = 19.2

5. The results of the anion gap show metabolic acidosis. The normal anion gap (using this calculation method) is 10 to 17 mEq/L. Arterial blood gas results will also find metabolic acidosis.

6. The following laboratory results are needed to calculate the corrected serum sodium:
   * Na+ 132, Glucose 644
   * CSS calculation: Serum Na$^+$ + {[(Serum glucose (mg/dL) − 100)/100] $\times$ 1.6}
     —$132 + \{[(644 - 100)/100] \times 1.6\}$
     —$132 + \{[544/100] \times 1.6\}$
     —$132 + \{5.44 \times 1.6\}$
     —$132 + 8.7 = 140.7$
     —Corrected serum sodium = 140.7

7. Based on the corrected serum sodium results, the nurse would expect to change IV fluids to 0.45% normal saline solution because the corrected serum sodium is within normal limits.

8. This client weighs 155 pounds. To calculate kilograms, 155 is divided by 2.2. Mrs. D weighs 70.45 or 70 kg. The 24-hour fluid replacement equals 100 mL/kg of weight, or 100 mL $\times$ 70 kg, or 7,000 mL in 24 hours. The nurse would anticipate giving one half of the total fluid volume in the first 8 hours, equal to 3,500 mL. Often, a fluid bolus of 1,000 cc is delivered in the first hour, leaving 2,500 mL to be administered in the remaining 7 hours. The hourly IV rate would be 357 mL/hr (2,500 ÷ 7 hours). The other 3,500 mL would be administered in the following 16 hours. The hourly IV rate would be 219 mL/hr (3,500 ÷ 16 hours).

9. a. The nurse would anticipate giving Regular insulin.
   b. The IV route is used for critically ill clients in DKA or HHNS.
   c. A common bolus dose is equal to 0.15 unit/kg. Because Mrs. D weighs 70 kg, the nurse would anticipate a bolus dose of 11 units of Regular insulin via the IV route (70 kg $\times$ 0.15 unit = 10.5 rounded to 11 units). Insulin infusions are often started at 0.1 unit/kg/hr. The nurse would anticipate giving 7 units of Regular insulin via the IV route per hour (0.1 unit $\times$ 70 kg per hour = 7 units per hour).
   d. The nurse would expect to adjust the insulin infusion after 1 hour based on hourly blood glucose results. The goal is to decrease blood glucose slowly to prevent complications by 50 to 70 mg/dL per hour.
   e. The nurse would assess potassium levels and level of dehydration prior to giving insulin. IV fluids should be initiated before starting an insulin infusion. If potassium levels are low, the nurse would anticipate replacing potassium before giving IV insulin.

10. It would be important to assess Mrs. D's basic knowledge of diabetes. The admission history includes an important clue that Mrs. D was in very good control of her diabetes prior to this acute illness. She reported that 2 months ago

her hemoglobin A_{1C} was 6.2. As a result, the focus of teaching during this hospitalization would include awareness of the specific precipitating factor that caused the present DKA episode and a plan to prevent future occurrences. Teaching would focus on the management of diabetes during acute illness and the importance of early communication with the physician during acute illness to prevent ketoacidosis or to treat it early.

Case 2

1. Mr. S's creatinine and BUN are both elevated, pointing to renal failure. With the presence of both renal failure and heart failure, the nurse will expect fluid intolerance and third spacing of fluid into the lungs and interstitial spaces. Fluid volume overload will be a problem even in the presence of severe dehydration. Because of this complication the nurse would anticipate placement of a Swan-Ganz catheter to accurately measure the outcomes of fluid volume replacement.

2. Albuterol causes bronchodilation by relaxing the smooth muscles of the respiratory tree. It is used to improve oxygenation. Dexamethasone is a glucocorticoid steroid. It has anti-inflammatory effects and is also used to improve oxygenation during pneumonia. Both albuterol and dexamethasone increase the blood sugar. The nurse would anticipate the use of increased doses of insulin to meet the goal of decreasing the blood glucose by 50 to 70 mg/dL per hour.

3. Based on a hemoglobin A_{1C} of 10.5, Mr. S's average blood sugar for the preceding 2 to 3 months ranged between 275 and 310 mg/dL. Mr. S is at significant risk for long-term complications such as retinopathy, peripheral and autonomic neuropathy, systemic vascular disease, and renal failure. Mr. S already has vascular complications, including a history of myocardial infarction, heart failure, and renal failure. The nurse would plan education and encouragement regarding the poor control of his blood glucose readings. A multidisciplinary approach would be helpful. The physician will review the prescribed medications. A certified diabetic educator (CDE), if available, would be very helpful to help with teaching and guiding decisions. It would also be very important to involve close family members or significant others in the teaching and coaching sessions.

4. The following complications are listed with rationales for their development and assessments that would indicate their presence:
   a. Fluid volume overload would be a common complication for Mr. S due to his preexisting heart failure and renal failure. Important assessments would be decreasing oxygen saturation, decreasing arterial oxygenation, high-pressure alarms on the ventilator, worsening lung sounds, decreased urine output, and changes on chest x-ray.
   b. Adult respiratory distress syndrome (ARDS) is a possibility due to pneumonia in addition to intracellular fluid shifts during rehydration. Either one of these conditions by themselves could predispose Mr. S to ARDS, though Mr. S has both problems. Initial assessments indicating the presence of ARDS include diffuse rales and diffuse infiltrates on chest x-ray. In contrast, pneumonia is detected by coarse rhonchi in a specific area of the lungs.
   c. Cerebral edema might develop as a result of intracellular fluid shifts during rehydration. The nurse would assess for headache, lethargy, confusion, and irritability to identify early signs of cerebral edema. A CT scan can also help to identify cerebral edema.
   d. Thrombosis is a complication that Mr. S might develop as a result of severely high serum osmolarity in addition to preexisting vascular disease (evidenced by prior heart attack, heart failure, and renal failure). Thromboses could cause a variety of problems including:
      • Myocardial infarction, identified by chest pain or pressure, and changes on the 12 lead ECG
      • Stroke, identified by inability to speak, one-sided facial droop, and/or one-sided muscle weakness
      • Deep vein thrombosis, evidenced by unilateral swelling of an extremity and abnormal peripheral vascular studies
      • Pulmonary embolism, evidenced by chest pain, hypoxia, and abnormal pulmonary vascular studies

Chapter 13: Answers to Critical Thinking Questions

1. Infection, conditions that induce stress (MI, CVA, trauma, or surgery), pregnancy, medications (especially steroids), and misuse of alcohol are the most common precipitating factors.

2. The patient with DKA often presents with metabolic acidosis, whereas the patient with HHNS usually does not. The patient with HHNS will often have visual disturbances such as blurred vision due to the increased blood osmolality.

3. The nurse must assess the patient's potassium level and prepare for potassium replacement. The nurse must also assess the patient's volume status and must have initiated volume replacement. In addition, the nurse checks the patient's pH, bicarbonate level, serum sodium, calcium, phosphate, and magnesium.

4. Medications that can increase the blood sugar include steroids, thiazide diuretics, calcium channel blockers, propranolol, phenytoin, and sympathomimetics.

5. Common complications following treatment of DKA and HHNS include hypoglycemia, hypokalemia, fluid volume overload with heart failure, cerebral edema, and ARDS.

6. The risk factors include central obesity, abnormal lipid panel, fasting blood glucose greater than 110 mg/dL, and hyperinsulinemia.

7. Hyperglycemia has been shown to cause an inflammatory response, resulting in damage to the endothelium of blood vessels. Even short periods of hypoglycemia during critical illness have been linked to poorer patient outcomes. Therefore, attempts are made to maintain the blood glucose between 80 and 110 mg/dL.

Chapter 14: Answers to Case Study Questions

1. She is dehydrated and requires immediate volume replacement.

2. Her BUN, creatinine, and potassium indicate that she is in renal failure.

3. Her CK might be so elevated from muscle breakdown due to her prolonged period on the floor.

4. The most likely cause of her renal failure is rhabdomyolysis, which can result in myoglobin blocking structures in the kidney and cause renal failure. However, her volume depletion and subsequent hypotension probably also contributed to the ARF.

5. Volume replacement (her H & H indicate that she is in need of volume replacement) would be the first essential collaborative management step and should also increase her BP.

   If her renal perfusion and urine output improved following volume replacement, then she would most likely be observed to determine that her BUN, creatinine, and CK returned to more normal levels. Hydration is key to management of rhabdomyolysis.

6. Renal replacement therapy would most likely be delayed until her response to hydration was determined and her BP increased.

Chapter 14: Answers to Critical Thinking Questions

1. In prerenal causes of ARF, urinalysis typically shows a concentrated urine with a high osmolality (greater than 500 mOsm/L) and a decreased urine sodium (less than 20 mmol/L). The fractional excretion of sodium (FENa), a test for assessing how well the kidneys can concentrate urine and conserve sodium, is usually less than 1%. There are rarely more than a few casts and/or a little sediment present in the urine. In intrinsic renal failure, urinalysis typically reveals an osmolality less than 350 mOsm/L, an increased urine sodium (greater than 40 mmol/L), and FENa greater than 1% with granular casts and sediment.

2. Intrinsic or intrarenal failure is primarily caused by a prolonged reduction in renal perfusion but may also be precipitated by other conditions, including nephrotoxic agents. By maintaining an adequate MAP and ensuring renal perfusion as well as avoiding administration of nephrotoxic agents, the nurse may help to prevent ARF.

3. • Hyperkalemia.
   • It may result in death from diastolic arrest or ventricular fibrillation.
   • Potassium may be counteracted with IV calcium or driven intracellularly with insulin and glucose or sodium bicarbonate. Longer term reductions in potassium might be achieved with a cation exchange resin or renal replacement therapy.

4. Peritoneal dialysis is often not speedy or efficient enough to adequately remove the midsized wastes such as urea that accumulate rapidly in catabolic ARF patients. Second, the volume of fluid that is placed in the peritoneum in PD tends to have a negative impact on respiratory function. Lastly, several studies have demonstrated poorer outcomes for patients who received PD rather than other modalities of treatment for AR.

5. Daily hemodialysis results in a higher rate of return of renal function and decreased mortality for critically ill patients in ARF. Excess fluid can be removed as quickly as the patient can tolerate and electrolyte imbalances may be returned to normal more quickly.

6. Dialysis disequilibrium is especially common in patients undergoing their first or second dialysis treatment who experience sudden, large decreases in their BUN. The most likely explanation for this syndrome is that the levels of urea do not drop as rapidly in the brain as the plasma because of the blood-brain barrier. The higher levels of urea in the brain result in an osmotic concentration gradient between the brain cells and the plasma. Fluid enters the brain cells by osmosis until the concentration levels equal that of the extracellular fluid, resulting in cerebral edema and the dialysis disequilibrium syndrome. Manifestations of the syndrome include:
   • Headache and mental impairment that may progress to confusion, agitation, and seizures
   • Nausea that may lead to vomiting

7. Convection occurs when replacement fluid flows through the filter at a fast rate (1,000 to 2,000 mL/hr), creating a "solute drag" that removes fluids and small to midsized molecules.

8. Rapid pulse of bounding quality.
   Skin that is pale and cool to the touch.
   An elevated BP, possibly with decreased pulse pressure.
   One of the earliest indications of fluid excess, occurring prior to the development of edema, may be a gradual increase in BP.
   Jugular venous distention and/or hepatojugular reflex.
   Nonpitting edema in dependent areas.
   Increased CVP or PAWP.
   Increased respiratory rate with shallow respirations.
   Dyspnea on exertion or in supine position
   Crackles in bases on auscultation.
   Increase in weight.

Chapter 15: Answers to Case Study Questions

1. Donation from a sibling would most likely provide David with a better match from a healthy donor. He would also be ensured of a kidney and most likely be able to receive the kidney at a much earlier date than if he were to receive one from a deceased individual. Donation from a live individual also allows for planning of the donation and immunosuppression to begin at the optimal time prior to donation.

2. David's sister is a better match because she is a O antigen mismatch. A person with B positive blood can donate to someone with AB positive.

3. The health status of the donor needs to be assessed, including:

   David was scheduled to receive a transplant. Immediately prior to surgery, his BP was 167/92. His lab studies revealed that his creatinine was 8.1 and BUN 83. His potassium was 5.5, and hematocrit 26. His donated kidney began working immediately and by later that day his creatinine had decreased to 6. On day 3, he was feeling well, was up and walking, and his creatinine was 1.3, BP 132/84. He was discharged home, taking prednisone, Cell-Cept, and tacrolimus.

4. David should be told to contact his health care provider or transplant center for signs and symptoms of rejection or

infection. Symptoms of acute rejection of a transplanted kidney include:
Weight gain, edema, and an increase in blood pressure
Fever, chills, and elevated WBC
Graft swelling and tenderness

5. Many transplant centers continue to instruct their patients to:
   • Wash their hands before putting anything in or near their mouth and after toileting
   • Wear a mask when in a crowd for the first few months post transplant
   • Remove plants and flowers in vases from their homes
   • Wash, peel, and/or cook all fruits and vegetables
   • Avoid exposure to live vaccines
   • Avoid environments contaminated by mold, fungus, or water damage
   • Obtain prophylactic antibiotics prior to dental procedures

6. The tremors are a common side effect of the tacrolimus that David is taking for immunosuppression.

7. David is most likely having an acute episode of rejection. He will need to consult his transplant center, will probably be hospitalized, will be provided with increased doses of immunosuppressant medications, and will probably require a change in his normal medication regimen.

8. Long-term use of steroids can result in aseptic necrosis of the hip.

Chapter 15: Answers to Critical Thinking Questions

1. An individual may "opt in" to the donor system by signing an organ donor card, stating that she desires to have her organs donated, if it is possible, after she dies. A system that uses "opting out" assumes that a potential donor would want to donate and proceeds with the donation unless the family objects.

2. Brain death is the irreversible loss of function of the brain, including the brainstem. The criteria for the clinical diagnosis of brain death include:
   —Evidence of an acute neurological catastrophe that is compatible with the clinical diagnosis of brain death
   —Exclusion of complicating medical conditions that may confound clinical assessment (no severe electrolyte, acid-base, or endocrine disturbance)
   —Absence of drug intoxication or poisoning
   —Core temperature of 32°C (90°F)
      The three cardinal findings in brain death are coma or unresponsiveness, absence of brainstem reflexes, and apnea.

3. When and how the family is approached about organ donation affects whether they will donate. Families are more likely to donate organs if:
   • They are **not** asked to donate at the same time that they are informed their family member has died
   • They perceive that the timing of the request is optimal
   • They view the requestor as sensitive to their needs
   • They are approached in a quiet, private place where they can consider their options

   • An organ procurement specialist from an organ donor bank makes the request

4. Tacrolimus (FK-506) is associated with fewer episodes of acute rejection 1 year after kidney transplant than cyclosporine.

5. The factor most responsible for the predisposition to infection in recipients of transplanted organs is the use of immunosuppressants, which alter the body's normal protective responses. Two other major contributing factors to the patient's immediate posttransplant likelihood of infection are the preoperative condition of the patient and nosocomial factors.

6. The development of CMV has been demonstrated to contribute to acute and/or chronic allograft injury and dysfunction as well as to an increased risk for opportunistic bacterial, viral, and fungal infections.

7. Hyperacute rejection usually results in loss of the transplanted organ.
   Accelerated rejection occurs when the recipient has been sensitized to some of the donor antigens resulting in immediate damage to the transplanted organ.
   Acute rejection is a cell-mediated immune response that results in T lymphocytes infiltrating the donated organ and damaging it by secreting lysosomal enzymes and lymphokines.
   Chronic rejection is a combination of humoral and cell-mediated immune responses that usually results in progressive deterioration in organ function. Chronic rejection is more likely to result in loss of an organ or death.

8. If at all possible, nutritional requirements are provided enterally because parenteral nutrition is associated with increased risk of infection in the transplant recipient.

9. Cardiac allograph vasculopathy (CAV), an aggressive diffuse form of arteriosclerosis, is common in heart transplant recipients, occurring in 40% to 50% of them 5 years after surgery. Unlike the stenoses that develop in CAD that are localized to one section of an artery, CAV can affect the entire length of an artery in the transplanted heart.

10. Health care providers have not been successful at identifying ways to predict a patient's compliance with the complex posttransplant regimens. Therefore, it is unclear which patients are most likely to be noncompliant post transplant. Noncompliance appears to be relatively common during the first year after transplantation and tends to worsen as time from transplantation increases. Nurses can help by working with the individual patient to determine what issues (e.g., changes in physical appearance, cost of medications, the complexity of the regiment, feeling of split personality or depression) may be making it difficult for the person to comply with therapy.

Chapter 16: Answers to Case Study Questions

1. Jon has no clothing on his upper body; the burn process has stopped. Attempting to cool him now may induce hypothermia.

2. Immediate signs of inhalation injury are changes to the mucosal lining of the oropharynx and larynx, including

the presence of soot, edema, or blisters. Symptoms of direct injury occur over the first 24 hours and include stridor, hypoxia, and respiratory distress.

3. The ED team will secure an airway and most likely intubate the patient if they suspect inhalation injury. Carboxyhemoglobin levels should be obtained for individuals burned within an enclosed space or with signs indicating inhalation injury. If inhalation injury is suspected, a bronchoscopy may be performed.

4. The location and appearance of all burn wounds should be assessed as to size and depth of injury. Patients with burns to the chest that are deep or circumferential are at increased risk for developing respiratory problems and may require eschartomies to ensure adequate respiration. All extremities should be assessed for circumferential burns to identify areas at risk for loss of perfusion as burn edema progresses. Peripheral nerve stimulation is difficult to do on edematous areas but should be attempted if circumferential extremity burns are present. A diagram of the burn injury should be drawn during the burn assessment using either the rule of nines or the Lund and Browder Chart (see Figures 16-1 and 16-2). The percentage TBSA of second- and third-degree burns, and the total % TBSA burned, should be calculated.

5. Lactated Ringer's is the preferred fluid for resuscitation because it is most like normal extracellular fluid. Normal saline contains a large amount of chloride and if a burn patient gets large amounts of chloride, there is a potential for metabolic acidosis. Fluid that contains dextrose is not used because it does not contain any electrolytes and the patient may be glucose intolerant. The amount of fluid that is required is calculated by whichever specific formula the burn unit recommends. Generally, adults and children with burns greater than 20% TBSA should undergo formal fluid resuscitation using estimates based on body size and surface area burned. "Common formulas used to initiate resuscitation estimate a crystalloid need for 2 to 4 ml/kg body weight/%TBSA during the first 24 hours."

   The nurse will know that fluid replacement is adequate by the amount of urine that Jon is producing. He should be maintaining a urine output of 100 mL/hr.

6. Jon most likely sustained these injuries when he jumped through his second floor window. Although they will require treatment, he is currently able to move all his extremities and they are not life threatening.

7. Ventilator settings
   Complete assessment, including a neurological assessment
   Estimation of extent of burn
   Calculation of fluid resuscitation needs
   Medications administered (pain, tetanus, etc.)
   History of the event
   Availability of family

8. Potential for renal failure
   Development of edema and potential need for an escharotomy
   Potential for pneumonia and ARDS
   Potential for development of peptic ulcer
   Risk of infection

9. Maintaining adequate fluid resuscitation
   Initiating prophylaxis for peptic ulcer
   Instituting VAP protocol
   Instituting CVC protocol
   Maintaining aseptic technique

Chapter 16: Answers to Critical Thinking Questions

1. The most common burns are thermal in nature and are caused by exposure to heat. Thermal burns include fire/flame injuries, scald injuries from exposure to hot liquids or steam, and contact/friction. Scald injuries are the most common form of burns, but fire/flame injuries account for the majority of deaths.

2. A partial-thickness, or second-degree, burn involves the epidermal and dermal layers of the skin, but the hair follicles, sebaceous glands, and epidermal sweat glands remain intact. A second-degree burn is further classified by the amount of dermis involved into either a superficial or deep second-degree burn. A superficial second-degree burn does not involve the entire depth of the dermis. The burn wound is often bright red in color and edematous. Capillary refill is near normal. The surface is moist and thin-walled; fluid-filled blisters appear within minutes. A superficial second-degree burn is very painful and sensation to even very superficial pressure, such as air currents, is increased. Healing occurs within 21 days with little to no scarring.

   A deep second-degree burn involves the entire dermis. The wound appearance is white and waxy and capillary refill is decreased. The surface may be wet or dry and blisters can range from large and fluid filled to flat. There is less pain and decreased sensation even to deep touch. A deep second-degree burn heals in approximately 3 weeks and scarring is likely. Initially, a deep second-degree burn may appear to be a full-thickness burn but after 7 to 10 days skin buds and hair growth will be noticeable, indicating that the skin appendages are intact. However, some burns that initially appeared to be deep second-degree burns may progress to full-thickness injuries due to decreased blood supply or infection.

   A full-thickness, or third-degree, burn involves all layers of the skin, including the hair follicles, sebaceous glands, and the epidermal sweat glands. The wound color ranges from very pale to bright red; but unlike a second-degree burn, there is little to no capillary refill and thrombosed blood vessels may be evident. The surface of the wound is dry and firm and may have a leathery feel. A third-degree burn has no sensation to deep pressure and there is no pain because the nerve endings have been destroyed.

3. Immediate signs of inhalation injury are changes to the mucosal lining of the oropharynx and larynx, including the presence of soot, edema, or blisters. Symptoms of direct injury occur over the first 24 hours and include stridor, hypoxia, and respiratory distress.

4. A burn injury can cause a variety of cardiovascular system changes, particularly in individuals with preexisting cardiovascular disease. The most common cardiovascular change is hypovolemic or burn shock. Other changes include alterations in cardiac rhythm and peripheral extremity vascular compromise.

Within minutes of a burn injury, increased capillary permeability in burned areas where the microcirculation is not destroyed results in edema formation. The extent of edema depends on burn severity and body parts affected. Burn edema is greatest over areas where the skin is less elastic, such as the face and genitals, and less over areas with increased elasticity, such as the extremities. Increased vascular permeability is present for approximately the first 24 hours after injury.

This increased capillary permeability explains the need for immediate fluid resuscitation and the potential for severe edema and altered tissue perfusion.

5. The immediate priorities when a burn victim arrives at a hospital are the same as for any trauma victim, the ABCs.

6. Full-thickness burn wounds require grafting.

7. Patients vary in how they respond to a burn injury depending on their previous coping skills and their social support. At first the burn survivor may not be aware of the seriousness of the injury. However, with realization may come fear, which can contribute to the patient's perception of pain. Patients may use disassociation, disintegration, and depersonalization to cope with the injury. As their body image changes and functional limitations become apparent, they may experience depression. Most patients recover from the emotional turmoil and return to leading productive lives.

8. Children are at increased likelihood for burn injury due to their impulsivity. Both children and older adults may be unable to move away from a burn source, making them more likely to be injured. They both also have thinner skin, making it more likely that they will suffer more severe burn injuries at lower temperatures. Finally older adults may be more likely to suffer burn injures due to cognitive and sensory impairments.

Chapter 17: Answers to Case Study Questions

1. a. Maintenance of adequate air exchange

   Check the patient's airway.
   Determine his ventilation (check his O_2 saturation, note the effect of PEEP on his ICP and BP, check his ABGs, position him appropriately).
   Check the functioning of his chest tube (note drainage and crepitus about the insertion site).
   b. Maintenance of adequate circulation and perfusion

   Monitor for blood loss (determine possible sites, check Hgb and Hct).
   Monitor BP, pulse, and urine output.
   Determine the appropriate position and level of HOB.
   Provide volume replacement as indicated.
   Provide pressors as needed.
   c. Assessment of neurological status

   Assess the level of neurological functioning (on and off sedation), compare to pre-op.
   Maintain HOB level.
   Check functioning of the Jackson-Pratt drain.
2. Pain relief
   Provision of adequate nutrition
   Prevention of infection
   Identification of potential alcohol withdrawal and prevention

Stabilization of leg and prevention of further injuries

3. Ensure accurate set-up.
   Monitor drainage, tidaling, bubbling in suction control chamber.
   Prevent dependent loops.
   Assess the insertion site for crepitus and drainage on the dressing
   Position the patient upright if possible; turn every 2 hours for air removal.

4. Ventilator bundle

5. Sinusitis
   Neurosurgical site
   Lungs from VAP
   Central lines
   Urinary catheter
   Left leg

6. • Temperature greater than 38°C (100.4°F) or less than 36°C (96.8°F)
   • Pulse greater than 90 beats per minute
   • Respiratory rate greater than 20 breaths/minute or $PaCO_2$ less than 32 torr
   • WBC greater than 12,000/mm³ or less than 4,000/mm³

7. Yes, he meets all of the criteria.

8. He meets the criteria. Severe sepsis occurs when dysfunction of two or more organ systems develops in response to hypoperfusion.
   • Acute lung injury indicated by tachypnea and/or hypoxemia
   • Coagulation abnormalities or thrombocytopenia
   • Neurological dysfunction indicated by a sudden change in mental status with possible confusion or psychosis
   • Renal dysfunction evidenced by a decreased urine output for at least 2 hours and an increase in serum creatinine greater than 0.5 mg/dL
   • Liver dysfunction indicated by jaundice, coagulopathy, decreased protein C levels, and increased D-dimer levels
   • Gastrointestinal injury indicated by stress ulceration, ileus (absent bowel sounds), and malabsorption
   • Cardiac dysfunction indicated by tachycardia, dysrhythmias, hypotension with decreased CVP or PA pressures, and either high or low cardiac outputs
   • Hypotension with lactic acidosis

   He also meets the criteria for septic shock. The most severe form of sepsis is defined as the presence of sepsis and refractory hypotension. Refractory hypotension is a systolic BP less than 90 mm Hg, a mean arterial pressure less than 65 mm Hg, or a decrease of 40 mm Hg in systolic BP that is unresponsive to a crystalloid fluid challenge of 20 to 40 mL/kg.

9. Xigris is inappropriate due to recent neurosurgery and would therefore not be used.

10. A continuous infusion of norepinephrine and/or low dose dopamine might possibly be useful to increase his blood pressure. Controversy surrounds their effects on kidney function.

11. PEEP might be increased with caution for ARDS to improve his oxygenation, but will likely affect his BP adversely so the nurse will need to monitor his blood pressure closely.

12. Rather than increasing his current sedation, which does not appear to be working, it might be worth trying a different sedative.

13. Yes, he has already developed ARDS (see Respiratory assessment) and most likely also has acute renal failure.

Chapter 17: Answers to Critical Thinking Questions

1. The majority of septic patients, approximately 70% of them, receive care in an intensive care, coronary care, or intermediate care unit. Sepsis affects the elderly disproportionately; more than half of all annual costs—$8.7 billion—were spent on care of septic patients 65 years or older. Because sepsis rates rise sharply with age, as the nation ages the incidence of sepsis will increase. There will be almost a million cases of sepsis in the United States by the year 2010.

2. Elevation of the head of the bed (HOB) to at least 30 degrees is recommended because it reduces the risk of aspiration of oropharyngeal contents.

3. The elements of the central line bundle are hand hygiene, maximal barrier precautions upon insertion, chlorhexidine skin antisepsis, optimal catheter site selection, and daily review of line necessity with prompt removal of unnecessary lines.

4. Evidence suggests that shaving a surgical site results in an increase in surgical site infections. Therefore, if the site must be cleared, either clipping the hair or using a depilatory is recommended.

5. • Temperature greater than 38°C (100.4°F) or less than 36°C (96.8°F)
   • Pulse greater than 90 beats per minute
   • Respiratory rate greater than 20 breaths/minute or $PaCO_2$ less than 32 torr
   • WBC greater than 12,000/mm³ or less than 4,000/mm³

6. • Does the patient have a cough or a change in the character of his sputum that might indicate a pulmonary source of infection?
   • Is the patient experiencing nausea, vomiting, or diarrhea? Does he have abdominal pain or rebound tenderness that might indicate an abdominal source of infection?
   • Has the patient been experiencing dysurea, frequency of urination, or pain at the costovertebral angle that could be indicative of a renal source of infection?
   • Does the patient have a new murmur or a change in a murmur, possibly indicating endocarditis?
   • Does the patient have a headache or a change in mental status or neurological findings that might indicate a neurological focus of infection?
   • Does the patient have redness, tenderness, or drainage at the sites of any implants, catheters, or medical devices?

7. Measure serum lactate.
   Obtain blood cultures prior to antibiotic administration.
   Administer broad-spectrum antibiotic within 3 hours of ED admission.
   In the event of hypotension or serum lactate greater than 4, deliver an initial crystalloid or colloid bolus and apply vasopressors if there is no response to volume repletion.

8. The following elements of the sepsis management bundle have had questions about their effectiveness by some practitioners:
   Administer low-dose steroids.
   Administer Drotrecogin Alfa.
   Maintain blood glucose greater than 80 but less than or equal to 150.

9. Unless a fever is severely elevated, the patient is very uncomfortable, or the patient is at risk for compromise from the fever, there may be no attempt to actively reduce the fever. Critical care nurses need to observe their patients with fever to determine if the fever is resulting in cardiovascular compromise or excessive metabolic demands. Fevers are more likely to result in compromise in very old patients, neonates, neurological patients with increased intracranial pressure or seizures, and patients with cardiovascular disease.

10. A trigger activates the coagulation cascade. Thrombin production, which should be balanced by chemical mediators, is not and continues unrestrained. The excessive thrombin production activates fibrinogen, resulting in the formation of fibrin. Fibrin is deposited throughout the microcirculation, leading to obstruction of blood vessels and ischemic tissue damage. As the fibrin deposits are formed, platelets and coagulation factors are consumed, leading to a deficiency of clotting factors and the patient begins to bleed. The bleeding may be intensified as the clots are lysed, resulting in fibrin degradation products (FDPs) because the FDPs are anticoagulants. Thus, the patient develops simultaneous thrombic and hemorrhagic complications.

Chapter 18: Answers to Case Study Questions

1. First, the nurse will need to establish trust with the son and the physician. Then, the nurse should attempt to gather the multidisciplinary team for a meeting. She should also ask social services to determine who is the legitimate spokesperson for Armand. In the meantime, she should be attentive to Armand, providing compassionate care and observing for any signs of returning consciousness.

2. The nurse needs to have an understanding of what Armand might have wanted, who the appropriate spokesperson is for him now, and what his physiological status is. How likely is he to benefit from the dialysis? What would be the burden of continuing care?

3. The nurse might agree that Armand's stepson was using substituted judgment to decide. In this case, the nurse would be persuaded that Armand's stepson understood Armand and was speaking honestly and authentically on his behalf. The nurse might weigh the benefits and burdens of the treatment and concur with Armand's stepson that the benefits did not outweigh the burdens or with the surgeon that the potential benefit (Armand's continued life) was worth the burden of dialysis.

4. The nurse can advocate at a multidisciplinary team meeting for what she believes Armand would have wanted or what was in his best interests. If she felt that the situation was not resolved after the team meeting, she could call for a meeting of the hospital ethics committee.

5. Learner's own position.

Chapter 18: Answers to Critical Thinking Questions

1. Yes, families should be able to be present IF they desire to be present and there are resources available for their support during the resuscitation. The benefits to the family in most situations clearly outweigh the discomfort experienced by some members of the health care team. Most studies reveal few, if any, untoward effects.

2. When an advance directive is in place that clearly delineates what the patient would want done in the specific situation and the patient has not changed her mind, the directive presents a clear indication of what care should be provided at the end of life.

3. The directive may be out of date, may not provide adequate guidance in the clinical situation, or the appointed health care proxy may not have a clear understanding of what the role entails or what the patient would have wanted to have done.

4. Families of patients dying in critical care units have identified needs to be helpful to the dying patient and to be assured of the patient's comfort. They want to be informed about the patient's condition as well as what is being done for the patient. They want to be comforted and allowed to ventilate their emotions. They need reassurance that their decisions are correct. Nurses can assist families by being present for the patient and the family and acting to meet the identified needs of the family.

5. If an ongoing medical treatment is not capable of benefiting the patient, most ethicists do not view withdrawing the treatment as the direct cause of the patient's death. The cause of death in such a circumstance would be the relentless progression of the patient's disease. Thus, when an intervention is neither enhancing the care of the patient nor promoting the patient's recovery, the intervention may be withdrawn.

6. Terminal weaning involves the gradual reduction in settings on the ventilator; a change to synchronized intermittent mechanical ventilation with pressure support, a decrease in the respiratory rate, a reduction in the FiO_2, and, finally, the discontinuation of the ventilator and provision of humidified room air by T piece. Terminal extubation involves removal of the endotracheal tube and discontinuation of the ventilator.

7. Withdrawal of a medical intervention has been classified as a "passive" action, allowing death to occur from the disease process. However, assisted death is an active process in which the health care provider takes an action that directly results in the patient's death. It is illegal in all states and most countries.

8. First, the nurse needs to establish trust among the patient, family, and other health care providers. Then they need to develop a common understanding of the patient's prognosis and the benefits and burdens of treatment. A multidisciplinary team meeting can help this to occur. If conflict continues, the nurse can suggest an ethics committee consultation.

Glossary

Absolute refractory period   The brief period during depolarization of the cardiac cell membrane when the cardiac cells will not respond to further stimulation.

Accelerated rejection   The recipient has been sensitized to some of the donor antigens.

Acute coronary syndrome   Umbrella term used to describe conditions that cause chest pain due to inadequate blood flow to the myocardium.

Acute lung injury (ALI)   Considered the pulmonary symptom of multiple organ dysfunction syndrome (MODS). The most severe form of ALI is **acute respiratory distress syndrome** (ARDS).

Acute rejection   A cell-mediated immune response that results in T lymphocytes infiltrating the donated organ and damaging it by secreting lysosomal enzymes and lymphokines.

Acute respiratory distress syndrome (ARDS)   The most severe form of acute lung injury.

Acute respiratory failure (ARF)   Failure of the pulmonary system to provide sufficient exchange of oxygen to supply the body's demands.

Advance directives   Allow competent patients to indicate in advance the kind of health care treatment they would desire should they become incapacitated at the end of their lives.

Adverse effect   Injury caused by medical management rather than the underlying condition of the patient.

Afterload   The pressure (resistance) against which the right or left ventricle has to pump to eject the blood.

Airways   (Nasopharyngeal or oropharyngeal); designed to hold the tongue away from the pharynx, preventing occlusion of the upper airway.

Alcohol withdrawal syndrome   Withdrawal of the depressant effects of alcohol that results in excitability of the central nervous system.

Alcoholic hallucinosis   The patient experiences perceptual disturbances—usually visual, auditory, or tactile phenomena—without sensorial alterations. The patient is fully conscious, aware of the environment, acknowledging that the hallucinations are related to the substance dependence and withdrawal.

Anabolic hormone   A hormone that synthesizes simple hormones into a more complicated hormone. Insulin is an anabolic hormone.

Angina pectoris   An oppressive pain or pressure in the chest caused by inadequate oxygenation and blood flow to the heart muscle.

Angioedema   Swelling of the skin and mucous membranes.

Anxiety   A subjective feeling of distress and anguish.

Ascites   The accumulation of a large amount of protein-rich fluid in the peritoneal cavity.

Astrocytomas   The most common types of malignant brain tumors.

Atherosclerosis   The most common form of arteriosclerosis marked by cholesterol-lipid-calcium deposits in the walls of the arteries.

Atrioventricular (AV) node   A pacemaker of the heart that is part of the electrical conduction pathway between the atria and ventricles and which, if not stimulated from the SA node, can spontaneously generate electrical impulses at a rate of 40 to 60 beats per minute.

Automaticity   The ability of certain cardiac cells to spontaneously initiate an electrical impulse.

Beck's triad   Signs seen with a pericardial tamponade that include hypotension, distended neck veins, and muffled heart sounds.

Brain death   The irreversible loss of function of the brain, including the brainstem.

Brain tumors   Classified as primary or metastatic. Most metastatic brain tumors arise from the lungs, breast, and skin. Primary brain tumors may be either benign or malignant.

B-type natriuretic peptide   A peptide released in response to increased ventricular filling pressures. Normal levels are 0 to 100 pg/mL.

Bundle of His   The initial part of the ventricular conduction system that penetrates the AV valves, and then bifurcates into the right and left bundle branches to bring electrical stimulation to the right and left ventricles.

Carbohydrates   Monosaccharides, disaccharides, and polysaccharides.

Cardiac cycle   The sequence of events related to the flow of blood from the beginning of one heartbeat to the beginning of the next.

Cardiac index   Cardiac output divided by the body surface area.

Cardiac output   The volume of blood ejected by the left ventricle every minute, determined by heart rate and stroke volume.

Cardiopulmonary resuscitation   Provision of ventilation and compressions in an effort to sustain life.

Cardioversion   Electrical shocks through the chest wall and heart that are synchronized with the QRS complex of the patient's cardiac rhythm.

Central venous pressure (CVP)   Measures the right-sided preload via a catheter placed in a central vein such as the subclavian or internal jugular. Normal CVP is 2 to 6 mm Hg (mean).

Cerebral perfusion pressure (CPP) The difference between the pressure of the incoming blood (best measured as the mean arterial pressure [MAP]) and the force opposing perfusion of the brain, the intracranial pressure (ICP). The formula is: CPP = MAP − ICP.

Cerebrospinal fluid leakages Occur when there is a tear in the dura, allowing an opening to develop between the subarachnoid space and the outside.

Chemoreceptors Central scrutinize the level of the hydrogen ion in the blood, while peripheral chemoreceptors monitor oxygen levels as well as carbon dioxide and hydrogen ion levels responding to these changes by stimulating acceleration or slowing of the ventilation rate.

Chronic rejection A combination of humoral and cell-mediated immune responses that usually results in progressive deterioration in organ function.

Closed ICU Patient care provided by a dedicated ICU team that includes a critical care physician.

Colloids Solutions that have protein in them, either natural or synthetic. Blood is a colloid.

Colonoscopy Involves the insertion of the endoscope into the anus to examine the colon or large intestine from the rectum to the ileocecal valve.

Compassion fatigue A "state of tension and preoccupation with the suffering of those being helped that is traumatizing for the helper."

Compliance The expansibility of the thorax and lungs as measured by the increase in lung volumes in comparison to increases in intra-alveolar pressure.

Conductivity The ability of cardiac cells to transmit an electrical impulse to adjacent cardiac cells.

Continuous renal replacement therapy (CRRT) An umbrella term for several methods of dialysis that allow for continuous fluid removal from the plasma (known as ultrafiltrate). The modalities differ in the principles, accesses, technology requirements, and nursing interventions.

Contractility The ability of cardiac cells to shorten in response to electrical stimulation.

Coronary artery bypass graft Surgical intervention that establishes collateral circulation from the aorta or internal mammary artery to a branch of a coronary artery at a point past an atherosclerotic lesion or blockage.

Cortical mapping Allows the surgeon to identify and avoid "eloquent" areas of the brain.

Creatine phosphokinase An enzyme that catalyzes the reversible transfer of high-energy phosphate and phosphocreatine. The specific isoform in cardiac muscle is CK-MB.

Critical care Direct delivery of medical care to a critically ill or injured patient.

Critical care nursing Specialty that deals specifically with human responses to life-threatening problems.

Critically ill patient A patient with an illness or injury that acutely impairs one or more vital organ systems such that the patient's survival is jeopardized.

Crossmatch The lymphocytes of the donor are mixed with the serum of the recipient. If the recipient has antibodies to the white cells of the donor, the cells are destroyed. This is called a "positive" crossmatch and means that the transplant is contraindicated.

Crystalloids Solutions of mineral salts or other water-soluble molecules. Normal saline is a crystalloid.

Dead space When an alveolus is not perfused and no gas exchange is occurring.

Defibrillation Unsynchronized electrical shocks administered through the chest wall and heart to depolarize myocardial cells in an attempt and restore sinus rhythm.

Delirium tremens (DTs) Also called alcohol withdrawal delirium; the most severe complication of withdrawal.

Depolarization The electrical state that exists at the cardiac cell membrane when the electrical charges are opposite the resting (polarized) state; the inside of the cell is more positively charged than the outside of the cell.

Diabetes insipidus Develops in 40% to 70% of deceased donors due to insufficient levels of antidiuretic hormone (ADH) and results in the production of large volumes of dilute urine.

Diabetic ketoacidosis (DKA) Caused primarily by insulin deficiency. Hyperglycemia is present (usually higher than 300 mg/dL). Although glucose continues to be absorbed into the bloodstream, the glucose is not transported into the cells because of the lack of insulin and cells "starve."

Diaphragm The primary muscle of ventilation.

Dicrotic notch A point on the arterial pressure waveform and the pulmonary artery pressure waveform that signals the end of systole.

Diffusion Solutes move across a semipermeable membrane from a solution where they are in higher concentration (the plasma) to a solution where they are in a lower concentration (the dialysate).

Disseminated intravascular coagulation or coagulopathy (DIC) Systemic intravascular activation of the coagulation cascade with fibrin formation and deposition in the microvasculature, resulting in simultaneous thrombic and hemorrhagic complications.

Diuretic phase of ARF Patients increase their urinary output, often producing up to 5 liters of urine each day but may not excrete wastes and regulate electrolyte or acid-base balance.

Diverticular disease Results from weak points on the intestinal wall that herniate to form a saclike projection called diverticula.

Do Not Resuscitate The decision not to provide cardiopulmonary resuscitation.

Dysphagia Difficulty swallowing.

Ejection fraction The percentage of blood ejected from the left ventricle with each contraction; normal is 55% to 75%.

Electrocardiogram A record of the electrical activity of the heart consisting of waves called P, Q, R, S, T, and sometimes U.

Electrophysiology   The study and intervention of cardiac dysrhythmias with the goal of restoring normal cardiac rhythm.

Embolic brain attacks or strokes   Particles arise from another part of the body and flow through the bloodstream, resulting in blockage of arterial blood flow to a particular area of the brain.

Endoscopy   A procedure that uses a flexible fiber-optic endoscope to directly visualize the inside of a hollow organ or cavity.

Endotracheal tubes   Tubes that are placed into the trachea via the nose or mouth in order to establish a patent and stable airway for patients.

Enteral nutrition   Delivery of nourishment by feeding tube into the gastrointestinal tract.

Epidural hematomas   Usually occur in conjunction with a skull fracture and result from a laceration of the middle meningeal artery, causing bleeding between the dura mater and the skull.

Epiglottis   Provides airway protection during ingestion of food and fluids by closing off the tracheal opening during swallowing.

Error   Failure of a planned action to be completed as intended or the use of a wrong plan to achieve an end.

Eschar   The hard crust that forms over the nonviable necrotic tissue.

Esophagogastroduodenoscopy   Upper GI endoscopy (EGD) that involves oral intubation with a flexible endoscope to visualize the esophagus, stomach, and proximal duodenum.

Ethical dilemma   A situation that gives rise to conflicting moral claims, resulting in disagreements about choices for action.

Excitability   A characteristic shared by all cardiac cells that refers to the ability to respond to an electrical impulse generated by pacemaker cells or other external stimuli.

Fats   Glycerides (such as triglycerides), phospholipids, and sterols (such as cholesterol).

Fractional excretion of sodium (FENa)   A test for assessing how well the kidneys can concentrate urine and conserve sodium, which is usually less than 1%.

Functional residual capacity (FRC)   The volume remaining in the lungs after a normal exhalation.

Futile treatment   Treatment that is without benefit (that provides neither palliation, restoration, nor cure) to the patient.

Glasgow Coma Scale   Scale used to determine a patient's level of consciousness; assesses both level of consciousness and motor response to a stimulus. Scores range from 3 to 15 based on the patient's ability to open the eyes, respond verbally, and move normally. Repeated assessments aid in determining if the patient's brain function is improving or deteriorating.

Glycogenesis   The conversion of excess glucose to glycogen.

Glycogenolysis   The formation of glucose from amino acids and fats when there is limited carbohydrate intake.

Glycosuria   Presence of glucose in the urine.

Heart failure   A clinical syndrome in which the ventricle is unable to fill or eject blood.

Helicobacter pylori   A highly mobile bacterium that avoids acid by burring underneath the mucosa. It causes the mucosa to be more susceptible to peptic acid.

Hematemesis   Vomiting of blood that is either bright red or has a coffee grounds appearance, indicating UGI bleeding.

Hematochezia   The passage of bright red blood from the rectum. It may or may not be mixed with stool. Hematochezia suggests a LGI bleed.

Hemodynamics   The study of forces that aid in the circulating blood throughout the body. These forces can be monitored by blood pressure, pulse rate, mental status, urinary output, and cardiac output.

Hemorrhage   Blood loss with organ compromise; threatens tissue perfusion or life.

Hepatic encephalopathy (HE)   Also known as portosystemic encephalopathy (PSE), HE is a condition characterized by a wide range of potentially reversible neuropsychiatric manifestations that occurs in patients with advanced liver disease and portal hypertension.

Hyperosmolar hyperglycemic nonketotic syndrome (HHNS)   Common in patients with type 2 diabetes. It is similar to DKA in that hyperglycemia is present. However, hyperglycemia is often more severe (usually greater than 600 mg/dL).

High-frequency oscillation (HFO)   Uses very small tidal volumes, allowing the lungs to retain higher volumes at end expiration.

Hollow organs   Organs that have a cavity or space inside (e.g., bladder or stomach).

Hydrocephalus   Blood in the subarachnoid space obliterates the arachnoidal villi, preventing absorption of cerebrospinal fluid (CSF), or blood within the ventricles blocks the foramen of Monroe, preventing drainage of CSF. It may lead to an increase in intracranial pressure and deterioration of the patient's neurological status.

Hydrolysis   Splitting of bonded fats and the addition of water to produce fatty acids and glycerol.

Hypercapnea   An elevated $PaCO_2$.

Hypercarbia   Elevation of pCO_2 above 45 mm Hg.

Hypovolemic shock   A shock state resulting from a loss of circulating volume.

Hypoxemia   A decreased PaO_2.

Infection   A pathologic process induced by a microorganism.

Informed consent   Has three components. The decision must be made voluntarily by a competent adult who understands his or her condition and the possible treatments.

Inotropic   Positive inotropes increase the contractility of the heart. Negative inotropes decrease the contractility.

Inspiratory reserve volume (IRV)   The volume of air one is able to inhale in addition to the V_T.

Intermittent hemodialysis (IHD)   Utilizes both ultrafiltration and diffusion to rapidly correct electrolyte imbalances, restore fluid balance, adjust acid-base balance, and remove wastes.

Intracerebral hemorrhage (ICH) Derived from bleeding of small arteries or arterioles directly into the brain, forming a localized hematoma that spreads along white matter tracts.

Intrarenal acute renal failure Commonly results from prolonged hypoperfusion of the kidney. The renal tubules respond to hypoxia with dysfunction, inflammation, and, possibly, necrosis.

Inverse ratio ventilation The normal ratio is reversed so that inspiration takes more time than expiration.

Involuntary euthanasia An action to end the patient's life is taken without the patient's consent.

Ischemia A temporary deficiency of blood flow to an organ or tissue.

Ketoacidosis Occurs as a result of buildup of fatty acids, metabolic acidosis happens when the blood becomes more acidic than body tissues.

Ketonuria Presence of ketones in the urine.

Ketosis More ketones are being formed than used for cellular metabolism, resulting in extra ketone bodies in the bloodstream.

Korsakoff's syndrome Selective memory disturbances and amnesia.

Kussmaul's respirations Deep and rapid respirations. The body's attempt to decrease carbon dioxide in order to compensate for metabolic acidosis.

Mean arterial pressure The average pressure over one cardiac cycle.

Mechanical ventilation Assists the breathing process in clients who cannot effectively ventilate independently.

Melena The passage of black tarry colored stool. It has a very characteristic foul odor.

Meningioma The most common type of benign brain tumor.

Meningitis Inflammation of the meninges and the underlying subarachnoid space that contains the cerebrospinal fluid. Depending on the development and duration of symptoms, meningitis may be classified as acute, subacute, or chronic.

Mild traumatic brain injury Head injury with patient having no or very limited loss of consciousness and GCS 13 or higher.

Moderate head injury (GCS 9–12); may be associated with a loss of consciousness for up to a day.

Moral distress Occurs when a nurse knows the right thing to do, yet institutional constraints prevent her from doing it.

Multiple organ dysfunction syndrome (MODS) The presence of altered organ function in an acutely ill patient such that homeostasis cannot be maintained without intervention.

Munro Kelly hypothesis Intracranial Volume (VIC) = Volume brain + Volume blood + Volume CSF + Volume lesion.

MVA Motor vehicle accident (aka MVC—motor vehicle crash).

Myocardial infarction The loss of living heart muscle as a result of coronary artery occlusion.

Myoglobin The iron-containing protein found in muscle cells that store oxygen for cells.

Necrosis The death of cells, tissues, or organs.

Negligence Composed of several specific elements, including a duty was owed, the duty was breached, the breach of the duty was the proximate cause of an injury to the patient, and damages resulted.

Non-heartbeating donor Donor who has sustained a devastating nonrecoverable neurological injury that did not result in brain death. The patient's proxy has determined in conjunction with the health care team that the patient would wish to have life-sustaining therapy withdrawn so that she could die and would want to donate her organs after death.

Nonoliguric acute renal failure Patient produces more than 400 mL of urine/day, usually about 1,000 mL/day, but does not excrete metabolic wastes and regulate electrolytes or acid-base balance.

Oliguric phase of acute renal failure The patient excretes less then 400 mL of urine/day.

Onset phase of acute renal failure Immediately follows the period of renal injury, the patient's urinary output typically decreases to 20% of normal and the BUN and creatinine may begin to increase.

Osmosis A solution (water) moves from an area of low solute concentration (the plasma) to an area of higher solute concentration (the dialysate).

Oxygen content The total amount of oxygen in the blood, including oxygen dissolved, hemoglobin level, and oxygen saturation.

Oxyhemoglobin dissociation curve The relationship between the two transport methods, the oxygen bound to hemoglobin and the oxygen dissolved in the serum.

P/F ratio The relationship between the PaO_2 and the FiO_2 (PaO_2/FiO_2) with normal values in healthy adults ranging from 400 to 500 mm Hg.

Pain "Whatever the person says it is, existing whenever he says it does."

Palliative care The goal of palliative care is the achievement of the best quality of life for dying patients and their families.

Pancreatitis A sudden inflammatory process of the pancreas.

Paracentesis The removal of fluid from the peritoneal space using a large-bore needle or catheter system.

Parenteral nutrition The infusion of nutrients using a venous catheter located in a large, usually central, vein.

Paroxysmal nocturnal dyspnea (PND) Dyspnea when the patient is lying flat; thought to be a sign of heart failure. Fluid that typically rests in the legs during the day when the individual is upright redistributes throughout the body (including the lungs) when recumbent.

Partial liquid ventilation The lungs are filled with 5 to 30 mL/kg of perfluorocarbon, a clear, odorless liquid with very low surface tension.

Peptic ulcer disease Ulcer in the stomach and the first part of the duodenum.

Percutaneous coronary intervention Any procedure in which catheters are placed within the coronary arteries to study them or open them when they are obstructed.

Peritoneal dialysis (PD) Uses osmosis and diffusion to produce a steady, gradual restoration of fluid, electrolyte, and acid-base balance while removing nitrogenous and other wastes.

Phlebostatic axis The reference point for the left atrium when leveling a pressure monitoring system. It is located at the fourth intercostal space halfway between the anterior-posterior diameter of the chest.

Polarization The electrical state that exists at the cardiac cell membrane when the cell is at rest; the inside of the cell is more negatively charged than the outside of the cell.

Portal hypertension Develops over time, is asymptomatic, and is responsible for an array of complications that can markedly reduce the life expectancy of the patient with chronic liver disease.

Postrenal acute renal failure Characterized by the sudden onset of anuria (production of less than 50 mL of urine/day) due to obstruction of the urinary tract.

Preload The stretch on the ventricular myocardium at end diastole.

Prerenal acute renal failure The nephrons and glomeruli are structurally and functionally normal and the glomerulofiltration rate decreases due to reduction in renal blood flow.

Primary survey Assessment of airway, breathing, circulation, and disability or neurological status.

Pruritus Itching.

Pulmonary artery wedge pressure The PAWP waveform is obtained when the balloon is inflated at the end of the PA catheter. This pressure reflects the left atrial pressure and indirectly the left ventricular end diastolic pressure. Normal PAWP is 8 to 12 mm Hg (mean).

Pulse pressure The difference between the systolic and diastolic blood pressure.

Purkinje fibers The terminal filaments of the electrical conduction system of the ventricles, which can generate electrical impulses at a rate of 20 to 40 beats per minute.

Recovery phase of acute renal failure Renal function returns to normal.

Refractory hypoxemia The decreased PaO_2 does not respond to increases in FiO_2.

Relative refractory period A brief period following the "absolute refractory period" of depolarization when some of the cardiac cells have repolarized; if they receive a stronger than normal stimulus, they may depolarize. It is also known as the "vulnerable period."

Remodeling Structural changes to the myocardium leading to chamber dilation and hypertrophy.

Repolarization The restoration of the polarized (resting) state at the cardiac cell membrane; the inside of the cell is more negatively charged than the outside of the cell.

Required request The regional organ donor bank must be notified when a patient is imminently dying so the organ bank can determine if the patient qualifies as an organ donor. If the patient does qualify but has not signed a donor card, the family must be asked if they are willing to donate the patient's organs.

Residual volume (RV) The volume of air that remains in the lungs following forced expiration beyond normal expiration, or the **expiratory reserve volume** (ERV).

Respiration The transport of oxygen and carbon dioxide between the alveoli and the pulmonary capillaries.

Right atrial pressure The RA pressure measures the right-sided preload through the proximal port of the PA catheter. Normal RA is 2 to 6 mm Hg (mean).

Rule of nines The body is divided into five areas, each with increments of 9% TBSA. These areas are the head and neck (9%), arms (9% each), anterior and posterior trunk (36%), anterior and posterior legs (18% each), and the perineum (1%).

SBAR A technique to guide nurses' communication to physicians in critical situations.

Secondary survey Head-to-toe assessment done to identify injuries.

Seizures Stereotyped behavior associated with electrographic abnormalities in the EEG.

Sepsis The development of SIRS accompanied by the presence or presumed presence of infection.

Septic shock The presence of sepsis and refractory hypotension (systolic BP less than 90 mm Hg, mean arterial pressure less than 65 mm Hg, or a decrease of 40 mm Hg in systolic BP that is unresponsive to a crystalloid fluid challenge of 20 to 40 mL/kg.

Severe head injury (GCS less than or equal to 8); usually associated with loss of consciousness for more than 24 hours.

Severe sepsis The presence of sepsis accompanied by one or more of the following organ dysfunctions: acute lung injury; coagulation abnormalities or thrombocytopenia; altered mental status; renal, liver, or cardiac failure; hypoperfusion with lactic acidosis.

Shock Syndrome marked by inadequate perfusion and oxygenation of cells, tissue, and organs usually as a result of markedly lowered blood pressure.

Shunt unit When an alveolus is inadequately ventilated in the presence of perfusion.

Sigmoidoscopy Involves only the inspection and visualization of the rectal-sigmoid area of the colon.

Silent unit When both ventilation and perfusion are impaired.

Sinoatrial (SA) node The dominant pacemaker of the heart, located in the upper posterior wall of the right atrium, that spontaneously generates electrical impulses at a rate of 60 to 100 beats a minute.

Spinal cord Part of central nervous system; extends from the medulla to the second lumbar vertebra within the spinal canal, protected by bone and enclosed in the meninges.

Spontaneous bacterial peritonitis (SBP) An infection of the ascitic fluid without indication of another intra-abdominal source such as a perforated viscus.

Square wave test A test performed on the pressure monitoring system to verify the ability of the pressure monitoring system to accurately reflect pressure values.

Stable angina   Angina that occurs with exercise and is predictable; usually promptly relieved by rest or nitroglycerin.

Stroke volume   The volume of blood ejected from each ventricle with each heartbeat.

Subarachnoid hemorrhage   Bleeding between the arachnoid and pia mater may result from rupture of a preexisting or a traumatic cerebral aneurysm.

Subdural hematomas   Usually are the result of countercoup injuries, occurring on the opposite side of the skull from the injury just below the dura. They are usually the result of venous bleeding, often originating with the stretching of bridging veins. Subdural hematomas are classified as acute, subacute, and chronic.

Supernormal period   The period during depolarization of the cardiac cell membrane that follows the relative refractory period; during this period a weaker than normal stimulus can cause depolarization of cardiac cells.

Symptom-triggered therapy   The preferred method of medication administration for AWS is administration of prescribed medications for clinically significant symptoms as established by the total CIWA-Ar score.

Systemic inflammatory response syndrome (SIRS)   The presence of two or more of the following: temperature greater than 38°C (100.4°F) or less than 36°C (96.8°F); pulse greater than 90 beats per minute; respiratory rate greater than 20 breaths/minute or $PaCO_2$ less than 32 torr; WBC greater than 12,000/mm^3 or less than 4,000/mm^3.

Tachyphylaxis   Tolerance to a medication over time; a decreasing response to a drug after initial doses were effective.

Thrombotic brain attacks or strokes   Occur when thrombus formation in an artery causes a stroke due to decreased blood flow.

Tidal volume (V_T)   The volume of one inhalation/exhalation cycle.

Tissue typing   Used to determine how much overlap exists between a potential donor's and the recipient's HLA antigens.

Total lung capacity (TLC)   The maximum volume the lungs can hold.

Trachea   The major tube connecting the upper and lower airways.

Tracheostomy   Involves an incision in the neck accessing the trachea and creation of a stoma through which a tracheostomy tube is inserted.

Transjugular intrahepatic portosystemic shunt (TIPS)   A minimally invasive radiological procedure in which a guidewire is passed through the wall of the hepatic vein through the body of the liver into the portal vein and an expandable metal mesh stent is inserted.

Trauma   Physical injury or wound caused by external force or violence; may be self-inflicted.

Trauma score   Numerical grading system that combines the Glasgow Coma Scale and measurements of cardiopulmonary function as a gauge of severity of injury and predictor of survival. The lowest score is 1 and the highest is 16.

Troponin   An inhibitory protein in the muscle fibers. Troponin I is a highly sensitive and specific indicator of recent myocardial infarction.

Type I respiratory failure   (Hypoxemic failure); stems from a breakdown of oxygen transport from the alveolus to arterial flow.

Type II respiratory failure   (Hypoxemic hypercapneic failure); originates in musculoskeletal or anatomical lung dysfunction or suppression.

Ultrafiltration (convection)   A pressure gradient is created between the sides of the semipermeable membrane. Solute is carried in solution across the semipermeable membrane in response to the pressure gradient, producing an ultrafiltrate.

Unstable angina   Angina that has changed to a more severe form. It can occur at rest and may be an indication of impending myocardial infarction.

Upper GI endoscopy   (Esophagogastroduodenoscopy [EGD]); involves oral intubation with a flexible endoscope to visualize the esophagus, stomach, and proximal duodenum.

Variant angina   Chest pain that results from the spasm of coronary arteries, rather than from exertion or other increased demands on the heart.

Vasospasm   An angiographic narrowing of cerebral blood vessel(s) that can lead to delayed ischemia.

Venous thromboembolism (VTE)   Deep vein thrombosis with the development of pulmonary embolism.

Ventilation   The mechanical act of moving air in and out of the respiratory tree.

Ventilator-associated pneumonia (VAP)   A new lung infection developing within 48 hours of intubation.

Ventricular remodeling   The reshaping of the walls of the myocardium after a myocardial infarction.

Vital capacity (VC)   The sum of the ERV, V_T, and IRV.

Voluntary euthanasia   A person requests an action be taken to end his life.

Weaning   The process of determining the patient's readiness to resume spontaneous breathing and concluding mechanical support.

Wernicke's encephalopathy   Confusion, abnormal gait, and paralysis of certain eye muscles.

Work of breathing (WOB)   The effort expended in the act of inspiration.

Zone of coagulation   Third-degree burns have all three zones, beginning with the inner zone of coagulation, which is the deepest part of the burn. The cells are nonviable and the microcirculation is destroyed, leaving the skin dark colored and leathery.

Zone of hyperemia   The outer zone of hyperemia is tissue with intact microvasculature that heals spontaneously within days. The area initially appears pink and capillary refill may be increased due to vasodilation induced by local inflammatory mediators.

Zone of stasis   The medial zone of stasis is composed of viable and nonviable cells. There is damage to the microcirculation, resulting in vasoconstriction and ischemia. The skin initially appears moist or blistered and is red in color.